Handbook
of
HIV/AIDS Nursing

Handbook
of HIV/AIDS
Nursing

Carl A. Kirton, MA, RN, ACRN, ANP-CS
Clinical Assistant Professor of Nursing and
Adult Nurse Practitioner, Division of Nursing
New York University
New York, New York
Clinical Nurse Manager/Nurse Practitioner
The Jack Martin Fund Clinic, AIDS Center
The Mount Sinai Medical Center
Mount Sinai–New York University Health
New York, New York

Dorothy Talotta, EdD, RN, FNP-CS
Professor, School of Nursing
College of New Rochelle
New Rochelle, New York

Kenneth Zwolski, EdD, RN, FNP-CS
Professor, School of Nursing
College of New Rochelle
New Rochelle, New York

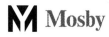 Mosby

A Harcourt Health Sciences Company

St. Louis   London   Philadelphia   Sydney   Toronto

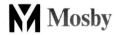

Mosby

A Harcourt Health Sciences Company

Editor-in-Chief: Sally Schrefer
Executive Editor: Barbara Nelson Cullen
Managing Editor: Sandra Clark Brown
Project Manager: Catherine Albright Jackson
Production Editor: Marc P. Syp
Designer: Judi Lang
Cover Designer: Kathi Gosche

Mosby, Inc.
A Harcourt Health Sciences Company
11830 Westline Industrial Drive
St. Louis, Missouri 63146

Printed in the United States of America

ISBN: 0-323-00336-2

01   02   03   04   05   TG/FF   9   8   7   6   5   4   3   2   1

This book is dedicated to all those who have fallen victim to AIDS and to those who continue to struggle daily with AIDS and HIV infection. It is also dedicated to their caregivers and to those whose work has led to more effective treatments and will, hopefully, in the future, lead to a cure and a vaccine.

In addition, the editors dedicate this book to the following individuals:

First to my loving family; my late father and brother John Sr. and John Jr. Thank you for being such positive influences in my life. To my mother Jackie, my sister Laura, and my niece Déja. I love each of you immensely; thank you for all of your continued love and support (even when I am difficult). Lance, thank you for your unending friendship, encouragement, and all of the laughter. Elizabeth, thank you for being such a great teacher and mentor; without you, pen would never have reached paper. Finally, Rick, thank you for being the first to teach me about HIV beyond the clinic and classroom.

Carl A. Kirton

To my late parents, Rose Ann and Robert Andrews Ross, for their unfailing and unquestioning love and support, and to my husband John for his steadfast love and his help, support, and encouragement throughout this project.

Dorothy Talotta

To my daughters, Audrey and Alexandra, who are a constant joy in my life, and to my wife, Joann, whose love has nourished me all these years.

Kenneth Zwolski

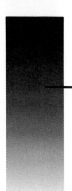

Contributors

Ann-Margaret Dunn, RN, MS, CPNP
Division of Pediatric Infectious Diseases
New York Presbyterian Hospital
New York, New York
Chapter 21   Children with HIV/AIDS

Jill Handel, MSN, ANP-C
Nurse Practitioner
Private Practice
New York, New York
Chapter 18   Dermatological Care of Clients with HIV/AIDS

Carl A. Kirton, MA, RN, ACRN, ANP-CS
Clinical Assistant Professor of Nursing and
Adult Nurse Practitioner, Division of Nursing
New York University
New York, New York
Clinical Nurse Manager/Nurse Practitioner
The Jack Martin Fund Clinic, AIDS Center
The Mount Sinai Medical Center
Mount Sinai–New York University Health
New York, New York
Chapter 2   Clinical Application of Immunological and Virological Markers
Chapter 3   Risk Assessment, Identification, and HIV Counseling
Chapter 4   Guidelines for the Initiation of Antiretroviral Therapy
Chapter 5   Clinical Trials
Chapter 6   Immunizations in HIV Care
Chapter 9   Hospitalized Clients with HIV/AIDS
Chapter 15   Oncologic Conditions
Chapter 16   Parasitic Infections
Chapter 24   Sexually Transmitted Diseases

Appendix B Internet Resources in HIV/AIDS
Appendix D HIV Drug Interactions
Appendix E Recommendations for the Prevention of Pneumococcal
Infections in HIV-Infected Children

Gail Kropf, RN, ACRN
Research Clinician
AIDS Research Consortium of Atlanta
Atlanta, Georgia
Chapter 12   Home Care Visitation: Nursing Assessment
and Interventions

Deborah Witt Sherman, PhD, RN, ANP-CS
Assistant Professor and Program Director
Advanced Practice Palliative Care Master's Program
Division of Nursing
New York University
New York, New York
Chapter 11   Palliative Care
Chapter 20   HIV/AIDS and Pregnancy

Neal Sherman, DO, FACOG
Attending Physician
Department of Obstetrics and Gynecology
Arden Hill Hospital
Goshen, New York
Chapter 20   HIV/AIDS and Pregnancy

Dorothy Talotta, EdD, RN, FNP-CS
Professor, School of Nursing
College of New Rochelle
New Rochelle, New York
Chapter 7   Tuberculosis Screening, Diagnosis, and Infection Control
Chapter 8   Gynecological and Cervical Disorders and Therapeutics
Chapter 10   Tuberculosis Control
Chapter 13   Bacterial Infections
Chapter 23   Health Care Worker Risk Reduction in HIV/AIDS Care

David D. Williams, MD
Staff Physician
Department of Family Practice
Bassett Healthcare
Stamford, New York
Appendix B: Internet Resources in HIV/AIDS

S. K. Glenda Winson, RN, MS, ACRN
Research Nurse, GI Immunology
St. Luke's Roosevelt Hospital Center
New York, New York

Kenneth Zwolski, EdD, RN, FNP-CS
Professor, School of Nursing
College of New Rochelle
New Rochelle, New York

Reviewers

Eileen Bailey, BSN, RN, MPH
Needlestick Coordinator
The Mount Sinai Medical Center
Mount Sinai–New York University Health
New York, New York

Joseph Colagreco, RN, MS, ANP-CS
Clinical Assistant Professor of Nursing
New York University
New York, New York

Michele Crespo-Fierro, RN, CRNI, MS/MPH
Nurse Consultant
New York, New York

Risa Denenberg, RN, NP, MSN
Family Nurse Practitioner
Nurse-Colposcopist
New York City, New York

Catherine Handy, RN, PhD, AOCN
Oncology Clinical Nurse Specialist
St. Vincents Hospital and Medical Center of New York
New York, New York

Lawrence Hitzeman, MD, BA, BSN
Attending Physician
Rivington House
Internal Medicine
Private Practice
New York, New York

Valery Hughes, RN, MS, CFNP
Research Nurse Practitioner
Cornell Clinical Trials Unit
The Center for Special Studies
New York–Presbyterian
New York, New York

Donald Kotler, MD
Associate Professor of Medicine
St Luke's Roosevelt Hospital
New York, New York

Wade Leon, RN, MA, ANP-CS, CRRN
Nurse Practitioner
St Vincents Hospital and Medical Center of New York
New York, New York

Kenneth J.A. Lown, RN, MSN, CPNP
Pediatric Nurse Practitioner
The Mount Sinai Medical Center
Mount Sinai–New York University Health
New York, New York

Lee Raden, RN, BA, BSN, ACRN
Manager of Client Health Services
Rivington House
45 Rivington Street
New York, New York

Laurie Sandman, RN, MPH, BA, BS
Research Nurse
New York University School of Medicine
New York, New York

Fran Wallach, MD
Assistant Professor of Infectious Disease
Assistant Medical Director
The Jack Martin Fund Clinic
The Mount Sinai Medical Center
Mount Sinai–New York University Health
New York, New York

Margaret Zak, PharmD
Clinical Specialist, Assistant Professor
University of Pittsburgh Medical Center
Pittsburgh, Pennsylvania

Preface

As more and better treatments for the human immunodeficiency virus (HIV) become available, more clients are living with HIV infection as a chronic illness. It is essential for nurses in all settings to be able to render the complex care needed by this client population.

This book was written to provide nurses with a portable reference for information essential to the nursing care of clients infected with HIV. It provides concise but thorough discussions of HIV/AIDS nursing in the ambulatory setting, the acute care setting, and the home. It also includes discussions of various opportunistic infections and of special topics that sometimes arise when the nurse is providing care to these clients.

Unit I includes discussions of the pathology of HIV infection and immunological and virological markers. This is followed by chapters related to the nursing care of clients in various settings. Units II, III, and IV discuss the care of clients in ambulatory settings, acute care settings, and homes, respectively. Unit V includes concise discussions of various opportunistic infections, including tables of recommended prophylaxis and treatment for quick reference. The final unit, Unit VI, includes special topics in HIV/AIDS care, such as nursing pediatric and pregnant clients, risk reduction for the health care worker, and complementary therapies that are used by many clients. As members of the HIV health care team, nurses play an important role in educating clients about their disease. Each unit concludes with a section titled "Frequently Asked Questions." This feature is a result of actual questions encountered in our clinical practice and provides nurses with appropriate answers. Because the care of clients with HIV continues to evolve, we have provided the nurse with important internet resources for updated HIV/AIDS information in Appendix B.

Clients infected with HIV and their caregivers, friends, and families need nursing care that is sensitive to the unique physical, psychosocial, and emotional issues raised by the nature of HIV infection. Access to appropriate information can help the nurse meet the complex care needs of this client population.

Acknowledgements

We thank all of the authors for their important and informative contributions to the first edition of this book; without them this project would not exist. We are grateful to all of the reviewers who have provided thoughtful analyses of each chapter and helpful suggestions for improvement. At Mosby we would especially like to thank Barry Bowlus, Barbara Watts, Robin Harris, and Stephanie Schutter, all of whom were involved in this project in its formative year. We would like to thank Barbara Nelson Cullen, whose oversight, suggestions, and vision for this project have been invaluable. A special thanks goes to Sandy Clark Brown, our managing editor, for her expert direction and supervision of the production process. And finally, a special thanks also goes to Marc Syp for his precise and thoughtful copyediting of the manuscripts. There are many persons at Mosby who we do not know but who certainly have played an important role in the development of this project. We thank them all.

Carl A. Kirton
Dorothy Talotta
Kenneth Zwolski

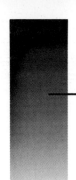

Contents

Unit III

Acute Care Nursing of Clients with HIV/AIDS, 155

Unit IV

Home Care Nursing of Clients with HIV/AIDS, 195

Unit V

Opportunistic Infections in HIV/AIDS,   227

13 Bacterial Infections,   229
Kenneth Zwolski
Dorothy Talotta

14 Fungal Infections,   254
Kenneth Zwolski

15 Oncologic Conditions,   271
Carl A. Kirton

16 Parasitic Infections,   281
Glenda Winson
Carl A. Kirton
Kenneth Zwolski

Unit VI

Unit I

Introduction to HIV:
Immunopathogenesis
and Clinical Testing

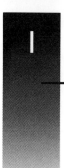

HIV Immunopathogenesis

Kenneth Zwolski

NATURAL HISTORY OF HIV INFECTION

TYPES OF RETROVIRUSES

Infection with the human immunodeficiency virus (HIV) frequently results in a progressive, debilitating, and eventually fatal disease, acquired immunodeficiency syndrome (AIDS). HIV belongs to a unique class of viruses, the retroviruses. The retroviruses are unusual because, unlike any other known living matter, they carry RNA rather than DNA and require an enzyme, reverse transcriptase, to transcribe RNA into double-stranded DNA.

The retroviruses include several types of viruses, some of which infect humans. Among these are the human T-cell lymphoma viruses, type I and type II (HTLV-I and HTLV-II), and the human immunodeficiency viruses, type 1 and type 2 (HIV-1 and HIV-2). Other retroviruses, not known to infect humans, include the simian immunodeficiency virus (SIV), equine infectious anemia virus, and feline immunodeficiency virus. SIV, equine infectious anemia virus, feline immunodeficiency virus, HIV-1, and HIV-2 belong to a subfamily of retroviruses, the lentiviruses. HTLV-I and HTLV-II, although retroviruses, do not belong to the subfamily of lentiviruses; rather, they are classified as oncoviruses.

HTLV-I and HTLV-II are very similar to HIV in their modes of transmission and in the cells that they target for infection once inside their human host. However, infection with either HTLV-I or HTLV-II does not cause AIDS. HTLV-I causes a variety of illnesses, including adult T-cell leukemia, chronic B-cell leukemia, polymyositis, infective dermatitis, uveitis, and immune deficiency syndromes (that may be AIDS-like in presentation). It is endemic in Southwestern Japan, the Caribbean, Melanesia, and parts of Africa. HTLV-II causes hairy cell leukemia, myelopathy, and a variety of miscellaneous clinical conditions. Infection with HTLV-I and HTLV-II can also be completely asymptomatic. HTLV-II is endemic to Native Americans and injection drug users. HTLV can be detected through blood bank screening assays that use whole HTLV virus lysates. If a client is identified as being HTLV-positive on this basis, it is important to assure the client that they are not infected with the "AIDS virus." Generally speaking, infection with HTLV does not inevitably result in disease complications, and compared to HIV, is not as readily transmittable via sexual encounters. However, infection with HTLV and HIV together may hasten the progression to AIDS.

HIV-1 and HIV-2 are members of the subfamily of retroviruses, the lentiviruses. All retroviruses contain the gag, pol, and env genes, but lentiviruses have more complex genomes than do other retroviruses. SIV (also a lentivirus, but which is only known to infect monkeys) has many varieties and is thought to be the source from which HIV originated. SIV, in its various forms, is present in African green monkeys, mandrills, and chimpanzees. HIV-1 and HIV-2 both cause AIDS, but there are important differences between these two strains of HIV.

HIV-2 is confined mostly to areas in Western Africa. When the nucleotide sequences are examined and compared to those in HIV-1, there is an approximate similarity of 40% to 50%. There are two major differences in genetic structure between HIV-1 and HIV-2: (1) HIV-1 contains a gene, vpu, not found in HIV-2, and (2) HIV-2 contains a gene, vpx, not found in HIV-1. Infection with HIV-2 is indistinguishable from infection with HIV-1 in terms of symptoms, although generally speaking infection with HIV-2 tends to be less virulent and disease progression occurs over a longer period of time. Current testing for HIV-1 and HIV-2 is discussed in Chapter 2.

HIV-1: STRUCTURE AND FUNCTION

The molecular structure of HIV-1 is icosahedral (Figure 1-1), measuring about 1×10^{-4} mm in diameter. The core of the virus, the nucleocapsid, contains four proteins, collectively referred to as the nucleocapsid proteins. These include: p24, which forms the inner shelf of the nucleocapsid; p17, which is associated with the inner surface of the virus' envelope; p7, which binds directly to the virus' RNA; and p9, which, together with p7, forms the nucleoid core. Besides these structural proteins the core also contains two copies of single-stranded RNA (the HIV-1 genome) and four enzymes. These enzymes are reverse transcriptase, RNase H, integrase, and protease.

These enzymes control and regulate several important aspects of the HIV-1 life cycle. Reverse transcriptase copies HIV-1 RNA into DNA in a two step process. First, it copies the RNA into a single-strand copy of DNA. Then, after RNase H has partially degraded the original RNA, reverse transcriptase synthesizes a second strand of DNA. Integrase imports this double-stranded DNA into the nucleus of the host cell and inserts it into the host's genome. Protease activates the gag and pol genes, resulting in the synthesis and assembly of new HIV-1 proteins.

The envelope of the HIV-1 virus is a lipid bilayer (which is actually acquired by the HIV-1 virus as it buds out of its human host cell) in which are embedded 72 external spikes and a variety of proteins also acquired

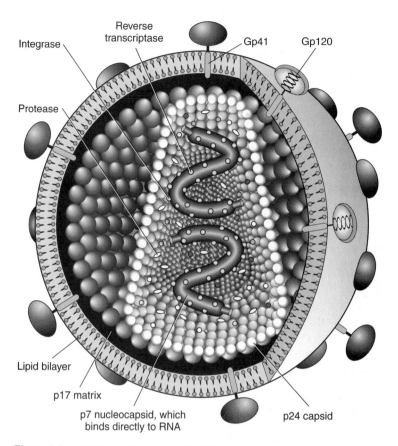

Figure 1-1. HIV Virion. (*From Greene W: AIDS and the immune system,* Scientific American Special Issue: Life and Death and the Immune System *269(3):100, Sept 1993.*)

from the host cell. Each spike is made up of two glycoproteins (gp), gp 41 and gp 120. The lipid bilayer is also likely to contain host proteins—Class I and Class II histocompatibility antigens—that the virus acquires in the course of budding from an infected cell.

The HIV-1 genome (Figure 1-2) is a 9 kilobase RNA strand; that is, it is 9,749 nucleotide bases long. It is comprised of nine genes and is flanked on either side by long terminal repeats (LTR), which are recognized by host transcription factors and serve as binding sites. The nine genes include two structural genes (gag and env), an enzymatic gene (pol), three regulatory genes (tat, rev, and nef), and three other genes (vif, vpr, and vpu). What is known about the function of these genes is summarized in Table 1-1.

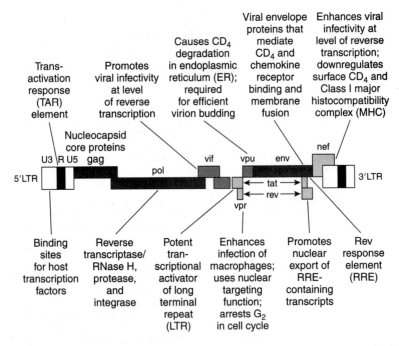

Figure 1-2.   Genomic structure of HIV-1. (*From Sande MA, Volberding PA: The medical management of AIDS, ed 6, Philadelphia, 1999, Saunders.*)

REPLICATION CYCLE OF HIV-1

HIV-1 is an obligatory intracellular parasite. Consisting only of an RNA genome and some structural and enzymatic proteins, it cannot reproduce without making use of the cellular organization and resources of a host cell. Its life cycle includes the following stages: attachment to a host cell, internalization (entering the host cell), reverse transcription and integration of its genome into the host cell's genome, assembly of new HIV-1 particles (virions) within the host cell (using the host cells organization and materials), and budding or exit of new virions from the infected host cell into surrounding tissue, in which these virions can begin the process anew by attaching to previously uninfected host cells.

The HIV-1 virus is able to readily attach itself to cells that contain a protein receptor on their surface identified as CD_4. CD_4 is found on the surface of helper T cells (commonly referred to simply as CD_4 cells) and monocytes/macrophages (when moving through tissue a monocyte is called a macrophage). In addition, HIV-1 may also be able to attach to and infect other types of cells within the human host, such as glial cells, which reside in the brain, gut epithelium, and bone marrow progenitors. CD_4 is considered to be a high-affinity cellular receptor for HIV-1. The gp 120 on

Table 1-1	HIV Genes and Associated Functions	

Gene	Function	Comment
Gag	Codes for the four nucleocapsid core proteins: p24, p17, p9, and p7	Structural gene; gag stands for *group-specific antigen*
Pol	Codes for the four enzymes found in HIV-1: reverse transcriptase, protease, integrase, and RNase H	Enzymatic gene
Vif	Promotes viral infectivity at the level of reverse transcription	Mutations of vif decrease yield of infectious particles from the cell and inhibit cell-to-cell transmission
Vpr	Weak transcriptional activator; arrests host cell cycle in postsynthetic gap (G2) phase	
Vpu	Degrades CD_4; required for efficient virion budding	When absent, the virion remains attached to the inside of the cell; not present in HIV-2
Tat	Potent transcriptional activator	Regulatory gene
Rev	Regulator of structural gene expression	Regulatory gene; induces transition into late phase of HIV life cycle
Env	Codes for envelope glycoproteins: gp 41 and gp 120	Structural gene; env stands for *envelope*
Nef	Enhances viral infectivity; down regulates surface CD_4	Regulatory gene; nef stands for *negative factor*

the surface of HIV-1 binds to the CD_4 receptor. The analogy frequently used to describe this process is that gp 120 fits the CD_4 receptor in the same manner that a key fits a lock. Without this affinity, HIV-1 would not be able to bind to the host cell and, subsequently, would not infect it.

Recent research has shown that receptors other than CD_4 may also play a role in enabling HIV-1 to infect human cells. These other receptors are referred to as coreceptors. Three have been identified so far: CCR-5, which is found on the surface of macrophages; CXCR4, also called fusin or LESTR, and which is found on the surface of T cells; and CCR3, which is found on the surface of microglia—monocyte-like cells of the central nervous system. These coreceptors normally recruit immune cells to sites of tissue damage or act as receptors for the binding of cytokines. Different strains of HIV-1 may have affinity for different coreceptors. This may help explain documented patterns of HIV-1 infectivity. One strain of HIV-1, referred to as non–syncytium-inducing (NSI) or sometimes macrophage-tropic (M tropic), seems to bind preferentially to cells with CCR-5 coreceptors (macrophages). NSI strains tend to occur early in the course of HIV infection. Another strain of HIV-1, referred to as syncytium-inducing

(SI), or sometimes T cell–tropic (T tropic), seems to bind preferentially with T cells. SI strains are more pathogenic and tend to occur later in the course of HIV infection. However, there is a hypothesis that one may be infected initially with an SI strain and would thereby progress rapidly to AIDS.

Once HIV-1 has successfully attached to a host cell by binding to a CD_4 receptor, the virus fuses with the cell membrane of the host cell. Internalization of the virus ensues. Internalization is facilitated because the envelope of the HIV-1 and the cell membrane of the host cell are both bilipid layers. The viral bilipid layer is actually part of the cell membrane of a previously infected host cell, which it acquired during the process of budding out of that cell.

Once internalized within a helper T cell, HIV-1 uncoats itself (sheds the bilipid layer) and begins the process of transcribing its RNA genome into DNA. Once the double stranded DNA is inserted into the host cell's genome it becomes a part of that genome. These viral genes persist for as long as the host cell lives. If the host cell divides into two daughter cells, the viral DNA will be duplicated with the rest of the cell's DNA and will be passed on to each of the daughter cells.

If the viral DNA within a helper T cell becomes activated, then it will result in the assembly of new virions. The assembly proceeds in a stepwise fashion. Viral DNA is translated into messenger RNA. The messenger RNA then brings about the synthesis and assembly of HIV-1 proteins in the cytoplasm of the helper T cell. Helper T cells are activated by exposure to antigens, certain cytokines (e.g., tumor necrosis factor, interleukin 1 [IL-1]), or other gene products from viruses (e.g., herpes simplex virus [HSV], Epstein-Barr virus [EBV], cytomegalovirus [CMV]). If the helper T cell is not activated, then the viral DNA will remain latent.

The concept of latency can be misleading, however. Infection with HIV-1 is a dynamic process. From initial infection to late infection there is a high amount of viral replication and CD_4 death occurring. Roughly 21 billion new virions are produced on a daily basis in lymph tissue, and the immune system produces 1 to 2 billion new CD_4 cells each day in order to replenish those that are killed by infection with HIV-1. Throughout HIV infection there is relentless destruction of CD_4 cells. A person not treated for HIV will have an entire supply of CD_4 cells turned over approximately every 15 days. As the disease progresses, the ability of the immune system to replace lost CD_4 cells adequately diminishes, and the overall CD_4 cell count gradually drops. And yet, despite dynamic viral activity, an infected person may be completely asymptomatic.

After the nucleocapsid of the virion is assembled in the cytoplasm of a helper T cell, the life cycle of HIV-1 is completed through a process called budding. The virion fuses with the host cell's membrane and then pushes itself out into the surrounding tissue, taking with it a part of the host cell's membrane, which it uses for its own envelope. During budding, the gp 120 and gp 40 proteins are attached to the envelope and the virion also takes with it some of the host cells own proteins, particularly Class I and Class II MHC proteins. These will aid the virion in its infection of other host cells.

IMMUNE SYSTEM RESPONSE TO HIV INFECTION

KEY ELEMENTS OF THE IMMUNE SYSTEM RELEVANT TO HIV INFECTION

To comprehend fully the pathological consequences of infection with HIV-1, certain elements of the immune system and its processes need to be understood. Immunity is protection. The immune system is a complex of cells, tissues, and molecules that protects the body against harm from foreign agents, such as microorganisms, viruses, chemicals, drugs, pollen, and other externally introduced substances. The immune system accomplishes this through recognition, memory, and activation of a variety of response mechanisms.

The cells of the immune system—leukocytes—can be divided into two major groupings: the polymorphonuclear (PMN) leukocytes, or granulocytes, and the mononuclear (MN) leukocytes. The PMN leukocytes include neutrophils (microphages), eosinophils, and basophils. When a basophil is positioned in tissue (as opposed to freely circulating in the blood stream) it is called a mast cell. The MN leukocytes are subdivided into two groups: lymphocytes and monocytes/macrophages. The lymphocytes, in turn, are comprised of two major subdivisions: the T cells and the B cells. T cells include subpopulations of helper T cells (CD_4 cells), Cytotoxic T cells (CD_8 cells), and natural killer cells.

All white blood cells derive from precursor cells located in the bone marrow. Some cells, such as neutrophils, have a high turnover rate, being replaced every 6 hours or so. Other cells, such as helper T cells normally have a low turnover rate. Lymphocytes are found in lymphatic tissue, although a small percentage can be found circulating in the blood stream. T cells mature in the thymus. B cells and other white blood cells mature in the bone marrow or in circulation.

Proteins on the surface of white blood cells are extremely important. They serve as receptors (e.g., to bind cytokines, other cells, and antibodies) and as recognition markers. Helper T cells have on their surface a protein, CD_4, which does not occur on other lymphocytes. Cytotoxic T cells have a surface protein, CD_8, which identifies them as unique. Two important proteins occurring on the surface of cells are Class I major histocompatibility complex (MHC) molecules and Class II MHC molecules. MHC refers to the series of genes that codes for these two classes of proteins. Class I and Class II MHC proteins differ from individual to individual, the difference being genetically determined. These proteins play an important part in enabling the immune system to distinguish self from nonself and also in activating and implementing a wide variety of immunological events, such as processing antigens by macrophages for presentation to other immune cells.

White blood cells communicate with each other by means of chemical mediators called cytokines. Cytokines are non–antigen-specific glycoproteins secreted by a wide variety of cells in the body. Cytokines produced by monocytes/macrophages are sometimes referred to as monokines. The same type of cytokine may be produced by several different types of cells. Cytokines are released by white blood cells into the circulation or surrounding tissue, where they can bind to an appropriate surface receptor on another cell. The binding of the cytokine to the specific receptor activates a specific physiological, genetically programmed response. Cytokines can have a large variety of different biological functions, depending on the particular target cell to which they bind. Sometimes a cytokine brings about an increased production of proteins by the target cell. These proteins are receptors, which are then inserted into the plasma membrane. (These newly formed receptors may be specific to the binding of other cytokines or they may serve to protect against infectious agents. An example of this latter response would be a receptor that can bind a portion of an antibody to itself. Often a cytokine will cause the growth, proliferation, or differentiation of the target cell. For example, a cytokine binding to a target cell in the bone marrow may stimulate the differentiation of hematopoietic blood cells.)

Cytokines that are produced by white blood cells are grouped into categories according to function. These five categories are:

1. Colony-stimulating factors (CSF)—These cytokines promote the maturation of early progenitor cells to committed cells, such as monocytes/macrophages. They include cytokines such as granulocyte CSF (G-CSF), granulocyte-macrophage CSF (GM-CSF) and macrophage CSF (M-CSF).

2. Proinflammatory cytokines—These include tumor necrosis factor alpha (TNF-α), IL-1, and IL-6. These cytokines are important in priming the immune system to respond to pathogens, and they are responsible for bringing about the acute phase response to infection (i.e., inflammation).

3. Antiinflammatory cytokines—These include IL-4 and IL-10; normally, these cytokines shut down the inflammatory response.

4. Interferons (IFN)—These include IFN-α and IFN-β, whose production is induced by viral infection and IFN-γ, which activates macrophages.

5. T cell growth factors (TC-GF)—these include IL-2, IL-12, and IL-15.

In addition to these five categories is another subset of cytokines, called chemokines. Chemokines are proteins with low molecular weight that are considered to be second-order cytokines because they act on fewer cells than other cytokines and because they have more distinct functions. Chemokines do not induce the proliferation of other cytokines. They play a role in both acute and chronic inflammation. Included among the chemokines are alpha chemokines and beta chemokines. Beta chemokines include macrophage inflammatory protein 1 alpha (MIP-1α), macrophage inflammatory protein 1 beta (MIP-1β), and RANTES. All beta chemokines are produced by CD_8 cells.

Some white blood cells are characterized by the types of lymphokines they produce. For example, among helper T cells there are two recognized subsets, Th 1 and Th 2. Th 1 cells produce IFN-γ, TNF-γ, and IL-2. Th 2 cells, on the other hand, produce IL-4, IL-5, IL-6, IL-9, and IL-10. Different cytokines affect different target cells and mediate different physiological responses; Th 1 cells, through the production of IL-2 and IFN-γ, activate CD_8 cells, natural killer (NK) cells, and macrophages. Hence, Th 1 cells are, for the most part, responsible for bringing about the cellular immune response. Th 2 cells, through the production of IL-4 and IL-5, activate B cells, stimulating the production of antibodies. Hence, Th 2 cells are mostly responsible for mediating the humoral immune response. Both Th 1 and Th 2 cells produce GM-CSF.

The leukocytes that are primarily involved in HIV/AIDS infection are summarized in Table 1-2.

The ability of a compound to induce an immune response is referred to as its *immunogenicity*. In the broadest sense, any foreign substance that is capable of inducing an immune response is considered an antigen. An antigen is often just a protein or saccharide on the surface of a cell. Almost any of the proteins of the HIV-1 virus can act as an antigen. The response, activated by exposure to an antigen, can include a variety of cellular and molecular events. This response can be classified as either natural (innate, or nonspecific) or acquired (adaptive, or specific).

A natural immune response is considered to be nonspecific because it always operates the same way, every time. This response is immediate. It involves granulocytes, macrophages, NK cells, and a variety of circulating serum proteins, particularly those series of proteins comprising the complement, clotting, and kinin systems of the body. Granulocytes and macrophages are capable of ingesting other cells and releasing physiologically active substances, such as histamines. When triggered, the natural immune response may produce fever. Very often it causes a series of tissue changes recognized as inflammation.

An acquired immune response is considered to be specific because it involves the production of substances (antibodies) and the proliferation of cells that target specific antigens. The acquired immune response uses specific information about the shape of the antigen to customize its response. This response involves a specific binding of an immune-produced protein (either an antibody or a receptor on the surface of an immune cell) to the antigen. Compared to the natural immune response, the acquired

Table 1-2	Leukocytes Involved in HIV/AIDS Infection	
White Blood Cell (WBC) Type	**General Profile**	**Involvement in HIV/AIDS Infection**
Neutrophils	Neutrophils normally constitute 50% to 75% of all circulating leukocytes and are capable of phagocytosis. They play an important role in inflammatory response and are the first line of defense against infection. They have a short life span.	Neutropenia commonly occurs in advanced stages of HIV infection. Drug-induced neutropenia is common (medications used to treat PCP, toxoplasmosis, CMV retinitis, CMV colitis, and zidovudine cause neutropenia).
Monocytes/ macrophages	In the circulating blood, monocytes constitute about 3% to 7% of all white blood cells. Macrophages are distributed throughout tissue and are capable of phagocytosis. They are involved in the inflammatory response. They are capable of processing antigens for presentation to T cells. They have CD_4 receptors and Class II major histocompatibility complex (MHC).	Monocytes/macrophages serve as a reservoir for HIV-1. Some strains of HIV (e.g., non–synctium-inducing [NSI]) have a greater preference for macrophages than other strains. When activated by stimulation with interferon they produce neopterin, a metabolite of guanosine triphosphate. Neopterin levels are increased in HIV infection.
Basophils/ mast cells	Basophils/mast cells are involved in acute inflammatory response, degranulation of mast cells releases histamine, SRSA, chemotactic factors and many other physiologically active substances.	In HIV infection, they may exhibit defective polymorphonuclear (PMN) chemotaxis, deficient degranulating response, and inhibition of leukocyte migration.
Helper T cells (Th cells, CD_4 cells, or T_4 cells)	Th cells contain CD_4 receptors. They are considered to be the master modulators of the immune response because of their secretion of cytokines, which modulate most aspects of immune response.	They are the major target of infection by HIV-1. Progressive infection gradually destroys the available pool of Th cells, so that the CD_4 cell count drops. A decreasing CD_4 cell count correlates with increasing immunodeficiency and onset of opportunistic infections. Infection with HIV-1 can impair Th cell function without killing the cell.

Table 1-2	Leukocytes Involved in HIV/AIDS Infection—cont'd	

White Blood Cell (WBC) Type	General Profile	Involvement in HIV/AIDS Infection
Cytotoxic T cells or Cytotoxic T lymphocytes (CTL/CD_8)	Cytotoxic T cells contain CD_8 receptors and produce cytokines in a more limited fashion than CD_4 cells. They regulate viral and bacterial infections and are involved in direct killing of target cells by binding to them and releasing a substance that can perforate the cell membrane.	Increased in HIV infection. They represent the cellular response to infection. The strength of this initial cellular response has been shown to be prognostic of progression to AIDS (better cellular response, slower progression). Cytotoxic T cells kill Th cells infected with HIV.
Natural killer (NK) cells	NK cells are large granular lymphocytes involved in antibody-dependent cell-mediated cytotoxicity (ADCC). Target cells are coated with antibody that binds to receptors on the surface of NK cells, hence allowing the NK cells to attach to the target cells and kill them. NK cells kill target cells by releasing a substance that triggers lysis of the cell.	NK cells remain numerically and phenotypically normal in clients with AIDS but they are functionally defective.
B cells	B cells produce antibodies specific to antigen. They are capable of being stimulated by Th cells.	B cells are involved in the humoral response to HIV infection and produce a variety of antibodies against HIV, which persist throughout the course of infection.

immune response is slower; it may take a few days before reaching its maximum functioning.

More specifically, if an antibody is involved in this binding, then its acquired immune response is referred to as humoral immunity. Antibodies are complex molecules produced by B cells. If a T cell is involved in the acquired immune response, then more specifically this is referred to as cellular immunity.

Once an antigen induces an acquired response, then immunization has occurred. When the body produces its own antibodies in response to an antigen, this is called active immunization. However, it is possible for immunization to be transferred from one individual to another. Passive immunization is defined as the transfer of antibodies from an immunized individual to a nonimmunized individual. A good example of passive immunization is the transfer of antibodies across the placenta from mother to infant.

RESPONSE OF IMMUNE SYSTEM TO HIV INFECTION

When the HIV-1 virus penetrates human tissue, the immune response is a dual response; that is to say, the immune system launches both natural and acquired mechanisms simultaneously. Of special consequence are the humoral and cellular immune mechanisms. This initial phase of infection is characterized by high levels of viremia. This is demonstrated in blood samples, obtained shortly after infection, that show high levels of plasma HIV RNA and p24 in the serum. However, as soon as cellular and humoral immune mechanisms have a chance to develop in response to HIV infection, the level of virus detectable in the blood begins to drop, indicating the partial effectiveness of these mechanisms in containing the virus (Figure 1-3).

Cellular and humoral immune mechanisms begin as soon as peripheral blood monocytes, infected with HIV, are carried from the site of initial infection (which is usually the genital mucosa) to the lymph nodes or spleen, where they come into contact with CD$_4$ cells. The cellular response is faster than the humoral response. CD$_8$ cells (cytotoxic T lymphocyte [CTL] cells) are mobilized. Their numbers increase. CTL

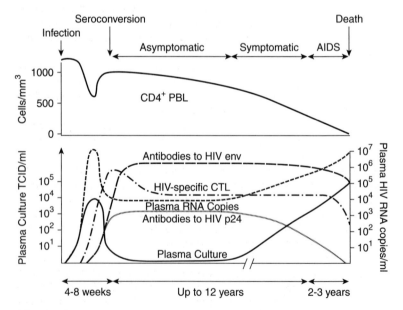

Figure 1-3. Natural history of HIV-1 infection. (*From Silvija S, Feinberg M: Natural history of immunopathogenesis of HIV-1 Disease. In Sande M, Volberding P, eds:* The medical management of AIDS, *ed 5, Philadelphia, 1997, Saunders.*)

cells can kill cells infected with HIV by recognizing fragments of HIV (proteins), which are extruded onto the surface of infected cells in combination with Class I MHC proteins. This combination of HIV protein fragments and Class I MHC proteins is not only a signal that the cell is infected but also allows for the CTL to attach to the infected cell and subsequently destroy it by delivering a lytic event. In this manner, many infected CD_4 cells are destroyed early in the course of HIV infection. Clinically, this is corroborated by an early and detectable decrease in the CD_4 cell count (see Figure 1-3).

This cellular response can be very vigorous in some individuals. Evidence indicates that the strength or weakness of this response is predictive of prognosis. Individuals who exhibit a weak CTL response at this stage of infection typically progress faster to AIDS. Part of the cellular response is also an increase in the amount of cytokines being released. Some cytokines increase and others decrease HIV-1 replication. TNF-α, IL-1, and IL-6 levels are often elevated. These are proinflammatory cytokines and their effect may be to actually increase HIV-1 replication at this point. CD_8 cells secrete beta chemokines at the sites of inflammation. These beta chemokines may block HIV replication by occupying coreceptor sites used for HIV attachment to CD_4 cells. Thus a strong CD_8 response may act to contain HIV infection early and portend a better prognosis. Increased levels of TNF, beta 2 microglobulin, and neopterin have been detected in blood and cerebral spinal fluid. High levels of these cytokines can cause fever, chills, myalgia, headache, and fatigue, which may account for many of the clinical manifestations experienced during early HIV infection (primary HIV infection).

The humoral response to HIV infection is the production of antibodies by B lymphocytes. Several neutralizing antibodies are produced. These include antibodies to the envelope glycoproteins and to the p24 protein of HIV. It typically takes 1 to 3 months after infection before these antibodies are detectable in the serum (see Figure 1-3). When antibodies can be detected by means of testing, the client is said to have seroconverted. By the time antibodies appear, the blood serum is already beginning to clear the virus, indicating that other immune mechanisms, particularly cellular mechanisms, are more important in the earliest control of HIV. Antibodies to HIV, however, can neutralize HIV present in the blood and, therefore, do play somewhat of a role in viral control. Most importantly, once made, these antibodies persist throughout the course of infection and serve as evidence that a person has been exposed to HIV.

Another response that occurs early in HIV infection and reflects aspects of both cellular and immune mechanisms is the occurrence of antibody-dependent cell-mediated cytotoxicity (ADCC). This involves cooperation between NK cells and antibodies. Antibodies that can mediate ADCC have been identified in the majority of HIV-positive individuals.

Both cellular and humoral immune mechanisms play an important role in limiting viral replication and slowing down disease progression.

These responses are able to temporarily contain HIV but are not able to eliminate it. In most individuals, an asymptomatic period ensues after infection. This asymptomatic period can last for as long as 10 or more years. Eventually, the ability to contain viral replication is lost and immune compromise severe enough to allow for the development of opportunistic infections occurs. The inability of cellular and immune mechanisms to continue to contain HIV is thought to be due to a variety of factors. Among these are the high rate of virus replication, which exhausts the ability of the immune system to keep pace, and the ability of the virus to remain latent for long periods of time.

CYTOPATHIC EFFECTS OF HIV-1

While the immune system of the host is trying to contain the HIV-1 virus, the virus itself is exerting a variety of cytopathic effects, which ultimately lead to the demise of CD_4 cells and alter the immune response to infection in other ways as well. Although the precise cytopathic effects involved are not completely known, the following are hypothesized to play a role.

1. Syncytia formation—A syncytium is two or more cells that have become fused together, forming a giant multinucleated cell, which eventually dies. It is thought that gp 120 of HIV, which can often be found clinging to the surface of an infected helper T cell, interacts with the CD_4 receptor of an uninfected helper T cell, resulting in the fusion, and, therefore, death, of these two cells. Some strains of HIV are more likely to mediate this effect than are others; these strains are syncytium-inducing (SI), as opposed to strains that are not likely to cause this effect, referred to as non–syncytium-inducing (NSI). In the early, asymptomatic, phases of HIV infection, NSI strains dominate. However, as the infection persists, SI strains often emerge, resulting in rapid progression to AIDS and death.

2. Disruption of cell functioning—Various HIV gene products expressed within an infected cell may disrupt the cell's normal function, causing cells to become arrested in the postsynthetic gap (G_2) phase of the cell cycle, interfering with mitotic cell division, or altering second messenger production within the cell.

3. Apoptosis—Apoptosis is a form of programmed cell death. Basically a cell destroys itself when certain cell surface receptors are activated. If the immune system needs to be down regulated or defective cells occur, then these cell surface receptors present on immune cells can be activated. It is postulated that chronic immune stimulation due to infection with HIV may lead some uninfected CD_4 cells to mistakenly initiate apoptosis.

4. Superantigen—A superantigen is a protein that binds to a receptor on the surface of a T cell; however, a superantigen binds to a part of the receptor that does not normally bind protein. Nonetheless, this binding activates the physiological response that occurs when the receptor is activated in the proper way. Superantigens often bind more

easily and readily than other antigens and can lead to chronic and inappropriate activation of cells. Chronic activation may lead to anergy. Inappropriate activation may lead to apoptosis. It is thought that HIV may release superantigens that can bind to uninfected cells, causing them to become anergic or to initiate apoptosis.

5. Single cell killing—A high-level replication of HIV may result in cellular death as a result of membrane injury from budding, accumulation of unintegrated viral DNA, altered membrane permeability, or inhibition of cellular protein synthesis.

6. Autoimmune destruction—Both ADCC mechanisms and activation of CTL cells lead to the destruction of infected CD_4 cells.

7. Suppression of immune functioning—The release of cytokines by infected cells can affect the ability of uninfected cells to mount an immune response or can lead to inappropriate cell signaling.

8. Infection of T cell precursors—HIV may infect T cell precursors in bone marrow, the thymus, and lymph tissue, resulting in their death and hence impairing the ability of the immune system to replace T cells.

9. Macrophage dysfunction—macrophages infected with HIV may have a compromised ability to process antigens for presentation to other immune cells, resulting in immune dysfunction.

CDC CLASSIFICATIONS OF HIV/AIDS

Shortly—approximately 1 to 3 months—after a person is infected with HIV they will develop antibodies to HIV that can be detected by a blood test. The person is now said to be HIV-positive. Being HIV-positive is not the same as having AIDS. There is a progression from HIV-positive to the onset of AIDS. In 1993, the Centers for Disease Control and Prevention (CDC), based on years of clinical observation and data, came out with a revised HIV classification system and expanded AIDS surveillance definition for adolescents and adults. The CDC system provides a clinically based definition of AIDS. But there are many other purposes for a classification system. By defining AIDS, it enables the CDC to track epidemiological data regarding the number of persons with AIDS. Further, by using clinical data to develop a classification system with several categories for HIV and AIDS, a more precise method of monitoring the progression of the disease and determining appropriate therapy is made available for use by clinicians and clients.

Table 1-3 presents the 1993 revised classification system. This classification system applies to anyone over 13 years of age who has tested HIV-positive by 2 or more reactive screening tests (usually the ELISA and the Western blot, although other reactive tests for HIV may be used) (see Table 2-1). An examination of Table 1-3 shows a system based on three ranges of CD_4 cell counts and three clinical categories, designated Clinical Category A, B, and C, respectively. The result is a matrix of nine categories.

Table 1-3	1993 Revised Classification System for HIV Infection and Expanded AIDS Surveillance Case Definition for Adults and Adolescents		
	Clinical Categories		
CD$_4$ Cell Count (cells/mm^3)	**A**	**B**	**C**
	(Asymptomatic, acute [primary] HIV, or persistent generalized lymphadenopathy [PGL])	(Symptomatic; no A or C conditions)	(AIDS indicator conditions)
>500	A1	B1	C1
200-500	A2	B2	C2
<200	A3	B3	C3

Note: Shading indicates AIDS-defining diagnoses. From Centers for Disease Control and Prevention: 1993 revised classification system for HIV infection and expanded surveillance case definitions for AIDS among adolescents and adults, *MMWR* 41(RR-17):1, 1992.

Clinical Category A includes anyone with any of the three following conditions: asymptomatic HIV infection, persistent generalized lymphadenopathy (PGL) (defined as nodes in two or more extrainguinal sites, measuring at least 1 cm in diameter and persisting for greater than 3 months), or acute primary HIV illness (acute retroviral syndrome).

Clinical Category B consists of a list of symptomatic conditions that are either directly attributable to HIV infection or have a clinical course or management complicated by the presence of HIV. Category B conditions are as follows:

- Bacillary angiomatosis
- Candidiasis, oropharyngeal (thrush)
- Candidiasis, vulvovaginal; persistent, frequent, or poorly responsive to therapy
- Cervical dysplasias (moderate or severe) or cervical carcinoma in situ
- Constitutional symptoms, such as fever (38.5° C) or diarrhea lasting more than 1 month
- Herpes zoster (shingles), involving at least two distinct episodes or more than one dermatome
- Idiopathic thrombocytopenic purpura
- Listeriosis
- Oral hairy leukoplakia
- Pelvic inflammatory disease, particularly if complicated by tubo-ovarian abscess
- Peripheral neuropathy

Clinical Category C comprises what are called AIDS indicator conditions. These include the following:

- Candidiasis of bronchi, trachea, or lungs
- Candidiasis, esophageal
- Cervical cancer, invasive
- Coccidioidomycosis, disseminated or extrapulmonary
- Cryptococcosis, extrapulmonary
- Cryptosporidiosis, chronic intestinal (of greater than 1 month's duration)
- Cytomegalovirus disease (other than liver, spleen, or nodes)
- Cytomegalovirus retinitis
- Encephalopathy, HIV-related
- Herpes simplex; chronic ulcer(s) (of greater than 1 month's duration); or bronchitis, pneumonitis, or esophagitis
- Histoplasmosis, disseminated or extrapulmonary
- Isosporiasis, chronic intestinal (of greater than 1 month's duration)
- Kaposi's sarcoma
- Lymphoma, Burkitt's (or equivalent term)
- Lymphoma, immunoblastic (or equivalent term)
- Lymphoma, primary of brain
- *Mycobacterium avium* complex or *Kansasii,* disseminated or extrapulmonary
- *M. tuberculosis,* any site (pulmonary or extrapulmonary)
- Mycobacterium, other identified or unidentified species, disseminated or extrapulmonary
- Pneumocystis carinii pneumonia (PCP)
- Pneumonia, recurrent
- Progressive multifocal leukoencephalopathy
- Salmonella septicemia, recurrent
- Toxoplasmosis of brain
- Wasting due to HIV

Based on the CDC classification system, a person has AIDS if either of the following two conditions is met: a CD_4 cell count less than 200, regardless of the presence or absence of symptoms, or an AIDS indicator condition, regardless of the CD_4 cell count. In the matrix, AIDS corresponds to anyone who fits into categories A-3, B-3, C-3, C-1, or C-2.

PRIMARY HIV INFECTION

ACUTE RETROVIRAL SYNDROME

The period immediately after infection with HIV is referred to as the period of *primary HIV infection.* It is characterized by high levels of viremia (see Figure 1-3). From about 2 to 6 weeks after infection with the HIV-1 virus, concurrent with high levels of viremia, approximately 50% of those infected develop an acute illness. This acute illness, if present, is called acute retroviral syndrome, although many authors also refer to it as primary HIV infection. The illness is usually acute in onset and can last from 1 to 2 weeks. Rarely, clients with acute retroviral syndrome may require hospitalization. Within weeks to months, the level of viremia drops considerably (see Figure 1-3). This is due to the success of both cellular and humoral immune mechanisms. The emergence of antibodies to HIV-1, which occurs during this time, is referred to as seroconversion.

At the peak of viremia it is estimated that up to 1% of all peripheral CD_4 blood cells are infected. As the viremia falls, with the resolution of acute symptoms, if they were present, the number of infected peripheral CD_4 cells also declines 10-fold to 1000-fold. However, during this phase, cell-to-cell spreading of HIV-1 has occurred and multiple lymph nodes have been seeded with HIV-1. By the end of this acute phase, the virus has firmly established itself in the lymph nodes where replication continues.

The nature and severity of the acute retroviral syndrome can offer clues as to prognosis. For example, those with severe clinical presentations before seroconversion are more likely to progress rapidly to AIDS than those who experience basically an asymptomatic primary infection. Other factors involved with primary infection may also be prognostic. An adverse prognosis is associated with the following: neurologic involvement, infection with an SI viral strain, infection with HIV-1 from an index case with late-stage HIV disease, persistent p24 antigenemia, higher than usual levels of viremia following seroconversion, low antibody titers to HIV-1, lower than usual CD_4 cell counts, and preexisting immunodeficiency prior to infection. The viral load that develops after the acute retroviral syndrome is called the *set point*. The higher the set point, the worse the prognosis.

Signs and Symptoms

Acute retroviral syndrome occurs only in adolescents and adults infected with HIV-1. The most common symptoms are detailed in Table 1-4.

Other symptoms do occur, but less frequently than those listed in Table 1-4. Splenomegaly can occur. Neurological symptoms can occur. The more common of these include headache and retroorbital pain, particularly exacerbated by eye movements and photophobia; less common neurological symptoms include meningoencephalitis, peripheral neuropathy, radiculopathy, brachial neuritis, Guillain-Barré syndrome, and disorders of cognitive or affective development. The client may present with mucocutaneous ulcerations on the buccal mucosa, gingiva, palate, esophagus, anus, or penis. These ulcerations are round or oval shaped and sharply demarcated. The presence of this mucocutaneous ulceration is a highly distinctive feature of primary HIV infection. Gastrointestinal symptoms, such as anorexia, nausea, vomiting, and diarrhea may also be present. Oral candidiasis may also occur.

According to the CDC, although acute retroviral syndrome is a distinct and recognizable clinical syndrome, it is often described as mononucleosis-like. The major differences between acute retroviral syndrome and EBV mononucleosis are shown in Table 1-5.

Table 1-4	Most Common Symptoms of Acute Retroviral Syndrome	

Symptom	Frequency	Comments
Fever	97%	Is a consistent sign and may or may not be associated with night sweats.
Myalgia or arthralgia	58%	Myalgia may be associated with muscle weakness and an increased level of serum creatinine kinase.
Lethargy and malaise	Common	Often severe; may persist for several months after resolution of other symptoms.
Lymphadenopathy	70%	Generally occurs in second week of illness. May be generalized but axillary, occipital, and cervical nodes are most commonly involved. May persist after the acute illness but tends to decrease with time.
Pharyngitis	73%	Sore throat and pharyngeal edema, with or without exudate.
Rash	70%	Mostly an erythematous, nonpruritic, maculopapular rash with lesions 5 to 10 mm in diameter, affecting the face or trunk but also sometimes the palms and soles; sometimes generalized. Other skin lesions include a roseola-like rash; diffuse urticaria; a vesicular, pustular exanthem and enanthem; desquamation of the palms and soles (typically 2 months after the onset of primary HIV and the resolution of other symptoms); alopecia (typically in the second month after onset of primary HIV and the resolution of other symptoms); and erythema multiforme.

Besides EBV, other possible diagnoses can mimic aspects of acute retroviral syndrome and need to be ruled out. These major differential diagnoses include: CMV, mononucleosis, toxoplasmosis, rubella, viral hepatitis, secondary syphilis, disseminated gonococcal infection, primary HSV infection, other viral infections (e.g., pityriasis rosea), and drug reactions. The skin rash that sometimes accompanies acute retroviral syndrome can be very useful in confirming the diagnosis, because skin eruptions are rare in cases of EBV and CMV infections (unless antibiotics have been given). Also, the skin rash of pityriasis rosea is scaly and may be pruritic; constitutional symptoms are most often absent in clients with pityriasis.

Laboratory Manifestations
Primary HIV infection is a time of intense immunologic activity. Many populations of white blood cells undergo fluctuation in their response to

Table I-5	Difference Between Acute Retroviral Syndrome and Epstein-Barr Virus (EBV) Mononucleosis	

Acute Retroviral Syndrome	EBV Mononucleosis
Acute onset	Insidious onset
Little or no tonsillar hypertrophy	Marked tonsillar hypertrophy
Exanthema on hard palate	Exanthema on border of both hard and soft palates
Exudative pharyngitis uncommon	Exudative pharyngitis common
Mucocutaneous ulcers possible	No mucocutaneous ulcers
Rash common	Rash rare in absence of ampicillin
Jaundice rare	Jaundice occurs in 8%
Diarrhea possible	No diarrhea

Adapted from Gaines H et al: Clinical picture of primary HIV infection presenting as a glandular fever like illness, *BMJ* 297:1363, 1988.

infection with HIV-1. Antibodies also appear. The following changes are most typical:

1. T cells decrease, initially—both CD_4 and CD_8, but CD_4 more dramatically. This lymphopenia, which is very transient, is soon followed by lymphocytosis, in which both CD_4 and CD_8 cells increase, although CD_8 cells increase more rapidly. Because of this rate imbalance, an inversion of the normal CD_4:CD_8 ratio occurs. This inversion can first be found during the second to third week of infection. Since CD_8 cells tend to remain higher throughout, this inversion persists throughout the course of infection. In some individuals, the decrease in CD_4 cells during primary HIV infection is so profound that the CD_4 cell count may go as low as is found in clients with advanced HIV disease.

2. B cells manufacture antibodies against HIV-1. These antibodies are made against both internal and surface proteins of HIV. The first antibodies appear within a few weeks of onset of the acute illness. First, antibodies of the IgM class are made, followed by antibodies of the IgG class. The IgM antibodies decline to undetectable levels within 3 months, whereas IgG antibodies, which appear anywhere from 3 to 6 months after infection, persist throughout the course of infection.

3. During the first week of illness there is an increase in the proportion of banded neutrophils and subsequently (in the third and fourth weeks) there is a decrease in segmented neutrophils.

    Other changes that can occur during primary HIV infection include:

1. Mild thrombocytopenia during the first 2 weeks of illness.

2. An elevated erythrocyte sedimentation rate (ESR) and increased C reactive protein (in approximately 50% of clients).

3. Elevated levels of hepatic transaminases (occasionally).

4. Presence of p24 antigen (typically this can be detected prior to sero-conversion).

CHRONIC HIV INFECTION

STAGES OF HIV INFECTION

The transition from the acute to the chronic stages of HIV infection is characterized by a decrease in the levels of viremia and the resolution of symptoms associated with acute retroviral syndrome (if present). Fluctuations in plasma HIV and CD_4 can occur for about 6 months until a period of stabilization of plasma HIV and CD_4 occurs. The point at which these stabilize is referred to as the set point. A client's set point depends upon the virulence of the HIV strain that he or she is infected with, the numbers of CD_4 infected cells, and the strength of the immune response. Plasma HIV set points vary from 100 to 10,000 copies per ml. Clients with higher set points are at higher risk for faster disease progression.

There is generally a period of clinical latency before the development of clinically apparent disease. In the clinical latency period the viral set point remains stable. Chronic HIV infection can be divided into three stages: early (CD_4 cell count ≥500), middle or intermediate (CD_4 cell count between 200 and 500) and late (CD_4 cell count ≤200). Late HIV infection is synonymous with AIDS. The staging of chronic HIV infection in this manner underscores the point that there is a progression from initial infection with HIV to the development of AIDS.

Table 1-6 summarizes the clinical, laboratory, and lymphatic changes characteristic of each stage.

The progression of HIV disease to AIDS is characterized by changes in the integrity and architecture of the lymphatic tissue, as well as changes in the rate of loss of CD_4 cells. In the earliest stages of chronic HIV infection, large numbers of HIV are trapped in the lymphatic tissue. This results in a decrease in plasma viral load and is accompanied by a hyperplasia of lymphatic tissue. The lymphatic tissue during this stage shows several changes typical of HIV infection, including irregular shape and larger size of germinal centers, the tendency for germinal centers to fuse, and abnormal locations of the germinal centers (e.g., invasion of the cortex). During this time most individuals experience few if any symptoms (the most likely are described in Table 1-6). If transaminase levels are elevated in an individual it is usually related to presence of a concomitant disease such as viral hepatitis, or to the side effects of various medications. By the middle stage of HIV infection, when the CD_4 cell count is between 200 and 500, there is a greater degree of immune impairment and an increased likelihood of symptoms. A significant event during this stage is the progressive destruction of lymphoid tissue. This results in the decreased ability to trap the virus and leads to an increase in the amount of virus found in peripheral blood.

Table 1-6	Stages of Chronic HIV Infection			
Stage	**CD$_4$ Cell Count (cells/mm³)**	**Clinical Features Most Likely Present**	**Typical Lab Features**	**Lymphatic Changes**
Early	>500	Persistent generalized lymphadenopathy (PGL), seborrheic dermatitis, shingles, folliculitis, recurrent aphthous ulcers	Leukopenia (mild), thrombocytopenia (may be severe), anemia (infrequent), increased transaminase levels	Hyperplasia of lymph tissue, sequestration of HIV in lymph tissue
Middle (intermediate)	200-500	Features present in early HIV often worsen: diarrhea; recurrent herpes simplex virus (HSV); oral or vaginal candidiases; increased incidence of bacterial infections of sinuses, respiratory tract, and skin	Similar to early HIV infection, levels of viral load increase in peripheral blood	Increased disruption of lymphoid tissue
Late (AIDS)	<200	Appearance of opportunistic infections (any or a combination of the AIDS indicator conditions, as described by CDC)	Substantial increase in virological parameters in peripheral blood and lymph nodes	Lymphoid tissue has been mostly replaced by fibroid tissue

By late stage AIDS, the progressive deterioration of the immune system allows for the occurrence of numerous opportunistic infections and the presence of severe or persistent constitutional symptoms. By now the lymphatic tissue is largely destroyed, virus trapping by the lymphatic tissue is minimal or absent, and the level of viral load increases even faster in the peripheral blood. During this period as many as 10^9 new virions are produced each day and as many as 2×10^9 CD$_4$ cells turn over each day. Often there is the appearance of more virulent SI virus strains. Without treatment, this stage of HIV infection is characterized by a 50% to 70% risk of developing a new AIDS-related condition, or dying within

2 years. In addition, there is a much greater probability of developing life-threatening side effects from drugs used for treatment.

Within late stage HIV infection (AIDS), clinical observation has led to a further stratification based on CD_4 cell count, sometimes spoken of as early AIDS and late AIDS. In early AIDS (CD_4 cell count between 200 and 100), the more likely opportunistic infections that tend to occur include PCP, cryptococcal meningitis, toxoplasmosis encephalitis, Kaposi's sarcoma, and lymphomas. In late AIDS, (CD_4 cell count <100), the more likely infections and situations that tend to occur include CMV, *M. avium-intracellulare* (MAI), progressive multifocal leukoencephalopathy, dementia, and wasting.

PROGRESSORS VERSUS NONPROGRESSORS

There is a significant variation among HIV-positive individuals in the rate at which they progress from early to late HIV infection. Three patterns have been identified: (1) typical progressors, (2) rapid progressors, and (3) long-term nonprogressors (LTNPs).

About 80% to 90% of all HIV-positive individuals fit the pattern of typical progressors. A typical progressor has a period of relative clinical latency, which lasts for several years, immediately following primary infection. Progression to AIDS takes an average of 8 to 10 years. By contrast, rapid progressors, which account for about 5% to 10% of all individuals infected with HIV, progress to AIDS within 2 to 3 years after seroconversion. Several features distinguish rapid progressors—their levels of antibodies against HIV are low or absent, the ability of CD_8 cells (cytotoxic T cells) to suppress HIV is impaired, and the viral load remains high.

LTNPs remain symptom-free for 10 years or more. They account for about 5% of all individuals infected with HIV. Many studies focusing on LTNPs have shown that they tend to have a vigorous immune response to their infection, both cellular and humoral, which results in an extremely low viral burden. Their CD_4 level shows minimal or no decline, and they have a high level of neutralizing antibody. Their lymph node architecture is preserved and their absolute number of CD_8 cells is significantly and consistently higher when compared to other HIV-positive individuals.

BIBLIOGRAPHY

Benjamini E, Sunshine G, Leskowitz S: *Immunology, a short course,* ed 3, New York, 1996, Wiley-Liss.

Cohen PT, Sande M, Volberding P: *The AIDS knowledge base,* ed 2, New York, 1994, Brown & Co.

DeVita VT, Hellman S, Rosenberg S: *AIDS: biology, diagnosis, treatment and prevention,* ed 4, New York, 1996, Lippincott-Raven.

Sande M, Volberding P: *The medical management of AIDS,* ed 5, Philadelphia, 1997, Saunders.

2

Clinical Application of Immunological and Virological Markers

Carl A. Kirton

Clinical markers can be used in practice to determine when a client is infected with HIV and the associated prognosis. Clinical markers in HIV practice fall into three categories: immunological markers, virological markers, and activated markers. There are a variety of immunological markers. The most common are those that are used to screen for HIV infection and those that are used to stage a client's illness. Virological markers are important in determining prognosis and initiating or changing therapy for HIV infection. Activated markers (e.g., β2 microglobulin, neopterin) were of value in the determination of progression to AIDS before the routine use of quantitative virological markers. Today, activated markers are rarely used.

IMMUNOLOGICAL MARKERS IN HIV

HIV-1 ANTIBODIES

Infection with an antigen, such as HIV, results in activation of B lymphocytes. When activated, B lymphocytes secrete antibodies into the serum that bind with the antigen and prepare it for elimination. The function of antibodies is further described in Chapter 1. When a person becomes infected with HIV, the first type of antibody produced is immunoglobulin M (IgM). The IgM antibody can be detected in a client's serum as early as 5 days after infection,[1] peaks after 2 weeks,[2] and then becomes undetectable after 3 months. Immunoglobulin G (IgG) antibodies appear during the second week of infection[3] in response to selected HIV structural genes and protein products. In most individuals these antibodies are detectable within 3 months after infection and remain detectable during the chronic period of infection. Antibody testing is based on the detection of antibodies of the IgG type.

Usefulness in Clinical Practice

Antibody testing remains the cornerstone of HIV diagnosis. Antibody testing, along with other tests, is used to screen the donated blood supply, as well as tissue and organ donors, for HIV infection. Antibody testing

Antibody Detection Tests	Antigen Detection Tests	Activated Immune Markers
Table 2-1 Tests Used in HIV Infection		
Screening Tests	**Nucleic Acid Determination Assays**	• Neopterin
• Enzyme-linked immunosorbent assay (ELISA or EIA)	• Reverse transcriptase–polymerase chain reaction (RT-PCR)	• β2 microglobulin
• Agglutination assays	• Branched DNA (bDNA)	• Absolute CD_4 count
• Oral fluid test (e.g., OraSure)	• Nucleic acid sequence–based analysis (NASBA)	• CD_4 percentage
• Urine screening test	• Qualitative PCR-DNA	• Absolute CD_8 count
Confirmatory Tests	**Viral Cultivation Methods**	• CD_8 percentage
• Western blot	• HIV culture	• CD_4:CD_8 ratio
• Indirect immunofluorescent antibody assay (IFA)		
• Radioimmunoprecipitation assay (RIPA)		

may be required when persons are applying for individual life, health, and disability income coverage.

Detecting HIV Infection with Antibody Tests

A variety of tests can be used to detect antibodies to HIV (Table 2-1). The enzyme-linked immunosorbent assay (ELISA) is the most widely used assay for the screening of people for HIV infection. This test is 99.9% reliable in determining those who have HIV infection. This means that the ELISA is a nearly perfect test for the detection of HIV antibodies. However, both false positive and false negative results can occur. A false positive result has occurred if a test is positive for HIV antibodies but the individual does not actually have HIV infection. To eliminate these false positives all positive test results, regardless of the antibody test used, are confirmed by additional testing (see the discussion of the Western blot test later in this chapter).

A false negative result has occurred when the test is negative for HIV antibodies but the individual actually is infected with HIV. In the majority of cases, the ELISA detects antibodies to HIV-1 approximately 6 to 12 weeks after exposure. However, testing before this time may result in a false negative because the client has not yet produced sufficient antibodies for detection by this assay. This period of time between the point of infection and seroconversion is referred to as the *window period*.

Most antibody tests are used to detect antibodies to HIV-1. In the United States, assays for the detection of HIV-2 were approved for use by

BOX 2-1 PRETEST AND POSTTEST COUNSELING ASSOCIATED WITH HIV-ANTIBODY TESTING

General Guidelines

Often people who test for HIV are fearful of the test results; therefore nurses should:

- Establish rapport with the client.
- Assess the client's ability to understand counseling.
- Determine the client's ability to access support systems.
- Explain the following benefits of testing:
  - Testing provides an opportunity for education that can decrease the risk of new infections.
  - Infected clients can be referred for early intervention and support programs.
- Discuss the following negative aspects of testing:
  - Breaches of confidentiality have led to discrimination.
  - A positive test affects all aspects of the client's life (e.g., personal, social, economic) and can raise difficult emotions (e.g., anger, anxiety, guilt, thoughts of suicide).

Pretest Counseling

- Determine the client's risk factors and when the last risk occurred. Counseling should be individualized according to these parameters.
- Provide education to decrease future risk of exposure.
- Provide education that will help the client protect sex partners and drug-use partners.
- Discuss problems related to the delay between infection and an accurate test. Testing will need to be repeated at intervals of 3 months after each possible exposure.
- Discuss the need to abstain from further risky behaviors during that interval.
- Discuss the need to protect partners during that interval.
- Discuss the possibility of false negative tests, which are most likely to occur during the window period.
- Explain that a positive test indicates HIV infection and not AIDS.
- Explain that the test does not establish immunity, regardless of the results.
- Assess support systems; provide telephone numbers and resources as needed.
- Discuss the client's personally anticipated responses to test results (positive or negative).
- Outline assistance that will be offered if the test is positive.

Posttest Counseling

If the test is negative, reinforce pretest counseling and prevention education. Remind the client that the test needs to be repeated at intervals of 3 months after the most recent exposure risk. If the test is positive, understand that the client may be in shock and not hear what is said. In addition:

- Provide resources for medical and emotional support, and help the client get immediate assistance.
- Evaluate suicide risk and follow up as needed.
- Determine the need to test others who have had risky contact with the client.
- Discuss retesting to verify results. This tactic provides hope for the client, but more importantly, it keeps the client in the system; while waiting for the second test result, the client has time to think about and adjust to the possibility of being HIV-positive.

BOX 2-1 PRETEST AND POSTTEST COUNSELING ASSOCIATED WITH HIV-ANTIBODY TESTING—CONT'D

Posttest Counseling—cont'd
- Encourage optimism.
- Remind the client that treatments are available.
- Review health habits that can improve the immune system.
- Arrange for the client to speak to HIV-positive people who are willing to share and assist the newly diagnosed client during the transition period.
- Reinforce that an HIV-positive test means that the client is infected, but a positive test does not necessarily mean that the client has AIDS.

Modified from Bradley-Springer LA, Fendrick R: *HIV instant instructor cards,* El Paso, Tx, 1994, Skidmore-Roth.

the FDA in April of 1990. Individual testing for HIV-2 is currently not routine practice, because of the lower prevalence of HIV-2 in the United States. Testing of donated blood for HIV-2, however, began in June of 1992.[4] Selected laboratories can test a single blood sample for both HIV-1 and HIV-2.

Nursing Implications for Antibody Testing

1. Before testing, the nurse or other qualified health care provider completes a risk assessment. (See Chapter 3 to determine a client's risk for infection with HIV.)
2. The client should understand the difference between confidential and anonymous testing. *Confidential testing* is often done in a health care facility and the process includes identifying the client with his or her blood sample. *Anonymous testing* is often done at a public health station or through a home HIV test. In this type of test, the client's name or any other identifying information is not sent along with the blood sample. The client is identified through a unique identification number. The client should be informed that regardless of the method used, test results will not be distributed to anyone except to local and state health departments where required.
3. The client should be informed that all states require that the names of clients with AIDS as defined by the Centers for Disease Control and Prevention (CDC) be reported to selfsame agency. Currently, 34 states conduct name-based HIV infection case surveillance as an extension of AIDS case surveillance, and such surveillance is being considered in other states.[5]
4. Informed consent is required for HIV testing. Pretest and posttest counseling is considered an essential component of HIV testing. Components of the pretest and posttest counseling session are listed in Box 2-1.

5. Clients who have recently been passively immunized (e.g., hepatitis A vaccine) or have received immunoglobulin (e.g., tetanus immune globulin) preparations should delay testing.[6]

6. Influenza vaccines do not appear to cause false positive ELISA results.[7,8]

7. Specimen collection—Blood is collected by venipuncture in a serum separator tube. Laboratory instructions for proper handling of the specimen must be followed.

8. Laboratory test results are reported as reactive (a positive test) or nonreactive (a negative test). All serum samples that are positive are tested several times. See testing algorithm for HIV antibody testing (Figure 2-1). Only reactive ELISA results are subjected to a confirmatory test such as a Western Blot. Some laboratories may report reactive tests as "repeatedly reactive." This means that the test has been performed several times.

9. Positive screening and confirmation tests should be interpreted with caution in clients with severe hepatic disorders; clients with cross reacting antibodies from pregnancy, blood transfusion, or organ transplantation; and clients with autoantibodies as produced by collagen-vascular disease, autoimmune diseases, and malignancy.[9] Follow-up with an antigen detection test (see the discussion of antigen detection later in this chapter) may be indicated.

10. The nurse should inform the client, if applicable (e.g., if the client asks), that the ELISA tests for antibodies to HIV-1. HIV-2 testing is not routinely performed. It is available, however.

11. Home HIV testing—In the summer of 1996 two tests were approved by the FDA for home use: the Confide HIV Testing Service and the Home Access Express Test. Specimens collected in this way undergo ELISA testing and, if necessary, Western blot and/or indirect immunofluorescent antibody assay (IFA) testing. Home testing kits contain a lancet that is used by the client to prick his or her finger to produce a drop of blood, which is placed on a special filter supplied by the manufacturer and allowed to dry. Nurses should teach clients to saturate each of the circles on the collection paper completely to ensure that the proper quantity of blood has been collected. The blood must be allowed to dry completely before the collection paper is placed into the shipping container. If the specimen is not allowed to dry completely, bacteria or fungus can grow within the media and cause inaccurate test results. Testing is anonymous because the client obtains his or her result using an anonymous code. The pros and cons of home HIV testing continue to be examined and debated.[10] Public acceptance of home HIV testing may not be as widespread as originally thought. About 1 year after receiving FDA approval, Johnson and Johnson, the maker of the *Confide* home HIV test, removed its product from the market due to lack of consumer demand. As of this writing *Home Access* is the only home HIV antibody test on the market.

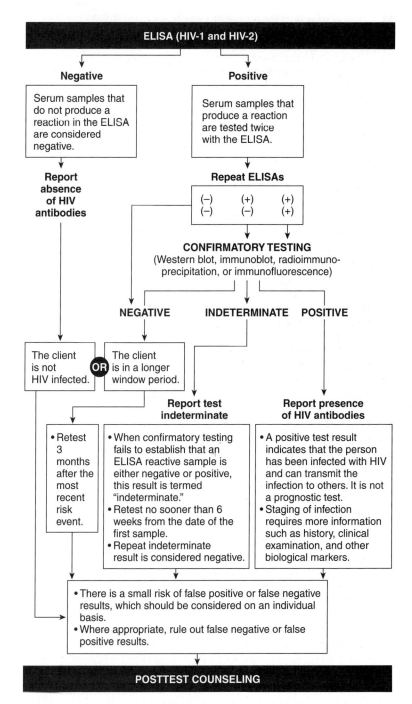

Figure 2-1. Interpretation of HIV testing. (*From Canadian Medical Association [CMA]: Counseling guidelines for HIV testing, Ottawa, Ontario, 1995, CMA.*)

The Western Blot Test

The Western blot is the test most widely used to confirm a positive screening test (i.e., ELISA). The Western blot detects antibodies to specific structural and internal particles of the HIV virus. Each of the viral proteins is separated and bound on paper. The client's serum is added and if antibodies are present, they react with the viral proteins. Reactions, called *bands,* to at least two of the following viral proteins are necessary for a positive determination to be made: p24, gp 41 or gp 160/120.* Samples that do not meet these criteria are labeled indeterminate and are then tested by another confirmatory test, such as the IFA (see Figure 2-1).

Nursing implications for Western blot testing

1. See the nursing implications for antibody testing.
2. Ensure that the client understands that the Western blot test is a confirmatory test for HIV. Only if the screening test (the ELISA antibody test) is positive is a Western blot or similar confirmatory test performed (see Table 2-1).
3. Indeterminate Western blot tests are followed by tests for the detection of HIV antigens, such as polymerase chain reaction DNA testing (PCR-DNA) (see the discussion of PCR-DNA testing later in this chapter). Nurses must ensure that clients understand the importance of follow-up testing after an indeterminate Western blot test.
4. Specimen collection: see the section on antibody testing earlier in this chapter.

Oral HIV-1 Antibody Testing

An alternative to invasive antibody testing is the oral HIV antibody test. This test uses the same technology and interpretive criteria used to detect antibodies to HIV in a serum sample (all reactive test screenings are subjected to confirmatory testing).[11]

The OraSure specimen collection device measures oral mucosal transudate (OMT), which contains high concentrations of IgG antibodies. OMT is a fluid that derives from plasma.

The OraSure pad is placed on the client's buccal mucosa for 2 minutes (Figure 2-2). The pad is then placed in a vial and sent to a lab for testing with an ELISA test. Those with positive results are then tested with the OraSure HIV-1 Western blot kit. The results of the test are sent to a health care provider.

Nursing implications for the use of OraSure for antibody testing

1. The nurse should ensure that risk assessment and informed consent have been obtained and the nature of testing has been explained to the client.
2. Specimen collection is currently limited to a trained individual on the order of a physician or nurse practitioner.

---

*Centers for Disease Control and Prevention/Association of State and Territorial Public Health Laboratory Directors' criteria.

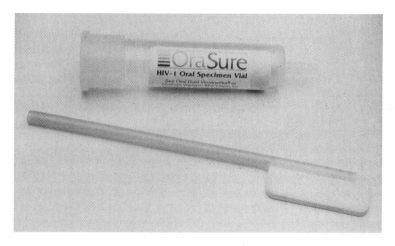

Figure 2-2.   The OraSure specimen collection device. *(Courtesy of Epitope.)*

3. Specimen collection is considered safe because the specially treated pad inactivates the virus within a few minutes after collection.
4. The technique used in collecting the specimen is important. Nurses should teach clients to distinguish saliva from oral fluids. Saliva contains a small number of immune related cells whereas oral fluids contain a large number of IgG antibodies. The specimen collection kit requires a sample of OMT, an oral fluid that has relatively high concentrations of serum-derived IgG antibodies. OMT is collected by placing the specially treated cotton fiber pad that is attached to a nylon stick between the lower cheek and gum for a minimum of 2 minutes.
5. After collection, the pad is placed in the vial contained in the kit and then shipped to the appropriate laboratory for processing.
6. The sample can remain at room temperature and is good for up to 3 weeks after collection.
7. Oral hygiene, oral ulcers, tobacco consumption, anticholinergic drugs, and food intake have been shown to have no effect on test results.[12]

Rapid HIV Testing
Rapid HIV tests use a technology different from the ELISA to detect antibodies to HIV and provide results in 10 to 15 minutes. The only rapid HIV test licensed by the FDA and commercially available in the United States is the Single-Use Diagnostic System for HIV-1 (SUDS). Accuracy of negative results is similar to that of the standard ELISA screening tests. Confirmatory testing is not necessary. Positive test results require that the client have a standard ELISA performed due to the test's low specificity.
Nursing Implications
1. See the implications for antibody testing discussed earlier in this chapter.

Table 2-2	Normal Lymphocyte Counts		
Age	CD$_4$ Absolute Count (mm or μl)	CD$_8$ Absolute Count (mm or μl)	CD$_4$:CD$_8$ Ratio
1 day-23 months	1600-2200	820-1600	1.3-2.6
2 years-6 years	900-1500	700-1200	0.9-1.4
7 years-17 years	640-1200	640-900	1.0-1.5
18 years-70 years	600-980	420-660	1.2-1.9

Urine HIV Testing

Urine HIV testing is performed by an FDA-approved ELISA test. Accuracy of negative results is similar to that of the standard ELISA screening tests. Further testing is not necessary. Positive test results require that the client have a standard ELISA performed due to the test's low specificity.

Nursing Implications
1. See the implications for antibody testing discussed earlier in this chapter.

ABSOLUTE CD$_4$ COUNT

The measurement of the absolute CD$_4$ cell count is an important measure in clients with HIV infection in that it correlates with the degree of the client's immunodeficiency. The normal CD$_4$ count varies with age (Table 2-2). This measure is used to stage the client's HIV illness and to determine the client's risk for the development of opportunistic infections. When reporting CD$_4$ cell counts, most laboratories report the absolute CD$_4$ cell count, the CD$_4$ percentage, the absolute CD$_8$ count and/or percentage, and the CD$_4$:CD$_8$ ratio. Table 2-3 lists common manifestations of HIV disease according to the absolute CD$_4$ cell count.

Usefulness in Clinical Practice

The CD$_4$ cell count, in addition to other markers, is used when making decisions about the initiation of antiretroviral therapy. It is no longer used as the sole measurement in the making of this decision.

Declines in the absolute CD$_4$ cell count are known to be indicative of a client's increasing risk for certain opportunistic infections. Decisions about the initiation of prophylactic therapies are often made on the basis of CD$_4$ cell count.

Nursing Implications of CD$_4$ Results

1. The CD$_4$ cell count should be measured at the time of the initial visit and then every 3 to 6 months thereafter, depending on clinical symp-

Table 2-3	Disease Manifestations of CD$_4$ T Lymphocyte Depletion

500 CD$_4$ Cells	200-500 CD$_4$ Cells	50-200 CD$_4$ Cells
• Low-grade fever • Night sweats	• Idiopathic thrombocytopenia • Progressive, disseminated histoplasmosis • Oral thrush • Intermittent diarrhea (due to *Giardia lamblia, Entamoeba histolytica, Campylobacter jejuni, Salmonella, Shigella*) • Folliculitis • Seborrhea • Psoriasis • Anemia	• Extrapulmonary TB • Lymphoma • HIV wasting syndrome • Oral aphthous ulcers • Esophageal candidiasis • Esophageal herpes • Severe diarrhea (due to *Mycobacterium avium* complex, cytomegalovirus [CMV], cryptosporidium, HSV, microsporidia) • Rectal and cervical dysplasia • Molluscum contagiosum • Human papilloma virus (warts) • Cryptococcal pneumonia • Pulmonary Kaposi's sarcoma • CMV or HSV pneumonia • CMV retinitis • Meningitis due to *Toxoplasma gondii, Cryptococcus neoformans* • CMV encephalitis • Progressive multifocal leukoencephalopathy (PML) • Advanced loss of motor control • Peripheral neuropathy • AIDS dementia complex • Toxoplasmosis • Histoplasmosis

Note: Disease manifestations are listed for the CD$_4$ cell count level at which they generally first occur. There may be a great deal of variation in the manifestations that any person may experience. From Grimes DE, Grimes RM: *AIDS and HIV infection*, St Louis, 1994, Mosby.

toms. The value of obtaining CD$_4$ cell counts once levels are below 50 cells/mm^3 has not been determined.

2. The CD$_4$ cell count remains the best single marker of the capacity of the immune system to prevent the development of opportunistic infections.[13] The nurse should evaluate the client's CD$_4$ cell count and ensure that prophylactic therapy is initiated, if necessary, for the following opportunistic infections.
   If CD$_4$ cell count is less than 200 cells/mm^3:
   - *Pneumocystis carinii* (see Chapter 16)
   - *Cryptococcus* spp. if antigen-positive (see Chapter 14)
   If CD$_4$ cell count is less than 100 cells/mm^3:
   - *T. gondii*, if antibody-positive (see Chapter 16)

If CD_4 cell count is less than 50 cells/mm^3:
  ■ *M. avium* complex (see Chapter 13)

3. Daily fluctuations can occur with CD_4 measurements. CD_4 measurements are typically higher in the morning than in the afternoon. Variations of up to 15% can be found in some individuals. Trends over time should be evaluated rather than isolated values.[14]

4. CD_4 counts should not be obtained during a period of acute illness. They may be lower during this period.

5. Specimen collection—Blood is collected by venipuncture in a lavender top tube containing ethylenediamine tetraacetic acid (EDTA). Nurses should follow laboratory instructions for proper handling of specimen.

6. CD_4 measures should be done by the same laboratory and should be drawn at the same time of the day.

7. On the laboratory report, the absolute CD_4 cell count may be expressed as follows: *T lymphocyte subset: Helper.*

8. An HIV-positive individual with a CD_4 cell count of 200 cells/mm^3 or less meets the CDC criteria for adult and adolescent AIDS.

CD_4 PERCENTAGE

The CD_4 percentage indicates the portion of lymphocytes that express the CD_4 protein receptor on the surface of the cell.

Usefulness in Clinical Practice

Clinically, this value is more important than the absolute CD_4 number and is preferred by most clinicians because it is a measure that is not subject to the same variation as the CD_4 cell count. The normal percentage range of immunocompetent persons is 30% to 60%. This measurement influences and is often used in conjunction with other markers to make decisions about the initiation of antiretroviral therapy both for suppression of HIV replication and for prevention of certain opportunistic infections.

Nursing Implications of CD_4 Percentage Results

1. The CD_4 percentage should be measured at the time of the initial visit and then every 3 to 6 months, depending on clinical symptoms.

2. A CD_4 percentage of less than 20% correlates with serious immunodeficiency. Considering the client's symptoms and other markers, such as viral load (see the discussion on viral load later in this chapter), the client may be considered for antiretroviral therapy.

3. A CD_4 percentage of less than 20% may indicate the need for prophylactic therapy against opportunistic infections.

4. A client with a CD_4 percentage of less than 14% is diagnosed as having AIDS, according to the 1993 CDC criteria for AIDS diagnosis.

5. Specimen collection—Blood is collected by venipuncture in a lavender top tube containing EDTA. Nurses should follow laboratory instructions for the proper handling of specimen.

CD_8 Count

CD_8 cells (also called cytotoxic T cells) mediate the direct killing of cells that have been infected with the HIV virus in two ways: (1) a CD_8 cell attaches itself to the HIV-infected cell and secretes substances into it that cause its death; and (2) a CD_8 cell attaches itself to and brings about changes in the genes of the HIV-infected cell so as to cause the cell to program its own death (apoptosis). These properties may explain the large increases seen in the CD_8 cell count during the first weeks of infection.[15] However, not all clients experience a large initial increase in CD_8 cell count. The clinical significance of this finding is described in Chapter 1. In HIV-positive individuals, the gradual decline in CD_8 cells may be related to progression of the disease. The normal CD_8 count varies with age (see Table 2-2).

Usefulness in Clinical Practice

The routine measurement of the CD_8 count is less common today because of the availability of measures that directly qualify and quantify particles of HIV (see discussion of virological markers later in this chapter). Some laboratories routinely include CD_8 measures along with measures of CD_4. On laboratory reports CD_8 measures may be expressed as follows: *T lymphocyte subset: Suppressor.*

Nursing Implications for CD_8 Results

1. The CD_8 count can increase twentyfold during acute infection. In end-stage infection, CD_8 cells decline concomitantly with CD_4 cells.
2. In adult clients a CD_8 count above 400 cells/mm³ is considered desirable.
3. Long-term nonprogressors (LTNPs) (i.e., clients with documented HIV infection for more than 7 years, stable CD_4 cell counts greater than 600 cells/mm³, no symptoms, and no antiretroviral therapy) have demonstrated vigorous CD_8 responses during acute infection and have consistently high CD_8 counts.
4. Specimen collection—Blood is collected by venipuncture in a lavender top tube containing EDTA. Nurses should follow laboratory instructions for the proper handling of specimen.

CD_4:CD_8 Ratio

The CD_4:CD_8 ratio compares the relative number of CD_4 cells to CD_8 cells. Immunocompetent adults have twice as many CD_4 cells as CD_8 cells, which yields a CD_4:CD_8 ratio approaching 2 (normal CD_4:CD_8 ratio is 1.2 to 1.9). In acute HIV infection the ratio is the opposite, with twice as many CD_8 cells as CD_4 cells.

Usefulness in Clinical Practice

The routine measure of CD_4:CD_8 ratio continues to decline with the availability of measures that qualify and quantify particles of the HIV virus.

Some laboratories routinely include $CD_4:CD_8$ ratio along with measures of T lymphocyte subsets.

Nursing Implications for Measures of the $CD_4:CD_8$ Ratio

1. Worsening of immunological status is associated with a $CD_4:CD_8$ ratio that is approaching zero (e.g., a CD_4 cell count of 250 cells/mm³ and a CD_8 cell count of 783 cells/mm³, with a ratio of 250:783, or 0.3).
2. Specimen collection—Blood is collected by venipuncture in a lavender top tube containing EDTA. Nurses should follow laboratory instructions for the proper handling of the specimen.

VIROLOGICAL MARKERS IN HIV

QUALITATIVE PCR OR PCR-DNA

This test uses a technique called *polymerase chain reaction,* which can be used to detect HIV infection. Once HIV internalizes within a helper T cell, it transcribes its RNA into DNA. This test can be used to measure whether or not this DNA has been incorporated into the host cell's DNA.

Usefulness in Clinical Practice

Qualitative PCR testing is clinically useful for the detection of HIV infection in the time before seroconversion. Not all laboratories have the ability to do this test. The test is most helpful in determining HIV infection in infants born to HIV-positive mothers. It can also be used to determine infection when the Western blot test is reported as indeterminate (see the discussion of Western blot testing earlier in this chapter).

Nursing Implications for PCR-DNA Testing

1. The PCR-DNA test will be positive at any stage of HIV infection. Its use is limited by the lack of widespread availability and the high cost of the test.
2. Specimen collection—Blood is collected by venipuncture in a serum separator tube. Nurses should follow laboratory instructions for the proper handling of specimen.
3. The PCR-DNA test is reported as "positive" if HIV-DNA is detected in the client's serum or "negative" if HIV-DNA is not detected in the client's serum.

NUCLEIC ACID MARKERS

Infection with HIV results in the integration of HIV into various cells. Using special laboratory techniques, nucleic acid of the virus can be detected, amplified, and quantified. Quantification of the amount of detected nucleic acids in the client's serum is commonly called the *viral load* or *viral burden.* This amount is highest during primary HIV infection and late stage AIDS. With highly effective antiretroviral therapy, HIV nucleic acids may become undetectable in the client's serum.

Quantification measures are not yet indicated as screening or diagnostic tests for HIV infection; the test has prognostic value and is used primarily to monitor the response to antiretroviral therapy in persons known to be infected with HIV. To date, there is only one test commercially approved by the FDA for nucleic acid determination assays—the Roche amplicor HIV-1 monitor test. This test uses the client's plasma from which ribonucleic acid (RNA) is isolated, reverse transcribed to DNA, amplified using polymerase chain reaction (PCR) technology, and then reported as the level of HIV-RNA. Two other nucleic acid tests are available (but have yet to receive FDA approval for commercial use as of this writing): branched DNA (bDNA) and nucleic acid sequence–based amplification (NASBA). While not used for screening and diagnosis of HIV infection, measurement and quantification of nucleic acids is now considered an essential standard of HIV care and should be offered to all clients diagnosed with HIV infection.

Usefulness in Clinical Practice

Measurement of the client's viral load is currently the critical marker in the management of a client's HIV disease. It is important in determining the client's risk for disease progression, whether to initiate therapy, the degree of initial antiretroviral effect achieved, and whether a drug regimen is failing.[16] Viral load measurements can vary from undetectable to several million viral particles. An undetectable viral load does not mean that the client has no absolute viral particles. Each of the tests has a *lower limit* below which the detection of viral particles is not possible. If the amount of particles in the client's serum is below this detection limit the results are reported as "undetectable." Manufacturers are constantly working to improve the technology to reach lower detection levels. The currently approved viral detection test is not sensitive enough to detect non–subtype B strains of HIV (i.e., types A, C, E, F, G, and O—strains uncommon in North America).[17]

Nursing Implications for Viral Load Testing

1. Assess the client's health status. Testing should be done at a time of clinical wellness.
2. Specimen collection varies by laboratory. The specimen is collected, however, in a tube that contains one of the following anticoagulants: acid citrate dextrose (ACD) or EDTA. In most testing situations the specimen is spun immediately to separate serum from plasma. The separated plasma is transferred into a plastic container and immediately frozen. To ensure the accuracy of results, *viral load specimens must always remain frozen even when being transported to the laboratory.*

3. Viral load measurements should be measured shortly after diagnosis. Determination of the client's viral load after seroconversion has prognostic value. Clients with over 100,000 copies/ml within 6 months after seroconversion have a poorer prognosis than do those with values below 5,000 copies/ml after seroconversion, unless treatment is initiated to control viral replication.

4. Viral load determination and CD_4 counts are important in determining whether to initiate treatment in HIV infection (see Box 4-1). There can be variability between viral load determinations due to several factors, including the taking of the specimen during a period of illness or improper handling. Therefore, decisions about initiating antiretroviral therapy should only be made after two subsequent viral load determinations, at least 1 to 2 weeks apart.

5. Viral load measurement is used to evaluate the effectiveness of antiretroviral therapy and to monitor disease progression. Determinations should be made every 3 to 4 months or 2 to 4 weeks after a change in any therapy.[18] Antiretroviral therapy should result in a large decrease in viral load as early as 2 months after initiation. If this response does not occur, the nurse should reassess client adherence and consider the possibilities of malabsorption of drugs, drug interactions, or drug failure (see the discussion of treatment failure in Chapter 4). The nurse works collaboratively with the primary health care provider in identifying factors that may have caused a poor viral reduction. A change in the drug regimen may be required. Most health care providers consider effective therapy as one that drives the viral load to undetectable levels at 4 to 6 months after the initiation of therapy.

6. Viral load determinations can be listed in two ways; both ways express the quantity of the genetic material of the virus detected in the client's serum. One way is *HIV-1 RNA QUANT PCR*—when the viral load is expressed this way the laboratory will report the absolute number of copies, in thousands, of HIV-1 RNA per milliliter of plasma tested by PCR. The laboratory gives a reference range that determines the lower limit of detection of the test. Some agencies are capable of providing ultrasensitive testing, meaning that the test used is able to detect HIV copies in the range of 20 to 25 particles. In agencies where ultrasensitive testing is not available, the lower limit of detection is generally at 400 copies/ml. The second way to express the viral load is in logarithmic form—a mathematical expression. In clinical practice, however, laboratories rarely report the viral burden in logarithmic form. Changes in the logarithms, rather than the absolute number of particles, are important indicators when monitoring a response to antiretroviral therapy. If therapy is effective, and the client is taking the medications as prescribed, a 1-log change in viral load should be seen in 4 weeks. Clients who do not have this type of response should be considered for a change in therapy if all other

causes for a lack of this response have been ruled out (e.g., poor compliance, malabsorption, laboratory error). A 1-log change in viral load represents a 10-fold change in the absolute number of viral particles, a 2-log change represents a 100-fold change in the absolute number of viral particles, and a 3-log change represents a 1000-fold change in the absolute number of viral particles.

REFERENCES

1. Bylund JD, Ziegner UH, Hooper DG: Review of testing for human immunodeficiency virus, *Clin Lab Med* 12(2):305, 1992.
2. Gaines H et al: Antibody response in primary human immunodeficiency virus infection, *Lancet* 1:124, 1987.
3. Gaines H et al: Immunological changes in primary HIV-1 infection, *AIDS* 4:995, 1990.
4. George JR, Schochetman G: Detection of HIV infection using serological techniques. In Schochetman, George, eds: *AIDS testing: a comprehensive guide to technical, medical, social, legal and management issues,* ed 2, New York, 1994, Springer-Verlag.
5. Centers for Disease Control and Prevention (CDC): HIV testing among population at risk for HIV infection—nine states, November 1995-December 1996, *MMWR* 47(50):1086, 1998.
6. Celum CL et al: Risk factors for repeatedly reactive HIV-1 EIA and indeterminate western blots: a population-based case control study, *Arch Intern Med* 154(10):1129, 1994.
7. MacKenzie WR et al: Multiple false-positive serological tests for HIV, HTLV-1, and hepatitis C following influenza vaccination, *JAMA* 268(8):1015, 1991.
8. Simonsen L et al: Multiple false reactions in viral antibody screening assays after influenza vaccination, *Am J of Epidemiol* 141(11):1089, 1995.
9. Bartlett JG: *Medical management of HIV infection,* Baltimore, 1999, Port City Press.
10. Anonymous: Critics voice concerns about counseling by telephone, *AIDS Policy Law* 11(10):10, 1996.
11. Gallo D et al: Evaluation of a system using oral mucosal transudate for HIV-1 antibody screening and confirmatory testing, *JAMA* 277(3):254, 1997.
12. Emmons WW et al: A modified ELISA and Western Blot accurately determines anti–human immunodeficiency virus type 1 antibodies in oral fluids obtained with a special collecting device, *J Infect Dis* 171:1406, 1995.
13. Masur H et al: CD_4 counts as predictors of opportunistic pneumonias in human immunodeficiency virus (HIV) infection, *Ann Intern Med* 111:223, 1989.
14. Curry JG: Interpreting laboratory data. In Muma R et al, eds: *HIV Manual for health care professional,* ed 2, Stanford, Conn, 1997, Appleton & Lange.
15. Haynes B: Immune responses to human immunodeficiency virus infection. In DeVita VT, Hellman S, Rosenber SA, eds: *AIDS: biology, diagnosis, treatment and prevention,* ed 4, Philadelphia, 1997, Lippincott-Raven.
16. Saag MS et al: HIV viral load markers in clinical practice, *Nat Med* 2(6):625, 1996.

17. Rouzioux C et al: Quantification of "Non B" subtype HIV-1 RNA: underestimation is frequent for all "non B" subtypes with Monitor and NASBA-QT test Fourth Conference on Retroviruses and Opportunistic Infections, Washington, D.C., 1997 (abstract 285).
18. Carpenter CCJ et al (for the International AIDS Society): Antiretroviral therapy for HIV infection in 1996: recommendation of an international panel, *JAMA* 276:146, 1996.

Unit 1   Frequently Asked Questions

Have subtypes of HIV-1 been identified? If so, what is known about these subtypes?

HIV-1 is a highly variable virus and, so far, has been further subdivided into two subtypes or clades, Group M and Group O. Group M consists of 10 genetically different subtypes (A-J). In Europe and North America, HIV-1 has spread mainly through subtype B, but in Africa (except Western Africa, which has HIV-2), Thailand, and India, initial epidemics of subtype B have been overwhelmed by the rapid spread of subtypes C and E. Group O (O stands for "outlier") viruses are extremely different from Group M viruses. They are so different that they cannot be detected by enzyme immunoassay tests, which are routinely used in the US and Europe. So far Group O has been detected in fewer than 100 people in Western and Central Africa. To date, only one case has been reported of Group O infection in the United States—this was in a woman who had immigrated from Africa. Furthermore, about 10% of viral isolates in HIV-1–positive people are hybrids (i.e., a combination of subtypes, such as A/E or B/F).

There are some differences in the activity of subtypes. Subtypes B, C, and E appear to grow equally well in monocytes and T lymphocytes, but subtypes C and E grow significantly more readily in Langerhans cells than does subtype B. Langerhans cells are precursors to antigen-presenting dendritic cells, which stimulate T lymphocytes to kill virus-infected cells. Langerhans cells also occur in great numbers in the reproductive tract. The implication is that subtypes C and E, with their propensity for Langerhans cells, may be more readily transmitted by heterosexual intercourse. One theory is that there is a higher rate of heterosexual spread of HIV-1 in Asia and Africa because subtypes C and E are more prevalent there.

Has HIV-1 ever been completely cleared from an infected individual?

No cases of this happening in adults have ever been confirmed. However, there is one well-documented case of this happening in an infant who was infected perinatally.[1] A child, identified shortly after birth as infected with HIV-1, has completely cleared the virus. Asymptomatic HIV-1 infection was diagnosed in the mother during the fourth week of pregnancy. She maintained a CD_4 cell count over 1000 cells/mm^3 during pregnancy and was asymptomatic of HIV-1 until 4 years after delivery. The infant was delivered vaginally at 36 weeks, received no blood products, and was not breast fed. HIV-1 was not detected at birth in the infant. HIV-1 was detected by culture of the infant's peripheral blood mononuclear cells at 19 and 51 days of age. At 51 days, HIV-1 was also detected by means of polymerase chain reaction (PCR) testing. At 12 months of age the infant was seronegative for HIV-1 and numerous subsequent cultures and tests by PCR have also been negative. The child has been followed for several years, remains seronegative, and has normal growth and development.

This case raises some interesting questions. How often does this happen? How does it happen? What does it mean for most HIV-1–positive pregnant women and their offspring? It seems likely (as the editors of the *New England Journal of Medicine* point out) that some infants of HIV-1–positive mothers who were declared uninfected may have been transiently infected. Perhaps an understanding of how this happens can help in the development of vaccines to prevent other types of transmission.

Why is it that some people remain uninfected with HIV-1 despite multiple high-risk sexual exposures to HIV-1?

One reason for this has to do with the integrity of the CCR-5 receptor. The CCR-5 receptor is a chemokine receptor found on macrophages. Normally it binds the beta chemokines RANTES, MIP-α, and MIP-β. However, it is also necessary as a coreceptor for the binding of HIV-1 to macrophages. CCR-5 is genetically determined. Some people have a faulty (mutated) gene for this receptor and, as a result, cannot express CCR-5 at all on the surface of macrophages. In a population of Caucasians (the mutated gene has not been found in African Americans or Asians) it is estimated that about 1.4% of this population are homozygous for the mutation (i.e., both alleles for this trait are mutated) and about 13.3% are heterozygous (i.e., they carry one normal allele and one mutated allele for this trait). It appears that those who are homozygous for the mutated gene are protected against infection through sexual transmission of HIV-1 since in these individuals HIV-1 cannot bind to macrophages at the site of entry and thus cannot be distributed throughout the body. (Initial infection with HIV-1 is usually with the non–syncytium-inducing [NSI] strain, which does not bind to T cells.) Those who are heterozygous for the trait are not resistant to HIV-1, but it seems that HIV-1 in these individuals does not replicate as efficiently as it does in people with two normal genes for CCR-5. Hence, heterozygotes for this receptor are more likely to be slow progressors. Evidence indicates that heterozygotes lose from 0 to 50 CD_4 cells per year compared to homozygous normals who lose 50 to 100 CD_4 cells per year.

What are the obstacles to developing an effective HIV-1 vaccine?

Since 1987, 15 experimental HIV-1 vaccines have been tested in the United States in 25 trials. Most of these vaccines were genetically engineered versions of proteins found in the viral coat of HIV-1. So far, though, no vaccine has been able to produce antibodies that consistently neutralize non–laboratory-adapted viral isolates (i.e., viral isolates that will replicate only in cultures of primary human peripheral blood with mononuclear cells).

The problem seems to be the incredible ability of HIV-1 to mutate. A large number of HIV-1 strains already exist. Because of the rapid turnover rate of HIV-1, new strains can arise within an infected individual and probably coexist with other strains. Antibodies produced by an individual can neutralize a significant portion of circulating virus, but there always seem to be some strains present that cannot be neutralized. To be effective, a prophylactic HIV-1 vaccine needs to be able to induce an immune state that will prevent infection of T cells by HIV-1, regardless of the strain. An effective vaccine will have to be able to neutralize all potential variations of HIV-1.

Are older people more vulnerable to being infected with HIV-1?

Yes. Older women are especially more susceptible to HIV-1 infection by sexual transmission. Two factors in the physiology of aging account for this. First, the immune systems of both men and women become less efficient with age. Second, women, after menopause, experience a thinning of the vaginal walls and decreased lubrication, which increases the likelihood of abrasions and therefore increases the risk of transmission of HIV-1.

To date, the Centers for Disease Control and Prevention (CDC) have reported 2500 cases of AIDS among women over 60 years of age and the rate of infection in this age group is increasing. In 1986 there were 102 cases of AIDS reported, and in 1996 there were 305 cases. There are probably many more cases than reported because health care workers do not typically look for HIV-1 infection in older clients; many are misdiagnosed or die before a diagnosis is made.

Does an increase in the CD_4 cell count always mean an improved immune system?

With the advent of new, more effective drug regimens, many people with HIV/AIDS are experiencing a dramatic increase in their CD_4 cell counts. Often, this also means a dramatic improvement in the overall functioning of their immune system. However, this is not true in every case. In some people this increase in CD_4 cell count does not return them to an immune status equal to what it once was at that particular level of CD_4 cells. This is especially true of those whose CD_4 cell counts have fallen below 200 cells/mm^3, and even more so for those whose CD_4 cell counts have reached 50 cells/mm^3 before beginning to rebound.

The reason for this has to do with the nature of CD_4 cells. The body has many clones of CD_4 cells—each clone is especially adapted to respond to a specific antigen. The large number of CD_4 clones is what gives the immune system such great diversity in its ability to recognize antigens. When CD_4 cells die, they are replaced by similar cells in the same clone, and the specific information to respond to a specific antigen is passed on to the newly formed CD_4 cells, so that no immunologic information is lost. However, if an entire clone has been lost, and if immature, naïve cells from the thymus cannot be programmed to replace the lost clone, then that particular immunologic information is lost. If the body is presented with an antigen that was specific to that clone, the immune system will not be able to respond to that antigen. CD_4 cells may be able to increase in numbers because of proliferation of existing clones, but a lost clone may never be replaced, and therefore defects in the immune system's ability to respond to certain antigens may continue despite a rising CD_4 cell count.

The implications of this are twofold. First, early diagnosis and treatment are paramount. Second, drugs to prevent opportunistic infections should be continued even when CD_4 cell counts are rising rapidly.

Can smoking during pregnancy by an HIV-positive woman increase the risk of the baby being infected with HIV?

Yes. In a recent study it was found that HIV-positive women who smoked and did not take prescribed drugs like zidovudine (ZDV) had an infant infection rate of 33%, compared to a rate of 22% for HIV-positive women who did not smoke during pregnancy and did not take ZDV.[2] The exact effects of smoking in HIV-positive women who take zidovudine have not been determined. However, smoking has a negative effect because nicotine is toxic to blood vessels and adversely affects the placenta, promoting premature rupture of the membranes surrounding the baby. This increases the baby's exposure to blood and other maternal secretions that contain the virus.

I saw an advertisement for an HIV test for which the results are obtained in 15 minutes. Why does the test that I am about to receive take one week to be reported?

There are several rapid tests for detection of HIV antibodies (e.g., single use diagnostic system [SUDS], RETROCELL, HIVCHEK, GENIE). The Food and Drug Administration (FDA) has licensed only one test of this type, SUDS (manufactured by Murex Corporation in Norcross, Ga), as a diagnostic test.[3] The sensitivity (99.9%) and specificity (99.6%) of this test are a few tenths of a point less than the standard ELISA/Western blot test. It is recommended that positive or indeterminate rapid test results be followed with a standard ELISA/Western blot confirmatory test to determine HIV infection.

Since 1996, a urine enzyme immunoassay (EIA) (Sentinel, manufactured by Seradyn) has been approved and is available for use. In 1998, the FDA approved a urine Western blot (Calypate, manufactured by Calypate Biomedical in Berkeley, Calif) for detection of HIV antibodies. These two tests are sufficiently accurate for screening in medical and public health facilities; however, the FDA recommends that positive screening tests be followed by testing of a blood sample.

If my viral load is at undetectable levels does it mean that I'm not infectious?

No. Undetectable viral load simply means that the number of viral particles has reached the lower limit of detection of the test used. However, let's assume that a highly effective drug regimen cleared the entire pool of virus from the blood. Only 2% of the body's HIV resides in the blood. The rest dwells in the body's lymphoid tissues and other sites such as the brain. It is thought that HIV may sequester itself in these sanctuary sites, waiting for the opportunity to emerge. Very little is known about how effective drug therapy is at these sanctuary sites. Moreover, HIV infection results in immune destruction that may never be wholly recovered. HIV is never cleared from the system (except in extremely rare cases) and a person should always be considered infectious despite laboratory results that show "undetectable" HIV.

REFERENCES

1. Bryson Y et al: Clearance of HIV infection in a perinatally infected infant, *New Engl J Med* 332(13):833, 1995.
2. Turner BJ et al: Cigarette smoking and maternal child HIV transmission, *J Acquir Immune Defic Syndr and Hum Retrovirol* 14(4):327, 1997.
3. George JR, Schochetman G: Detection of HIV infection using serological techniques. In Schochetman G, George JR, eds: *AIDS testing: a comprehensive guide to technical, medical, social, legal, and management issues,* ed 2, New York, 1994, Springer-Verlag.

Unit II

Ambulatory Nursing Care of Clients with HIV/AIDS

3

Risk Assessment, Identification, and HIV Counseling

Carl A. Kirton

RISK ASSESSMENT

Risk assessment in HIV care refers to the process of identifying clients who are at risk for infection with HIV. Transmission of HIV most commonly occurs through unprotected sexual intercourse, through needle sharing associated with intravenous (IV) drug use, and perinatally. Uncommon modes of HIV transmission include transfusion- or transplant-related transmission, household transmission (e.g., razor sharing,[1] contact with bloody lesions[2]), and transmission in the health care setting.[3] Combined, uncommon modes of HIV transmission account for approximately 0.01% of the AIDS cases reported to the Centers for Disease Control and Prevention (CDC).[4] Uncommon modes of transmission and perinatal transmission are described elsewhere in this text. This chapter focuses on assessing the risk of infection in relation to injection drug use and sexual practices.

INJECTION TRANSMISSION

Sharing of injection equipment contaminated with HIV-infected blood is the primary way in which HIV is transmitted to injection drug users. The majority of HIV-positive women have acquired HIV through unprotected sex with an HIV-positive partner or through injection drug use. In the United States, drug injection is often considered a personal weakness rather than a disease and, therefore, the injection drug user often encounters negative responses from health care providers. All clients who present for health-related care should be asked directly about drug use. The best means of screening for substance abuse is by history.[5] However, the ability of providers to recognize clients who abuse alcohol, prescribed medications, or illegal drugs is typically poor.[6] If a client has been identified as having a substance abuse problem, a careful review of the client's drug-related activities is essential in determining the client's risk for HIV. This cannot be done without understanding drug injection behaviors and terminology that may be used by the client. Box 3-1 lists some commonly used terms related to drug use.

BOX 3-1 INTRAVENOUS DRUG USER TERMINOLOGY

Angel dust	Slang for phencyclidine (PCP)
Balloon	A unit of measure similar to a bag
Bag	A unit of measure: ¼ g
Base	To smoke a specially prepared form of cocaine in a water pipe (very fast and addictive high)
Belushi (i.e., John Belushi)	Alternated injections of cocaine and heroin; a speedball
Boot	To draw up blood into syringe and mix with substance—usually cocaine
Boost	To inject drugs; also to steal
Clean, clean up	To be drug free; to stop using
Cooker	A bottle cap or spoon used to heat and dissolve heroin in water
Cotton	Heroin and other drugs are drawn into the syringe through a piece of cotton for filtration; well-used cottons are boiled during scarce times
Crashing	A state of physical discomfort and depression caused by stopping speed use, especially after an extended period of use
Cut	A substance added to a drug that acts as an extender
Detox	Medical management of withdrawal from heroin—usually refers to 21-day methadone treatment
Dillies	Prescription synthetic morphine (very addictive)
Dirty	Using heroin or speed, especially after being clean
Eight ball	⅛ oz of cocaine
Fix	To inject drugs, especially heroin; an injection of drugs
Freebase	To smoke a form of cocaine in a water pipe; a smokeable form of cocaine
Getting off	Getting high; the initial awareness of pleasure after injection
Guzzle	To inject drugs—usually heroin
Horn	To snort or snuff—usually refers to stimulants
KJ	Killer joint; marijuana cigarette with PCP
Needle	Usually refers to the entire syringe/needle combination

Sharing of needles is the behavior that is most frequently associated with transmission of HIV; however, other drug paraphernalia or "works" (e.g., cookers, rinse waters, and cotton swabs) are known to serve as vehicles of transmission.[7] One method of reducing HIV transmission is to focus on reducing or changing risky behaviors. A framework for this approach is known as the Harm Reduction Model. This public health strategy is surrounded by controversy. It acknowledges that abstinence from drug injection is not always achievable; rather than stressing abstinence it focuses on teaching clients ways to prevent the transmission of HIV. It focuses on user-friendly services for drug injectors, such as an informal atmosphere at meetings (held in community-based locations), needle exchange programs, and peer education. Critics of the harm reduction approach purport that it promotes drug injection

BOX 3-1   INTRAVENOUS DRUG USER TERMINOLOGY—CONT'D

Nod, nodding	A dreamlike state induced by heroin
OD	Overdose; ranges from unconsciousness to death
Outfit	Syringe/needle
Overamp	Overdose of speed—usually in the sense of overly intense sensation
PCP	Phencyclidine; a hallucinogen that was used originally for battlefield anesthesia and is currently used as a horse tranquilizer
Point	Syringe/needle
Redi-rock	A small piece of specially prepared cocaine, often inserted in a cigarette for instant availability
Rig	Syringe/needle
Rush, rushing	The initial intense sensation felt when injecting drugs
Script	Prescription
Shoot up	To inject drugs
Sick	The intensely painful period during withdrawal from opiates
Slam	To inject drugs
Snort	Inhalation of a substance via the nostrils (e.g., cocaine, crystal, Persian heroin)
Speedball	A mix of cocaine (or speed) and heroin in a syringe
Speed, speeding	Amphetamines, using amphetamines
Spoon	A utensil for dissolving and heating substances before injecting
Stick	To inject drugs
Strung out	Heavily addicted
Track	An injection mark
Tweaking	A level of speed intoxication reached after 1 or more days of constant use, characterized by obsessive behavior
Well	A state of well-being achieved by injecting heroin after being sick
Works	Syringe/needle

use. The claims of this argument, however, have not been demonstrated empirically.

Nurses who work with clients who inject drugs must be holistic in their approach; they must focus not only on reducing the risk of HIV infection but also on economic and social problems that clients often face, such as poverty and homelessness.

TRANSMISSION BY SEXUAL CONTACT

All clients who are sexually active, regardless of age, gender, sexual orientation, or race, are at risk for infection with HIV, although each person's individual risk is markedly different. Identification of clients at risk for HIV begins by taking a sexual history. The sexual history is done as part of the health history and is one of the most overlooked elements of the history, even in cases where the risk for acquiring HIV infection was self-identified as being medium to high.[8,9] The traditional nursing history often excludes an examination of sexual issues; however, sexual issues can result from a variety of chronic illnesses or treatments, and if problems or potential problems are left unidentified, the client's self-concept can be affected and adjustment to altered body image or altered bodily function can be difficult.[10] In one particular study, more than 90% of clients thought that nurses were appropriate providers with whom to discuss sexual concerns.[11] Disease prevention and health promotion are an essential part of nursing practice, and must include HIV risk assessment and the promotion of a healthy sexual lifestyle. Each client encounter, regardless of setting, offers the clinician an opportunity to discuss sexual activities. Taking a sexual history, as a rule, should occur regardless of the nursing care setting. Box 3-2 lists essential questions that should be included in the sexual history.

Taking a Sexual History

Clinicians and clients have difficulty in initiating discussions and communicating about sex and AIDS.[8] One of the techniques that a nurse should employ at the beginning of a history is, after a cordial greeting, to ask the client's "permission" to take a sexual history. Attention to the particulars of the setting reduces communication barriers and promotes an atmosphere of trust and healthy intimacy that allows information to be exchanged in both directions. In the ambulatory setting, this discussion is done in a confidential and safe place, without interruption, and with the client in street clothes. Removal of physical barriers, such as a desk, between the clinician and client often facilitates communication about uncomfortable subjects. For hospitalized clients, a quiet time of the day should be selected for the interview and, if a roommate is present, the client's curtain should be drawn and a subdued tone of speech should be used during the discussion.

While taking a sexual history, the clinician must be prepared for various emotional responses such as avoidance, tears, anger, or transference. Emotional responses are important clues for the clinician and may lead to the revelation of sexual assaults, sexual abuse, a history of childhood incest, or ongoing sexual violence in a current relationship. Referral to a clinician more skilled in handling sexual issues of this nature is often warranted.

The clinician should be aware that judgment and ridicule are the most feared responses, and so the clinician must clearly convey that neither is occurring. The clinician must be aware that clients often feel judged by both verbal and nonverbal communications. Clients may often reveal participation in sexual activities that differ from the provider's own; nevertheless, the clinician must always treat the client with positive regard. *Positive regard* is the ability to appreciate and respect another person's worth and dignity with a nonjudgmental attitude. Clinicians who respect their clients value their individuality and accept them re-

BOX 3-2 SEXUAL HEALTH HISTORY

Questions

Do you have any problems in the genital area, such as sores or lesions, or have you had these in the past? If so, how were these treated?

Do you currently have any vaginal discharge? If so, describe its color, odor, and consistency.

Has the onset of the vaginal discharge been sudden or gradual?

Does your sexual partner have any discharge?

Do you have any associated symptoms, such as itching; tender, inflamed, or bleeding external tissues; a rash; dysuria or burning during urination; abdominal pain; or pelvic fullness?

Do you have any abdominal pain?

Have you had a sexual relationship with someone who has a sexually transmitted disease (STD), such as gonorrhea, herpes, HIV infection, AIDS, chlamydial infection, venereal warts, or syphilis? If so, when?

Have you ever been treated for any of these problems? If so, was the treatment successful? Were there any complications? Do you use any precautions to prevent the transmission of AIDS or other STDs? Do you have any questions or concerns about these diseases?

For women: Have you ever had surgery on the uterus, vagina, or ovaries? If so, what was done? When? Why? How do you feel about having had the surgery? How has it affected you?

For men: Have you had any surgery on the penis, prostate, or scrotum?

Are you currently in a relationship that involves sexual intercourse?

Do you have one or multiple partners?

How many sexual partners have you had in the past 12 months?

Do you prefer relationships with men, women, or both?

For men: Have you ever had sex with another man, even once?

How frequently do you engage in sexual activities?

Are you and your partner(s) satisfied with the sexual relationship?

Do you and your partner(s) use any contraceptive/protective methods? Which ones? Are they satisfactory to you? Do you have any questions about methods? Do you communicate comfortably about sex?

Adapted from Thompson J, Wilson S: *Health assessment for nursing practice,* ed 4, St Louis, 1996, Mosby.

gardless of the information conveyed. Clients can sense a positive regard in the clinician's demeanor, attitude, and verbal and nonverbal communication.[12] Being attentive to the forms of communication serves to place the client at ease and allow free expression of the matter at hand. Should the client decline to provide a sexual history, this should be respected, noted, and kept in mind. The nurse should express to the client the importance of the sexual history in determining factors that may affect the client's health. Should the client continue to refuse, the sexual history should be brought up at a later time when there is more trust between the client and the clinician.

BOX 3-3 CLINICAL TERMS FOR VARIOUS SEXUAL EXPRESSIONS

Fellatio	Oral-penile contact, with or without ejaculation
Oral insertive intercourse	Giving oral sex (putting the mouth on someone else's genitalia)
Oral receptive intercourse	Receiving oral sex (someone else putting the mouth on the genitalia)
Cunnilingus	Oral-vaginal contact, with or without a dental dam
Anal insertive intercourse	Anal-penile contact, with or without ejaculation*
Anal receptive intercourse	Anal-penile contact, with or without ejaculation*
Vaginal sex	Vaginal-penile contact, with or without ejaculation*
Anilingus	Oral-anal contact
Brachioanal/brachiorectal contact	Digital or whole-hand contact with rectum
Brachiovaginal contact	Digital or whole-hand contact with vagina
Coprolagnia	Sexual behavior involving feces
Deep kissing	Oral-oral contact, in which the tongue is inserted and/or oral fluids are exchanged
Frottage	Sexual gratification that can occur by rubbing the genital area against the genital area of another person while clothed
Tribadism	Vaginal-vaginal frottage
Urolagnia	Sexual behavior involving urine

*Protected: with a condom; unprotected: without a condom.

Dealing with embarrassment. The sexual history is a particularly sensitive area of discussion for clients and may at times embarrass them. The nurse must acknowledge this embarrassment. Showing understanding of the client's embarrassment may not eliminate it but may help further the discussion of this particularly difficult subject.

Finding appropriate language. Using language that is formal and scientific may alienate clients because of lack of comprehension. It may also act as a barrier to obtaining an accurate sexual history. The nurse must allow the client to use colloquial terms when discussing sexual matters. There are no rules as to language that is appropriate. The nurse must take cues from the client. To get the best sexual history, the nurse must use the client's terms when discussing sexual activities. Because sexual terms can often have several connotations, the nurse must clarify with the client the exact meaning of terms. When the client is vague or the nurse does not understand the meaning of the term, the nurse must seek clarification. For example, the client may tell the nurse that she and her partner were "going at it." For some people this can mean heavy petting and for others it can mean sexual intercourse.

To communicate effectively with the client, nurses must be knowledgeable about different sexual practices and sensitive to different personal expressions about sex. Box 3-3 list various sexual practices and com-

> ## BOX 3-4   Clients Who Should Be Offered HIV-Antibody Testing
>
> - Men who have sex with men
> - Persons who have multiple sexual partners
> - Any person who uses drugs or alcohol at the time of sexual activity
> - Persons with a current or remote history of injection drug use
> - Persons who received blood products between 1978 and 1985
> - Persons who have a history of any sexually transmitted diseases (STDs)
> - Sex workers and their sexual partners
> - Sexual partners of those who are at risk for HIV infection
> - Children born to HIV-positive mothers
> - Women who report unprotected sex
> - Any person who considers himself or herself at risk

mon colloquial expressions used to describe them. Nurses should bear in mind that colloquial expressions vary greatly among different genders, races, and age groups. Regional variations can also occur.

HIV COUNSELING AND TESTING

It is a well-known fact that HIV, although it is a preventable disease, is a continuing problem among sexually active adolescents and adults and injection drug users in the United States. Identifying clients at risk because of their behaviors and transferring knowledge about methods of reducing risk is no longer a matter of choice for health care providers—each clinical encounter should be viewed as a potential opportunity to assess risk for HIV infection and to offer prevention information.[13] Clients at risk for HIV infection should be offered HIV counseling and testing. The purposes of HIV counseling and testing are: (1) to help the person initiate behavioral change to prevent infection or, if the person is already infected, to prevent transmission to others; and (2) to help persons obtain referrals to receive additional prevention services, HIV-related medical care, assistance with drug and alcohol withdrawal, or other needed services.[13] Box 3-4 lists clients who should be offered HIV antibody testing.

The process of antibody testing for HIV begins with a session of counseling by a person trained in the key components of pretest and posttest counseling (see Box 2-1). This person may be a nurse, physician, or lay person. Regardless of the type of provider, the following are the key components of the interview.

DETERMINATION OF SEXUAL EXPERIENCES

The interviewer should try to establish the client's sexual experiences in the past and at the present time. Modes of sexual expression can change throughout a person's life. Sexual expression is often influenced by various cultural, environmental, and spiritual mores. Labels such as

BOX 3-5   DRUG NAME AND STREET TERMS

Amphetamines	Uppers, Speed, Meth, Whites, Dexies, Black Beauties, Crank
Cocaine	Coke, Crack, White Candy, Nose Candy, Snow, Toot, Blow, Free Base, C, Flake, Gold Dust
Marijuana	Dope, Pot, Reefer, Joint, Grass
Opiates	Codeine (school boy), Heroin (smack, horse, junk), Hydrocodone, Morphine ("M," "Miss Emma")
Phencyclidine	Angel Dust, Devil Stick, PCP, Dummy Dust, Elephant Juice, Hog
Barbiturates	Downers, Dolls, Reds, Rainbows, Yellows, Tunia, Goof Balls, Blues
Benzodiazepines	Downers
Methadone	Done, Dolophine, Methadose
Methaqualone	Ludes, Soapers, Quads

"gay," "heterosexual," and "straight" are not reliable indicators of sexual activity, and the client's description of his or her current activities does not always serve as an indicator of past sexual activity. To ask only if one is "straight" or "gay" can limit data gathering and lead to inappropriate determination of risk. To determine the client's full spectrum of sexual activity, the interviewer should ask clients whether they have ever had any sexual contact with either men or women or both. If there has been sexual contact, the practices in which the client has engaged should also be explored.

DETERMINATION OF DRUG USE

Clients should be asked directly about their use of alcohol, prescription drugs, or any illegal drugs in the past and presently. Commonly abused drugs and their street names are listed in Box 3-5. The counselor should use language that is appropriate to the client. The counselor should ask about injectable drugs as well as noninjectable drugs. The use of any mood-altering substance can cause loss of inhibitions and may lead to unsafe sexual activity.

DETERMINATION OF RISK

During the interview, the counselor should encourage an open and free-flowing discussion about the client's sexual and drug activities. Doing so prevents the counselor from missing—because of preconceived notions about the client based on gender or sexual orientation stereotypes—any details about drug or sexual activities that may put the client at risk. Common preconceived (and incorrect) notions include that heterosexual women do not engage in anal intercourse and older adult clients do not engage in sex or use illicit drugs.

Abstinence, dry kissing, hugging, holding hands, and massage never transmit HIV from one individual to another. Any type of sexual activity confers a risk of transmission of HIV, however, the actual risk of particular sexual activities follows a continuum of low risk to high risk. Any client who reports a history of drug use should be considered at high risk for HIV infection.

During the determination of risk, the counselor is also afforded the opportunity to evaluate the client's sexual health. The information obtained is used to create a risk reduction plan for the client. The counselor should inquire as to the number of sexual partners a client has had in a specific period of time. This information is important because the number of partners a person has is proportionally related to risk for HIV infection. It is important to explore with clients whether or not they know their sexual partners and are concerned about any drug or sexual behaviors in which their partners are engaged or have engaged in the past. The professional counselor* should explore with clients the existence and quality of their sexual and personal relationships. The quality and nature of sexual experience may reveal a sexual dysfunction. Clients should be asked questions about sexual activities that may put their physical health in jeopardy such as rough sex, autocratic sex, sex in the open, or forced sex. The professional counselor needs to ascertain clients' abilities to set boundaries and to maintain boundaries with varying degrees of intimacy with their partners. This knowledge is important to the development of the risk reduction plan. Specific strategies of the sexual risk reduction plan are described in the following sections.

HIV EDUCATION AND RISK REDUCTION

One of the most important components of the counseling and testing process is to provide education about HIV transmission and ways to reduce the risk of infection. At the time of antibody testing, clients may be anxious about talking to the counselor about activities of which they feel ashamed and about the outcome of the test. To be effectual, the HIV education message must be short and simple. Clients' capacity to recall instruction and advice has been empirically demonstrated to be poor.[14] Four methods of instruction seem to increase recall: (1) short words and sentences, (2) categorization, (3) repetition, and (4) use of concrete-specific rather than general-abstract statements (e.g., "anal sex without a condom transmits HIV" rather than "various sex-related behaviors transmit HIV").[14]

The client must know that transmission occurs in one way: through the exchange of body fluids. Exchange of body fluids can occur in three ways: (1) direct injection (with contaminated drugs, needles, syringes, blood, or blood products), (2) sexual intercourse and other activities in

---

*A health care provider or other person specifically trained in the identification of sexual dysfunction.

which body fluids are exchanged, and (3) from mother to fetus. When teaching clients about sexual transmission, mnemonics can be helpful for both the counselor and the client. For sexual transmission, the OVA mnemonic teaches that sexual transmission occurs through unprotected **O**ral, **V**aginal, and **A**nal sex. The risk of infection is ordered from lowest to highest. For risk reduction, the ABC mnemonic teaches the client that risk reduction is achieved by: **A**bstaining from sex, the use of a latex **B**arrier, or being involved in a **C**ommitted relationship with someone who is HIV-negative.

Other elements of education and risk reduction should be individualized to the client based on the drug and sexual history.

Risk Reduction for Injection Drug Users

Clients should not share needles or any other "works." Not all injection drug users are needle sharers. Factors that seem to favor needle sharing are poly-drug use and injection of drugs in "shooting galleries."[15] Peer behavior has also been shown to influence needle sharing. Injection drug users, in one study, were more likely to share needles if they thought that their drug-injecting friend would be insulted by their refusal. The authors also demonstrated that clients who shared needles knew of the consequences of their behaviors.[16]

Clients who continue to inject drugs should be taught how to clean their "works" before and after injecting drugs. Lay counselors should refer such clients to agencies or other appropriate health care providers that can assist the client with drug treatment or rehabilitation.

Clients who inject drugs should know that they could also contract infections other than HIV (e.g., hepatitis, endocarditis) or develop abscesses. Clients should be referred to appropriate health care providers if indicated.

Risk Reduction for Clients Who Use Drugs During Sexual Activities

The client should be taught that the use of illicit drugs such as amyl nitrate (poppers) or alcohol may impair judgment and lead the client to take sexual risks that he or she would otherwise not take. The client should be instructed that these substances may also impair the immune system, making the client more susceptible to HIV infection.

Risk Reduction for Clients at Risk for Sexual Transmission of HIV

The client should be taught to always use latex condoms and not sheepskin condoms for sexual activities. Dental dams should be used to cover areas that may contain body fluids (e.g., the vulva during cunnilingus) or that serve as potential routes of transmission (e.g., areas of broken skin).

The counselor should review with the client his or her history of sexually transmitted diseases (STDs), such as herpes, hepatitis B and C, gonorrhea, chlamydia, and others. STDs, particularly ulcerative genital diseases, facilitate the transmission of HIV. Infection with syphilis, chancroid, or herpes increases the risk of getting HIV 10 to 20 times. In the case of gonorrhea or chlamydial infection the risk increases three to four times.[17]

The counselor should review with the client the use of water-based lubricants. Their use should be encouraged; lubricants such as Forplay, Wet, and AstroGlide reduce the friction and tearing of mucosa that can occur during sexual intercourse.

Use of spermicidal agents such as nonoxynol 9 may confer some protection from HIV. Nonoxynol 9 has been demonstrated to kill HIV in vitro,[18] but there are many questions surrounding its possible use in prevention of HIV transmission. Clients should be taught that nonoxynol 9 should never be used as a substitute for latex condoms. There is concern that nonoxynol 9 may promote the transmission of HIV because it may be toxic to the epithelium of the genital tract and irritation of the vaginal mucosa may provide a portal of entry for HIV.[18,19] To some persons nonoxynol 9 is an irritant and may cause irritated tissue to serve as a portal of entry for HIV (see Chapter 8).

DISCUSSION OF ANTIBODY TESTING

The knowledge needed by the counselor about antibody testing is discussed in Chapter 2. The counselor uses this information to discuss with the client the purpose of antibody testing and the meaning of a positive and negative test result. A careful review of the client's most recent drug use and sexual activity will help to determine if the client is in the window period of testing. The counselor should ensure that the client understands the meaning of the window period and should advise further testing if indicated. For clients who have been previously tested, it is prudent to review their sexual and drug activity 3 months prior to the last HIV test; at the point of last testing the client may have been in the window period. The client should understand the difference between HIV and AIDS.

CONCLUDING THE TESTING SESSION

The counselor should explore with the client what it would mean to the client to be both HIV-negative and HIV-positive. This serves as a way of evaluating the client's understanding of information that was conveyed and may indicate a need to provide further education. The counselor should ask clients about their support mechanisms and also what they think it would be like if they were tested and found to be antibody positive. The client should be offered the opportunity to ask questions. Instructions on returning for results should conclude the session.

PROVIDING TEST RESULTS

Test results, regardless of the outcome, must be communicated in person. Providing test results in person ensures that the proper person is receiving the test results. "In person" communication also allows the counselor to assess the client's response and understanding of the result and take appropriate action if the client has an adverse psychological reaction.

When providing test results it is important to do so immediately. Clients are often fraught with anxiety about the test outcome and delays in giving results only add to the client's stress. ELISA results are often recorded as reactive (antibody positive) or nonreactive (antibody negative). The counselor may need to clarify the meaning of a reactive or nonreactive test.

Negative Test Results

When clients are told of a negative test result, the counselor should anticipate a reaction that can vary from indifference to tears. The counselor must be certain that the client understands the meaning of a negative result. It means that the client is either not infected with the HIV virus or that the client is so recently infected that ELISA testing could not detect antibodies. The counselor must review the client's sexual and drug history to determine which one of the above circumstances applies to the client. Clients in the latter category should return for follow-up testing 3 months after the most recent suspected exposure. Clients with negative results should be given information that focuses on behaviors important to HIV risk reduction.

Positive Test Results

If a client has reactive (positive) samples, the client should be told right away that the results are positive. The counselor should expect that emotional responses may include tears, disbelief, and sometimes anger. Ensure that the client understands that the results indicate that the client is infected with HIV. Allow the client to ask questions about the information that has just been provided. Clients will often ask if the counselor is sure that the results are positive. The client should be given a brief explanation about ELISA and Western blot testing. Unless results are reported as indeterminate, rarely is further testing indicated.

A newly diagnosed HIV-positive client requires several referrals (Box 3-6). This initial meeting period may not be the most appropriate time to make referrals; the client may be unable to absorb information. The counselor focuses this session on client support; however, an immediate mental health referral is warranted if the client expresses a desire to inflict personal harm. All clients should be scheduled for a follow-up session. These secondary sessions should focus on the importance of medical follow-up, discussion of ways to stay healthy, arrangement of social support services and psychological services. In situations in which it is unlikely that the client will return for follow-up or in which telephone follow-up may not be feasible, prompt medical referral is warranted.

BOX 3-6 POTENTIAL REFERRALS FOR THE NEWLY DIAGNOSED HIV-POSITIVE CLIENT

- Infectious disease specialist, nurse practitioners, physician assistants
- Free clinics for the indigent client
- Social Service agencies (e.g., public assistance programs, drug assistance programs)
- Hospitals with and without dedicated AIDS units
- For pregnant women: Prenatal clinics
- Family planning clinics, if indicated
- Mental health centers and professionals
- AIDS service organizations (see Chapter 12 for further discussion)
- HIV/AIDS community-based organizations (see Chapter 12 for further discussion)
- Substance abuse treatment facilities
- Religious institutions

REFERENCES

1. Centers for Disease Control and Prevention: HIV transmission between two adolescent brothers receiving intravenous therapy for hemophilia, *MMWR* 42:228, 1992.
2. Centers for Disease Control and Prevention: Human immunodeficiency virus transmission in household settings: United States, *MMWR* 43:347, 1994.
3. Fitzgibbon JE: Infrequent patterns of HIV transmission: infection control implications, *AIDS Reader* 5(3):80, 1995.
4. Centers for Disease Control and Prevention: Statistics from the Centers for Disease Control and Prevention, *AIDS* 8:399, 1994.
5. Hyman SE: Approach to the substance-abusing patient. In Gorell AH, May LA, Mulley AG, eds: *Primary care medicine*, ed 3, St Louis, 1995, Lippincott.
6. Potter PA: Physical examination and health assessment. In Potter PA, Perry AG, eds: *Fundamentals of nursing*, ed 4, St Louis, 1997, Mosby.
7. Shah SM et al: Detection of HIV-1 DNA in needle/syringes, paraphernalia and washes from shooting galleries in Miami: a preliminary report, *J Acquir Immune Defic Syndr Hum Retrovirol* 11(3):301, 1996.
8. Gerbert B, Bleecker T, Bernzweig J: Is anybody talking to physicians about acquired immunodeficiency syndrome and sex? A national survey of patients, *Arch Fam Med* 2(1):45, 1993.
9. Ross PE, Landis SE: Development and evaluation of a sexual history taking curriculum for first- and second-year family practice residents, *Fam Med* 26(5):293, 1994.
10. Wilson RE: The nurse's role in sexual counseling, *Ostomy Wound Management* 41(1):72, 1995.
11. Waterhouse J, Metcalfe M: Attitudes toward nurses discussing sexual concerns with patients, *J Adv Nurs* 16(9):1048, 1991.
12. Sims LK et al: *Health assessment in nursing*, ed 1, Redwood, Calif, 1995, Addison & Wesley.

13. Centers for Disease Control and Prevention: Technical guidelines on HIV counseling, 1993, *MMWR* 42:11, 1993.
14. Ley P: Memory for medical information, *Br J Soc Clin Psychol* 18:245, 1979.
15. Dolan MP et al: Characteristics of drug abusers that discriminate needle-sharers, *Public Health Rep* 102(4):395, 1987.
16. Magura S et al: Determinants of needle sharing among intravenous drug users, *Am J Public Health* 79(4):459, 1989.
17. Stine G: *Acquired immune deficiency syndrome: biological, medical, social, and legal issues,* ed 2, Englewood Cliffs, NJ, 1996, Prentice Hall.
18. Martin HL et al: Safety of a nonoxynol-9 vaginal gel in Kenyan prostitutes: a randomized clinical trial, *Sex Transm Dis* 24:279, 1997.
19. American Health Consultants: No stones unturned in major push to develop microbicides, *AIDS Alert* 11(12):133, Atlanta, Ga, 1996, The Association.

4 Guidelines for the Initiation of Antiretroviral Therapy

Carl A. Kirton

Several factors determine the decision to start a client on antiretroviral therapy: the degree of immunodeficiency (i.e., CD_4 cell count), the amount of viral replication (viral load), the presence of certain opportunistic infections (e.g., thrush, pneumocystic carinii pneumonia), and the client's willingness and ability to adhere to a complex medication regimen. To date, there is no universally accepted standard regarding the optimal time to begin antiretroviral therapy. Recommendations vary among expert panels and agencies. Box 4-1 lists the recommendations for the initiation of antiretroviral therapy cited by most health care professionals.

Medical providers base HIV treatment decisions on currently understood HIV pathogenesis and immune system functioning. Viral load value and absolute CD_4 cell counts are important criteria for treatment decisions. In addition, clients should be initiated on antiretroviral therapy when symptoms of HIV disease, such as thrush, unexplained fever, or any one of the AIDS defining illnesses, are present. Most providers agree that absolute viral suppression is a desirable goal; however, many providers report that at least 50% to 60% of their clients are unable to achieve this goal, or that the clients achieve this goal and then fail.[1]

Viral eradication through antiretroviral therapy is desirable but has only been conceptualized in mathematical models. The best clinical strategy to date has been to protect the immune system from further destruction by HIV through sustained suppression of viral replication, using antiretroviral therapy. Theoretically, adequate viral suppression may allow the immune system to strengthen itself and prevent the emergence of life-threatening opportunistic infections. Viral replication is represented by the amount of plasma HIV RNA or viral load. Immune system functioning is represented by the CD_4 cell count or percentage.

DRUG THERAPY IN HIV

When considering the use of antiretroviral therapy, one popular approach is to initiate therapy as early as possible and with strong enough combinations to suppress all viral replication. The best method to achieve this

> ### BOX 4-1   GUIDELINES FOR THE INITIATION OF ANTIRETROVIRAL THERAPY
>
> **International AIDS Society—USA Panel (IAS-USA)**
>
> - Therapy is generally recommended for all clients with confirmed HIV RNA levels >30,000 copies/ml, regardless of CD_4 count.
> - Therapy is generally recommended for clients with CD_4 counts <350 cells/mm^3, regardless of HIV RNA level.
> - Therapy is recommended for clients with both plasma HIV RNA levels of 5000-30,000 copies/ml and CD_4 counts of 350-500 cells/mm^3.
> - Therapy should be considered in clients with CD_4 counts around 500 cells/mm^3 with confirmed HIV RNA levels in the 5000-30,000 copies/ml range.
> - Clients with CD_4 counts >500 cells/mm^3 and HIV RNA levels <5000 copies/ml are at low risk for clinical progression. It is reasonable to defer treatment but continue monitoring of these clients.
> - Therapy is recommended for all clients with symptomatic HIV infection.
>
> From Carpenter CJ et al: Antiretroviral therapy in adults: updated recommendations of the International AIDS Society—USA Panel, *JAMA* 283(3):381, 2000.

goal is through the use of a combination of potent drugs. The goal of this approach is to reduce the client's viral burden to nondetectable levels and is commonly called highly active antiretroviral therapy (HAART). The combination of a drug in the protease inhibitor class and two nucleoside drugs is a highly effective combination that inhibits viral replication. Two nucleoside reverse-transcriptase inhibitors (NRTIs) in combination with one nonnucleoside reverse transcriptase inhibitor (NNRTI) or combinations of two protease inhibitors have also been shown to suppress viral replication effectively.[2] Drugs commonly used to treat HIV infection are listed in Table 4-1.

DRUG RESISTANCE

Viral replication can be suppressed with any of the current antiretroviral drugs. What has become apparent over time is that *monotherapy,* using a single drug, is less efficacious than using *combination therapy,* using multiple drugs at the same time. As a result, combination therapy is the current standard of care for all HIV-positive persons. Although combination therapy is a highly effective treatment strategy, the virus has the ability to become resistant to one or more of the drugs in the combination. Resistance is the ability of some variants of HIV to replicate fairly well, even when a drug is preventing replication of other variants.[3] Combination therapy, ideally, suppresses all HIV replication. However, mutant HIV arises because of clients' poor compliance to regimens, drug absorption problems, drug-drug interactions, or suboptimal drug po-

Table 4-1	Drugs Used to Treat HIV Infection	
Class	**Action**	**Examples**
Nucleoside reverse transcriptase inhibitors (NRTIs)	NRTIs inhibit the reverse transcriptase enzyme from changing viral RNA to DNA	Zidovudine (AZT, Retrovir) Didanosine (ddI, Videx) Zalcitabine (ddC, Hivid) Stavudine (d4t, Zerit) Lamivudine (3TC, Epivir) Abacavir (Ziagen)
Nonnucleoside reverse transcriptase inhibitors (NNRTIs)	NNRTIs inhibit reverse transcriptase, but by a different mechanism than NRTIs	Nevirapine (Viramune) Delavirdine (Rescriptor) Efavirenz (Sustiva)
Protease inhibitors (PIs)	PIs prevent the protease enzyme from splitting large viral proteins into smaller structural proteins and enzymes necessary for viral assembly	Saquinavir (Fortovase) Ritonavir (Norvir) Indinavir (Crixivan) Nelfinavir (Viracept) Amprenavir (Agenerase)

tency. A mutant strain that is drug-insensitive can reproduce rapidly and subsequently cause a rise in the client's viral load. This is known as clinical resistance. When a client is receiving combination therapy and clinical resistance develops, it is difficult to know to which drug or drugs in the regimen the virus is resistant. Therefore, it is possible that some or all of the drugs in the regimen must be replaced (see "Treatment Failure" later in this chapter).

Resistance assays are tests that can be used to detect loss of antiretroviral activity.[4] There are two assay types: phenotypic and genotypic. Phenotypic assays determine drug susceptibility by actively growing the virus population in the presence of antiretroviral drugs. Essentially, the virus is isolated from the client's serum and allowed to grow in the presence of one or more antiretroviral drugs. Viral replication indicates drug resistance and a lack of growth indicates drug susceptibility. In theory, the drugs that have been shown to inhibit viral replication should be included in the client's antiretroviral regimen. Genotypic assays, on the other hand, isolate the viral population and search for mutations in certain amino acid sequences. One or more amino acid mutations imply reduced drug susceptibility. Results of genotypic assays must be interpreted with caution since the current generation of tests only have the ability to give information about the most predominant variant or the level of resistance in actively replicating virus.[4]

BOX 4-2   CROSS-RESISTANCE

Nucleoside Drugs

- Resistance testing that demonstrates mutation at codon* 151 along with three or more other mutations leads to resistance to all nucleoside RT inhibitors.
- Resistance testing demonstrates that a mutation at codon 69 leads to resistance for this entire class; however, this mutation is difficult to identify in genotypic testing.
- Clients taking 3TC can develop a mutation at codon 184. This mutation may lead to cross-resistance to ddC and ddI and may also contribute to abacavir resistance.
- Viruses resistant to ddC are cross-resistant to ddI and vice versa.†

Nonnucleoside Drugs

- Resistance testing that demonstrates mutations at codon 103 and 181 leads to cross-resistance to all of the drugs in this class.

Protease Inhibitors Drugs

- Protease inhibitor cross-resistance is not completely understood. A client on a protease inhibitor develops mutations over time. Many of these mutations are overlapping, thus conferring a great deal of protease inhibitor cross-resistance. This does not necessarily mean that a person who has resistance to one protease inhibitor will get no benefit from another protease inhibitor. Some therapies including one or two protease inhibitors that have not been taken before can be effective regardless of resistance to another protease inhibitor. This is because cross-resistance may not be complete. Even with cross-resistance there may be some anti-HIV effect, though the drugs may not be as effective as if there were no resistance.

---

* A codon is a sequence of three nucleotide bases that codes for an amino acid.
† Kurtizkes D: Reverse transcriptase inhibitor resistance, *National AIDS Treatment Advocacy Reports* 1(3):30, January 1998.
Adapted from Bartlett JG: *Medical management of HIV infection,* Baltimore, 1999, John Hopkins University, Department of Infectious Disease.

As of this writing, resistance assays are not currently approved by the Food and Drug Administration (FDA). They are, however, beginning to emerge as important clinical tools, and will be approved in the near future. (See Appendix A for further information on resistance testing). An accompanying, nonpreventable phenomenon that results from viral mutation is the development of drug cross-resistance. Cross-resistant virus is resistant to one or more and sometimes all drugs in a similar therapeutic class, which further limits the armamentarium available for the treatment of HIV. Genotypic testing can be useful in determining when a client's virus is resistant to drugs in a similar class. Understanding and determining cross-resistance patterns is a field of continuing investigation. Key points in cross-resistance are listed in Box 4-2; treatment strategies should be designed with cross-resistance patterns in mind.

Table 4-2	Recommended Antiretroviral Agents for the Treatment of Established HIV Infection

Choose one drug from Column A and a combination of drugs from Column B.

Column A	Column B
Indinavir (Crixivan)	AZT (Retrovir) + ddI (Videx)
Nelfinavir (Viracept)	d4T (Zerit) + ddI (Videx)
Ritonavir (Norvir)	AZT (Retrovir) + ddC (HIVID)
Ritonavir + saquinavir (Fortovase)	AZT (Retrovir) + 3TC (Epivir)
Retrovir + indinavir	ddI (Videx) + 3TC (Epivir)
Efavirenz (Sustiva)	d4T (Zerit) + 3TC (Epivir)
Nevirapine (Viramune)	
Delavirdine (Rescriptor)	
Abacavir (Ziagen) + one other NRTI	
Amprenavir (Angenerase)	

Note: Drugs are listed in random, not priority, order. Other combinations are under evaluation.

TREATMENT REGIMENS

Combination therapy for HIV necessitates the simultaneous administration of drugs with different sites or mechanisms of action and with no overlap of toxicities. Antiretroviral drugs attack HIV by inhibiting several processes necessary for its replication, such as: (1) viral attachment to and penetration of the host cell, (2) viral transcription and integration, (3) viral assembly, and (4) release of the virus from the host cell. Nucleoside reverse transcriptase inhibitors (NRTI), nonnucleoside reverse transcriptase inhibitors (NNRTI), and protease inhibitors (PI) are the three classes of currently approved drugs. NRTIs and NNRTIs work by inhibiting viral transcription and integration and PIs prevent HIV assembly in the host cell.

An initial drug treatment regimen preferably consists of two nucleoside drugs and one protease inhibitor (depending on HIV RNA and CD_4 count). Other combinations, such as one NNRTI and two NRTIs may provide adequate suppression, but long-term efficacy is less clear. The combination of efavirenz and two nucleosides has been shown to compare favorably in regard to viral suppression to a regimen containing protease inhibitor. This combination is also recommended as the initial combination for the treatment of established HIV infection.[5] Table 4-2 outlines currently recommended approaches for the use of antiretroviral agents in the treatment of established HIV infection; they are based on the recommendations of the Department of Health and Human Services.[5]

Most experts advise clinicians to treat early, using the most potent combination therapies first—specifically, combination therapy that includes a protease inhibitor instead of a protease inhibitor–sparing regimen. The rationale for this strategy is that potent therapy restores immune function and decreases viral replication, and therefore it decreases mutations. Restoration of immune function is reflected by increases in the client's CD_4 cell counts. This strategy has also led to dramatic decreases in the incidence of opportunistic infections, hospitalizations, and deaths from HIV.[6]

Nurses and clients should know that the long-term durability of viral suppression with HAART is currently unknown and is thought to be time limited. When viral load becomes repeatedly detectable after initial suppression (i.e., after treatment with a combination of drugs),* treatment failure is said to have occurred. Further discussion and management of treatment failure is discussed later in this chapter.

INITIATING THERAPY—NURSING CONSIDERATIONS

The evaluation of candidacy for antiretroviral therapy is guided primarily by, though not limited to, an evaluation of viral load and CD_4 cell count or percentage. Although quantitative clinical data are indispensable and essential to the design of a treatment plan, the client's willingness and ability to accept, participate in, and adhere to the medication regimen must be the chief consideration. In the absence of compliance, antiretroviral therapy will fail as drug-resistant strains of HIV are allowed to develop.

Various factors influence the client's decision to accept antiretroviral therapy. These include social stress, the client–healthcare provider relationship, cultural factors, social support, and substance use.[7] Clients who are unable to commit to the demanding management tasks associated with HAART should receive counseling and education about the treatment plan and should delay the initiation of their therapy until they are willing and able to comply. A client's inability to adhere fully can lead to the emergence of drug-resistant virus strains and perhaps limit the client's future pharmacological options. The nurse, as an HIV treatment team member, fulfills the pivotal role of assessing clients' ability to manage the complex treatment regimen and educating clients about the importance of adhering to the prescribed therapy. The nurse identifies clients' strengths and weaknesses related to the ability to manage the medication regimen and empowers clients to design strategies to manage their own treatment plans. Specific items to be included in the nursing plan of care are discussed in the following section.

READINESS ASSESSMENT

When a client is prescribed antiretrovirals, the provider should schedule a face-to-face nurse-client assessment and teaching session. At this session the nurse can determine the client's educational needs and assess the client's affect, attitude, motivation, and competence related to the self-

---

*The degree of plasma HIV RNA increase must be considered. Low detectability in a client (500 to 5000 copies/ml) could, in effect, be carefully monitored.

administration of a complex medication regimen. Clients who are unwilling or unable to manage such a regimen would benefit from the deferral of antiretroviral therapy until they are willing and able to adhere. The following are some factors that may indicate that a client is unwilling or unable to participate or adhere fully[8]:

- The client is unable to accept his or her HIV/AIDS diagnosis.
- The client expresses skepticism of the treatment or providers of care.
- The client has concurrent mental health problems or demonstrates continued use of illicit substances.
- The client's social situation does not support adherence (e.g., having no domicile, no health insurance, or a lack of disclosure to family).
- The client's work or other activities of daily living do not support the client's ability to manage the disease (e.g., travel, erratic work schedule, competing priorities, need to hide medications from coworkers).

When a client begins antiretroviral therapy, particularly during the first few weeks, the nurse should follow the client closely. Face-to-face encounters in the home or clinic setting are best. The purpose of these encounters is to ensure that the client understands the instructions for medication administration, to determine if any questions have arisen about the medicine, and to assess if any side effects have developed that may affect adherence or necessitate adjustment or change of the regimen. During an encounter, the nurse should have the client verbally recall the medications that they are taking and the times at which they are taking them. Restatement or recall is a simple and important tool that has long been used in client education. It can be used to assess the client's understanding of HIV medications.

DOSING CONSIDERATIONS

The frequency of administration and the absolute number of medications a client is required to ingest are known to affect adherence to prescribed treatment. The nurse must prepare the client for antiretroviral therapy by adequately communicating the requirements of the prescribed regimen. Table 4-3 lists all of the currently available antiretroviral drugs, and the number of pills that must be taken within a 24-hour period.

When providers ask clients to take multiple medications, errors in self-administration can occur, such as missed doses, double dosing, or underdosing. Double dosing or overdosing can lead to an increase in adverse side effects, which in turn may cause clients to discontinue their medications. Missed doses (failure to take medication at the prescribed time) or underdosing (not taking the suggested dose of medication) can lead to the emergence of resistant virus.

The ideal dosing frequency for all medications is once a day. Of the 16 currently approved antiretroviral drugs, only one, efavirenz (Sustiva), is approved for once a day dosage. Didanosine (Videx), though not approved by the FDA, has been demonstrated to be effective as once daily dosages.

Table 4-3	Daily Dosage			

Medication	Daily Dosage	Usual Administration	Frequency	Number of Pills Daily
Zidovudine (Retrovir, AZT)	600 mg	2 caps × 100 mg 1 tab × 300 mg	q8h q12h	6 2
Lamivudine (Epivir, 3TC)	300 mg	1 tab × 150 mg	q12h	2
Zidovudine + Lamivudine (Combivir, AZT + 3TC)	600 mg + 300 mg	1 tab × 300 mg + 150 mg	q12h	2
Didanosine (Videx, ddI)	400 mg	4 tabs × 100 mg	qhs	4
Zalcitabine (Hivid, ddC)	2.25 mg	1 tab × 0.75 mg	q8h	3
Stavudine (Zerit, d4T)	80 mg	1 cap × 40 mg	q12h	2
Abacavir (Ziagen, 1592)	600 mg	1 tab × 300 mg	bid	2
Delavirdine (Rescriptor)	1200 mg	4 tabs × 100 mg	tid	12
Nevirapine (Viramune)	400 mg	1 tab × 200 mg	q12h	2
Efavirenz (Sustiva)	600 mg	3 caps × 200 mg	qhs	3
Saquinavir (Fortovase)	3600 mg	6 caps × 200 mg	q8h	18
Nelfinavir mesylate (Viracept)	2500 mg	5 tabs × 250 mg	bid	10
Indinavir mesylate (Crixivan)	2400 mg	2 tabs × 400 mg	q8h	6
Ritonavir (Norvir)	1200 mg	6 tabs × 100 mg	q12h	12
Agenerase (Amprenavir)	2400 mg	8 caps × 150 mg	bid	16

The Nursing Role in Dosing Considerations

The nurse should teach clients that adherence to recommended dosing schedules is important in ensuring that the medications achieve their therapeutic effect. Medication schedules should fit a client's lifestyle—not the opposite. The nurse should teach clients that they can be somewhat flexible with medication administration times. For example, medications designed for administration three times daily should be taken at the same time everyday; however, it is acceptable to take the medication an hour or two before or after the routine scheduled time.[9] Nurses should be certain that medications designed for administration every 8 hours (e.g., indinavir) or every 12 hours (e.g., nevirapine) are spaced appropriately to avoid any prolonged drug-free periods. This is particularly important for hospitalized clients. In the institutional setting, nurses should ensure that medications designed for administration every 8 hours or every 12 hours are not subject to institutional three times daily (i.e., 10 AM, 2 PM, and 6 PM) or twice daily (i.e., 10 AM and 6 PM) schedules.[10]

If a client misses a dose and it is close to the next regularly scheduled time (within 2 hours), the client should take the next dose at the regularly scheduled time and not double the dose. It may be helpful to have clients keep diaries of missed doses and the circumstances surrounding the missed doses. Nurses can use this information to help clients modify their circumstances or behavior to ensure that they miss as few doses as possible.

ADHERENCE

Drug therapy for HIV is a life-long endeavor using complex drug combinations at the onset and therapies of increasing complexity as the disease progresses. Adherence to these medical regimens is inversely proportional to the length of therapy, the number of drugs administered, the frequency of drug administration, and the overall complexity of the treatment regimen.[11] Nurses and clients should work together to develop a plan that provides the client with specific, mutually agreed upon goals and that facilitates adherence to the prescribed regimens.

No one method or tool has been shown to be superior in facilitating adherence; related factors are complex and not well understood. Traditional strategies such as partner participation, pill counting, telephone calling, and pharmacy review and tracking are often used, but have not been demonstrated to be beneficial.[12] In a review of the literature on strategies for completion of tuberculocidal therapy, investigators found that the greatest completion rates of therapy were in the groups that were under supervised therapy with multiple incentives. The completion rate in these groups ranged from 86% to 95%. The completion rate in groups that were unsupervised was 42% to 86%.[13] One implication that can be gleaned from this study is that rewards and incentives may play some role in a client's adherence.

Before therapy is initiated, the nurse must counsel clients on the frequency of dosing for each of their medications. It may be helpful to rehearse a typical day and see how the medication schedule fits into the client's daily routine. One monograph that examined motivators and barriers to antiretroviral therapy found that half of those who declined antiretroviral therapy were concerned about the effect of the treatment regimen on their lives.[14]

When preparing a client to take medications throughout the day, the nurse should be particularly sensitive to social situations in which the client may feel uncomfortable taking medications—at work or school, for instance. Clients who are concerned about taking medications in public places should be encouraged to carry their medications in containers that are less conspicuous than the traditional brown pill containers supplied by the pharmacy. "Pill containers" are often available from pharmacies at a small charge and sometimes may be supplied free of charge by drug companies. When clients carry their medications in pill containers, nurses should ensure that clients are able to identify each medication, the proper administration time, and the proper method of administration (e.g., with food) since medications mixed in one pillbox can often lead to administration errors.

Adherence is inversely related to the complexity of the regimen. As more pills are added to a client's regimen the client will experience more difficulty in adhering to the plan. The nurse should develop a plan with the client that outlines how logistically to manage the large number of pills prescribed. In some cases, the nurse must ensure that clients understand that some antiretrovirals require special storage and handling to prevent inactivating the medication.

The adherence plan is most valuable if it is revisited regularly. When asked directly about whether or not they are adhering to their prescribed regimen, clients are often honest about their behaviors.[15] Asking regularly about adherence will reinforce its importance to clients.[16] An ideal time to review the adherence plan is concurrently with viral load assessment. Nurses should ask questions in a nonjudgmental manner and in the spirit of helping clients find strategies that will facilitate adherence. Box 4-3 compares appropriate and inappropriate interviewing techniques.

DIETARY RESTRICTIONS

Certain antiretrovirals require the presence or absence of food or acid in the stomach to achieve maximal absorption in the gastrointestinal system. Therefore, nurses must ensure that clients fully understand the dietary instructions for each medication. Detailed written instructions should be provided to the client—visual cues or pictorials should be provided for clients who cannot read. Table 4-4 outlines dietary and other special considerations for currently available antiretrovirals. Drugs without dietary restrictions (those that can be taken with or without food) are not included.

MEDICATION STORAGE AND HANDLING

With the exception of ritonavir (Norvir), all of the current antiretrovirals can be stored at room temperature. Nurses should instruct clients to keep the entire bottle of ritonavir capsules in the refrigerator (i.e., 36° to 46° F) until completed. One dose of the drug may be left at room temperature for up to 12 hours. Clients who travel or work in areas where refrigeration is not available may find it easier to use the ritonavir oral solution (80 mg/ml). Refrigeration of ritonavir oral solution is recommended, but not required if the solution is used within 30 days of opening and stored

BOX 4-3   ASSESSING ADHERENCE: HELPFUL AND NOT-SO-HELPFUL QUESTIONS

Helpful

- A lot of my clients find sticking to a schedule really hard and they sometimes miss doses. Does that ever happen to you? If it does, what do you do?
- How do you feel things are going with your ability to take your medications?
- Tell me a little about how you are fitting your medications into your day. What reminders do you use to help yourself remember your pills during the day?
- Is anything making it hard for you to take your pills (e.g., nausea, diarrhea, work schedule, children)?
- What kinds of things keep you from taking your medicine?
- Is the schedule we have come up with affecting your eating habits?
- Do you feel we need to talk about rescheduling your medication dosing times to make it easier for you?
- When did you last get your medications refilled?
- Can you tell me what your pills look like, how many you take, and when you take [the blue ones?]
- Show me on this chart which pills you are taking and how many times each day. Is there anyone in your life who knows your medication schedule and helps you to remember your pills?
- Do you have any side effects to the medicine? What do you take to help control the side effects?
- Are you taking any over-the-counter medications?

Not-So-Helpful

- You're taking your pills, aren't you?
- You haven't missed any, have you?
- I hope you are being compliant and not missing any doses at all. Do we need to go over this again?
- Everything is going great, right? Missed no doses?
- I will be really disappointed if you aren't taking these medications right—any problems?
- I thought we discussed this last time. Why are you unable to do this right?
- You are taking these correctly, right? You know how important this is!
- This looks really easy to me—what's the problem here?
- Come on, it can't be that bad, can it?

Adapted from Hecht FM: Measuring HIV treatment adherence in clinical practice, *AIDS Clin Care* 10(8), 1998.

below 77° F. It should be stored in the original container. Exposure to excessive heat should be avoided and the cap should be kept tightly closed.[13]

Clients using saquinavir (Fortovase) should keep their supply in the refrigerator; however, this is not a strict recommendation. A 3-month supply can be kept out of the refrigerator. If traveling for less than 3 months at a time, the client can safely maintain the medication without refrigeration.

Table 4-4	Dietary Considerations for Current Antiretroviral Medications		
Medication	**With Food**	**Without Food**	**Special Considerations**
Didanosine (ddI, Videx)		Take at least 30 minutes before or 1 hour after a meal.	Alcohol and antacids should be avoided when taking this medication.
Delavirdine (Rescriptor)			Should be taken 1 hour before or after an antacid.
Saquinavir (Fortovase)	Take with high fat meal; when taken with grapefruit juice, may increase absorption.		Must be taken within 2 hours of a hefty meal.
Ritonavir (Norvir)	Preferably.		
Nelfinavir (Viracept)	Take with a meal or light snack.		
Indinavir (Crixivan)		Take 1 hour before or 2 hours after a meal.	Can be taken with a no-fat or low-fat light snack, such as: • Toast, jelly, juice, and coffee with skim milk • Cereal with skim milk and sugar Can be taken with other beverages, such as coffee or juice. A minimum of six 8-ounce glasses of water should be drunk daily to prevent nephrolithiasis.
Abacavir (Ziagen)			Alcohol increases the level of the drug and should be avoided.
Amprenavir (Agenerase)			High fat meals should be avoided. Should be taken at least 1 hour apart from ddI and from antacids. Vitamin E supplements should not be taken with amprenavir.

POTENTIAL SIDE EFFECTS AND MANAGEMENT

Because all HIV-related medications have side effects, it is important to make sure that clients understand those that are most common. A client who is poorly prepared may feel compelled to stop some or all medications when a common side effect occurs. Such interruption in therapy may lead to inadequate viral suppression and drug resistance.

One of the most common and early side effects associated with antiretrovirals is the development of gastrointestinal upset. This may manifest as nausea, bloating (excessive gas), or diarrhea. Nurses should make clients aware that, for most people, these effects are transitory and subside after several weeks of therapy. If symptoms persist, medical providers should suspect a cause, such as infection or lactose intolerance (lactose is found in saquinavir, indinavir, stavudine, and zalcitabine). Common side effects of the currently approved antiretrovirals are listed in the drug guide (see color insert). Some antiretrovirals also have drug-drug interactions. Nurses should make clients aware of these interactions. Drug-drug interactions are detailed in Appendix D.

When a client experiences side effects, the nurse should take a history of the onset, duration, and severity of the symptoms to determine if the effect is severe enough to recommend a change in therapy. Some side effects are time limited (e.g., diarrhea with Combivir, nightmares with Efavirenz) and often disappear with prolonged use of the medications. In this case, the nurse should help the client work through them by informing the client that the effects are likely to disappear within a specified time frame. However, the nurse runs the risk that the client will skip doses of medication if the client feels that sufficient attention has not been paid to his or her symptoms. To combat this, the nurse should ask frequently about symptoms and work with the client and his or her health care provider to develop a plan for managing the disruptive ones. A plan might include eating or avoiding certain foods, using vitamins or herbal preparations, using over-the-counter remedies, or using prescription medications. Strategies such as a "Hotline," in which clients can talk to a nurse or case manager about medication effects (outside of regularly scheduled appointments), may help achieve adherence to the medication plan.

Some antiretrovirals result in secondary clinical conditions, such as dyslipidemia and endocrine abnormality. Health care team members must be alerted to these conditions. They should monitor clients at regular intervals for dyslipidemia and endocrine abnormality. With the exception of lipodystrophy, if a new clinical condition arises as a result of antiretroviral therapy, the offending drug should be eliminated from the regimen. Known clinical conditions that result from antiretroviral therapy are listed in Table 4-5.

If a client has intolerable side effects the offending drug should be replaced. The replacement drug should be from the same class, but with a different side effect profile. For example, a client who is receiving a

Table 4-5	Clinical Conditions Warranting a Change in Antiretroviral Therapy	

Clinical Condition	Drug	Signs/Symptoms/Laboratory
Hepatitis	Various antiretroviral medications	Increased AST, ALT, LDH, GGT
Diabetes	All protease inhibitors	Polyuria, polydipsia, polyphagia, increased fasting glucose levels, glycosuria
Lipodystrophy (change in therapy not always warranted)	Thought initially to be related to protease inhibitors. Other metabolic disturbances and drugs have been implicated; however, the actual cause is unknown and may be multifactorial.	Lipomas on the back of neck, central obesity, gynecomastia (breast enlargement)
Dyslipidemia	Various protease inhibitors	Increases in total cholesterol, low density lipoproteins, increased triglycerides
Pancreatitis	Didanosine Zalcitabine Stavudine Ritonavir	Increase in amylase or lipase
Hemolytic anemia	Zidovudine (Retrovir) Indinavir	Fatigue, jaundice, hematomas
Peripheral neuropathy	Didanosine Zalcitabine Stavudine Lamivudine	Pain or paresthesia in the feet or hands
Nephrolithiasis/ Nephrotoxicity	Indinavir Ritonavir	Low back pain, hematuria
Stevens-Johnson syndrome	Nevirapine Delavirdine	Severe exfoliation of the skin
Myopathy	Zidovudine (Retrovir)	Proximal muscle weakness, myalgias, fatigability, elevated CPK
Hypersensitivity reaction	Abacavir All NNRTIs Some protease inhibitors	Fever, malaise, possible rash, gastrointestinal upset
Hepatotoxicity	Delavirdine Efavirenz Nevirapine All NRTIs Protease inhibitors	

three-drug combination including didanosine (ddI) and who develops severe peripheral neuropathy should not be switched to another drug that also causes peripheral neuropathy, such as d4T or ddC.

Intolerance of a medication due to side effects should not be confused with treatment failure. In treatment failure the drugs are no longer able to cause viral suppression, which requires changing one or all of the drugs in the regimen.

MONITORING ANTIRETROVIRAL THERAPY

Some health care providers define effective antiretroviral therapy as a decrease in viral load to as low a level as possible for as long as possible. Others define effective antiretroviral therapy as a decrease in viral load below the limit of detection levels by current assays. In short, currently there is no consensus as to what constitutes effective antiretroviral therapy. Nevertheless, the first definition acknowledges that the target viral load is contingent on the pretreatment value. The pretreatment value, often called the baseline or set-point, is the plasma HIV RNA level that is detected after seroconversion occurs. In a client who has a very high pretreatment viral load (e.g., 10^7 HIV RNA copies/ml) it may not be possible to achieve undetectable levels of HIV RNA, even with effective therapy. The pretreatment value is an important determinant of a client's risk for disease progression. It has been demonstrated that with higher levels of pretreatment HIV RNA the client is likely to progress more rapidly to AIDS.[17] To slow progression many clinicians have adopted a treatment strategy of aggressive drug combinations to reduce the viral load to as low as possible, as quickly as possible.

When a client begins a potent antiretroviral regimen, a significant decline in viral load can be detected as early as 2 weeks after initiating therapy. Current standards dictate that viral load measurement should be obtained after 4 weeks of therapy. A client who demonstrates a greater than 1.0 log reduction in viral load and is tolerating therapy is defined as having a favorable treatment response (see Chapter 2 for a discussion of viral load).[9] Decreases in viral load should be accompanied by increases in the absolute CD_4 cell count. A persistently declining CD_4 cell count or percentage and an inadequate decline in viral load indicates worsening immune status and treatment failure, which warrants a change in therapy.

TREATMENT FAILURE

Treatment failure, simply defined, is a lack of response to therapy. The plasma RNA and the client's clinical conditions are the two most important factors in determining treatment failure. Box 4-4 lists specific criteria indicative of treatment failure.

Treatment failure is thought to occur as a result of one or more of the following factors: (a) the development of drug resistance; (b) drug malabsorption; and (c) client nonadherence. If treatment failure occurs, a

BOX 4-4   CRITERIA FOR TREATMENT FAILURE

- *Less than a 0.5- to 0.75-log reduction in plasma HIV RNA by 4 weeks after the initiation of therapy, or less than a 1.0-log reduction by 8 weeks.*
- *Failure to suppress plasma HIV RNA to undetectable levels within 4 to 6 months of initiating therapy.* In this regard, the degree of initial decrease in plasma HIV RNA and the overall trend in decreasing viremia should be considered. In some clients, for example, a level of 10^6 viral copies/ml prior to therapy that stabilizes after 6 months of therapy at an HIV RNA level that is detectable but less than 10,000 copies/ml may not warrant an immediate change in therapy.
- *Repeated detection of virus in plasma after initial suppression to undetectable levels, suggesting the development of resistance.* However, the degree of plasma HIV RNA increase should be considered—the clinician may consider short-term observation of a client whose plasma HIV RNA increases from undetectable to low-level detectability (e.g., 500 to 5000 copies/ml) at 4 months of initial therapy. In this situation the client should be observed very closely. It should be noted, however, that most clients in this situation subsequently show progressive increases in plasma viremia that require a change in the antiretroviral regimen.
- *Any reproducible significant increase, defined as threefold or greater, from the nadir of plasma HIV RNA not attributable to intercurrent infection, vaccination, or test methodology.*
- *Persistently declining CD_4 T cell counts,* as measured on at least two separate occasions.
- *Clinical deterioration.* A new AIDS-defining diagnosis acquired after the initiation of treatment suggests clinical deterioration but may or may not suggest failure of antiretroviral therapy. (For a discussion of AIDS-defining diagnoses see Chapter 1.) If the antiretroviral effect of therapy has been poor (e.g., less than tenfold reduction in viral RNA), then a judgment of therapeutic failure can be made.

Modified from US Department of Health and Human Services: *Guidelines for the use of antiretroviral agents in HIV-infected adults and adolescents,* May 5, 1999, developed by the Panel on Clinical Practice for Treatment of HIV Infection, convened by the Department of Health and Human Services (DHHS) and the Henry J. Kaiser Family Foundation.

change in the current antiretroviral therapy is warranted. Given the limited number of drugs available, the clinician must rule out all factors that can cause increases in HIV RNA before diagnosing treatment failure. Small increases in viral load can be caused by factors other than treatment failure, such as upper respiratory infection or immunization. Increases should be confirmed as "sustained" by repeating the viral load test after 1 to 2 weeks.

Whenever possible, all drugs in a failing regimen should be changed. Careful consideration must be given to the possibility of cross-resistance between drugs in the same class (see Box 4-2). Treatment failure in a client who has been on multiple antiretrovirals is a complex management issue, as there are limited published standards or sets of empirical evidence to guide clinicians in treatment decisions. One strategy is to combine five, six, or seven different antiretrovirals with the hope that adequate viral suppression will occur. Some of these drugs will be new to the client's treatment, while other drugs will be recycled (previously used). This type of strategy is often referred to as "Mega-HAART." Another strategy is to offer the client "intensification" of therapy. With this strategy an additional agent or agents are added to a partially successful regimen—one which is suppressing viral replication but which has either not brought the viral load to undetectable levels using an ultrasensitive assay or has resulted in low-level viral rebound following complete suppression. Yet another strategy for a failing regimen is structured treatment interruption, or a "drug holiday." This strategy, theoretically, reverts a drug resistant viral population to a wild type of viral population that responds to antiretroviral therapy when it is reintroduced. The benefit of such a strategy has not been well studied and at this time should not be attempted by providers or clients except for those in well-designed studies. Clients with limited options can also be referred to clinical trials, which may include new or novel therapies or treatment strategies designed for highly experienced clients (see Chapter 5).

REFERENCES

1. Bartlett JG: Major controversies in the DHHS guidelines for use of antiretroviral agents in HIV-Infected adults, *The Hopkins HIV Report,* January 1998.
2. Gallant JE: Antiretroviral Strategies and Controversies. In Phair, King, eds: *Medscape HIV/AIDS: annual update,* New York, 1999, Medscape.
3. Richman DD: *Resistance to drugs in HIV infection: what you can do to keep your HIV treatment working,* Booklet, May 1998, IAPAC.
4. Carpenter CJ et al: Antiretroviral therapy in adults: updated recommendations of the International AIDS Society—USA Panel, *JAMA* 283(3):381, 2000.
5. US Department of Health and Human Services: *Guidelines for the use of antiretroviral agents in HIV-infected adults and adolescents,* May 5, 1999, developed by the Panel on Clinical Practice for Treatment of HIV Infection, convened by the Department of Health and Human Services (DHHS) and the Henry J. Kaiser Family Foundation.
6. Centers for Disease Control and Prevention: Update: trends in AIDS incidence, deaths, and prevalence—United States, 1996, *MMWR* 46(8): 165, 1997.
7. Crespo-Fierro M: Compliance/adherence and care management in HIV disease, *J Assoc Nurses AIDS Care* 8(4):43, 1997.
8. Katzenstein DA et al: HIV therapeutics: confronting adherence, *J Assoc Nurses AIDS Care* 8:46, 1997.
9. Merck & Co, Inc: Patient information about Crixivan, 972607-(4)-(502)-CRX (pamphlet).
10. Ungvarski PJ, Rottner JE: Errors in prescribing HIV-1 protease inhibitors, *J Assoc Nurses AIDS Care* 8(4):55, 1997.
11. Chaulk PC, Kazandjian VA: Directly observed therapy for treatment completion of pulmonary tuberculosis, *JAMA* 279:943, 1998.

12. Haynes RB, McKibbon KA, Kanani R: Systematic review of randomized trials of interventions to assist clients to follow prescriptions for medications, *Lancet* 348:383, 1996.

13. DeBell S: *Mosby's complete drug reference: physicians' GenR$_x$*, ed 9, St Louis, Mosby, 1999.

14. Richter B et al: Motivators and barriers to use of combination therapies in patients with HIV disease, *Center for AIDS Prevention Studies Monograph Series*, occasional paper #5, January 1998.

15. Sackett D et al: Randomized clinical trial of strategies for improving medication compliance in primary hypertension, *Lancet* 1:1205, 1975.

16. Hecht FM: Measuring HIV treatment adherence in clinical practice, *AIDS Clin Care* 10(8), 1998.

17. Mellors JW et al: Plasma viral load and CD$_4$$^+$ lymphocytes as prognostic markers of HIV-1 infection, *Ann Intern Med* 126:946, 1997.

5 Clinical Trials

Carl A. Kirton

Current therapy for HIV is based on the understanding of the dynamics of HIV as it enters the human body and embarks on a highly destructive course. Current treatment is based on adequate viral suppression, to protect the already weakened immune system. This goal is achieved through the use of a highly active combination of drugs to suppress viral replication. The appropriate use of antiretrovirals and other therapies has in large part been learned through controlled clinical studies. These studies are the only true way of knowing whether a drug is effective, ineffective, or harmful. It is important for nurses to understand clinical drug studies—often called clinical trials—for several reasons. Nurses may be asked by clients, for instance, about participation in a specific trial; or clients may already be enrolled in clinical trials, in which case nurses need to understand the trial components. Moreover, if a client is failing approved therapies, participation in a clinical trial may be the only choice left for therapy.

HIV/AIDS AND CLINICAL STUDIES

Advances made in the knowledge of pharmacological management are achieved through the use of well-designed clinical studies that document substantial benefits of a drug in the treatment of a particular disease under study. Until the emergence of HIV/AIDS, clinical studies were not very well understood by most health care providers, and even less so by those most affected by the disease or treatment being studied. In fact, the process used to study and approve drugs had undergone very little change, since its inception, prior to the HIV/AIDS epidemic. To understand the effect of the HIV/AIDS epidemic in the United States, one must understand the traditional drug development process.

THE DRUG DEVELOPMENT PROCESS

The Food and Drug Administration (FDA) is a public health agency charged with protecting American consumers by enforcing the Federal Food, Drug, and Cosmetic Act and several related public health laws. Assessing the risk of drugs and medical devices and weighing the risks against benefits is the core of FDA's public health protection duties. Within the FDA is the Center for Drug Evaluation and Research (CDER), best known for its evaluation of new drugs—both prescription and over-the-counter. The CDER doesn't test that drugs are safe and effective. It is the responsibility of the company seeking to market a drug to test it and submit evidence that it's safe and effective. A team of CDER physicians, statisticians, chemists, pharmacologists, and other scientists reviews the sponsor's new drug application (NDA), which contains the data and proposed labeling.

Before a drug can be considered for use in humans it must be extensively tested in the laboratory and in animals. This is called preclinical research. If the preclinical research data is favorable, the sponsor submits an investigational new drug (IND) application to the FDA. After a successful review, the drug can enter Phase I clinical studies. In Phase I clinical studies the drug is given to human subjects for the first time and the FDA requires that only a small number of subjects be tested. The drug is often given to healthy individuals—those not affected with the disease under study—with the purpose of determining the most common acute adverse side effects and the size of doses that clients can take safely without a high incidence of side effects. Phase I studies also illustrate what happens to the drug in the human body—whether it changes (metabolism), how much of it permeates the blood and various organs (distribution), how long it stays in the body (half-life), how the body gets rid of the drug (elimination), and its side effects. The study of these factors is called pharmacokinetics. Phase I trials can vary but typically last for a few weeks to 1 year.

After the drug has successfully completed Phase I, Phase II clinical trials can begin. The goal of Phase II trials is to further determine safety, to monitor efficacy, and to determine correct drug dosages. In Phase II clinical trials the drug is given to persons who have the clinical condition for which the drug is intended. Phase II studies can vary but typically last for 6 months to 2 years. If the drug shows some clinical benefit in Phase II studies, Phase III studies can begin. The core of the phase III study is a comparison of the drug to the "gold standard" treatment or to a placebo. Phase III testing typically lasts for 3 to 4 years or longer, primarily to determine if there are any long-term effects of the medication which were not uncovered in the shorter Phase I and II studies.

On average, the drug development process takes 7 to 8 years to complete; for persons with life-threatening illnesses, this time period is unacceptable. Under pressure from AIDS activists and scientists, the FDA changed its policy, streamlined the process of drug review, and created the *accelerated approval process,* which gives top priority to the review of drugs for AIDS and other life-threatening illnesses. The accelerated approval allows drugs to be available after Phase II testing has been completed and the drug under study has shown some benefit. In 1991, the FDA began a new drug approval process called *parallel tracking.* In parallel tracking, a drug is released for practitioner use, often after Phase I testing has occurred. In order to use the drug, the practitioner must collect clinical data about the client using the drug and supply the FDA with this information.

WHEN CLIENTS ASK ABOUT CLINICAL TRIALS

Increasingly, news about potential new therapies for HIV reaches the lay public by way of the media even before the therapies have been adequately evaluated as having any clear benefit. Clients may inquire about such studies, their availability, and whether or not they should consider participating in them. Nurses should encourage clients to obtain details about the study from the study coordinator; however, clients should be informed about specific benefits and risks associated with study participation.

BENEFITS

The benefit of any drug or therapy cannot be touted by the drug developer during a study phase; however, a client who participates in a clinical trial may develop a sense of self-actualization by participating in a study which may potentially advance the treatment of HIV/AIDS. Participation in the trial may also give the client access to expert nurses and physicians in HIV/AIDS care, who carefully monitor study participants. Participation may include access to technology that is not otherwise available to the general public for monitoring the disease (e.g., ultrasensitive assays for HIV antigen detection). The company sponsoring the study usually incurs the cost of such technology.

RISKS

Clients who participate in drug studies should understand that there might be risks associated with participation. First and foremost, the client must understand that, especially with new drugs, there may be no benefit to the therapy under study and that the treatment under study may actually be harmful. Side effects associated with the therapy may be unpleasant or even life threatening. Drugs under study may be less efficacious than treatments that have already been approved as therapies. They may lead to inadequate viral suppression and cause viral mutation. The drug under study may cause the virus to become resistant to future therapies. As client advocates, nurses must ensure that the client has a full understanding of the possible effects of participation in the study. Box 5-1 lists questions that the client should ask of the study investigators.

THE RESEARCH PROCESS

To determine the benefit of any drug or therapy, the study must be carefully constructed, adhering to strict principles of research design. It is not essential that the client understand all elements of the research process, but the client must have a basic comprehension of the process and how it affects the client's participation in a trial. For example, clients may think

**BOX 5-1   KEY QUESTIONS TO ASK
WHEN CONSIDERING PARTICIPATION
IN A CLINICAL TRIAL**

- Will I need to alter—or stop—my current treatment? (Be sure to bring to your first meeting with the study organizers a list of all drugs you are taking.)
- What is the evidence that this treatment might work against HIV?
- What are the potential risks? Are there any side effects? Who will take care of my side effects? Will I have 24-hour access to a doctor involved in the study, in case I have an emergency that could be related to the experimental drug?
- How long will the study last?
- How often do I need to come in for visits, and how many blood samples or other specimens will be needed? Are evening and weekend appointments available?
- Will I incur any costs?
- Can I be reimbursed for travel expenses or childcare? Will I have access to the drug after the study is over, and will I be eligible for future studies of the drug?

From Armington KJ: Should you participate in clinical trials? *AIDS Care* 1(6):86, 1997.

that their participation in a trial ensures access to "better drugs" or "better treatment" when, in fact, the client may be assigned to a group in which no new treatment or the standard treatment is given. Clients should also understand that they and their providers may be "blinded" to their group assignment. This means that neither the client, nor his or her health care provider, is aware of whether the client is receiving experimental medications, standard medications, or in some cases a placebo (an inactive substance given so that the client will have the perception of receiving medication). Clients should also understand that participating in an experimental drug study might potentially have a negative effect on their ability to respond to other available therapies. See Box 5-2 for common terms used in research studies.

Clients should also understand that not all studies are accessible to everyone. Study investigators may have "eligibility criteria" or "inclusion criteria" for study participation to control for specific circumstances and thereby understand a drug's effect fully. These criteria may include such factors as race, gender, CD_4 cell count, viral load levels, previous therapies, concurrent illnesses, sexual activity, and client availability.

Well-designed clinical trials will require clients to give their consent for participation in the study. Clients should be discouraged from participating in a trial for which no consent is required. The consent process requires that the study coordinators fully explain the study, including the benefits and risks both real and potential, the study length, and exactly what is expected of the client if he or she signs the informed consent. Clients should understand that although they have given consent, it could be withdrawn at any time during the study process. Obtaining informed

BOX 5-2 TERMS ASSOCIATED WITH **HIV/AIDS** CLINICAL TRIALS

Arm	All of the study subjects taking a particular drug or drug dose are said to be in that "arm" (or "cohort") of the study
Bioavailability	How much of the drug is absorbed into the bloodstream
Blinded	Without the knowledge of arm assignments (i.e., without the knowledge of drugs or drug doses received)
Control group	The trial participants who do not receive the experimental treatment
Crossover	A trial in which the experimental and control groups switch treatments
Data Safety Monitoring Board (DSMB)	A group of independent researchers who review the data while the trial is being conducted, to determine if one drug or drug dose is markedly safer or more effective than another
Double-blinded study	A study in which neither the trial participants nor the researchers know who is receiving which drugs or drug doses
Exclusion criteria	A list of reasons why some prospective participants should not be included in the study (e.g., a trial may not want people with CD_4 counts above 500 cells/mm^3, pregnant women, or clients who have previously used the drug being studied)
Experimental group	The trial participants who receive the experimental treatment
Half-life	The time it takes for the body to eliminate half of the drug that reaches the bloodstream
Inclusion criteria	A list of conditions (clinical state, blood values, etc.) that every participant must satisfy at time of entry to a clinical trial
Open-label	A trial in which all study participants receive the experimental treatment
Pharmacokinetics	The study of a drug's metabolism, absorption, and half-life in the human body, as well as other variables
Placebo	A drug that looks like the experimental drug but that does not contain any active ingredients
Protocol	The overall design or blueprint of the study
Randomized	A study in which each person has an equal chance of being selected

From Armington KJ: Should you participate in clinical trials? *AIDS Care* 1(6):86, 1997.

consent from people who cannot read or write is particularly challenging. Cohen suggests that when obtaining consent from such individuals, comprehension can be verified by having the client repeat the explanations as they understand them. She also suggests that, in these circumstances, the researcher should not obtain consent on the same day as giving the explanation. The client should return on another day and repeat their understanding of the research.[1]

BOX 5-3   COMMUNITY PROGRAMS FOR CLINICAL RESEARCH ON AIDS (CPCRA)

The CPCRA, founded in 1989, is a network of research units composed of community-based health care providers who offer their clients the opportunity to participate in research where they get their health care. The 15 CPCRA units comprise a variety of clinical settings, including private physicians' practices, university and veterans' hospital clinics, drug treatment centers, and freestanding community clinics. Clients at these clinics are eligible for participation in CPCRA studies. The CPCRA, funded by the National Institute of Allergy and Infectious Diseases (NIAID), an institute of the National Institutes of Health (NIH), is designed to serve populations underrepresented in previous clinical trials efforts. The research focus and scientific agenda of the CPCRA is to identify and improve treatment options in the day-to-day clinical care of people with HIV.

Mission of the CPCRA

- To test, by scientifically sound methodology, interventions that are in wide use or that are of potential use, in primary care settings, incorporating underserved populations, and emphasizing studies that assess clinical hypotheses with easily measured and clear clinical endpoints.

Nurses must teach clients that clinical trial participation may not be easy. The clinical trial visits do not replace follow-up care by a primary care provider; therefore clients may be subjected to additional clinic appointments and blood work, and in certain trials, clients may have to fill out detailed, lengthy questionnaires regarding the phenomena of interest.

The researchers attempt to control factors that may influence study results to ensure the validity of the study findings, and therefore often have very strict rules that the client must follow to maintain study eligibility. These may include keeping appointments within a certain period of time; eating or not eating certain foods; or making certain lifestyle changes, such as the cessation of alcohol or tobacco use, taking drugs exactly as prescribed, and recording or reporting all symptoms experienced.

CLIENTS FAILING APPROVED THERAPIES

To date, there are 15 drugs approved as antiretroviral agents against HIV, which can be used in various combinations. The durability of viral therapies is known to be time limited, and therefore sometimes novel drug regimens must be considered. Such regimens may include "Mega-HARRT" regimens in which clients are placed on six to eight different drugs. Because such strategies may not be effective, a clinical trial offering new and experimental therapies may be a client's best treatment option. Clients can be referred to a study site, such as those conducted by the AIDS Clinical Trials Group (ACTG) or the Community Programs for Clinical Research on AIDS (CPCRA) (Box 5-3). These multicenter sites, under the

**BOX 5-3   COMMUNITY PROGRAMS
FOR CLINICAL RESEARCH ON AIDS (CPCRA)—
CONT'D**

Purpose of the CPCRA
- To conduct research that expands the clinical knowledge of the day-to-day management of HIV disease and its manifestations
- To integrate research into the primary care of persons with HIV disease
- To develop research questions that are relevant to community settings in general, as well as to individual communities
- To extend opportunities to conduct scientifically sound HIV clinical research to primary care providers in community settings
- To bring opportunities to participate in clinical HIV research to those currently underrepresented in research (e.g., African Americans, Hispanics, women, drug users).

auspices of the National Institute of Allergy and Infectious Diseases (NIAID), are involved in all phases of HIV/AIDS drug research. Nurses and clients can also obtain clinical trials information by contacting the AIDS Clinical Trials Information Service (ACTIS) by calling 1-800-TRIALS-A (1-800-874-2572). ACTIS has a fax service that can be accessed in the United States by calling 1-301-519-6616. Online information may be obtained at http://www.actis.org/. The NIAID also provides clinical trials information. They can be contacted at 1-800-AIDS-NIH (1-800-243-7644) or online at http://www.niaid.nih.gov.

CLINICAL TRIALS NURSING

The role of the clinical research nurse (CRN) is best known in the area of cardiovascular and cancer nursing. The HIV/AIDS epidemic however, has significantly increased the number of nurses involved in clinical trials and perhaps has made this role emerge as a desirable career for nurses. In an effort to document CRN activities clearly, investigators surveyed several CRNs' perceptions of their day-to-day work—two main roles of the nurse have emerged:[2] that of the study coordinator and that of the direct care provider.[3] These roles are not mutually exclusive, however, and overlap is the rule rather than the exception.

Study coordinator.   The study coordinator works closely with the principal investigator and is often responsible for the day-to-day operation of the study. He or she may also have a supervisory role over all other study members. The coordinator supervises all grant-related activities, such as budgeting and quality control and assurance. He or she attends appropriate study meetings and works directly with the company or organization sponsoring the study.

Direct care provider.   The actual direct care provider role varies, according to the intended purpose of the research, but may include the roles of recruiter, teacher, counselor, data collector, and data manager. Clinical activities include taking client histories, performing physical examinations, administering medication, and performing medically indicated procedures.

The CRN must learn to collaborate with the participant's primary care provider to ensure that the participant maintains study eligibility at all times. This may include reviewing and sharing the client's clinical and laboratory data. Frequent negotiation with other departments, such as radiology, dietary, physical therapy, and social services, may be necessary to meet study and participant needs.

Recruitment of study participants is often one of the responsibilities ascribed to the CRN and can be one of the most difficult to fulfill. The nurse must work within the confines of a clinical agency to recruit participants and must often rely on primary care providers or other agency staff for the participant referral. Unfortunately, clinical research is often not a top priority for agencies engaged in the day-to-day care of clients. The research nurse must be highly visible to the agency staff to facilitate recruitment, regularly explicating the studies available and seeking referrals. This requires a great deal of flexibility and creativity. Strategies that have worked in the past include presentations at regular staff meetings, research "lunch and learn" gatherings, and general educational sessions.

Another difficult aspect of clinical trial work is the maintenance of study cohorts. Because participating in clinical trials can require a great deal of effort on the part of the client (e.g., frequent travel, frequent duplication of services such as blood drawing), the nurse must be creative in devising ways to keep participants from "dropping out" or leaving the study. Incentives such as travel money, childcare, food vouchers, and parties have been demonstrated to be highly effective. Home care visitation may be effective in studies that require very little use of health care facilities.

Although the HIV/AIDS CRN role is an exciting opportunity to be involved in HIV/AIDS nursing, there are several barriers to overcome. Nurses are often not involved at the start of protocol development. Experienced CRNs are skilled in identifying problems in the area of study design so as to avoid later amendments to protocols. More importantly, nurses who have experience in working with study clients will often have a sense of what it is reasonable to expect from study participants. Involvement from the study's initiation may help to avoid modification of a study that is already in progress. Nursing involvement also ensures that funding is secured for research nurses to attend coordinating meetings, which are often a part of multicenter research protocols.

CRNs must also take the opportunity to involve themselves and their colleagues in the research process. This involvement may take the form of ancillary studies, in which additional and distinct questions are asked about intervention; retrospective analyses of previously collected data; or "substudies," which are similar to ancillary studies but which differ in that their question of study is complementary to the main research.[3]

In most cases, additional nursing research requires permission of the principal investigator or funding agency to use data or subjects from the original work.

REFERENCES

1. Cohen HL et al: Coordinating a large multicentered HIV research project, *J Assoc Nurses AIDS Care* 8(1):47, 1997.
2. Xanthos GJ, Carp D, Geromanos KL: Recognizing nurses' contributions to the clinical research process. *J Assoc Nurses AIDS Care* 9(l):39-48, 1998.
3. Hill MN, Schron EB: Opportunities for nurse researchers in clinical trials, *Nurs Res* 41(2), 1992.

BIBLIOGRAPHY

Department of Health and Human Services Food and Drug Administration: *The CDER Handbook,* March 1998, Center for Drug Evaluation and Research.

6

Immunizations in HIV Care

Carl A. Kirton

In the United States, vaccination against certain illnesses is a very important component of the routine care of children; however, in routine adult care, vaccination has not achieved the same level of importance. HIV infection places a client at greater risk for infection with many vaccine-preventable diseases. Immunization against these diseases is a very important component of the ongoing care of an HIV-positive person.

Immunization of an HIV-positive person is similar to that of an immunocompetent client. However, there are some basic tenets to vaccination of HIV-positive adults that should be noted:

- Clients with low CD_4 counts may not respond to vaccines of the usual adult doses—additional doses may be necessary.
- Clients receiving live vaccines are at risk for contracting the disease from the vaccine, and therefore this type of vaccine should be avoided. In situations where a live vaccine is required (e.g., for travel), the risk of acquisition of a life-threatening infection and the sequela of illness must be weighed against the risk associated with vaccination. The current live vaccines are measles, mumps, rubella, polio, yellow fever, and varicella. The MMR vaccine (for measles, mumps, and rubella) is the only live vaccine that is recommended for persons with HIV infection who do not demonstrate serologic evidence of immunity.
- Vaccination may transiently increase the client's viral burden,[1,2] however there are conflicting data in the literature[3] regarding this finding. Generally, most providers would recommend that vaccination and viral load testing be separated by at least 3 to 4 weeks.
- Two inactivated vaccines can be given simultaneously at separate injection sites, as can an inactivated vaccine and a live vaccine.[4]
- Administering a vaccine to children[5]:
    - Intramuscular injections (IM)
        - Infants (less than 12 months of age)—The anterolateral aspect of the thigh provides the largest muscle mass and is therefore the recommended site. The deltoid can also be used with the thigh, however, when multiple vaccines must be administered at the same visit, for example. In most cases, a ⅞- to 1-inch, 22- to

25-gauge needle is sufficient to penetrate the muscle in the thigh of a 4-month-old infant. The free hand should bunch the muscle, and the needle should be directed inferiorly along the long axis of the leg at an angle appropriate to reach the muscle while avoiding nearby neurovascular structures and bone.

- Toddlers and older children—The deltoid may be used if the muscle mass is adequate. The needle size can range from 22- to 25-gauge and from ½ to 1 inch, based on the size of the muscle. As with infants, the anterolateral thigh may be used, but the needle should be longer—generally from ⅞ to 1¼ inches.
- Subcutaneous (SC) injections
  - Subcutaneous injections are usually administered into the thigh of infants and in the deltoid area of older children. A ⅝- to ¾-inch, 23- to 25-gauge needle should be inserted into the tissues below the dermal layer of the skin.

PNEUMOCOCCAL PNEUMONIA VACCINATION

Pneumococcal pneumonia, a disease caused by the *Streptococcus pneumoniae* bacteria, is a significant cause of morbidity and mortality in the United States. The effect of pneumococcal infection can be severe—approximately 30% of clients with pneumococcal pneumonia develop bacteremia.[6] Even with adequate treatment, pneumococcal bacteremia is a serious manifestation of this infection with a high rate of mortality in the elderly and HIV-positive populations. Among all persons, pneumococcal pneumonia is the sixth leading cause of death in the United States. Clients with HIV are 150 to 300 times more likely to contract pneumococcal pneumonia than non–HIV-positive individuals.[7] The organism is transmitted from person to person and may occur through direct contact.

Infection with *S. pneumoniae* results in an abrupt onset of fever, rigors, productive cough with mucopurulent sputum, dyspnea, and generalized malaise. Penicillin is the drug of choice for acute infection.

NURSING CONSIDERATIONS

1. Two vaccines are available in the United States: Pneumovax 23 by Merck and Co. and Pnu-Immune 23 by Lederle Laboratories.
2. According to the United States Preventative Service Task Force,[6] immunocompetent persons should be immunized at least once with pneumococcal vaccine. Routine revaccination is not recommended unless the client is at risk for significant morbidity or mortality. Immunodeficient clients may not have the same antibody response as immunocompetent clients and therefore should be revaccinated every 5 years.
3. The current vaccine is 23-valent pneumococcal vaccine, which contains antigens for at least 85% to 90% of the serotypes of *S. pneumoniae* that cause bacteremia. The vaccine is administered as a 0.5 ml IM or SC injection, using a 1- to 1½-inch, 20- to 25-gauge needle.

BOX 6-1 PEDIATRIC CONSIDERATIONS
Pneumococcal vaccination

Pneumococcal infections are very common in children and cause otitis media, bacteremia, pneumonia, sinusitis, and meningitis. Invasive pneumococcal disease may present as the first clinical manifestation of HIV infection in children. Clients with pneumococcal meningitis or other bacteremic disease have the highest mortality rate.* Therefore, immunization of HIV-infected children is an important component of their primary care.

Heptavalent pneumococcal conjugate vaccine (PCV 7 or Prevnar) was approved by the FDA in February 2000 and is recommended for universal use in children 23 months of age and younger. To expand serotype coverage, recommendations have also been made for use of 23-valent pneumococcal polysaccharide (23 PS) vaccine in children at high-risk.

See Appendix E.

---

* American Academy of Pediatrics: Pneumococcal infections. In Peter C, ed: *Red Book: report on the Committee on Infectious Disease,* ed 24, Elk Grove Village, Il, 1997, Academy of Pediatrics.

4. Protection from the vaccine may not occur until 2 to 3 weeks after injection. The nurse should teach clients that illness can occur during this period.
5. Vaccination does not confer complete immunity from pneumococcal disease. At best, the vaccine has a protective efficacy of approximately 60%.[6] In clients with HIV, antibody response is lower than in clients without HIV infection. It is also known that in immunodeficient clients, protective antibodies decline more rapidly than in immunocompetent clients.
6. The nurse should teach the client that although the vaccine is considered safe, the client may have some mild pain at the injection site.
7. Pneumococcal vaccine should not be given to pregnant women.
8. For pediatric considerations see Box 6-1.

HEPATITIS B VACCINATION

Hepatitis is caused by a virus that affects primarily the cells of the liver. This virus is primarily transmitted as a result of blood or sexual contact. The known hepatotropic viruses are hepatitis A, hepatitis B, hepatitis C, hepatitis D–associated, and the hepatitis E, hepatitis F, and hepatitis G viruses. Vaccines exist only for hepatitis B and hepatitis A.

When infection occurs with the hepatotropic B virus, the immune system responds to it by attempting to eliminate the virus. It is actually the immune system response that causes damage to liver cells, as a result of inflammation and necrosis. Clinical manifestations of disease occur in three stages: *prodromal,* in which the client has anorexia, nausea and vomiting, abdominal pain, and myalgia; *icteric,* which is characterized by jaundice, light colored stools, and hepatomegaly; and *convalescence,* in which malaise and fatigue continue. About 50% of adults who have infection never have any clinical evidence of disease. Clearance of the virus results in protective immunity, as evidenced by the appearance of hepatitis B surface antibody (anti-HBs) in the client's serum. Clients who are unable to clear the virus from their system are chronically infected and have detectable levels of hepatitis B surface antigen (HBsAg). Chronic infection may lead to cirrhosis of the liver, liver failure, and hepatocellular carcinoma. HIV-positive clients are less likely to clear the virus and more likely to become chronic carriers.

NURSING CONSIDERATIONS

1. Hepatitis B vaccination is considered 95% effective. Vaccination provides protection from hepatitis B for a period of approximately 10 years.
2. All HIV-positive individuals should be tested for evidence of previous infection with hepatitis B. Clients who have been previously exposed to the virus will have detectable anti-HBs. Clients without evidence of antibodies to hepatitis B should be offered a vaccine.
3. The recommended dosage is given in a series of three injections. Immunocompetent individuals almost always develop immunity after the series of three injections. Additional doses may be necessary for immunodeficient individuals.
4. The recommended schedule for vaccination is at 0, 1, and 6 months.
5. Two types of vaccines are available: Recombivax HB and Engerix-B. Both vaccines can be used interchangeably. However, the nurse should be alerted to the fact that for immunocompromised clients the recommended Recombivax dose is 10 μg in 1 ml and the Engerix-B dose is 20 μg in 2 ml.
6. Both vaccines are given as IM injections into the deltoid muscle using a 1- to 1½-inch, 20- to 25-gauge needle.
7. Gluteal injections should be avoided since immunogenicity is decreased with this route.[8]
8. The nurse should teach the client that side effects from the medications are rare but that fever and myalgia can occur. The client may also experience some discomfort at the injection site. The application of heat to the affected area may ameliorate the discomfort.
9. Antibody testing should be performed 30 to 60 days after vaccination.
10. For pediatric considerations see Box 6-2.

BOX 6-2   PEDIATRIC CONSIDERATIONS
Hepatitis B vaccination

Infants born to hepatitis B surface antigen–negative mothers	Infants born to hepatitis B surface antigen–positive mothers
1. The first dose of the vaccine for hepatitis B can be given at birth or up to 60 days after birth.	1. The first dose of the vaccine for hepatitis B must be given within 12 hours after birth.
2. The second dose is administered at least 1 month after the first dose.	2. The infant should also receive 0.5 ml of hepatitis B immune globulin (HBIG) as an IM injection within 12 hours after birth.
3. The third dose should be administered at least 4 months after the first dose and at least 2 months after the second dose, and not before the age of 6 months.	3. The vaccine and the HBIG must be given at separate injection sites.
	4. The second dose is administered 1 to 2 months after the first dose.
	5. The third dose should be administered at age of 6 months.

Note: Infants born to mothers whose hepatitis B surface antigen status is unknown should be vaccinated in a manner similar to infants born to HBsAg-positive mothers.

HEPATITIS A VACCINATION

Hepatitis A is a hepatotropic virus that is transmitted via the fecal-oral route. Infection with this virus rarely results in disease but can cause hepatitis and sometimes death. Particularly, clients with HIV are at high risk for infection; drinking contaminated water or milk and eating shellfish from infected waters are fairly common routes of transmission.[9] Most hepatitis A infections go unrecognized. Clinical illness with hepatitis A is similar to that of hepatitis B. It differs in that the hepatitis A virus does not progress to a chronic carrier state or result in cirrhosis of the liver.

NURSING CONSIDERATIONS

1. Vaccination provides protection from hepatitis A for a period of approximately 20 years.
2. All HIV-positive individuals should be tested for evidence of previous infection with hepatitis A. Clients who have been previously exposed or vaccinated will have detectable levels of hepatitis A antibodies (anti-HAV IgG). Clients who do not have this protective immunity should be offered a vaccine.
3. The recommended dosage is given in a series of two injections. Almost all clients develop immunity after the first dose; the second dose almost always confers immunity.
4. The recommended schedule for vaccination is at 0 and 6 months.

BOX 6-3 PEDIATRIC CONSIDERATIONS
Hepatitis A vaccination

Hepatitis A vaccination is currently not recommended as a routine vaccination for children. The primary modes of contraction of hepatitis A in children are personal contact (24%) and attendance at daycare (15%) and are secondary to contamination with feces because of poor toileting habits of others. The primary care provider should consider vaccination of children as a preventative measure in children in communities that have high rates of hepatitis A and periodic hepatitis outbreaks. Some HIV care providers consider routine vaccination of children against hepatitis A if the child is also infected with hepatitis C. This measure may protect the liver from further insult from a vaccine-preventable hepatotropic virus.

Nursing Considerations

1. Children over the age of 2 years should be considered for hepatitis A vaccination.
2. The HAV vaccine comes in two types of pediatric formulations:
   - Havrix (2 units—360 EL U and 720 EL U):
     - 360 EL U—Given as three doses: at 2 years of age, 1 month after, and 6 to 12 months after the first dose
     - 720 EL U—Given as two doses: at 2 years of age and 6 to 12 months after the first dose
   - Vaqta: 25 U
     - Given as two doses: at 2 years and 6 to 18 months after the first dose
3. Regardless of the type or units administered the dose is 0.5 ml.

---

* Harris N, Edwards K: A progress report on hepatitis A vaccination, *Contemp Pediatr* 15(12):64, 1998.

---

5. Two types of vaccines are available: Havrix and Vaqta. It is unknown whether or not these vaccines are interchangeable. The recommended Havrix dose is 1,440 ELISA in 1 ml and the recommended Vaqta dose is 50 units in 1 ml.
6. Both vaccines are given as IM injections and can be given at almost any site using a 1- to 1½-inch, 20- to 25-gauge needle.
7. The nurse should teach clients that discomfort at the injection site is expected. The application of heat may ameliorate the discomfort.
8. Pregnancy is not a contraindication to vaccination.
9. For pediatric considerations see Box 6-3.

INFLUENZA VACCINATION

Influenza is a viral illness contracted by direct contact with or inhalation of infected droplets. There are three subtypes of the influenza virus: influenza A, influenza B, and influenza C. Influenza A commonly affects adults and can cause a severe viral illness. Influenzae B and C rarely affect adults.

Influenza A is primarily confined to the respiratory tract. It results in a sudden onset of chills, internal temperature of 101° to 104° F, headache, myalgia, dry cough, and laryngitis. Symptoms generally subside in 5 days or less. High fevers that last more than 5 days are a serious sign that infection could lead to viral pneumonia.

NURSING CONSIDERATIONS

1. There are two types of influenza vaccines available: whole and split. Whole-virus vaccines are prepared by using chick embryos. Split-virus vaccines are prepared using organic solvents or detergents. Vaccines are prepared annually and are formulated based on the suspected circulating strain.
2. Influenza vaccination is highly effective in young, healthy adults but much less effective in ill clients such as the frail elderly and the severely immunosuppressed. The effectiveness of the vaccine also depends on how close the vaccine matches the circulating strain.
3. The vaccine is most effective when it precedes the influenza season (which, in the United States, is in December) by 2 months. In some cases, the vaccine can be administered up to 4 months after the influenza season.
4. HIV-positive adults should be vaccinated annually between September and mid-November.
5. Persons that are severely ill should defer vaccination.
6. Clients can receive whole- or split-virus vaccines. Dosage is 0.5 ml by IM injection using a 1- to 1½-inch, 20- to 25-gauge needle.
7. Local reactions can occur at the injection site, including erythema, pain, and induration.
8. Rare allergic reactions can occur in clients who are allergic to eggs. Vaccination should be deferred in clients who have documented or self-identified allergic reactions to eggs.
9. Clients with severe immune deficiency (CD_4 <100 cells/mm^3) may have a poor antibody response to the vaccine.[10] Severely immunodeficient clients or clients in whom the vaccine is contraindicated can be offered amantadine or rimantadine. These antiviral drugs have specific activity against influenza A virus. These drugs must be administered within 48 hours of flulike symptoms to be effective.
10. The client should be taught that influenza can occur despite vaccination. The nurse instructs the client about the importance of bedrest and hydration, especially with fever, during illness. Gargling with and drinking warm fluids such as teas will soothe the sore throat that accompanies illness. Acetylsalicylic acid (ASA) or Tylenol can relieve fever and myalgias.
11. The vaccine is safe for pregnant women.
12. For pediatric considerations see Box 6-4.

BOX 6-4   PEDIATRIC CONSIDERATIONS
Influenza vaccination

The influenza vaccine should be administered annually each fall to children who are HIV infected or who reside with HIV-positive household members. Vaccination should begin at the age of 6 months; efficacy has not been evaluated in infants vaccinated in the first 6 months of life. Influenza immunization is an IM injection and the dose and schedule are age specific, as indicated below. The duration of protection is thought to be less than 1 year, and for this reason annual revaccination is necessary.

Schedule

Age	Recommended vaccine	Dose	No. of doses
6 to 35 months	Split virus only	0.25 ml	1-2*
3 to 8 years	Split virus only	0.5 ml	1-2*
9 to 12 years	Split virus only	0.5 ml	1
>12 years	Whole or split virus	0.5 ml	1

Nursing Considerations

1. The influenza vaccine may be administered simultaneously with other routine vaccinations, including pertussis vaccine, at separate sites. However, it is important to note that both the influenza and whole cell pertussis vaccines can cause fever; if both must be administered at the same time, acellular pertussis vaccine should be used.
2. Children with a history of anaphylaxis to chicken or egg protein can experience a similar reaction to killed influenza vaccine. Although influenza vaccination has been safely administered to such children after skin testing and desensitization, they generally should not receive influenza vaccination because of the risk of such a reaction.
3. Only a split virus vaccine should be administered to children aged 12 years and younger, because whole virus immunizations are associated with higher rates of adverse reactions in young children.
4. Adults in close contact with HIV-infected children (e.g., household contacts) should be encouraged to receive annual influenza vaccination. This is especially important for adults who are household contacts of HIV-infected infants of less than 6 months of age, who are not yet candidates for influenza vaccination.
5. Febrile reactions to influenza vaccination are infrequent, especially after receiving split virus; however, fever is most likely to occur 6 to 24 hours after vaccination in children of less than 24 months of age.

---

* Two doses, administered 1 month apart, are recommended for children who are receiving the influenza vaccine for the first time at the age of 6 months to 8 years.

HAEMOPHILUS INFLUENZAE TYPE B VACCINATION

Haemophilus influenzae (Hi) is a bacterium that can cause a whole host of diseases including meningitis, sepsis, epiglottitis, pneumonia, and osteomyelitis. There are six subtypes (a-f) of Hi; type b (Hib) accounts for 95% of all infections. Transmission of the bacterium is almost exclusively through the nasopharynx. This organism primarily causes disease in children but HIV-positive adults are at high risk for Hi pneumonia. The role of vaccination in HIV-positive adults has not been clearly established.

NURSING CONSIDERATIONS

1. The following vaccines are available: ProHIBiT, HibTITER, Pedvax-HIB, ActHib, and OmniHIB; as well as Tetramune—a combination of Hib, diphtheria, tetanus, and pertussis vaccinations.
2. The nurse should question the client about childhood vaccination against Hib (and verify, if possible). Previously vaccinated adults do not require a series of injections, as does an unvaccinated child. Unvaccinated adults should receive one dose of one of the aforementioned vaccines (except Tetramune).
3. The recommended dosage is 0.5 ml given as an IM injection using a 1- to 1½-inch, 20- to 25-gauge needle.
4. Adverse reactions are uncommon. Instruct the client that he or she may experience mild fever, redness, or swelling at the injection site.
5. For pediatric considerations see Box 6-5.

TETANUS VACCINATION

Tetanus is a serious disease that is caused by an endotoxin produced by the bacillus *Clostridium tetani* and can result in painful spasms of the muscles. The organism is found in soil, street dust, and the intestines of various animals. Human skin also harbors the bacillus. Consequently, clients with soft tissue injuries and intravenous drug users are at high risk for infection. Drug users who inject heroin SC are at particularly high risk for infection with *C. tetani;* such users often dilute the heroin using a substance called quinine, which is known to promote the growth of *C. tetani* and may cause infection of the subcutaneous tissue.

In the United States, there are fewer than 50 cases of tetanus annually. The majority of these cases occur in adults over 50 years old who have not been previously immunized or whose immunization statuses are unknown. The small number of annual infections is undoubtedly due to a successful childhood vaccination program.

Infection with *C. tetani* almost always initially results in trismus (i.e., spasm of masticatory muscles with difficulty opening the mouth), or what is commonly known as "lockjaw." Trismus also stimulates the autonomic nervous system and results in an increase in temperature, tachycardia, diaphoresis, and high blood pressure. Various complications can also occur

BOX 6-5 PEDIATRIC CONSIDERATIONS
Haemophilus influenzae type b (Hib) vaccination

Immunocompromised children should receive Hib conjugate vaccines in the same dosage and schedule as immunocompetent children.
- The first dose of Hib is administered at 2 months of age. Immunization can be initiated as early as 6 weeks of age.
- The second dose of Hib is administered at 4 months.
- The third dose of Hib is administered at 6 months unless Pedvax HIB or COMVAX (PRP-OMB–type vaccines) are used.
- Antibody levels decline after the primary series and a booster vaccine is required at 12 months (or greater) of age.

Nursing Considerations

1. Any combination of the available conjugated vaccines is thought to provide an antibody response. However, the nurse should use the same vaccine for immunization at the ages of 2, 4, and 6 months; any conjugated vaccine can be used for the fourth dose at 12 to 15 months of age.
2. The vaccine is administered by 0.5 ml IM injection.
3. The vaccine should be administered using a separate syringe and at a separate site from other vaccines administered at the same visit.
4. Infants that are vaccinated with PedvaxHIB or COMVAX should receive a vaccine at 2 and 4 months of age. A third dose is administered at 12 to 15 months of age. The nurse should use the same vaccine for the first two doses. Any conjugated vaccine can be used for the third dose at 12 to 15 months of age.
5. If a child has an infection prior to vaccination, the vaccine does not confer immunity. Vaccination should continue once the child is well.

as a result of infection, including laryngospasm, coma, and even death. Unlike with other infections, protective immunity does not develop if a client is infected with *C. tetani*. There is no laboratory manifestation of this disease.

NURSING CONSIDERATIONS

1. There are two tetanus preparations: absorbed tetanus toxoid and tetanus toxoid fluid. Both are equally effective, but the absorbed preparation is most commonly used today because of longer lasting immunity.
2. The nurse should question the client about previous immunization. Childhood vaccination programs generally administer tetanus in combination with diphtheria (DT or Td), or in combination with diphtheria and pertussis (DTP or DTaP). If the adult has never been vaccinated, he or she should receive the full series of three injections. After initial vaccination, the second dose should be given 1 to 2 months later and the third dose 6 to 12 months later.

3. Adults who have received the full childhood series may be protected for life, however in some adults protective immunity may decline over time, and therefore a booster of tetanus-diphtheria (Td) is recommended every 10 years (preferably at age 15, 25, and so forth).

4. The recommended dosage for all adult tetanus and diphtheria vaccines is 0.5 ml, given via IM injection, preferably in the deltoid muscle using a 1- to 1½-inch, 20- to 25-gauge needle.

5. The nurse should teach clients that local reactions may occur at the injection site, such as pain, redness, or induration. The nurse should also inform clients that a nodule may be palpable at the injection site for several weeks.

6. Clients who have severe adverse reactions to the vaccination (e.g., febrile illness) may be given tetanus immune globulins instead. The recommended dosage is 250 units, given via IM injection using a 1- to 1½-inch, 20- to 25-gauge needle.

7. A careful history of vaccination is required prior to the administration of the vaccine. Clients should not receive the vaccine more than every 10 years. Frequent administration can lead to an exaggerated localized Arthus reaction, which manifests as painful swelling from the shoulder to the elbow 2 to 8 hours after injection.

8. Women who are pregnant should not receive the vaccine during the first trimester of pregnancy.

9. For pediatric considerations see Box 6-6.

DIPHTHERIA VACCINATION

Diphtheria is a contagious disease that is caused by the bacillus *Corynebacterium diphtheriae*. There are three biotypes of *C. diphtheria*: gravis, intermedius, and mitis. Disease caused by *C. diphtheria* can be mild or severe, depending on whether the particular strain of *C. diphtheria* produces toxins; it is the toxin that actually produces the manifestations commonly associated with diphtheria. Any strain may produce toxins; however, the most severe disease is thought to occur with the gravis strain.

C. diphtheria is spread to others by the secretions of an infected person. The toxin is spread by the bloodstream and distributed to tissues of the body, causing damage to organs such as the heart and kidneys. Cutaneous disease with *C. diphtheria* is very common in homeless persons and results in a scaling rash or ulcers with clearly demarcated edges. Cultures of lesions and mucous membranes can be tested to confirm a suspected case of the disease. The most common complications of this disease are myocarditis and neuritis; death occurs in 5% to 10% of these cases.

Nursing Considerations

The vaccine for diphtheria is always given in combinations with tetanus. Refer to the nursing considerations for tetanus vaccination (see Box 6-6).

BOX 6-6 PEDIATRIC CONSIDERATIONS
Tetanus vaccination

The tetanus vaccine is always administered in combination with diphtheria and pertussis. This combination vaccine is available in two forms: a whole cellular vaccine (DTP) and an acellular vaccine (DTaP). Concerns about the safety of the whole cellular vaccines have led to diminished use. The acellular vaccine is the preferred vaccine. There are currently four approved DTaP vaccines: Acel-Immune, Certiva, Infanrix, and Tripedia.

- The first dose of DTaP is usually administered at 2 months of age but can be given as early as 6 weeks.
- The second dose of DTaP is administered at 4 months.
- The third dose of DTaP is administered at 6 months.
- The fourth dose (a booster) of DTaP is administered at 12 months of age if 6 months have elapsed since the third dose and if the child is unlikely to return at 15 to 18 months of age. Otherwise, the fourth dose is given at 15 to 18 months.
- The fifth dose (a booster) of DTaP is administered between 4 and 6 years of age. In children who receive their first booster dose after their fourth birthday, a second booster is not necessary.

Nursing Considerations

1. Any combination vaccine that includes pertussis should not be given to children aged 7 years or older.
2. The vaccine is administered by 0.5 ml IM injection.
3. The vaccine should be administered using a separate syringe and at a separate site from other vaccines administered at the same visit.
4. Infants that have been vaccinated with Tetramune (DTP + Hib) have received whole cell pertussis in this combination. Any of the above acellular vaccines can be used to complete the five-dose series.
5. Tetanus toxoid (Td) is recommended at 11 to 12 years of age if at least 5 years have elapsed since the last dose of DTaP.

MEASLES VACCINATION

Measles is an acute systemic viral illness. It is a highly contagious illness that is spread to others by the respiratory droplets of an infected person. The virus replicates in the respiratory tract and gains access to the other organs by way of the lymphatic tissue. The hallmark of this disease is the appearance of a maculopapular rash. Approximately 1 week prior to the appearance of the rash, the client may have flu-like symptoms with a very high fever—103° to 105° F. About 1 to 2 days before the appearance of the rash the client may also develop Koplik's spots. These are blue-white spots on a bright red background and are located on the buccal mucosa.

A measles rash usually begins in the hairline and then proceeds downward and outward, finally reaching the hands and feet, and typically remains for approximately 1 week. Initially, discrete lesions blanch with pressure, but by day 4 this blanching disappears. There may also be a fine desquamation of the lesions. The rash disappears in the same order that it appeared. Clients are most infectious 4 days prior to and 4 days after the appearance of the rash.

Mortality for measles is rare; the majority of such deaths are related to complications such as encephalitis or pneumonia. In HIV-positive adults, the course of measles may be prolonged and illness may be more severe. Any client who presents with rashlike symptoms and a fever should be suspected of having measles. A serum specimen containing IgM antibodies indicates active infection with the measles virus.

NURSING CONSIDERATIONS

1. Previous exposure or vaccination should be confirmed by the presence of IgG measles antibodies. Clients with IgG greater than 1:40 by immunofluorescence assay (IFA) have measles immunity. Vaccines are contraindicated in these clients.
2. Measles vaccine is a live attenuated vaccine. Only one strain of measles virus vaccine (Moraten) is currently available in the United States. The measles vaccine, given in combination with mumps and rubella vaccines, is the only live vaccine that should be given to HIV-positive individuals.
3. Antibody response with the vaccine is generally good; lifelong immunity is expected.
4. The vaccine is given as a 0.5 ml SC injection (commonly as MMR) using a ⅝- to ⅞-inch, 25- to 27-gauge needle.
5. An immune globulin preparation is available for clients who have been exposed to measles. This preparation must be given within 6 days of exposure.
6. Fever and rash are the most common side effects associated with vaccination. Because the vaccine is grown in chick fibroblast culture, it may contain a minute quantity of egg protein. Egg-allergic clients should receive vaccination with caution. Protocols are available for vaccine administration to egg-allergic clients. The vaccine should also be given with caution to clients who have demonstrated an allergic reaction to gelatin or neomycin.
7. The vaccine should not be administered to clients who have received high doses of prednisone or its equivalent (i.e., the vaccine is safe when prednisone dosage is 2 mg/kg, not to exceed 20 mg) until at least 3 months after discontinuation of the corticosteroid.
8. The vaccine should be given at a time of clinical wellness.
9. The vaccine should not be given to pregnant women.

MUMPS VACCINATION

Mumps is an acute viral disease that causes a systemic illness. The majority of people infected with the virus that causes mumps rarely have severe disease. In approximately 50% of cases the only manifestations are nonspecific respiratory symptoms; about 20% of clients have asymptomatic disease. The virus is transmitted via respiratory droplets. The clinical manifestations of this infection are varied; the most common manifestation is parotitis. It occurs within the first 2 days of infection and lasts for as long as 10 days. Complications from mumps include aseptic meningitis, orchitis, oophoritis, deafness, and myocarditis. In addition to clinical findings, serology studies show IgM antibodies against the mumps virus during the first few days of illness.

Nursing Considerations

1. The presence of IgG measles antibodies indicates previous exposure or vaccination; vaccination is contraindicated in these clients.
2. Adults born in 1957 or later, regardless of HIV status, should have at least one dose of the measles-mumps-rubella (MMR) vaccine if serological immunity is not present. Persons born before 1957 are considered immune.
3. Serological results may be reported as immune, nonimmune, or equivocal. Clients who do not demonstrate immunity or who have equivocal results are candidates for vaccination.
4. The vaccine is given as a 0.5 ml SC injection (commonly as MMR) using a ⅜- to ⅝-inch, 25- to 27-gauge needle.
5. Mumps vaccination is considered safe. Mumps is always administered in combination with measles and rubella; adverse events are more likely attributable to one of those components rather than the mumps antigen.
6. The vaccine should be given with caution to clients who have demonstrated an allergic reaction to eggs, gelatin, or neomycin.
7. The vaccine should not be given to pregnant women.

RUBELLA VACCINATION

Rubella is a viral disease caused by the *Rubivirus*. In adults, respiratory inhalation of the virus causes infection and results in viremia, occurring 5 to 7 days after exposure. About 50% of infections are subclinical. Manifestations of illness include rash, lymphadenopathy, arthralgia, and arthritis. Complications such as hemorrhage and encephalitis occur rarely. Evidence of acute infection is demonstrated by the presence of rubella IgM antibodies in the client's serum. The presence of rubella IgG antibodies indicates previous infection or vaccination. Persons born before the year 1957 are considered immune. Immunity, indicated by the presence of IgG antibodies, should be checked even when the risk of infection with rubella is high, as in HIV-positive clients.

Nursing Considerations

1. Rubella vaccination is indicated for women of childbearing age, health care workers, and adults entering college.
2. The presence of IgG rubella antibodies indicates previous exposure or vaccination; vaccination is contraindicated in these clients.

BOX 6-7 PEDIATRIC CONSIDERATIONS
Measles, mumps, and rubella (MMR) vaccination

MMR vaccination is the only live vaccine administered to children with HIV-infection who are not severely immunocompromised. The risks of measles are far greater than the risks associated with MMR immunization in HIV-infected children without severe immunosuppression. Children with symptomatic HIV disease should not receive this vaccine, as there is the potential for measles to occur.

Nursing Considerations
1. The MMR dose is 0.5 ml, administered SC.
2. For unvaccinated children aged 12 to 15 months with no history of measles, a 2-dose schedule is recommended.
   - The first dose is administered at 12 to 15 months of age.
   - The second dose is administered at 4 to 6 years of age.
3. Before the administration of an MMR vaccine, it is important to assess for any recent receipt of immune globulin or blood products. Immune globulin preparations interfere with the serologic response to measles vaccination (for variable periods, depending on the dose administered). For example, the suggested intervals between varicella zoster immune globulin (VZIG) administration and MMR vaccination and between intravenous immune globulin (IVIG) administration (doses larger than 400 mg/kg) and MMR vaccination are 5 months and 8 months, respectively. If hepatitis B immune globulin (HBIG) is given, a period of 3 months should elapse before MMR is administered.
4. Tuberculin skin testing should not be performed until 4 to 6 weeks after MMR vaccination; measles vaccination may temporarily suppress tuberculin skin test reactivity, and a false negative result may occur.

Measles Exposure
All HIV-infected children should receive prophylaxis with immune globulin after exposure to measles, regardless of whether or not they have been vaccinated against measles.

Nursing Considerations for the HIV-Positive Child after Exposure to Measles
1. IM immune globulin is administered within 6 days of suspected exposure.
2. Immune globulin is administered by 0.5 ml/kg IM injection; maximum dose is 15 ml.
3. All nonimmune contacts in the family, even those that are not HIV-positive, should also receive immune globulin. The dose in the noninfected host is 0.25 ml/kg, given IM.
4. Children receiving monthly IVIG infusions whose last doses were received within 3 weeks of measles exposure may not need an additional dose of IVIG. However, some experts recommend that an additional dose be considered if 2 or more weeks have elapsed since the last dose of IVIG.

3. Serological results may be reported as immune, nonimmune, or equivocal. Clients who do not demonstrate immunity or who have equivocal results are candidates for vaccination.
4. The vaccine is given as a 0.5 ml SC injection (commonly as MMR) using a ⅝- to ⅞-inch, 25- to 27-gauge needle.

BOX 6-8 PEDIATRIC CONSIDERATIONS
Polio vaccination

Inactivated poliovirus vaccine (IPV) is the only polio vaccine recommended for HIV-positive persons. IPV should be given to the household contacts of infected children. If oral polio vaccine (OPV) is inadvertently administered to a household contact of an HIV-infected child, close contact between the child and the OPV recipient should be minimized for approximately 4 to 6 weeks after immunization. In healthy recipients of OPV, the virus persists in the throat for 1 to 2 weeks and in the feces for several weeks; immunodeficient clients may excrete the virus for prolonged periods.

- The first dose of IPV is administered at 6 to 8 weeks of age.
- The second dose of IPV is administered at 4 months.
- The third dose of IPV should be given 12 to 18 months after the second dose.
- A supplemental dose is administered before school entry at 4 to 6 years of age.

Nursing Considerations

1. OPV is contraindicated in children with HIV infection because of the theoretical or known risk of vaccine-associated paralytic illness.
2. The IPV dose is 0.5 ml, administered SC.

5. Rubella vaccination is considered safe. Because rubella is always administered in combination with measles and mumps, adverse events are more likely attributable to one of these components rather than the rubella antigen. Arthralgia and arthritis may be associated with the rubella component of the MMR vaccine.
6. Persons with a history of anaphylaxis to neomycin should not receive the rubella vaccine. The vaccine should be given at a time of clinical wellness.
7. The vaccine should not be given to pregnant women.
8. For pediatric considerations see Box 6-7.

POLIO VACCINATION

Poliovirus enters a susceptible host via contaminated drinking water or contact with contaminated feces (e.g., on hands). The virus establishes itself in the cells of the intestines. In most cases, the virus results in transient, self-limiting diarrhea; it may be completely asymptomatic.

In approximately 1% of infections, the virus spreads from the intestine into the central nervous system, eventually reaching motor neurons and causing paralysis or, in extreme cases, death. Widespread vaccination against polio has effectively eliminated its natural occurrence in the Western Hemisphere. Adults who have not been immunized as children do not need to be immunized. Polio vaccination is contraindicated in HIV-positive adults. For pediatric considerations see Box 6-8.

BOX 6-9 PEDIATRIC CONSIDERATIONS
Varicella virus vaccine

Until very recently, varicella vaccination was considered contraindicated in HIV-infected children. It has now been recommended that children with asymptomatic HIV infection be considered for varicella vaccination. Children who are considered candidates for this vaccine include those with asymptomatic infection (i.e., a CD$_4$ percentage of greater than 25).

Nursing Considerations
1. The vaccines are administered preferably as a subcutaneous (SC) injection. The intramuscular (IM) route may also be used. The vaccine is administered as a 0.5 ml dose.
2. Eligible HIV-infected children should receive 2 doses of varicella vaccine. The first dose is given between the ages of 12 to 18 months. The second dose should be administered 3 months after the first dose.
3. Parents should be instructed to return the child to the health care provider if a post-immunization rash develops.

BOX 6-10 PEDIATRIC CONSIDERATIONS
Administration of varicella zoster immune globulin

The varicella vaccine is contraindicated in symptomatic HIV-infected children. However, prevention, via vaccination, may be attempted for household contacts of an HIV-infected child who cannot receive the vaccine. No precautions are needed for healthy vaccinees who are living with an unvaccinated HIV-infected child and do not develop a rash. Vaccinees who develop a rash should avoid direct contact with a varicella-susceptible immunocompromised child for the duration of the rash. Varicella zoster immune globulin (VZIG) may be administered to varicella-susceptible HIV-infected infants and children after varicella exposure in an attempt to prevent the disease.

Nursing Considerations
1. Teach the parents of HIV-infected children to notify the provider of possible exposure to varicella as soon as possible.
2. VZIG is administered within 96 hours of exposure.
3. The dose of VZIG is a 125 U intramuscular (IM) injection for each 10 kg of body weight. The minimum suggested dose is 125 U and the maximum suggested dose is 625 U (5 vials).
4. Each vial contains 125 U, which is approximately 1.25 ml in volume.
5. Local discomfort after the IM injection is the most common adverse effect, and this may be lessened if the VZIG is room temperature when administered.
6. Children receiving monthly high-dose intravenous immune globulin (IVIG) probably will not require VZIG if the last dose of IVIG was given 3 weeks or less before the exposure.

VARICELLA VACCINATION

Varicella-zoster virus (VZV) is a herpesvirus. Primary infection with varicella results in chickenpox, a very common childhood illness. In adults, primary infection is more severe, often with systemic symptoms. Varicella infection often starts as localized erythematous macules and progresses to a vesicular eruption along one dermatome. In HIV-positive adults VZV infection can be severe enough to be a life-threatening illness. Transmission occurs via direct contact with infection lesions or inhalation of aerosolized droplets. Treatment of VZV infections is discussed in Chapter 17. VZV vaccination is contraindicated in HIV-positive adults. For pediatric considerations see Box 6-9 and 6-10.

REFERENCES

1. Staprans SI et al: Activation of viral replication after vaccination of HIV-1–infected individuals, *J Exp Med* 182:6, 1727, 1995.
2. Ho D: HIV-1 viraemia and influenza, *Lancet* 3(9):1549, 1992.
3. Fowke KF et al: Immunologic and virologic evaluation of influenza vaccination of HIV-1–infected patients, *International Conference on AIDS* 11(1):7, July 17, 1996. (Abstract No.: Tu.A.385.)
4. Simon BB: Immunization. In Gorell A, May LA, Mulley AG, eds: *Primary care medicine: office evaluation and management of the adult patient,* ed 3, Philadelphia, 1994, Lippincott.
5. Centers for Disease Control and Prevention: General recommendations on immunization recommendations of the Advisory Committee on Immunization Practices (ACIP), *MMWR* 43(RR-1):1, 1994.
6. US Department of Health and Human Services, Public Health Service Office of Public Health and Science, Office of Disease Prevention and Health Promotion: *Clinician's Handbook of Preventive Services,* ed 2, Washington, DC, 1998, US Government Printing Office, Superintendent of Documents, Mail Stop: SSOP, Washington, D.C., 20402-9328, ISBN: 0-16-049227-0.
7. Keller DW, Breiman RF: Preventing bacterial respiratory tract infections among persons infected with human immunodeficiency virus, *Clin Infect Dis* 21(Suppl 1):S77, 1995.
8. Dolan SA: Vaccines for hepatitis A and B, *Postgrad Med* 102:6, 1997.
9. Porth CM: *Pathophysiology: concepts of altered health states,* Philadelphia, 1998, Lippincott.
10. Kroon FP et al: Antibody response to influenza, tetanus and pneumococcal vaccines in HIV-seropositive individuals in relation to the number of CD_4^+ lymphocytes, *AIDS* 8(4):469, 1994.

7

Tuberculosis Screening, Diagnosis, and Infection Control

Dorothy Talotta

The history of tuberculosis (TB) as a disease and epidemic is a fascinating one. Some form of the disease has affected humans since at least 4000 B.C.[1] TB was the leading cause of death in Europe and the United States until the early part of the twentieth century.[2] During the industrial revolution, people began migrating into cities where conditions such as poverty, malnutrition, and crowding were suitable for the growth and spread of the organism that causes TB. The result has been referred to as the "great white plague" in Western Europe.[3] A German physician named Robert Koch isolated the bacillus that causes TB in 1882; but it was not until 1944 that streptomycin was isolated in Selman Waksman's laboratory by a graduate student named Albert Schatz. Streptomycin proved effective against TB, but its clinical usefulness was limited by the emergence of drug resistance. The development of streptomycin was followed closely by that of paraaminosalicylic acid (PAS) and isonicotinic acid hydrazide (INH). PAS was the first drug available that, when given concurrently with streptomycin, prevented the emergence of streptomycin resistance. By 1952, INH was also available and was used in combination with streptomycin or PAS.[4] Between 1953 and 1985, the number of TB cases reported annually in the United States decreased by 74%.[5] The use of drug therapy contributed to this decrease as did improvements in living conditions, natural resistance, and public health measures.[3]

Between 1985 and 1991, the downward trend in reported cases reversed. A number of factors have been cited as contributing to this reversal.[3] However, HIV infection has been singled out as a major factor in the resurgence of TB[6] and as the greatest risk factor for the development of active TB ever identified.[7] In 1989, reported TB cases had increased approximately 5% from 1988 and cases continued to rise, reaching a peak in 1992. The resurgence of TB prompted more effective TB control programs that resulted in annual decreases in reported cases in the United States since 1992. A record low number of reported cases was reached in 1998.[5]

Clinicians must not relax their vigilance, however, in the face of this decline; there continue to be approximately 18,000 new cases of TB in the United States annually, and approximately 15 million people have latent TB infection, which puts them at risk for future disease. In addition, multidrug resistant TB (MDR TB) continues to spread.[5] (See Chapter 13 for a discussion of latent and active TB infection and MDR TB.) Recently the Advisory Council for the Elimination of Tuberculosis (ACET) reaffirmed its commitment to the elimination of TB in the United States.[5]

It is difficult to determine the true rate of coinfection with HIV and TB in the United States. In 1997, only 50% of TB case reports in the 25- to 44-year-old age group included information about HIV status; only 15 states reported HIV test results for at least 75% of TB cases in this age group. According to the CDC, of all TB cases reported in 1993/1994, 14% also appeared in the AIDS registry.[8]

The nurse plays an important role in screening clients for TB, preventing the spread of the organism, and educating clients about the disease and its implications. This chapter describes the standard screening test for TB (the Mantoux test) and sputum collection for sputum studies, which are used in diagnosing TB. This chapter also describes infection control procedures for ambulatory settings. (See Chapter 13 for a discussion of TB and TB diagnosis and see Chapter 10 for infection control in acute care settings.)

SCREENING CLIENTS FOR TB—THE MANTOUX TEST

Tuberculin skin testing is the standard means of identifying people infected with *Mycobacterium tuberculosis* (MTB), the organism that causes TB. Skin testing uses a purified protein derivative (PPD) of TB, which acts as an antigen. The ability of the client's immune system to respond to the injected antigen is the basis for the test results. The skin test, known as the Mantoux test, is the cornerstone of MTB infection identification.[9] In the past, multiple puncture tests such as the Tine test were also used. Today, these should not be used as they are fraught with problems related to administration and standardization.[10]

PROCEDURE FOR THE MANTOUX TEST

To perform a PPD test using the Mantoux method, the nurse injects 0.1 ml of PPD tuberculin containing 5 tuberculin units (TU) intradermally. The nurse may use the following procedure:

1. Gather the appropriate equipment needed for the administration of the injection. This includes:
   - A vial, containing 5 TU per 0.1 ml of PPD tuberculin.
   - A disposable tuberculin syringe with a short (¼- to ½-inch), 26- or 27-gauge needle. The TB syringe has a long, thin barrel with a preattached needle, is calibrated in minums and hundredths of a milliliter, and has a capacity of 1 ml.
   - Alcohol pads, disposable gloves, skin pencil.
2. Position the client's elbow and forearm on a flat surface.

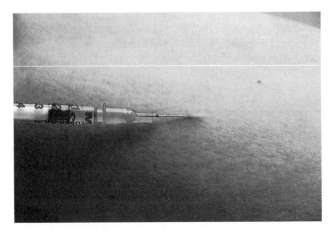

Figure 7-1. Advancing the needle. (*From Perry AG, Potter PA:* Clinical skills and techniques, *ed 4, St Louis, 1998, Mosby.*)

3. Select an area on the forearm that is free of hair and lesions so that results can be seen easily and interpreted correctly.
4. Prepare the medication—withdraw 0.1 ml of solution.
5. Apply gloves.
6. Cleanse the site with alcohol. Make sure alcohol dries before administering injection.
7. With the needle almost against the client's skin, bevel up, advance the needle slowly at a 5° to 15° angle until resistance is felt. Then advance the needle through the epidermis to approximately 3 mm (⅛ inches) below the skin surface. The needle tip should be seen through the skin (Figure 7-1).
8. Inject medication slowly. Normally, resistance is felt. If it is not, the needle is too deep; remove and begin again.
9. While injecting medication, a small bleb resembling a mosquito bite should appear on the skin's surface (Figure 7-2). This bleb should be approximately 6 to 10 mm in diameter.
10. Withdraw the needle while applying an alcohol or gauze pad gently over the site.
11. Do not massage the site; this may disperse the medication into underlying tissue and alter test results.
12. Use the skin pencil to draw a circle around the perimeter of the injection site. Instruct the client not to remove the circle until after the test results have been read.
13. Instruct the client to return to the clinic 48 to 72 hours later for interpretation of the skin test results.[11]

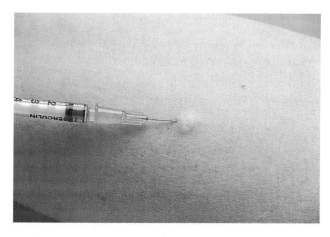

Figure 7-2. A small bleb appears while injecting. (*From Perry AG, Potter PA:* Clinical skills and techniques, *ed 4, St Louis, 1998, Mosby.*)

INTERPRETING RESULTS OF THE TUBERCULIN SKIN TEST

The test is read after 48 to 72 hours. To interpret the test, the nurse observes and palpates the injection site. If there is no palpable induration, the test is considered negative, even if there is an area of erythema or ecchymosis.[9]

If a nurse is able to palpate an area of induration, the size of the induration should be measured. To ensure accuracy in interpreting the test, the nurse should use a measuring ruler like the one located on the inside back cover. In a client with HIV infection, an induration of 5 mm or more is considered positive.[12] The size of the induration that indicates a positive skin test result varies in different groups. Table 7-1 indicates the size of the induration defined as positive in various groups of clients.

A client whose tuberculin skin test results change from a known negative to a known positive reaction but who has no evidence of the disease is known as a "tuberculin converter."[13]

False Positive Results

The PPD test is not 100% sensitive, nor is it 100% specific for TB; therefore, false positive and false negative results occur.[12] A *false positive result* is when the client is actually TB negative but the test is positive. False positive results can occur from errors in test administration or in result interpretation. A common error in interpretation is the measurement of erythema instead of the area of palpable induration.[9]

Another cause of false positive results is previous vaccination with bacille Calmette-Guérin (BCG), a TB vaccine.[12] In some countries indi-

Table 7-1	**Interpretation of Skin Test Results**

Induration	Considered Positive if:
≥5 mm	HIV infection is present
	The client's HIV status is unknown but risk factors for HIV infection are present
	There has been recent close contact with known case of active TB
	Chest X-ray studies are consistent with healed TB
≥10 mm	The client is known to be HIV seronegative but is an IVDU
	The client has a medical condition (e.g., diabetes mellitus, chronic renal failure, certain malignancies that increase the risk of progressing from latent to active TB)
	The client is an employee or resident in a crowded living condition such as a prison, nursing home, or homeless shelter
	The client was born in and arrived within last 5 years from a country with a high incidence of TB
	The client belongs to a low-income, medically underserved population (e.g., homeless persons, migrant farm workers)
	The client belongs to a locally defined high-risk racial or ethnic minority population
	The client is a child under 4 years of age
	The client is an infant, child, or adolescent exposed to a high-risk category adult
≥15 mm	The client meets none of the above criteria

Adapted from Bloch AB: Screening for tuberculosis and tuberculosis infection in high-risk populations: recommendations of the Advisory Council for the Elimination of Tuberculosis, *MMWR* 44(RR-11):24, September 8, 1995.

viduals are vaccinated with BCG, which can produce a false positive result but is not a contraindication for PPD testing.[9] However, when a tuberculin skin test is administered to a client who has previously been vaccinated with BCG, the health care provider has the difficult task of distinguishing between a reaction caused by BCG vaccination and one caused by infection with MTB. The likelihood that the reaction results from MTB infection rather than BCG vaccination increases both as the reaction size increases, and as the time interval between vaccination and PPD testing increases—the reactivity induced by BCG vaccination decreases with time. The likelihood of infection with MTB also increases when the client is a contact of an infected person, when the client is from a country with a high prevalence of TB, or when there is a family history of TB.[12]

False positive results can also occur due to infection with mycobacteria other than MTB. It is also difficult to distinguish between reactions caused by MTB and those caused by other mycobacteria. However, the larger the area of induration, the greater the likelihood of MTB infection.[12]

PPD results can also be misinterpreted as a result of the "booster effect," which can give the false impression that a person is a tuberculin converter. Repeated skin testing of uninfected persons does not sensitize them to PPD and will not result in future false positive PPD results. However, if a person has been infected with MTB in the past or has received the BCG vaccine, the resulting hypersensitivity may gradually diminish over time, and therefore a PPD test may produce negative results. The stimulus of a first PPD test, however, can increase or "boost" the size of the reaction to a subsequent test administered during a period of 1 week to 1 year after the first test—the first test stimulates the immune system to recall that it was previously infected. The increase in the size of the reaction can give the false impression that the person is a tuberculin converter. In populations that are frequently tested with the Mantoux test, such as health care workers, initial two-step testing can be used to decrease the possibility that a boosted reaction will be interpreted as a conversion. If the result of a first Mantoux test is negative, the person is retested 1 to 3 weeks later. If the result of the second test is positive, it probably means that boosting from a past infection or prior BCG vaccination has occurred. Individuals with boosted reactions should not be classified as converters but as reactors. If the result of the second test is negative, the individual is probably not infected; however, if this individual tests positive on a subsequent test, a true conversion has occurred.[12,14]

False Negative Results

A *false negative result* is when the test is negative but the client is infected with TB. This can occur for a number of reasons, including inadvertent subcutaneous administration of the PPD and the use of PPD that has been stored improperly. The PPD solution must be kept in the refrigerator and should be injected soon after it is drawn up, otherwise the solution will be adsorbed by the plastic of the syringe.[9]

False negative results can also result from immune system anergy. Immunocompromised clients may be anergic (i.e., the immune system is not able to produce a positive response), and because the Mantoux test depends on the body's ability to mount a hypersensitivity response to the PPD, a negative PPD under such circumstances could be a false negative.[9] In one study, HIV-positive subjects with CD_4 cell counts below 400 cells/mm^3 were more likely to be anergic than HIV-negative control subjects. HIV-positive subjects with CD_4 counts below 200 cells/mm^3 were most likely to be anergic.[15] Therefore, some clinicians may choose to perform an anergy panel, which involves administering two or three other antigens in addition to the PPD, such as mumps, candida, and tetanus toxoid.[9,16] Most people will have a positive response to several of these antigens. If the response to all of the antigens is negative, the client is probably anergic. The use of an anergy panel helps to determine the validity of the response to the PPD.[16]

The clinical usefulness of the information obtained from anergy testing has been questioned, however.[9] The CDC has cited several limitations in the use of anergy testing, including the variability in available testing methods, and no longer recommends routine anergy testing in HIV-infected people. The CDC does indicate that clinicians may find the results of anergy testing useful in individual situations when used as part of a multifactorial assessment of a person's risk for TB. The results of such testing must be supplemented with information concerning the person's risk of exposure to and infection with MTB.[17] Some experts recommend repeat PPD testing on clients who were previously anergic but whose immune systems have responded to antiretroviral therapy.[18] HIV-positive clients who are close contacts of individuals with infectious TB should receive prophylactic therapy (after active disease has been excluded) regardless of PPD test results.[19]

SPUTUM SPECIMEN COLLECTION IN THE DIAGNOSIS OF TB

Sputum studies are used in the diagnosis of TB. (See Chapter 13 for a complete discussion of TB diagnosis.) Once a screening test is positive, culture of the client's sputum is essential in confirming a diagnosis of TB. Collecting a "good" sputum specimen is essential. However, the infectiousness of a person with TB correlates with the number of organisms expelled into the air. Coughing or other forceful expiratory maneuvers increase the degree of infectiousness since they increase the number of organisms expelled into the air.[20]

When obtaining sputum specimens from a client with suspected TB, precautions to prevent transmission of the organism must be taken. The nurse should follow state and local health department guidelines and agency policies regarding TB infection control. Because of the danger of spread of MTB, there are CDC guidelines[21] that address the performance of procedures that are cough inducing and aerosol generating on clients who may have infectious TB. The guidelines recommend that such procedures be performed only if absolutely necessary and with appropriate precautions. Cough-inducing procedures should be performed in areas with local exhaust ventilation devices such as booths or special enclosures, or in a room which meets the ventilation requirements for TB isolation. Health care workers present in the room must wear respiratory protection.[21] (See Chapter 10 for a more complete discussion of the guidelines.)

Cough-inducing procedures for clients with infectious TB should not be done in the client's home unless absolutely necessary. When cough-inducing procedures such as diagnostic sputum induction must be performed for the TB client, they should be done in a health care facility in a room or booth, as described in Chapter 10. Health care workers should wear respiratory protection when entering the homes of clients with suspected or confirmed infectious TB.[21]

OBTAINING A SPUTUM SPECIMEN VIA COUGHING

To obtain an adequate sputum specimen, the nurse must adhere to the following principles:

1. Sputum specimens are best collected in the early morning before eating or brushing teeth.
2. The client should rinse his or her mouth with water before coughing to minimize contamination of the sample with normal flora or food debris.
3. The nurse should provide the client with a sterile, wide-mouthed jar with a screw top. The client should press the rim of the container under his lower lip, rather than inside his lips, to prevent contamination of the jar.
4. Specimens should be obtained on at least three different days. Explain to the client that two teaspoons of sputum (5 to 10 ml) are needed, and that saliva and nasopharyngeal secretions aren't useful.[22]

OBTAINING A SPUTUM SPECIMEN VIA SPUTUM INDUCTION

If the client cannot produce an adequate amount of sputum spontaneously, a sputum induction may be done using aerosolized hypertonic saline. The client is instructed to take several normal breaths of the aerosol mist and then to take a deep breath, cough, and expectorate. It usually takes about fifteen minutes for a specimen to be produced.[23] Sputum induction may cause transient nausea in some clients or bronchospasm in clients with reactive airway disease. The sputum induction procedure is one that produces large numbers of infectious aerosolized organisms, which are potentially dangerous to the health care worker.[24]

INFECTION CONTROL—AMBULATORY CARE SETTINGS

In health care facilities, transmission of MTB is a recognized risk to health care workers and clients. Transmission is most likely to occur when clients have unrecognized pulmonary or laryngeal TB and are not in isolation or are not undergoing effective therapy.[21] In ambulatory care settings, clients may be seeking care for symptoms of TB but may not yet have been diagnosed. The early identification, isolation, and effective treatment of individuals with active TB are important goals in an effective TB control program.[21]

In outpatient areas, the nurse should make vigorous efforts to identify clients with active TB promptly to minimize the amount of time that such clients spend in ambulatory-care areas. TB precautions should be followed while the diagnostic process is being carried out. These clients should not be placed in open waiting areas but should be in a separate area apart from other clients. Ideally, they would be placed in a room or enclosure meeting TB isolation requirements. (See Chapter 10 for a discussion of infection control.) Tissues should be given to the client, with instructions to cover the mouth and nose with tissues when coughing or sneezing. The client should be given a surgical mask to wear and should be instructed to keep the mask on. If a client is known to have active TB and has not completed therapy, TB precautions should be followed until it is determined that the client is noninfectious.[21]

In ambulatory care areas where clients who are at high risk for TB are treated, ventilation should be designed and maintained to reduce the risk of transmission of the organism. The use of air-disinfection techniques such as ultraviolet germicidal irradiation (UVGI) or high efficiency particulate air (HEPA) filters or enhanced general ventilation may be useful.[21] (See Chapter 10 for discussion of UVGI and HEPA filters.) Ideally, ambulatory care settings in which clients with TB are frequently seen should have a TB isolation room or rooms available. In ambulatory care settings where TB clients are seen infrequently, such rooms are not necessary; however, the facility should have a written protocol for early identification of clients with TB symptoms and referral to a setting in which the person can be evaluated and managed appropriately.[21]

In medical offices, TB infection control policies should be based on periodic risk assessments and should include methods for identifying and managing clients who may have active TB that is not yet diagnosed. Medical office policies should also include provisions for managing clients with active TB and for educating, screening, and counseling health care workers. All clients should be asked routinely about a history of TB or symptoms that suggest TB. Those clients with a history and suggestive symptoms should undergo appropriate diagnostic testing and be evaluated promptly for infectiousness. Such an evaluation should ideally be done in a facility with TB isolation capability. At a minimum, the client should be separated as much as possible from other clients, should be given and asked to wear a surgical mask, and should be taught to cover the mouth and nose with tissues when coughing and sneezing. Those medical offices that provide evaluation or treatment for clients with TB should follow the above recommendations regarding ambulatory care settings. The appropriate precautions must be followed if cough-inducing procedures are conducted in a medical office for clients who may have active TB.[21]

REFERENCES

1. Haas F, Haas SS: The origins of mycobacterium tuberculosis and the notion of its contagiousness. In Rom WN, Garay SM, eds: *Tuberculosis,* Boston, 1996, Little, Brown & Co.

2. Bloom BR: Foreword. In Rom WN, Garay SM, eds: *Tuberculosis,* Boston, 1996, Little, Brown & Co.
3. Waxman S, Gang M, Goldfrank L: Tuberculosis in the HIV-infected patient, *Emerg Med Clin North Am* 13(1):179, 1995.
4. Harris HW: Chemotherapy of tuberculosis: The beginning. In Rom WN, Garay SM, eds: *Tuberculosis,* Boston, 1996, Little, Brown & Co.
5. Centers for Disease Control and Prevention: Tuberculosis elimination revisited: obstacles, opportunities, and a renewed commitment—Advisory Council for the Elimination of Tuberculosis (ACET), *MMWR* 48(RR-9):1, August 13, 1999.
6. Barnes PF et al: Tuberculosis in patients with human immunodeficiency virus infection, *N Engl J Med* 324(23):1644, 1991.
7. Scharer LL, McAdam JM: *Tuberculosis and AIDS: the epidemiology of tuberculosis and human immunodeficiency virus,* New York, 1995, Springer.
8. US Department of Health and Human Services: Tuberculosis morbidity—United States, 1997, *MMWR* 47(13):253, 1998.
9. Leiner S, Mays M: Diagnosing latent and active pulmonary tuberculosis: a review for clinicians, *Nurse Pract* 21(2):86, 1996.
10. Frieden TR: *Tuberculosis at a glance: a reference guide for practitioners covering the basic elements of tuberculosis care,* 1995, New York City Department of Health, Bureau of Tuberculosis Control.
11. Kirton CA: Administering intradermal injections. In Perry A, Potter A, eds: *Clinical nursing skill and techniques,* ed 4, St Louis, 1998, Mosby.
12. Bloch AB: Screening for tuberculosis and tuberculosis infection in high-risk populations: recommendations of the Advisory Council for the Elimination of Tuberculosis, *MMWR* 44(RR-11):19, September 8, 1995.
13. Cronin SN: Nursing care of clients with disorders of the lung parenchyma and pleura. In Black JM, Matassarin-Jacobs E, eds: *Medical-surgical nursing: clinical management for continuity of care,* Philadelphia, 1997, WB Saunders.
14. Jones SG: Tuberculin testing in patients with HIV/AIDS, *AACN Clinical Issues* 7(3):378, 1996.
15. Markowitz N et al, for the Pulmonary Complications of HIV Infection Study Group: Tuberculin and anergy testing in HIV-seropositive and HIV-seronegative persons, *Ann Intern Med* 119:185, 1993.
16. Calianno C, Pino T: Getting a reaction to anergy panel testing, *Nurs 95* 25(1):58, 1995.
17. Centers for Disease Control and Prevention: Anergy skin testing and preventive therapy for HIV-infected persons: revised recommendations, *MMWR* 46(RR-15):1, September 5, 1997.
18. Centers for Disease Control and Prevention: Prevention and treatment of tuberculosis among patients infected with Human Immunodeficiency Virus: principles of therapy and revised recommendations, *MMWR* 47(RR-20):1, October 30, 1998.
19. Centers for Disease Control and Prevention: 1999 USPHS/IDSA guidelines for the prevention of opportunistic infections in persons infected with human immunodeficiency virus, *MMWR* 48(RR-10):1, 1999.
20. Centers for Disease Control and Prevention: Guidelines for preventing the transmission of tuberculosis in health-care settings, with special focus on HIV-related issues, *MMWR* 39(RR-17), 1990.

21. Centers for Disease Control and Prevention: Guidelines for preventing the transmission of mycobacterium tuberculosis in health-care facilities, *MMWR* 43(RR-13):1, October 28, 1994.
22. Finkelstein L: Sputum testing for TB: getting good specimens, *Am J Nurs* 96:2, 1996.
23. Boutotte J: TB: the second time around . . . and how you can help to control it, *Nurs 93* 23(5):42, 1993.
24. Serkey JM: Multi–drug-resistant tuberculosis: a new era in prevention and control, *Dimensions of Critical Care Nursing* 14(5):236, 1995.

8

Gynecological and Cervical Disorders and Therapeutics

Dorothy Talotta

Women now constitute the group in which the AIDS epidemic is growing most rapidly.[1] Among AIDS cases reported annually in adults and adolescents, the proportion of women increased from 7% in 1985 to 18% in 1994.[2] By 1999, the proportion of women, which has continued to increase steadily, reached 23%.[3] In the United States, most HIV-positive women become infected through heterosexual contact or injection drug use. The proportion of women infected through heterosexual contact has been increasing and in 1994 surpassed the proportion of women infected through injection drug use.[3] Heterosexual intercourse with an infected male has become the most common mode of transmission among women.[4]

HIV is more easily transmitted from men to women than from women to men. In one study, male-to-female transmission was approximately eight times more efficient than was female-to-male transmission.[5] The reason for this difference in susceptibility is not known. However, certain differences may contribute towards the increased susceptibility of women. The surface area of the female reproductive tract that is exposed to infected semen is significantly larger than that of the male urethra exposed to infected vaginal fluid, and following sexual intercourse the duration of exposure to fluids containing the virus is greater for women.[6] The vaginal secretions of an HIV-infected woman may be less infectious than the semen of an HIV-infected man for several reasons including the low pH of the vagina during reproductive years. This acidic environment is unfavorable for HIV. Also, the female reproductive tract is extremely susceptible to the attachment of HIV due to the types of cells present and the permeability of the mucosa.[7]

In 1997, the incidence of AIDS decreased in all groups when compared with the 1996 incidence, mostly as a result of effective therapies. However, the decrease was smaller among women than among men (8% and 16%, respectively). Between 1996 and 1997, AIDS deaths declined but, as with AIDS incidence, the decrease was smaller among women than among men (32% and 44%, respectively).[8] HIV infection is the third leading cause of death among women aged 25 to 44 years.[9]

At the beginning of the HIV epidemic, the disease was primarily seen in men. Therefore, most information about AIDS was based on data collected from males.[10] However, with the exception of disorders of the female reproductive tract, it is likely that, on the whole, women experience the same opportunistic infections that men do and that the disease follows a similar clinical course.[11]

Overall differences between men and women in the incidence rates of opportunistic infections and malignancies appear to be minimal, with a few exceptions.[12] For example, Kaposi's sarcoma is one opportunistic infection that is more common in men because of its high prevalence among men who have sex with men.[13] (See Chapter 15 for a discussion of Kaposi's sarcoma.) Esophageal candidiasis appears to be more common in women.[14,15] (See Chapter 14 for a discussion of candidiasis.)

Some early studies indicated that the survival rate (the interval from AIDS diagnosis to death) of women might be lower.[16,17] Women were found to be diagnosed later in the course of the disease.[18] It has been suggested that differences in outcomes for women may be related to less access to health care, less utilization of health care for HIV infection,[19] and socioeconomic disadvantage.[20] Moreover, even though a woman may present with symptoms similar to those of HIV-infected men, the health care provider may evaluate the symptoms differently because he or she may not expect a woman to have HIV infection.[21]

In 1993, the Centers for Disease Control and Prevention (CDC) revised the AIDS case definition for reporting purposes. The classification system now includes invasive cervical cancer as an AIDS-defining (Category C) illness. It also includes as Category B illnesses (those attributable to or complicated by HIV): vaginal candidiasis that is persistent, frequent, or poorly responsive to therapy; moderate or severe cervical dysplasia; and pelvic inflammatory disease.[22] These gynecological problems are discussed in this chapter with the exception of vaginal candidiasis which is discussed in Chapter 14. Menstrual problems and contraception are also addressed in this chapter.

GYNECOLOGICAL PROBLEMS

The prevalence of gynecological disease has been reported to be as high as 42% among women infected with HIV.[20] The gynecological health of such women is more affected when immunosuppression is greater.[23] Gynecological infections can be an early sign of HIV progression.[13]

The kinds of infections seen in HIV-positive women are also common in HIV-negative women. However, HIV-positive women often have infections that are recurrent and tend to be more severe and refractory to treatment.[1] The infections that will be discussed are pelvic inflammatory disease, and human papilloma virus (HPV), which is the causative agent of condyloma acuminata (anogenital warts) and also associated with cervical dysplasia, preinvasive disease, invasive carcinoma, and vulvar intraepithelial neoplasia (VIN).[1,24]

Pelvic Inflammatory Disease

■ DEFINITION AND ETIOLOGY

Pelvic inflammatory disease (PID) consists of a spectrum of inflammatory disorders of the female upper genital tract. It may include any or all of the following: endometritis, salpingitis, tuboovarian abscess, and pelvic peritonitis. In the majority of cases in the general population, sexually transmitted organisms, particularly *Neisseria gonorrhoeae* and *Chlamydia trachomatis,* are the offending organisms. However, organisms that can be part of normal vaginal flora, including a number of anaerobic organisms, can also cause PID.[25] Both HIV and the organisms associated with PID can be transmitted sexually. However, there is some indication that, in HIV-positive women, PID may frequently be caused by endogenous pathogens (that are no longer controlled by local immunity) ascending from the lower genital tract.[23]

■ CLINICAL OVERVIEW

Symptoms of PID most commonly begin within a week of the onset of menses. The risk of PID is increased in adolescents, women with multiple sexual partners, and those with a previously diagnosed sexually transmitted disease (STD). The use of an intrauterine device (IUD) and douching also increase risk.[26] Within the general population of women there is a wide variation in signs and symptoms of PID. Symptoms may be subtle or mild and not readily recognized.[25] There have been conflicting reports regarding clinical presentation of immunocompromised women with acute PID. Some have reported that immunocompromised women present with fewer symptoms than immunocompetent women, while others have reported that HIV-positive women present with more severe symptoms.[13]

In the general population the most typical presentation of PID is continuous bilateral pain in the lower abdomen or pelvis, which may be accompanied by fever, nausea, and vomiting.[26] However, some clients may have atypical PID, which consists of mild or nonspecific signs or symptoms, such as abnormal vaginal bleeding, vaginal discharge, or dyspareunia; others may have asymptomatic PID.[25]

■ DIAGNOSTIC TESTING

The CDC has made recommendations to assist clinicians in diagnosing PID. The criteria for diagnosing PID are classified as minimum, additional, and definitive criteria.[25]

The CDC recommends three minimum diagnostic criteria: the presence of lower abdominal tenderness, adnexal tenderness, and cervical motion tenderness (i.e., pain when the cervix is moved from side to side during a gynecological examination). If these minimum criteria are present in sexually active young women and others at risk for STDs, and no other cause for the illness can be identified, the CDC recommends initiating empiric treatment for PID.

Since incorrect diagnosis or management of PID may cause unnecessary morbidity, additional diagnostic evaluation is often needed. Additional criteria that support a diagnosis of PID include an oral temperature of greater than 101° F (38.3° C), abnormal cervical or vaginal discharge, elevated erythrocyte sedimentation rate (ESR), elevated C-reactive protein, and laboratory documentation of cervical infection with *N. gonorrhoeae* or *C. trachomatis*.[25] (Both the ESR and C-reactive protein are nonspecific tests that indicate the presence of inflammation.) In an HIV-positive woman with a low CD_4 cell count, there may not be an elevated white blood cell count (WBC) in response to infection, and the ESR may already be elevated in response to chronic illness. In such a case, the diagnostic value of these tests is reduced.[13]

Definitive criteria for diagnosing PID are warranted in selected cases. These criteria involve additional diagnostic testing with results consistent with PID. Criteria considered definitive by the CDC include:

1. Histopathologic evidence of endometritis by endometrial biopsy,
2. Transvaginal sonography or other imaging techniques that show thickened, fluid-filled tubes, with or without free pelvic fluid or tuboovarian complex, and
3. Laparoscopic abnormalities consistent with PID.[25]

Other tests that aid in the diagnosis of PID include a wet mount or Gram stain of endocervical secretions. A pregnancy test is also indicated.[26] An ectopic pregnancy can produce symptoms similar to those of PID; the results of a sensitive pregnancy test are useful in evaluating this possibility.

■ MEDICAL MANAGEMENT

The CDC recommends that immunosuppressed, HIV-positive women with PID be managed aggressively, using a parenteral regimen. Immunodeficiency is one of the criteria for hospitalizing women with PID. For all women with PID, antibiotic regimens must provide empiric, broad-spectrum coverage of likely causative organisms and all regimens should be effective against gonorrhea and chlamydia as well as anaerobes. It is important to begin treatment immediately once the presumptive diagnosis has been made to prevent long-term sequelae. There are two parenteral antibiotic regimens for inpatient treatment of the general population of women with PID, the effectiveness of which have been demonstrated in multiple trials. These regimens have also been recommended for HIV-positive women (Table 8-1). In most trials, parenteral treatment was continued for at least 48 hours after the client demonstrated substantial clinical improvement. However, the decision about transition to oral therapy should be guided by clinical experience and may be accomplished within 24 hours of clinical improvement.[25]

There are also oral and intramuscular antibiotic regimens available for outpatient treatment of PID. They provide coverage against the organisms that frequently cause PID; data supporting their use is limited, however. If a client does not respond to oral therapy within 72 hours, she should be reevaluated to confirm the diagnosis and should receive parenteral therapy[25] (Table 8-2).

Table 8-1	Parenteral Regimens for the Treatment of PID	
Parenteral Regimen A	**Parenteral Regimen B**	**Alternative Parenteral Regimens**
Cefotetan 2 g IV q12h **or** cefoxitin 2 g IV q6h *Plus* Doxycycline 100 mg IV **or** PO q12h Parenteral therapy may be discontinued 24 hours after clinical improvement. It should be followed by: Doxycycline 100 mg PO bid × 14 days*	Clindamycin 900 mg IV q8h *Plus* Gentamicin loading dose IV or IM (2 mg/kg of body weight), followed by a maintenance dose of 1.5 mg/kg q8h (single daily dosing may be substituted) Parenteral therapy may be discontinued 24 hours after clinical improvement. It should be followed by, for a total of 14 days of therapy†: Doxycycline 100 mg PO bid *Or* Clindamycin 450 mg PO qid	(Less data supporting their use is available.) Ofloxacin 400 mg IV q12h **plus** metronidazole 500 mg IV q8h *Or* Ampicillin/sulbactam 3 g IV q6h **plus** doxycycline 100 mg IV or PO q12h *Or* Ciprofloxacin 200 mg IV q12h **plus** doxycycline 100 mg IV or PO q12h **plus** metronidazole 500 mg IV q8h

*If tuboovarian abscess is present, clindamycin or metronidazole is often used with doxycycline for continued therapy for improved anaerobic coverage.
†If tuboovarian abscess is present, clindamycin may be used for continued therapy for improved anaerobic coverage.
Adapted from Centers for Disease Control and Prevention: 1998 guidelines for treatment of sexually transmitted diseases, *MMWR* 47(RR-1):1, January 23, 1998.

It may sometimes be necessary to treat PID surgically with laparotomy. If an abscess ruptures, peritonitis occurs and it may be necessary to remove the uterus, ovaries, and fallopian tubes.[27]

It is imperative that sexual partners of women with PID be evaluated and treated for infection if they have had sexual contact during the 60 days before the onset of symptoms. There is risk of reinfection and a high likelihood that the partner has urethral gonococcal or chlamydial infection.[25] Male partners of women whose PID is caused by chlamydia or gonorrhea are often asymptomatic. Rescreening for *C. trachomatis* and *N. gonorrhoeae* 4 to 6 weeks after therapy is completed is recommended by some experts.[25]

■ NURSING IMPLICATIONS

1. Psychosocial care of clients with PID and significant others is important. If PID is caused by an STD, the woman may have feelings of embarrassment, guilt, or anger. She may encounter conflict with sexual partners and significant others related to her having contracted an

Table 8-2	Outpatient Regimens for the Treatment of PID

Regimen A	Regimen B
Ofloxacin 400 mg PO bid × 14 days *Plus* Metronidazole 500 mg PO bid × 14 days	Ceftriaxone 250 mg IM × 1 dose **plus** doxycycline 100 mg PO bid × 14 days *Or* Cefoxitin 2 g IM **plus** probenecid 1 g PO concurrently in a single dose **plus** doxycycline 100 mg PO bid × 14 days *Or* Other parenteral third generation cephalosporin (e.g., ceftizoxime, cefotaxime) **plus** doxycycline 100 mg PO bid × 14 days

Adapted from Centers for Disease Control and Prevention: 1998 guidelines for treatment of sexually transmitted diseases, *MMWR* 47(RR-1):1, January 23, 1998; Uphold CR, Graham MV: *Clinical guidelines in family practice,* ed 3, Gainesville, Fla, 1998, Barmarrae Books.

STD.[27] Loss of fertility may be associated with PID because of inflammation and scarring, or the need for hysterectomy or oophorectomy in severe cases. Infertility can represent a great loss for a woman and her sexual partner. The nurse needs to make provisions for the expression of feelings. (See the nursing implications for menstrual disorders later in this chapter.)

2. The client should be taught good perineal hygiene, including the following[28]:
   - Tight fitting and synthetic clothing below the waist should be avoided.
   - Underwear with a cotton crotch should be worn.
   - The perineum should be wiped from front to back.
   - Douching or using feminine hygiene products should be avoided.
   - Only unscented, nondeodorized tampons, pads, or panty liners should be used; pad and tampon use should be alternated; tampons should not be worn overnight and tampons or sanitary pads should be changed every few hours. Hands should be washed before and after changing tampons or pads.
3. The nurse should assess the presence and severity of pain. Analgesics may be required.
4. The client should be counseled regarding the following:
   - The infection itself
   - Risk factors
   - Safer sexual practices
   - The importance of partner treatment
   - How to identify PID if it recurs and the need to seek treatment immediately

- The need to seek treatment immediately if she suspects she may have an STD, or if a sexual partner is treated for an STD
- Avoiding douching
- Avoiding the use of an IUD
- The possible sequelae of PID, which include infertility, ectopic pregnancy, and chronic pelvic pain[29]
- The importance of completing the full course of antibiotic therapy even if feeling better, and of reporting signs of allergic reaction or superinfection

5. Doxycycline can decrease the effectiveness of oral contraceptives that contain estrogen. The nurse should advise clients that use such contraceptives to use another method of contraception during treatment and until their next menstrual period.[30] The CDC advises that because Doxycycline is painful when infused, it should be administered orally when possible even when the client is hospitalized. If it must be given IV, measures to reduce complications (e.g., use of lidocaine, extension of infusion time) should be used.[25] For complete information on doxycycline and other medications, the reader is referred to a nursing drug reference.

HUMAN PAPILLOMA VIRUS–ASSOCIATED CONDITIONS OF THE LOWER GENITAL TRACT: GENITAL WARTS AND DYSPLASIAS AND NEOPLASMS OF THE LOWER GENITAL TRACT

There are more than 20 types of human papilloma virus (HPV) that can infect the genital tract. HPV types 6 and 11 are usually the causes of visible genital warts. They also can cause warts on the cervix as well as in the urethra, vagina, and anus. Subclinical genital HPV infection occurs more frequently than visible warts in clients of both genders, and is usually diagnosed in women by Pap smear, colposcopy, or biopsy. On the vulva or other genital skin, it may be diagnosed by the appearance of white areas after acetic acid is applied (see the discussion of diagnostic testing later in this section). On rare occasions HPV types 6 and 11 are also associated with invasive squamous cell carcinoma (SCC) of the external genitalia.[25]

Other HPV types (including types 16, 18, 31, 33, and 35) occur in the anogenital region and occasionally result in visible genital warts. These types are associated with vaginal, cervical, and anal intraepithelial dysplasia, as well as with SCC. Squamous intraepithelial neoplasia of the external genitalia (the vulva, penis, and anus) is also associated with these types of HPV.[25]

Immunosuppression causes an increased risk of genital warts and HPV-associated neoplasms.[31] Some data suggest that HPV disease in HIV-positive women may be more likely to be multicentric involving the vulva, vagina, and cervix.[24] Women who are HIV-positive are more likely to demonstrate signs of HPV infection than women who are not HIV-positive. As the CD_4 cell count decreases, the likelihood of demonstrating signs of HPV infection increases.[1,32]

Genital Warts

■ DEFINITION AND ETIOLOGY

HPV types 6 or 11 are usually the causes of visible genital warts and they can also cause warts on the cervix and in the urethra, vagina, and anus. Intraanal warts (as opposed to perianal warts) are seen primarily in persons who have had receptive anal intercourse, whereas perianal warts occur in persons of both genders who do not have a history of anal sex.[25] Anogenital warts are also known as condylomata acuminata or condyloma acuminata.

■ CLINICAL OVERVIEW

Genital warts are quite contagious and condylomata acuminata is currently at epidemic proportions. It is the most common symptomatic viral STD in the United States.[33] Most anogenital HPV infections are asymptomatic, subclinical, or unrecognized.[25] The incubation period is unknown but is estimated to be from 3 months to several years. Immunosuppression can stimulate the growth of warts.[26]

Genital warts are often asymptomatic and appear as small, white, or skin-colored growths. They may occur singly or in clusters. Warts can become confluent and appear as a large, single lesion. They are usually not painful but can cause dyspareunia; they may also be friable and bleed easily. Some clients may complain of pruritus. Reactivation of subclinical infection is more likely to cause a recurrence than is reinfection by a sexual partner.[34]

■ DIAGNOSTIC TESTING

Diagnosis of anogenital warts is usually made on the basis of clinical manifestations. The external genitalia and rectal area are examined for the characteristic lesions. Application of a 3% or 5% acetic acid solution assists in visualizing warts because it causes "acetowhitening" of the lesions. The diagnosis of genital warts can be confirmed by biopsy. Biopsy should be performed in cases of atypical presentations, which could represent dysplasia or neoplasia. It may be required more frequently among immunosuppressed persons because of the greater danger of SCC resembling or arising in genital warts.[25]

A newer technique for improving Pap smear accuracy can also be used for HPV testing. The clinician collects the cells and transfers them to a liquid that is sent to the laboratory. The Pap smear is prepared in the laboratory and HPV testing can be done from the liquid in the vial.[35]

■ MEDICAL MANAGEMENT

There is no therapy that eradicates HPV nor is there any evidence that currently available treatments affect the natural history of HPV infection. It is not known whether the removal of warts decreases infectivity. If untreated, visible genital warts may resolve, remain unchanged, or increase

Table 8-3	Treatment of External Genital Warts		
Client-Applied Treatments	**Provider-Administered Treatments**		**Alternative Treatments**
Podofilox 0.5% solution or gel Imiquimod 5% cream	Cryotherapy with liquid nitrogen or cryoprobe Podophyllin resin (usually 10%-25%) in compound tincture of benzoin Trichloroacetic acid (TCA) 80%-90% Bichloracetic acid (BCA) 80%-90% Surgical removal		Interferon (intralesional) Laser surgery

Adapted from Centers for Disease Control and Prevention: 1998 guidelines for treatment of sexually transmitted diseases, *MMWR* 47(RR-1):1, January 23, 1998.

in number or size. Treatment of genital warts should be guided by the client's preference, the resources available, and the provider's experience. Because the role of reinfection in HPV is probably minimal and there is no curative therapy, examination of sexual partners is not necessary. However, the partners may benefit from assessment of their STD status and counseling regarding the implications of having a partner with genital warts.[25]

External Genital Warts

Treatments for external genital warts are classified by the CDC as therapies applied by the client and therapies applied by the provider. Those applied by the client include podofilox and imiquimod. Those administered by the provider include cryotherapy, podophyllin resin, trichloroacetic acid (TCA), bichloracetic acid (BCA), and surgical removal. Other treatments include intralesional interferon, and treatment with carbon dioxide laser (Table 8-3). Factors that might influence treatment selection are the size and number of warts, the anatomic site and morphology of warts, client preference, cost, convenience, adverse effects, and the experience of the provider. A course of therapy, rather than a single treatment, is required by most clients.[25]

Vaginal Warts

TCA or BCA can be used. A small amount is applied only to the warts and allowed to dry, at which point a white "frosting" develops. If an excess amount of medication is applied, powder with talc or baking soda can be used to remove unreacted acid. The treatment can be repeated weekly if necessary. Vaginal warts can also be treated with cryotherapy with liquid nitrogen. The use of a cryoprobe is not recommended due to the risk of vaginal perforation and fistula formation. Some experts caution against vaginal application of podophyllin because of concern about the potential for systemic absorption.[25] (Podophyllin has the potential to produce myelotoxic and neurotoxic effects.[36]) Referral to an expert has been recommended for clients with vaginal warts.[26]

Anal Warts
Anal warts can be treated with cryotherapy with liquid nitrogen, with TCA or BCA 80% to 90%, or by surgical removal. Clients with warts on the rectal mucosa should be referred to an expert for treatment.[25]

Urethral Meatal Warts
Urethral meatal warts may be treated with cryotherapy with liquid nitrogen or podophyllin.[25] Referral to an expert is recommended for clients with urethral meatal warts.[26]

Cervical Warts
In women with cervical warts, high-grade squamous intraepithelial lesions (HSIL) must be ruled out before treatment is begun. The CDC recommends consultation with an expert for the management of cervical warts.[25]

■ NURSING IMPLICATIONS

Client-Applied Treatments for External Genital Warts
Clients who are to apply medication to warts themselves must be able to identify and reach the warts that are to be treated. Hands should be washed before and after application. Both Podofilox and Imiquimod can cause local skin reactions with pain and burning.[37,38] These reactions are usually of mild to moderate severity.

1. Podofilox—available as a gel (0.5%) or a topical solution (0.5%). Some important nursing and teaching implications for clients using podofilox are listed in Table 8-4. For complete information the reader is referred to a nursing drug reference.
2. Imiquimod—available as a cream (5%). Imiquimod is an immune modulator that increases cytokine activity and activates the cell-mediated immune system.[35,39] Some important nursing and teaching implications for clients treated with Imiquimod cream are listed in Table 8-5. For complete information the reader is referred to a nursing drug reference.

Provider-Administered Treatments for External Genital Warts
1. Cryotherapy—using liquid nitrogen or a cryoprobe. Cryotherapy destroys tissue by exposing it to extreme cold. (Substantial training is required for its proper use or warts may be overtreated or undertreated, with an increased likelihood of complications.) The nurse should be aware that pain, followed by necrosis and sometimes blis-

Table 8-4	Some Nursing Implications of Podofilox Administration
Adverse Effects	In clinical trials, adverse reactions of the gel included local skin reactions such as inflammation, pain, burning, itching, and erosion.
	Bleeding (usually mild) is a local reaction associated with podofilox gel. The most common systemic adverse effect of the gel is headache.
	Topically applied podofilox may be absorbed systemically with the potential for neurotoxic and myelotoxic effects.
	Topical overdosage should be treated by washing the skin free of any drug that remains and by supportive and symptomatic therapy.
Administration	The client can apply the solution with a cotton swab or the gel with a finger to visible genital warts. (The topical solution is not indicated for treatment of perianal warts.)
	The medication (solution or gel) should be allowed to dry before allowing opposing skin surfaces to return to their normal position.
	The medication is applied twice daily for 3 days. This is followed by 4 days of no therapy. The cycle can be repeated up to 4 times. The total volume of podofilox used should not exceed 0.5 mL/day. The total wart area treated should not exceed 10 cm^2.
	The provider should apply the initial treatment in order to identify which warts are to be treated and demonstrate the proper technique of application.
Client Teaching	Proper method of administration should be taught and demonstrated.
	The medication should be kept away from the eyes.
Pregnancy	Topical podofilox is contraindicated during pregnancy because of the potential for myelotoxic and neurotoxic effects.
	It must not be used in nursing mothers because of the potential for serious adverse reactions in the infant.

Note: Not an exhaustive list. Adapted from Centers for Disease Control and Prevention: 1998 guidelines for treatment of sexually transmitted diseases, *MMWR* 47(RR-1):1, January 23, 1998; Downing PE: Nursing care of clients with sexually transmitted diseases. In Black JM, Matassarin-Jacobs E, eds: *Medical-surgical nursing: clinical management for continuity of care*, ed 5, Philadelphia, 1997, Saunders; Mosby: *GenRx: the complete reference for generic and brand drugs*, ed 9, St Louis, 1999, Mosby; Delmar: *Physician's desk reference: nurse's handbook*, Montvale, NJ, 1999, Delmar.

tering, can occur after the application of liquid nitrogen. Local anesthesia, while not used routinely for cryotherapy, may be used if the area of warts is large or there are many warts.[25]

2. TCA and BCA (80% to 90%)—TCA is a commonly used treatment. Both TCA and BCA are caustic agents. They destroy warts by chemical coagulation of the proteins. A small amount should be applied, only to warts, and allowed to dry before the client sits or stands.

Table 8-5	Some Nursing Implications of Use of Imiquimod Cream
Adverse Effects	The most frequent adverse effects are local skin reactions such as erythema, erosion, excoriation/flaking, and edema. Such reactions are usually mild to moderate in intensity; however, severe reactions have occurred. Severe remote skin reactions in women have been reported, such as erythema, ulceration, and edema.
	In addition to local and remote skin reactions, some systemic reactions possibly or probably related to Imiquimod have been reported, including fatigue, fever, headache, flu-like symptoms, diarrhea, and myalgia.
Administration	The cream should be applied at bedtime with a finger, three times a week, and left on the skin for 6 to 10 hours. A thin layer of cream should be applied to the wart area and rubbed in until no longer visible.
	No occlusive type of dressing or covering should be used on the site.
	After 6-10 hours, the cream should be washed off with mild soap and water.
	The treatment should be continued until genital/perianal warts are totally cleared or for a maximum of 16 weeks.
	If local skin reaction is severe, or a client is experiencing severe discomfort, a rest period may be taken for several days with treatment resuming once the reaction subsides.
Client Teaching	The cream is for external use only. The client should avoid getting cream in the eyes.
	The client should be advised to avoid sexual contact (genital, oral, anal) while the cream is on the skin.
	The cream may weaken condoms and vaginal diaphragms.
	The client should report severe reactions to the provider.
Pregnancy	Imiquimod should not be used during pregnancy. The safety of Imiquimod during pregnancy and lactation has not been established.

Note: Not an exhaustive list. Adapted from Centers for Disease Control and Prevention: 1998 guidelines for treatment of sexually transmitted diseases, *MMWR* 47(RR-1):1, January 23, 1998; 3M Pharmaceuticals: *Aldara (Imiquimod) Cream 5%*, Northridge, Calif, 3M Pharmaceuticals.

When dry, a white "frosting" is apparent. If an excess amount of the agent is applied, powder with talc or baking soda can be used to remove unreacted acid. If the client has intense pain, the acid can be neutralized with baking soda or soap.[25]

3. Podophyllin—used much less frequently today than 10 years ago.[35] Preparations of podophyllin resin differ in concentration of active components and their stability and shelf life are unknown. If it is used, some important nursing implications for its use are as follows[25,36,40]:

   ■ Excessive application of the medication must be avoided. A small amount should be applied to the lesion with a cotton swab.

- Contact of podophyllin with healthy tissue should be avoided. Petroleum jelly can be used to protect unaffected areas. The medication must be allowed to air dry before the treated area comes in contact with clothing. Otherwise, the podophyllin can spread to adjacent areas resulting in local irritation.
- The volume of podophyllin resin should not exceed 0.5 mL in volume and the area treated should not exceed 10 cm^2 per session in order to avoid the possibility of complications from systemic absorption and toxicity. The medication should be washed off thoroughly in 1 to 4 hours to decrease local irritation.
- The treatment can be repeated weekly if necessary.
- Topical podophyllin is potentially toxic. It has the potential to produce myelotoxic and neurotoxic effects. Signs of toxicity include nausea, vomiting, lethargy, coma, and paralysis.
- Podophyllin is contraindicated during pregnancy.

4. Surgical removal—has the advantage of usually rendering the client wart-free in a single visit but substantial training, a longer office visit, and additional equipment are required.[25]
5. Interferon—injected directly into warts. It is thought to reduce HPV lesions by improving the immune system. Side effects include flu-like symptoms, fever and malaise.[40]

Other Nursing Implications

1. Immunosuppressed clients may not respond as well to treatment for genital warts as immunocompetent clients and may have more frequent recurrences after therapy.[25]
2. The client should be cautioned that treatment of genital warts does not eliminate the HPV infection and that she remains infectious. (It is not known whether clients with subclinical HPV infection are as contagious as those with warts.) Condoms should be used but there is no evidence that their use diminishes HPV spread. It is possible that HPV is transmitted manually during foreplay, nonvaginal sex, and on the outside of the condom.[35]
3. It is critically important for the nurse to teach clients with HPV the importance of regular Pap smears.
4. The chemotherapy cream 5-fluorouracil has been used in treatment but has become much less popular due to the occurrence of painful vaginal ulcers and scarring, as well as a high recurrence rate.[35]

HPV-Associated Dysplasias and Neoplasias of the Lower Genital Tract

■ DEFINITION AND ETIOLOGY

In addition to causing genital warts, HPV is associated with an increased risk of intraepithelial cancer precursor lesions and genital tract squamous cancers. Immunosuppression places a person at increased risk for HPV-associated neoplasms.[31] In a recent study, both HPV infection and immunodeficiency associated with HIV were found to be strong risk factors for abnormal cytology.[41] HPV types 16, 18, 31, 33, and 35 occur in the anogenital region and are associated with vaginal, cervical, and anal intraepithelial dysplasia, as well as SCC. Squamous intraepithelial neoplasia of the external genitalia (i.e., vulva or penis, anus) is also associated with these types of HPV.[25]

Dysplasia is an alteration in the shape, size, organization, and regularity of cells. Cells in this state may revert to normal or may transform into a neoplasia. A neoplasm (usually synonymous with tumor) is a new, abnormal growth of tissue, which does not serve a useful purpose and may be harmful to the organism. Carcinoma is a form of cancer, composed of epithelial cells that can infiltrate surrounding tissue and spread to distant sites.[42]

The association of HIV with cervical dysplasia and neoplasia is clear. The frequency of abnormal Pap smear results in HIV-positive women is 4 to 10 times greater than it is in HIV-negative women.[43] Cervical dysplasia in HIV-positive women is more likely to progress rapidly and recur after therapy than in noninfected women.[23]

In one study comparing the long-term outcomes of HIV-positive and HIV-negative women after treatment for cervical intraepithelial neoplasia (CIN), 62% of HIV-positive women developed recurrent CIN by 3 years after treatment, as opposed to 18% of HIV-negative women. In HIV-positive women whose CD_4 cell counts were less than 200 cells/mm^3, recurrence rates reached 87%. The same study also found that there was progression to higher-grade neoplasia in 25% of HIV-positive women and in 2% of HIV-negative women. One HIV-positive subject developed invasive cancer.[44] There is also evidence suggesting that HIV positivity may place women at increased risk for vulvovaginal lesions, including vulvar intraepithelial neoplasia (VIN), a precursor of vulvar carcinoma.[24,45]

■ CLINICAL OVERVIEW

There are no symptoms of cervical dysplasia, carcinoma in situ, or early cervical cancer. It is not until later in the course of the disease that the client may develop symptoms, such as vaginal discharge and bleeding. Bleeding can occur initially as spotting from cervical trauma after sexual intercourse or douching. Bleeding increases as the disease progresses. Bleeding between menses, increased frequency of menstrual bleeding, and postmenopausal bleeding can occur. Vaginal discharge may become foul-smelling and dark as the cancer progresses.[27] Because of the lack of early symptoms, regular Pap smears are critical.

■ DIAGNOSTIC TESTING

The Pap smear is the screening test done to detect cervical dysplasia, neoplasia, and carcinoma in situ. Early detection increases the likelihood of cure. The significant drop in the death rate from cervical cancer that has occurred over the last 40 years has been attributed largely to the widespread use of the Pap smear.[46] The Pap smear test is critical because it is able to detect precursor lesions, so that early treatment can be initiated.

The classification system used for the interpretation of Pap smears is the 1988 Bethesda System for Reporting Cervical/Vaginal Cytological Diagnoses.[46] According to this system, epithelial cell abnormalities are characterized as *squamous cell* or *glandular cell*. (Most cervical cancers are of the squamous cell type.[47]) Squamous epithelial cell abnormalities are classified as atypical squamous cells of undetermined significance (ASCUS), squamous intraepithelial lesions (SILs), or SCC. SILs are further categorized as low-grade or high-grade. Low-grade squamous intraepithelial lesions (LSILs) include cellular changes consistent with HPV infection and mild dysplasia/cervical intraepithelial neoplasia grade 1 (i.e., CIN 1). High-grade squamous intraepithelial lesions (HSILs) include moderate dysplasia/cervical intraepithelial neoplasia grade 2 (i.e., CIN 2), severe dysplasia/cervical intraepithelial neoplasia grade 3 (i.e., CIN 3), and carcinoma in situ (i.e., also CIN 3).[46,48] (There are also categories related to abnormalities of glandular cells. These include atypical glandular cells of undetermined significance (AGCUS) and endocervical, endometrial, and extrauterine adenocarcinoma.[49] These will not be discussed in this text.)

Colposcopy is used as a diagnostic test. This is the use of a magnifying instrument called a *colposcope* to examine the vulva, vagina, and cervix. The instrument is able to magnify the area under observation from 4 to 40 times. During the procedure, a 3% or 5% solution of acetic acid is applied to the cervix and vagina. The solution has a temporary dehydrating effect which causes abnormal cells to appear white (i.e., acetowhitening). Biopsy specimens are taken from tissue that appears abnormal.[50] After the biopsy, Monsel's solution or silver nitrate may be applied to stop bleeding. Colposcopy can be used to diagnose both cervical and noncervical lesions (lesions of the vulva, vagina, or perianal areas). It is sometimes used to screen women who are expected to be poorly compliant with medical appointments. The disadvantages of colposcopic screening are its cost and the need for a trained clinician to perform the examination.[23]

There are data suggesting that the sensitivity of the Pap smear in HIV-positive women is similar to that in HIV-negative women.[51] However, the adequacy of Pap smears as a screening method to detect cervical neoplasia in HIV-positive women has been questioned. A recent study highlighted what the authors termed "significant limitations" of the Pap smear in HIV-positive women because of the high prevalence of abnormal cytology and CIN in this population.[41]

Some newer techniques for cervical cancer screening include PAPNET and speculoscopy. PAPNET is a computerized, automated system used to rescreen negative smears, identifying fields of cells that may have been misinterpreted.[35] Images of the most abnormal appearing cells are presented to screeners in a convenient, interactive way. In one study of PAPNET-assisted screening, there was a significantly lower percentage of false-negative results than with the conventional method.[52] In another study, it was found that the use of PAPNET identified a few more cases of ASCUS than manual rescreening, but the cost was relatively high.[53] PAPNET is FDA-approved.

In speculoscopy, a disposable light is attached to the inner surface of the upper speculum blade before insertion. The light is chemiluminescent; that is, it does not produce heat. The light is not toxic to tissues. The examiner dims the room lights and inspects the cervix and vagina through a magnifying lens. Acetic acid solution (3% or 5%) is applied to the vagina and cervix, and the examiner inspects for the presence of any acetowhitened lesions. The chemiluminescent light is "blue-white" and is reflected more strongly by neoplastic tissue, which appears to be bright white. Normal epithelium appears bluish. When used with a Pap smear, speculoscopy is more effective in identifying women with CIN than a Pap smear alone.[54]

HPV typing can be helpful as an adjunctive test if used properly by a knowledgeable clinician. An improved HPV typing test may soon be available that will identify more HPV types.[35]

The CDC recommends that a complete history of cervical disease and a comprehensive gynecological examination, including a Pap smear, be done as part of the initial medical evaluation for women who are HIV-positive.[25,55] The CDC further recommends that a Pap smear be obtained twice during the first year after diagnosis of HIV infection. If the results are normal, Pap smears can be done annually thereafter. If the results are abnormal, the Interim Guidelines for Management of Abnormal Cervical Cytology published by the National Cancer Institute Consensus Panel[49] should be followed.[25] These interim guidelines do not specifically address the issue of managing low-grade lesions in immunosuppressed women. Currently the CDC recommends their use for HIV-positive women, but the nurse should bear in mind that other management options may be used in clinical practice. Because of the increased risk for CIN and for rapid progression of cervical dysplasia in HIV-positive women, some clinicians may repeat Pap smears more frequently and use colposcopy more readily in HIV-positive women.

The Interim Guidelines for Management of Abnormal Cervical Cytology suggest that there are several options for the management of women whose Pap smears are interpreted as ASCUS.[49] The option selected depends on clinical circumstances and whether interpretation of ASCUS is further qualified. An interpretation of ASCUS may be unqualified or qualified, for example, by a statement indicating that a reactive process is favored or that a neoplastic process is favored. Reactive changes can be associated with inflammation, atrophic vaginitis (i.e., vaginitis related to lowered estrogen levels), and other causes.

According to the guidelines, a possible management option, particularly when the diagnosis of ASCUS is not further qualified or when the cytopathologist favors a reactive process, is to follow up with Pap smears every 4 to 6 months for 2 years until three consecutive tests have been negative. Clients to be managed in this way must be selected carefully and must be considered reliable to return for follow-up. If, during the 2-year period, a second report of ASCUS occurs, colposcopy should be considered.

The guidelines recommend that if a client has a diagnosis of unqualified ASCUS associated with severe inflammation, she should be reevaluated after 2 to 3 months. If specific infections are identified, they should be treated, and reevaluation should be done after appropriate treatment. If a diagnosis of ASCUS is qualified by an indication that a neoplastic process is favored, management should be the same as for a low-grade squamous intraepithelial lesion (LSIL). In a client who is postmenopausal, a diagnosis of ASCUS may result from the appearance of atrophic cells. In such cases, a course of topical estrogen therapy may assist in making the diagnosis. The interim guidelines recommend that colposcopy be considered for any client with a diagnosis of ASCUS who is considered to be at high risk for cervical cancer.

The guidelines recommend several management options for women with LSIL. These include follow-up with Pap tests every 4 to 6 months for 2 years, which is an option for carefully selected clients. Other options, according to the guidelines, include colposcopy, endocervical curettage (ECC), and directed biopsy.[49] (Elsewhere, however, it is recommended that optimally a woman with LSIL should have colposcopic examination within 4 weeks of the LSIL diagnosis.[56]) If a woman has a cytologic diagnosis of HSIL or SCC, both colposcopy and directed biopsy are indicated.[49] In cases of HSIL, these evaluations should be performed as soon as possible.[56]

There are clinicians, however, who perform Pap smears and colposcopies on a somewhat different basis than the above recommendations. Because lower genital tract neoplasia is very common in HIV-positive women and may be refractory to usual treatment, some clinicians recommend semiannual Pap smears with colposcopy if dysplasia or atypia is present.[23] Others consider CD_4 cell counts when scheduling Pap smears. Some clinicians, for example, perform annual Pap smears for women with CD_4 cell counts above 400 cells/mm^3 and semiannual Pap smears for women with CD_4 cell counts below 400 cells/mm^3.[13] Another recommendation based on CD_4 cell counts is to increase Pap smears to every 6 months in women with CD_4 cell counts below 500 cells/mm^3, and certainly for counts below 200 cells/mm^3.[57] The Public Health Service has recommended Pap smears every 6 months for women with symptomatic HIV infection, prior abnormal Pap smears, or signs of HPV infection.[58]

There are also differing recommendations regarding the use of colposcopic examination. It has been suggested that a colposcopy be done when HIV or AIDS is first diagnosed and then, if negative, follow-up with Pap smears is recommended. Another suggestion is that the clinician give strong consideration to primary colposcopic examination if the client is expected to be poorly compliant with medical care.[23,51] It has also been stated that colposcopy may be indicated for all HIV-positive women with condyloma, regardless of Pap smear results, because of the increased incidence of CIN in such cases.[24] Other investigators have suggested that all clients with persistent inflammatory atypia or ASCUS might benefit from colposcopy.[56]

When indicated, biopsies can be obtained by conization, in which a cone-shaped section of the cervix is excised with a scalpel or by a loop electrosurgical excision procedure (LEEP). Conization is necessary if areas are involved that are not readily visualized.

■ MEDICAL MANAGEMENT

Therapy for CIN may include cryotherapy, laser therapy, or LEEP.[59] Cryosurgery consists of freezing abnormal cells and tissues locally. Cell death results and dead tissue sloughs off. In laser therapy, a laser beam is directed at abnormal tissues where its energy is absorbed by the fluid in the tissues, causing them to vaporize. A LEEP involves the use of a thin wire loop and electrical current to remove and destroy abnormal tissue. It can allow for both diagnosis and treatment in selected clients. When a biopsy is performed by conization, this procedure also may serve as both diagnosis and treatment if analysis of the tissue indicates that an excised malignancy is surrounded by a wide area of normal tissue.[27] Complications of conization include hemorrhage, which may be immediate or delayed; perforation of the uterus; cervical stenosis; incompetent cervix; and infection.[60] Should the client develop invasive cancer, treatment may include radical hysterectomy or more extensive surgery, chemotherapy and radiation therapy.

Women with dysplasia who are HIV-positive may have frequent recurrences and may need second or third procedures.[23] Because of higher recurrence rates in HIV-positive women and shorter intervals to recurrence and death, there must be meticulous follow-up surveillance after therapy to prevent invasive cervical cancer.[59]

■ NURSING IMPLICATIONS

1. Many women find gynecological examinations embarrassing and uncomfortable. Insensitive treatment by the examiner and memories of an unpleasant examination may cause a woman to avoid gynecological care. Therefore, it is critical that the nurse provide teaching, support, and encouragement to make the client as comfortable as possible, both physically and psychologically. Comfort can be increased if the room and equipment is comfortably warm, the client voids prior to the examination, proper draping is used, and the client's privacy and dignity is maintained at all times.[47] The woman's permission must be requested for any observers (e.g., students) to watch the procedure. Each step in the examination should be explained and the client should be encouraged to verbalize any discomfort. If the client

is to undergo colposcopy, pretreatment with an analgesic should be offered.

2. Many women have only sketchy knowledge of their anatomy and physiology and may have misconceptions and misunderstandings about their bodies' functioning. The use of models for teaching is helpful. Also, a mirror can be used during the examination, which helps to make the client an active participant in learning about her body. The head of the examining table is raised and the client holds the mirror above the examiner's hands to observe her external genitalia, her cervix, and the examination procedure. The use of a mirror is also helpful to the client in visualizing abnormalities, which she can then monitor if necessary.

3. Clients should receive an explanation of the Pap test and the possible range of results at the time the test is done so that they will be better prepared if there is an abnormal result.[61] Clients should understand the difference between precursor lesions and cancer.

4. The nurse should teach clients that Pap smears cannot be performed during menstruation and that the best time to schedule the test is around midcycle.[62] For best results, the woman should not douche, have sexual intercourse, or put anything into the vagina for 24 to 48 hours before the test.[63,64]

5. Colposcopy and other diagnostic and treatment procedures require written, informed consent.

6. Clients scheduled for colposcopy are likely to be quite anxious. There may be fear of dying or loss of fertility, a perceived threat to sexuality, and concern about further treatment.[61] In addition, clients may worry that the procedure itself will be painful or embarrassing. A complete explanation of the procedure should be given, including that it consists of careful observation under magnification of the genital area and cervix. The observation is painless but does involve a period of time while the speculum is left in place in the vagina. Clients should also be told that cervical biopsy specimens will likely be taken during the procedure and that these may be somewhat painful.[47] As noted above, pretreatment with an analgesic should be offered prior to colposcopy. During the procedure, the client should be told when the examiner is about to take any biopsy specimens. An ECC may also be done if the woman is not pregnant. In an ECC, endocervical cells are obtained with a small curette from the endocervical canal. After the procedure, the woman should be allowed to rest for a short time. Before leaving, clients should be told that they may have a small amount of blood-tinged vaginal discharge but should report any excessive bleeding immediately. Usual further instructions include avoidance of vaginal sexual activity, use of tampons, and douching for several days to 2 weeks.[47,65] Clients should be told when and how they will receive results, and who to contact in the event that they experience any adverse effects.

7. After procedures such as cryotherapy, laser surgery, and conization, clients should be instructed to report any excessive pain, bleeding, or fever to the provider. Clients should be told if discharge is expected and what type to expect, as well as be advised to avoid sexual intercourse, the use of tampons, and douching for 4 to 6 weeks, depending upon the procedure performed.[56,65,66] Clients should be told when to return for follow-up.

8. In a study of HIV-positive and HIV-negative women who were treated with laser therapy, cold knife cone biopsy, or cryotherapy,[67] a significantly higher rate of bleeding that required unscheduled visits to the clinic or emergency room occurred in the HIV-positive group. The authors suggest that platelets be monitored prior to treatment. The same study found a significantly higher rate of cervicovaginal infections in the HIV-positive women after treatment by laser or cone biopsy. Infection was more prevalent in subjects with low CD_4 counts. The authors recommend closer monitoring after treatment for women with severely depressed CD_4 counts. The authors also stress the need to caution HIV-positive women about being prone to complications and to provide them with information about what to do in the event that serious symptoms occur. Women must know who to call and where to go if problems arise.

9. Women who are HIV-positive need teaching regarding the critical importance of regular Pap smears. If abnormalities are detected, the client needs to understand the importance of follow-up care. In counseling the client, the nurse needs to discuss individual situations and circumstances that might make it difficult for clients to keep follow-up appointments. Employment, child care responsibilities, caregiving responsibilities for other family members, lack of transportation, drug or alcohol use, a partner who does not know the client's HIV status, and various other circumstances may make it difficult for a client to access care. The nurse can help clients access social or other services according to their individual needs.

10. The nurse must address client concerns about fertility, sexuality, her partner's response, follow-up care, and recurrence, among others.

Menstrual Disorders

■ DEFINITION AND ETIOLOGY

Abnormal uterine bleeding includes the following disorders:

- Menorrhagia—prolonged or excessive uterine bleeding that occurs at regular intervals.
- Metrorrhagia—uterine bleeding that occurs at irregular intervals.
- Polymenorrhea—uterine bleeding that occurs at regular intervals of less than 21 days.
- Dysfunctional uterine bleeding (DUB)—abnormal uterine bleeding with no identified organic cause. It is most often associated with anovulation.

- Oligomenorrhea—infrequent uterine bleeding that occurs with intervals of 35 days to 6 months between menstruation.[68]
- Amenorrhea—absence of menses. It can be primary (i.e., no menses by the age of 16 years) or secondary (i.e., the absence of menses for at least 6 months in a woman who previously had regular cyclic bleeding).[27] The time period criterion for secondary amenorrhea is controversial; it is sometimes considered to be absence of menses for 3 months.[26]

There are many possible causes of abnormal uterine bleeding, which include disorders of the outflow tract (e.g., cervical stenosis) and ovarian, pituitary, and hypothalamic disorders.[69] These disorders are not discussed in detail in this text; the reader is referred to a gynecological text for further information.

There is a need for further study of menstrual disorders in HIV-positive women. Theoretically, there is a basis for the possibility of menstrual irregularities in such women. Heavier than normal bleeding could result from platelet disorders. Wasting, stresses, and other systemic illnesses could cause oligomenorrhea or amenorrhea.[23] Menstrual abnormalities, usually spotting or irregularities in cycle length, are common in women with HIV infection. However, they are not seen more often in HIV-positive women than in HIV-negative women with a history of chronic illnesses or drug use.[70]

Amenorrhea, however, has been associated with HIV infection, reportedly occurring 3 times more commonly than expected in HIV-positive women.[70] In one study, women with CD_4 cell counts below 50 cells/mm^3 were more likely to report amenorrhea than women with higher cell counts or women who were not HIV-positive.[58] Amenorrhea is also more likely if serum albumin is less than 3 grams, if a woman had a live birth within the past year, or if she is using heroin or amphetamines.[70] Another study found the overall prevalence of amenorrhea to be higher in HIV-positive women with weight loss than in asymptomatic women.[71]

■ CLINICAL OVERVIEW

Reproductive capacity is of central concern to most women. Many women find the regular appearance of menstrual flow reassuring in terms of their reproductive health. Therefore, the absence of menses can be very distressing. When amenorrhea occurs, there may be fear of pregnancy, infertility, premature menopause, or serious illness.[72]

■ DIAGNOSTIC TESTING AND MEDICAL MANAGEMENT

Currently, there are no data suggesting that the diagnosis or treatment of menstrual disorders in HIV-positive women should be different than for HIV-negative women.[73] Simply to attribute a woman's amenorrhea to her HIV status is to do the woman a disservice and has the potential to lead to significant problems.[74] For information on diagnosis and treatment of menstrual disorders, the reader is referred to a gynecological nursing reference.

■ NURSING IMPLICATIONS

1. Women respond to menstrual problems in differing, individual ways. Some women seek health care promptly, while others do not. Some women find it difficult to discuss menstruation because they view it as a personal, intimate, and private matter. Others may have been told that menstrual problems are to be expected and, therefore, dismiss their problems as unimportant. Some women may not seek advice because they fear the treatment or doubt whether relief is possible. The nurse needs to be skillful and sensitive in the assessment of clients.

2. Gynecological disorders have the potential to cause alterations in a woman's self-concept (e.g., body image) and sexuality. These can have major effects on her feelings of femininity. Shame, embarrassment, and other negative reactions can occur in response to gynecological disorders and their treatments.

3. Women hold beliefs about their bodily functions that are culturally defined and learned. In many cultures, fertility is still considered to be the primary function of women. Fertility may be linked to a woman's social status. Amenorrhea, which is related to infertility, may signify that a woman is unable to fulfill her culturally sanctioned role and therefore she may lose the support of her family or society. Personal and social crises can result from a woman's failure to fulfill her reproductive role and meet expectations within social culture.[27] The nurse needs to be sensitive to the cultural meanings and consequences of amenorrhea for each individual client.

4. Because spontaneous ovulation can occur in functional amenorrhea, the need for a mechanical means of contraception should be stressed if a client does not wish to become pregnant.[72]

CONTRACEPTION

There are no definite guidelines for counseling HIV-positive women on birth control.[10] Condoms with spermicides, when acceptable to both partners, are an excellent contraceptive choice. However, education in the correct use of condoms is of critical importance and there is the possibility of allergy to latex or spermicide.[12] The possibility of condom failure also exists and the use of lubricants with an oil base can damage latex.[75]

Norplant and medroxyprogesterone acetate (Depo-Provera) provide effective contraception, but there is uncertainty about their possible interactions with medications commonly used in HIV infection treatment.[12] Also, they offer no STD protection for either partner. A diaphragm with spermicide or a cervical cap can also provide effective contraception but does not prevent (though it may limit) STD transmission. The IUD is not a good contraceptive choice for women who are immunocompromised, as it may place them at increased risk of infectious disease.[12] It also does not protect either partner against STDs.

Oral contraceptives are an effective contraceptive method and have a number of advantages, which include menstrual regulation and decreased dysmenorrhea, premenstrual symptoms, and menstrual blood loss. There are also disadvantages, however, such as a number of contraindications for their use and interactions with other medications. Some of these interactions may not yet be known.[12] It is known that there are interactions between some protease inhibitors and ethinyl estradiol and norethindrone, which are contained in oral contraceptives. Indinavir causes a modest increase in Ortho-Novum levels but no dosage change is indicated. Both ritonavir and nelfinavir decrease ethinyl estradiol levels, and nelfinavir also decreases norethindrone levels. If a client is receiving ritonavir or nelfinavir, an alternative contraceptive method or an additional contraceptive method is recommended. In addition, there is suspicion that the nonnucleoside reverse transcriptase inhibitor (NNRTI) nevirapine interacts with oral contraceptives; if given together, careful monitoring is required.[76]

A number of reports have emphasized the need for a female-controlled method of HIV prevention.[77,78] The female condom is available and provides an effective mechanical barrier to HIV[79] but it cannot be used without a partner's knowledge. Chemical barriers are also needed which would be easy to apply and unobtrusive to the sexual partner.[77] The spermicide nonoxynol 9 kills HIV in vitro,[80] but there are many questions surrounding its possible use in the prevention of HIV transmission. Nonoxynol 9 may be toxic to the epithelium of the genital tract,[80] and irritation of the vaginal mucosa may provide a portal of entry for the virus.[77] It is possible that the dose and frequency of use of nonoxynol 9, as well as the type of product containing it (e.g., gels, suppositories, films, creams) may play a role in genital irritation and HIV transmission.[80,81] Findings of a recent study indicated that daily short-term use of nonoxynol 9 in a low-dose gel was safe with regard to toxicity to the genital epithelium.[80] However, another recent study did not demonstrate that the use of a vaginal contraceptive film containing nonoxynol 9 affected HIV transmission rates.[82]

Other microbicides are being developed, and the question arises as to whether the highest priority is to develop a microbicide that is not a contraceptive or a contraceptive spermicide that is also a microbicide. A woman might want to have children but also want protection against HIV, for instance.[81]

◼ NURSING IMPLICATIONS

1. The nurse should emphasize the importance of condom use in preventing HIV transmission. Since condom use requires the sexual partner's cooperation, the nurse should determine if there are circumstances that may discourage the client from discussing condom use with a partner. Appropriate counseling, referrals, and support services will be needed if, for example, disclosure of HIV status is an issue or if the client is, or fears becoming, a victim of domestic violence or abuse.

2. In order to use condoms effectively, the user must understand how to use them properly. The nurse should instruct clients to keep a supply of latex condoms (unless allergic to latex) easily available for use at every intercourse. Condoms should be kept in a cool, dry place and should never be reused. Condoms should not be tested by inflating or stretching them. They should be handled gently and kept away from sharp objects (e.g., long fingernails). The condom should be applied before genital contact. A spermicide containing nonoxynol 9 can be placed inside the condom, if desired, unless either partner is allergic to it. The rolled up condom is placed on the head of the erect penis and the end is pinched to create a space to accommodate the ejaculate. The condom is placed with the rolled portion out so that it will unroll properly. The condom is unrolled until the fingers reach the base of the penis. The outside of the condom may be lubricated, if desired, using water-soluble lubricant or contraceptive jelly. (Oil-based lubricants such as petroleum jelly, baby oil, and cooking oil can damage the condom.) After ejaculation, the condom must be held firmly at the base of the penis to prevent it from becoming dislodged. The penis should be withdrawn while still erect.[36,83]

3. The nurse should counsel the client using oral contraceptives about use of an alternative or additional contraceptive method if ritonavir or nelfinavir is prescribed.[76]

ONGOING STUDIES OF WOMEN AND HIV/AIDS

Two of the ongoing studies of women with HIV/AIDS are the Women's Interagency HIV Study (WIHS) and the HIV Epidemiology Research Study (HERS). WIHS is a multicenter, prospective cohort study that was established in August, 1993 to study the natural history of HIV infection in women in the United States. The study is co-sponsored by the National Institute of Allergy and Infectious Diseases (NIAID) and other institutes of the National Institutes of Health (NIH). The HERS study is also a multicenter, prospective cohort study of HIV infection in women and is a companion study to WIHS. HERS is sponsored by the CDC and NIAID.[84] As additional results from these two ongoing studies become available, more will be learned about women and HIV/AIDS.

RESOURCES—WOMEN AND HIV

A number of internet sites provide information about resources for those living with HIV. Two practical sites for accessing information about women and HIV are:

■ http://www.womenhiv.org/
   WORLD (provides information and support for women with HIV)
   PO Box 11535
   Oakland, CA 94611
   (510) 658-6930

■ http://www.thebody.com/wa/wapage.html
Women Alive (by and for women living with HIV/AIDS)
1566 Burnside Avenue
Los Angeles, CA 90019
(213) 965-1564

REFERENCES

1. Larkin J et al: HIV in women: Recognizing the signs, *Medscape Women's Health* 1(11):1, 1996.
2. Centers for Disease Control and Prevention: *Facts about women and HIV/AIDS,* CDC National AIDS Clearinghouse, Document No. 290, February 13, 1995.
3. Centers for Disease Control and Prevention: *HIV/AIDS Surveillance Report* 11(2):1, 1999.
4. ARHP Advisory and Editorial Committee, eds: Treatment strategies for HIV-infected women—introduction, *ARHP Clinical Proceedings: A Publication of the Association of Reproductive Health Professionals,* p 3, October 1998.
5. Padian NS et al: Heterosexual transmission of human immunodeficiency virus (HIV) in northern California: Results from a 10-year study, *Am J Epidemiol* 146(4):350, 1997.
6. Staprans SI, Feinberg MB: Natural history and immunopathogenesis of HIV-1 disease. In Sande MA, Volberding PA, eds: *The medical management of AIDS,* ed 5, Philadelphia, 1997, Saunders.
7. Nicolosi A et al: The efficiency of male-to-female and female-to-male sexual transmission of the human immunodeficiency virus: A study of 730 stable couples, *Epidemiology* 5(6):570, 1994.
8. Centers for Disease Control and Prevention, *HIV/AIDS Surveillance Report* 10(1):4, 1998.
9. National Institute of Allergy and Infectious Diseases, National Institutes of Health: *Fact sheet—HIV infection and women,* May 2000, United States Department of Health and Human Services, Public Health Service. http://www.niaid.nih.gov/fact sheets/womenhiv.htm
10. Newmann RE, Nishimoto PW: Human immunodeficiency virus update for the primary care provider, *Nurse Pract Forum* 7(1):16, 1996.
11. Abercrombie PD: Women living with HIV infection, *Nurs Clin North Am* 31:97, 1996.
12. Anastos K, Denenberg R, Solomon L: Human immunodeficiency virus infection in women, *Med Clin North Am* 81:533, 1997.
13. Anastos K, Denenberg R, Solomon L: Clinical management of HIV-infected women. In Wormser GP, ed: *A Clinical Guide to AIDS and HIV,* Philadelphia, 1996, Lippincott-Raven.
14. ARHP Advisory and Editorial Committee, eds: Treatment strategies for HIV-infected women—HIV disease, *ARHP Clinical Proceedings: A Publication of the Association of Reproductive Health Professionals,* p 5, October 1998.
15. Cadman J: Candidiasis in immune-compromised women, *GMHC Treatment Issues: Newsletter of Experimental AIDS Therapies* 11(7/8):18, 1997.
16. Rothenberg R et al: Survival with the acquired immunodeficiency syndrome: experience with 5833 cases in New York City, *N Engl J Med* 317:1297, 1987.

17. Freidland GH et al: Survival differences in patients with AIDS, *J Acquir Immune Defic Syndr Hum Retrovirol* 4(2):144, 1991.

18. Smeltzer SC, Whipple B: Women and HIV infection, *Image J Nurs Schol* 23(4):249, 1991.

19. Hirschhorn LR: HIV infection in women: is it different? *AIDS Reader* 5:99, 1995.

20. Hankins CA, Handley MA: HIV disease and AIDS in women: current knowledge and a research agenda, *J Acquir Immune Defic Syndr Hum Retrovirol* 5(10):957, 1992.

21. Smeltzer SC, Whipple B: Women with HIV infection: the unrecognized population, *Health Values* 15(6), 1991.

22. Centers for Disease Control and Prevention: 1993 revised classification for HIV infection and expanded surveillance case definition for AIDS among adolescents and adults, *MMWR* 41(RR17):1, 1992.

23. Korn AP, Landers DV: Gynecological disease in women infected with human immunodeficiency virus type 1, *J Acquir Immune Defic Syndr Hum Retrovirol* 9(4):361, 1995.

24. Chiasson MA et al: Increased prevalence of vulvovaginal condyloma and vulvar intraepithelial neoplasia in women infected with the human immunodeficiency virus, *Obstet Gynecol* 89:690, 1997.

25. Centers for Disease Control and Prevention: 1998 guidelines for treatment of sexually transmitted diseases, *MMWR* 47(RR-1):1, January 23, 1998.

26. Uphold CR, Graham MV: *Clinical guidelines in family practice,* ed 3, Gainesville, Fla, 1998, Barmarrae Books.

27. Carlson E: Nursing care of women with gynecological disorders. In Black JM, Matassarin-Jacobs E, eds: *Medical-surgical nursing: clinical management for continuity of care,* ed 5, Philadelphia, 1997, Saunders.

28. Williams AB et al: Factors associated with vaginal yeast infections in HIV positive women, *J Assoc Nurses AIDS Care* 9(5):47, 1998.

29. McIntyre-Seltman K, Matson CC: Gynecology. In Rakel RE, ed: *Textbook of Family Practice,* ed 5, Philadelphia, 1995, Saunders.

30. Deglin, JH, Vallerand AH: *Davis's drug guide for nurses,* ed 5, Philadelphia, 1997, Davis.

31. Kiviat N B: Human papillomavirus and hepatitis viral infections in human immunodeficiency virus-infected persons. In DeVita VT, Jr, Hellman S, Rosenberg SA, eds: *AIDS: etiology, diagnosis, treatment, and prevention,* Philadelphia, 1997, Lippincott-Raven.

32. Schafer A et al: The increased frequency of cervical dysplasia-neoplasia in women infected with the human immunodeficiency virus is related to the degree of immunosuppression, *Am J Obstet Gynecol* 164:593, 1991.

33. Robinson K M: Sexually transmitted infections. In McCance KL, Huether SE, eds: *Pathophysiology: the biologic basis for disease in adults and children,* ed 3, St Louis, 1998, Mosby.

34. Centers for Disease Control and Prevention: Sexually transmitted diseases treatment guidelines, 1993, *MMWR* 42 (RR-14):72, 1993.

35. Sedlacek TV: Advances in the diagnosis and treatment of human papillomavirus infections, *Clin Obstet Gynecol* 42(2):206, 1999.

36. Downing PE: Nursing care of clients with sexually transmitted diseases. In Black JM, Matassarin-Jacobs E, eds: *Medical-surgical nursing: clinical management for continuity of care,* ed 5, Philadelphia, 1997, Saunders.

37. Mosby: *GenRx: the complete reference for generic and brand drugs,* ed 9, St Louis, 1999, Mosby.

38. Delmar: *Physician's desk reference: nurse's handbook,* Montvale, NJ, 1999, Delmar.

39. 3M Pharmaceuticals: *Aldara (Imiquimod) Cream 5%,* Northridge, Calif, 3M Pharmaceuticals.

40. Schaffer SD: Vaginitis and sexually transmitted diseases. In Youngkin EQ, Daris MS, eds: *Women's health: a primary care clinical guide,* ed 2, Stamford, Conn, 1998, Appleton & Lange.

41. Maiman M et al: Prevalence, risk factors, and accuracy of cytologic screening for cervical intraepithelial neoplasia in women with the human immunodeficiency virus, *Gynecol Oncol* 68:233, 1998.

42. Petty J: Basic concepts of neoplastic disorders. In Black JM, Matassarin-Jacobs E, eds: *Medical-surgical nursing: clinical management for continuity of care,* ed 5, Philadelphia, 1997, Saunders.

43. Denenberg R: Cervical cancer and women with HIV, *GMHC Treatment Issues: Newsletter of Experimental AIDS Therapies* 11(7/8):10, 1997.

44. Fruchter RG et al: Multiple recurrences of cervical intraepithelial neoplasia in women with the human immunodeficiency virus, *Obstet Gynecol* 87(3):338, 1996.

45. Korn AP, Abercrombie PD, Foster A: Vulvar intraepithelial neoplasia in women infected with human immunodeficiency virus–1, *Gynecol Oncol* 61:384, 1996.

46. National Cancer Institute Workshop: The 1988 Bethesda System for reporting cervical/vaginal cytological diagnoses, *JAMA* 262:931, 1989.

47. Carlson E, Matassarin-Jacobs E, Carpenter LC: Assessment of clients with reproductive disorders. In Black JM, Matassarin-Jacobs E, eds: *Medical-surgical nursing: clinical management for continuity of care,* ed 5, Philadelphia, 1997, Saunders.

48. U.S. Department of Health and Human Services: *Clinical practice guideline no. 7: evaluation and management of early HIV infection,* AHCPR Publication No. 94-0572, Rockville, Md, 1994, The Association.

49. Kurman RJ et al: Interim guidelines for management of abnormal cervical cytology: the 1992 National Cancer Institute workshop, *JAMA* 271:1866, 1994.

50. Worthington S, Rubin M: Nurse-midwifery evaluation and management of cervical pathology and the colposcopic examination, *J Nurse Midwifery* 38(Suppl 2):36S, 1993.

51. Korn AP et al: Sensitivity of the Papanicolaou smear in human immunodeficiency virus–infected women, *Obstet Gynecol* 83(3):401, 1994.

52. PRISMATIC Project Management Team: Assessment of automated primary screening on PAPNET of cervical smears in the PRISMATIC trial, *Lancet* 353(9162):1381, 1999.

53. O'Leary TJ et al: PAPNET-Assisted rescreening of cervical smears: cost and accuracy compared with a 100% manual rescreening strategy, *JAMA* 279:235, 1998.

54. Carrico, D J: Speculoscopy: A tool to enhance the detection of abnormal vaginal and cervical cells, *Nurse Pract* 21(5):14, 1997.

55. Centers for Disease Control and Prevention: 1997 USPHS/ISDA Guidelines for the prevention of opportunistic infections in persons infected with human immunodeficiency virus, *MMWR* 46(RR-12):25, 1997.

56. Rubin MM: Management of the abnormal Pap test and colposcopy. In Wallis LA, ed: *Textbook of women's health,* Philadelphia, 1998, Lippincott-Raven.
57. Baker DA: Management of the female HIV infected patient, AIDS Patient Care 9(2):78, 1995.
58. National Institute of Allergy and Infectious Diseases, National Institutes of Health: *Fact sheet—women and HIV,* April, 1997, U.S. Department of Health and Human Services, Public Health Service. http://www.niaid.nih.gov/factsheets/womenhiv.htm
59. Maiman M: HIV infection and cervical neoplasia, *Resident and Staff Physician* 42(7):34, 1996.
60. Stovall TG, Ling FW: *Atlas of benign gynecological and obstetric surgery,* London, 1995, Mosby-Wolfe.
61. Smith T: Colposcopy, *Nursing Standard* 11(45):49, 1997.
62. Jaffe MS, McVan BF: *Davis's laboratory and diagnostic test handbook,* Philadelphia, 1997, Davis.
63. Bates B, Bickley LS, Hoekelman RA: *A guide to physical examination and history taking,* ed 6, Philadelphia, 1995, Lippincott.
64. Jarvis C: *Physical examination and health assessment,* ed 2, Philadelphia, 1996, Saunders.
65. Sanchez R: Premalignant lesions of the cervix. In Leppert PC, Howard FM, eds: *Primary care of women,* Philadelphia, 1997, Lippincott-Raven.
66. Gant NF & Cunningham FG: *Basic gynecology and obstetrics,* Norwalk, Conn, 1993, Appleton & Lange.
67. Cuthill BS et al: Complications after treatment of cervical intraepithelial neoplasia in women infected with the human immunodeficiency virus, *J Reprod Med* 40(12):823, 1995.
68. Levine DW, Hillard PJA: The menstrual cycle and abnormal uterine bleeding. In Wallis LA, ed: *Textbook of women's health,* Philadelphia, 1998, Lippincott-Raven.
69. McIntyre-Seltman K, Matson CC: Gynecology. In Rakel RE, ed: *Textbook of family practice,* ed 5, Philadelphia, 1995, Saunders.
70. ARHP Advisory and Editorial Committee, eds: Treatment strategies for HIV-infected women—clinical manifestations and management of HIV-related conditions, *ARHP Clinical Proceedings: A Publication of the Association of Reproductive Health Professionals,* p 14, October 1998.
71. Grinspoon S et al: Body composition and endocrine function in women with acquired immunodeficiency syndrome wasting, *J Clin Endocrinol Metab* 82:1332, 1997.
72. Goroll AH, May LA, Mulley AG Jr: *Primary care medicine: office evaluation and management of the adult patient,* ed 3, Philadelphia, 1995, Lippincott.
73. Newman MD, Wofsy CB: Gender-specific issues in HIV disease. In Sande MA, Volberding PA, eds: *The medical management of AIDS,* ed 5, Philadelphia, 1997, Saunders.
74. Ball SC: Clinical challenge—amenorrhea in an HIV-infected woman, *AIDS Reader* 8(3):92, 1998. http://www.medscape.com/SCP/TAR/1998/v08.n03/a4150.ball/a4150.ball-01.html
75. O'Connell ML: The effect of birth control methods on sexually transmitted disease/HIV risk, *J Obstet Gynecol Neonatal Nurs: Principles & Practice* 25:476, 1996.

76. Centers for Disease Control and Prevention: Guidelines for use of antiretroviral agents in HIV-infected adults and adolescents, *MMWR* 47(RR-5):42, 1998.

77. No stones unturned in major push to develop microbicides, *AIDS Alert* 11(12):133, Atlanta, Ga, 1996, American Health Consultants.

78. Potts M: The urgent need for a vaginal microbicide in the prevention of HIV transmission, *Am J Public Health* 84:890, 1994.

79. Centers for Disease Control: Update: Barrier protection against HIV infection and other sexually transmitted diseases, *MMWR* 42(30):589, Aug 1993.

80. Martin HL et al: Safety of a nonoxynol 9 vaginal gel in Kenyan prostitutes: a randomized clinical trial, *Sex Transm Dis* 24(5):279, 1997.

81. Council calls for guidance on spermicide use, *AIDS Alert* 11(3):27, Atlanta, Ga, 1996, American Health Consultants.

82. National Institute of Allergy and Infectious Diseases: NIAID evaluates N-9 film as microbicide, *NIAID News*, April 3, 1997.
http://www.niaid.nih.gov/newsroom/n9.htm

83. Thomas CL: *Taber's cyclopedic medical dictionary*, Philadelphia, 1993, Davis.

84. Office of Communications, National Institute of Allergy and Infectious Diseases, National Institutes of Health: *NIAID Resources for studying HIV/AIDS in women*, Bethesda, Md, 1997, Public Health Service, U.S. Department of Health and Human Services.
http://www.4woman.org/owh/pub/hiv-aids/niaidresources.htm

Unit II   Frequently Asked Questions

I was told that oral sex is a high-risk behavior and I also read that it was hard to get HIV from oral sex, I am confused. What are the risks of oral sex?

You are not alone. Experts and expert agencies do not agree on the actual risk of infection from oral sex. Some experts state that oral sex is a low-risk behavior while others indicate the exact opposite. The reason for the confusion is that transmission of HIV by the oral route has never been proven; however, there are many reports that indicate individuals have become infected after having only oral sex. Common sense tells us that there is some risk associated with oral sex and that the actual risk is determined by several factors. Some of these factors include whether or not the person providing the oral sex takes ejaculate in the mouth; the amount of virus, if present, in the ejaculate (i.e., seminal viral load); and the healthiness of the gums and other oral tissue.

Some persons feel that any risk is too great and they may choose not to perform oral sex at all on any partners. Others choose to reduce their risk by limiting their oral activities. Using a condom or dental dam can help limit risk.

I have been taking two nucleoside drugs with an undetectable viral load and a near normal CD_4 count. My new doctor is concerned about this and is changing my therapy. I thought my HIV was well under control. Why is it indicated to change my drugs?

Your HIV is well under control and you are very fortunate to have such a great response to this therapy. There are many unanswered questions about the most appropriate combination therapy in persons with undetectable viral loads and near normal CD_4 counts. The benefit of two nucleoside drugs used alone is unknown. Two important principles, however, seem to suggest that combination therapy with different classes of antiretrovirals is preferred. First, the two drugs you are taking belong to a class of drugs called nucleoside reverse transcriptase inhibitors (NRTIs). These drugs work before the virus' genetic material infects the nuclei of cells. There is no way to know or to determine how many of your cells' nuclei had been infected before you started therapy. NRTIs are ineffectual in cells in which HIV RNA has already been incorporated into cellular DNA. Other classes of drugs work in different ways. Protease inhibitors (PI), for example, work by inhibiting virus assembly, a process that occurs after the virus is released from the nucleus. Therefore, if some of your cells' nuclei were already infected, the PI will help prevent viral replication in these cells. Taking drugs that have different sites of action minimizes viral replication; a potent regimen is one that attacks the virus at various sites of its reproduction.

Second, although there is an emphasis on limiting viral replication, there is an equal emphasis on maintaining viral suppression for as long as possible. HIV eventually develops resistance to all antiretrovirals. Resistance to the NRTIs when used alone can occur as early as 1 month after taking medications. Although you had a good response to the double NRTI strategy, your new physician probably wants to switch your medication because he may be concerned that resistance to the two nucleoside drugs could soon develop. Simply adding a PI to the regimen would allow the drug-resistant virus to replicate, and adequate viral suppression would not be obtained. Resistance testing is now available to determine if there is resistance to specific drugs. You could discuss this with your physician.

I am traveling to a developing country. What preparations must I make and what precautions should I follow?

Gastrointestinal infections that result in diarrhea are among the most common infections that occur in HIV-positive travelers. They are caused by ingesting food or water that has been contaminated by any of a wide array of pathogens. To protect yourself, make sure that your food is well prepared and cooked thoroughly. Do not eat raw, uncooked vegetables or fruits. Be alert to hidden sources of infected water, such as ice cubes, showers, and recreational water. If diarrhea does occur, be sure to replace lost fluids adequately with boiled water. Before your trip, you should ask your health care provider to supply an appropriate amount of antibiotic to treat common enteric infections. Carry it with you in case infection develops.

If you develop diarrhea, loperamide or bismuth subsalicyate, both available over the counter, can be used but should be avoided if you have fever or a bloody diarrhea. Upon returning from travel you should be evaluated by your health care provider, regardless of whether or not you experienced an episode of diarrhea.

Certain vaccines that are not routinely given to HIV-positive individuals may be required before entry into certain countries. These may include typhoid (Latin America, Africa, Asia), meningococcus (Nepal, Saharan Africa, New Delhi), rabies (India, Asia, Mexico), Japanese B encephalitis (Asia), and yellow fever (parts of Africa and South and Central America). You should inform your health care provider about your travel plans as early as possible; there may be some risk of illness involved with certain vaccines. Depending on the vaccine, your state of health, and the risk involved, your health care provider may elect to administer the vaccine, omit the vaccine and provide a letter of waiver, or ask that you change or reconsider your travel plans. You and your health care provider can obtain information and assistance from the International Association of Medical Assistance to Travellers at (519) 836-0102.

I am HIV positive and was told that I should not let my child receive the vaccine against chicken pox because it can harm me. Should the varicella vaccine be administered to my healthy child?

Expert groups such as the American Academy of Pediatrics (AAP) recommend that healthy household contacts of immunocompromised persons be vaccinated. There is, however, a small risk of household transmission of the virus contained in the vaccine. If your child develops a vaccine-related rash you should avoid contact with your child while the rash is present.

I am in a foreign country for a holiday vacation and accidentally left my protease inhibitor at home. My doctor mailed a new prescription to me, but the pharmacy said they will not have the medication for a week. Should I continue to take my two nucleoside drugs?

It is probably best to stop taking all your antiretrovirals until you are able to continue taking them as prescribed. Stopping your antiretrovirals will more than likely raise your viral load to pretreatment levels in as little as 2 weeks. However, the virus that will replicate will be of the same type; that is, it will not become resistant to the two nucleoside drugs in the way that it would if you continued to take them without the protease inhibitor. However, repeated interruptions in treatment could lead to drug-resistant virus and should be avoided.

In general it is a good idea to find out information beforehand about HIV care in the city or country to which you will be traveling. Although most people don't plan on getting sick while on vacation, a little preparation may be extremely helpful. You may want to call a clinic, a hospital, or a provider of HIV services. Inquire about provisions or referrals they can make for you as a visitor to their country or city. Be sure to bring enough medications. It may also be wise to carry emergency funds for medication purchase if the bag containing your medications becomes lost or stolen or if the medications spoil. You may want to carry medications with you rather than packing them in a bag that will be "checked" and could be lost. You may also want to consider having a friend hold a supply of medications that could be shipped to you overnight or in several days in the event of an emergency.

I was told that I could not join an advertised antiretroviral clinical trial because I was not "treatment naïve." What does that mean?

Treatment-naïve individuals are those that have never used any antiretrovirals. Treatment experienced individuals are those that have taken several antiretroviral drugs. To determine the true value of a drug in clinical investigation, the drug's efficacy must be differentiated in clients who are treatment naïve and clients who are treatment experienced. Some people refer to treatment-experienced individuals as moderately experienced or highly experienced. A highly experienced individual is someone who has taken several drugs in various classes. These labels are arbitrary and have no scientific definitions.

It is believed that treatment naïve individuals respond better to antiretroviral therapy because the virus is more homogeneous (wild type) and little drug resistance is present (some pretreatment resistance occurs as a result of errors in viral replication, the clinical significance of this remains unknown). Treatment experienced individuals generally have a more diverse viral population with several mutations, which may limit the usefulness of one or all drugs in a particular class.

Although today it is rare, some clinical trials may first limit participation to treatment naïve individuals to determine the effectiveness and durability of viral suppression.

My partner lives with me and sleeps in the same room as me. I am concerned about his catching my recently diagnosed tuberculosis. How can I protect my partner from catching tuberculosis from me?

First, your partner should see his health care provider and have a tuberculosis test to determine if he has contracted TB. Cases of TB are reported to the health department and your partner may have already been contacted regarding the need for the test. If he has not, but is also HIV-positive, the provider may prescribe medication to prevent him from contracting the disease. In addition, you can reduce exposure by following some very simple steps. Since the organism is spread when you cough or sneeze, you should always do this in a tissue. Infected tissues should be discarded promptly by flushing them down the toilet. You should wash your hands promptly after coughing or sneezing. You should keep your home well ventilated, allowing free flow of air. If possible, you and your partner should consider sleeping in separate rooms until it has been determined that your TB has become noninfectious with treatment. This happens for most people after they have been on antituberculous medication for a period of time. The period of time can vary; your health care provider will determine when your TB is no longer infectious. Until that time, it is necessary to use these and other precautions to prevent spread of the infection.

Why is everyone so concerned about my getting a Pap smear?

Pap smears are important for every woman for the early detection of cervical cancer. In addition, it has been found that certain women are at greater risk of having an abnormal Pap smear. Women who are immunosuppressed or HIV-positive are among those who are at greater risk. When abnormal cells are found early, a number of methods are available to treat the abnormality. However, if not found early, abnormal cells can progress to cervical cancer. Therefore, it is critical to have regular Pap smears done so that, if an abnormality is present, it will be detected and treated. Your health care provider will determine how frequently a Pap smear is necessary; you should follow this recommendation. Some women are also infected with human papilloma virus (HPV). If you have this infection, you are also at greater risk of having an abnormal Pap smear. The use of screening with Pap smears has greatly decreased the death rate from cervical cancer in the United States; you should take advantage of this relatively easy method of decreasing your risk of developing cervical cancer.

Unit III

Acute Care Nursing of Clients with HIV/AIDS

9

Hospitalized Clients with HIV/AIDS

Carl A. Kirton

One of the most important events in the timeline of the HIV epidemic has been the development of highly active antiretroviral therapy (HAART) because of the effects it has had on the health of HIV-positive individuals. Before the availability of protease inhibitors, most individuals infected with HIV were cared for primarily in acute care settings, and the resulting mortality from complications of this disease was often as high as 70% to 90%. The need for dedicated and willing providers to care for infected individuals, as well as the need for a new comprehensive model of caregiving, led to the formation of AIDS-dedicated units (ADUs). Clustering of clients with HIV is the ideal care model; client care improves when there are providers that have chosen to work in a specialized area with a special population.[1] ADUs often provide high-acuity nursing to HIV-positive individuals and require that nurses be especially skilled in symptom assessment and intervention, crisis intervention, and grief work. Nurses who work in ADUs are required to incorporate knowledge about clinical drug research, unconventional or complementary therapies, and end-of-life care into their daily plans of care.

Since the late 1990s, HIV has evolved into a chronic, manageable disease. Improved care of HIV-positive individuals is undoubtedly related, in part, to the understanding of how to use drugs in the most effective combinations, minimizing adverse effects, and keeping opportunistic infections at bay. These improvements have caused the site of care provision to shift from the acute care setting to the ambulatory setting. This shift has been validated by researchers and is thought to be directly attributable to the medication regimens containing protease inhibitors.[2] The decline in acute care admissions has forced institutions that once supported AIDS specialty units to shift from clustering infected clients to scattering clients among the general medical population.

Although these improvements have led to less acutely ill clients, the strategies used to keep clients healthy have become more complex and can be particularly challenging for individuals unfamiliar with these complexities. For example, frequently there are drug-drug interactions that occur with antiretroviral drugs and commonly prescribed antibiotics or other medications. Nurses in general medicine units or specialty care units may be unaccustomed to the care needs of HIV-positive individuals.

ADMISSION TO THE ACUTE CARE FACILITY

Opportunistic infections associated with HIV continue to be responsible for the largest number of hospitalizations of clients with HIV. It is difficult to determine the predominant cause of hospitalization today, because much of the data that examined the causes of hospitalization of HIV-positive individuals were collected before or at the advent of protease inhibitor (PI) combination therapy. Moreover, these data were almost always based on an individual facility's experience rather than regional or national databases. Nonetheless, such data are useful as a framework for determining the predominant needs of an HIV-positive individual in the acute care setting.

Studies demonstrate that clients are primarily admitted for pulmonary symptoms, followed by gastrointestinal and neurological symptoms. Therapeutic interventions such as chemotherapy and blood transfusion also account for a significant number of hospitalizations of HIV-positive clients.[3,4] While the number of hospital admissions in the post-HAART era has diminished significantly, one study has determined that the reasons for hospital admissions (e.g., opportunistic infections, HIV-related illnesses, non–HIV-related illnesses) and types of opportunistic infections requiring hospitalization have not changed significantly.[5]

THE NURSING ASSESSMENT

The nursing admission database is important in determining the type and level of nursing care required for a client infected with HIV. The standard admission database often does not include all data that are relevant to the infected person. Certain HIV-specific information is important in that it has the potential to influence the care that will be given in the acute care facility. Aside from standard information, the following items should be gleaned from the client so that appropriate care can be planned.

FAMILY ASSESSMENT

HIV does not occur in isolation; it also affects those who are close to the infected person, such as family and friends. Because others are often involved in the care of a client and will most likely continue the care once that person returns home, it is essential for the nurse to explore who the client considers family. Family in this context can often be defined as partners and/or friends who provide primary support. When obtaining the nursing history, it is essential that the nurse ask the client the following questions:

- Who do you consider to be your family?
- Who knows about your diagnosis?
- Have you told anyone in your immediate family? If so, who have you told and will they come to visit you?
- What have you told your visitors about the reason for this hospitalization?

The nurse should inform clients that confidentiality about their present and past health history, as well as their HIV status, will be strictly maintained. Information regarding the current hospitalization must not be shared with any visitors. It is important to explore with the client how he or she plans to deal with family and friends who come to visit; the client should be advised that it is necessary to ask these questions so that appropriate hospital and discharge care can be planned.

Some clients may harbor guilt, shame, or anger about their HIV status and choose not to disclose their HIV status to others. The nurse may choose to explore with clients who have decided not to disclose their status the reasons for this decision. These issues may warrant interventions by a nurse specializing in HIV or a mental health professional.

ALLERGIES AND ADVERSE REACTIONS TO MEDICATION

During the course of their disease, clients are exposed to a variety of different medications. Many of these are likely to be antiretrovirals, which have an extensive adverse reaction record. It is not common practice to change antiretrovirals while a person is hospitalized; however, the "allergies and reactions history" serves as a database for prescribers involved in the client's care. A careful review of the client's known allergies and reactions to previously administered medications is essential. Prominent notation in the medical record reduces the possibility that clients may be exposed to a drug or drugs that may negatively affect health. A history of reactions to drugs used for opportunistic infection (OI) prophylaxis should be included.

MEDICATION HISTORY

The nurse should record all of the medications that clients currently take. It is particularly important to note which medications clients are taking as preventive or maintenance therapy for OIs and when the last dose was taken. Some of these medications are administered on an "every other day" or "three times a week" basis. In particular, azithromycin, a drug used in *Mycobacterium avium-intracellulare* prophylaxis is administered once weekly (1200 mg/wk). Trimethoprim-sulfamethoxazole (TMP-SMX) (Bactrim), a drug used to prevent *Pneumocystis carinii* pneumonia (PCP) can be effectively administered three times weekly. The nurse should ensure that clients' medication patterns continue at admission so as to prevent underdosing or overdosing.

TUBERCULOSIS HISTORY

Even if a client is admitted to the hospital for non–pulmonary-type symptoms, it is essential to document the client's tuberculosis (TB) history in the medical record. The client should be asked about his or her purified protein derivative (PPD) of tuberculin status; if unknown, PPD testing may be required. Any client suspected of pulmonary TB should be placed in respiratory isolation until pulmonary TB has been ruled out (see Chapter 10).

BOX 9-1 EXPECTED MEDICATIONS BASED ON CD₄ CELL COUNT

CD₄ <200 Cells/mm³
Prophylaxis against *Pneumocystis carinii*
Trimethoprim/sulfamethoxazole—the drug of choice for prevention is one double-strength (DS) or single-strength (SS) tablet qd or three times a week. Clients who have adverse reactions to this drug may take an alternative regimen such as dapsone 100 mg qd or aerosolized pentamidine (see Chapter 16).

CD₄ <100 Cells/mm³
Prophylaxis against *Toxoplasmosis gondii*
Trimethoprim/sulfamethoxazole—Clients who take trimethoprim/sulfamethoxazole daily, as above, receive simultaneous protection against this pathogen. Alternative regimens are available (see Chapter 16).

CD₄ <50 Cells/mm³
Prophylaxis against *Mycobacterium avium* complex
Clarithromycin 500 mg PO bid or azithromycin 1200 mg PO weekly (see Chapter 13).

Note: Review client's history for previous opportunistic infections (OIs). Clients may be on suppressive therapy for certain OIs (e.g, herpes simplex, cryptococcal disease).

IMMUNOLOGICAL AND VIROLOGICAL DATA

Immunological data (i.e., CD₄ cell count) and virological data are not routinely monitored during the course of a client's hospitalization. This is based on the fact that when clients are acutely ill, generally the viral load count increases and the CD₄ count decreases. However, the nurse should inquire about the client's most recent values, prior to the current illness, and record them in the medical record. Clients can usually be the source of this data, as they often know their most recent CD₄ and viral load counts. (For a discussion of CD₄ and viral load see Chapter 2.) This information is also important so that the nurse will know what medications to expect clients to be continuing during their hospitalization. Box 9-1 indicates expected medications based on CD₄ counts.

ADVANCED DIRECTIVES

The nurse or other health provider should ask clients whether they have completed any advanced directives, such as a *living will* or *health care proxy*. A copy of these documents should be obtained and entered into the medical record. For discussion of advanced directives see Box 11-13.

THE ACUTE CARE STAY

FEVER OF UNKNOWN ORIGIN

Fever of unknown origin (FUO) in HIV clients continues to account for a significant number of hospitalizations. The definition of HIV-

BOX 9-2 MEDICATIONS LIKELY TO CAUSE FEVER

- Sulfonamides
- Dapsone
- Amphotericin B
- Phenytoin

- Penicillin
- Barbiturates
- Bleomycin
- Carbamazepine

- Thalidomide
- Pentamidine
- Clindamycin

associated FUO is fever of 38.3° C or higher on several occasions, persistent fever for 3 weeks (in an outpatient setting) or 3 days (in an inpatient setting); and an uncertain diagnosis despite 3 weeks of evaluation (in an outpatient setting) or 3 days (in an inpatient setting).[6] If the origin of a fever is unknown, the nurse admitting the client should be alert to the fact that a pathogen may be causing the fever and may have the potential of being spread to other clients or even staff members. Prevention of the spread of infection through the use of hospital infection control practices must be instituted immediately. This often includes, but is not limited to, placing the client in a private room, especially when pulmonary TB is suspected (see Chapter 10). Other organisms that have the potential to be transmitted to others are those causing infectious diarrhea and zoster infections. A discussion of these can be found, respectively, in Chapters 16 and 17.

The etiology of fever in HIV-positive adults is varied. For example, HIV itself may cause fever, though this usually occurs with acute HIV infection; persistent fever attributable to the virus itself is uncommon. In addition, HIV-related medications (Box 9-2), opportunistic infections, or malignancies may cause fever. Nurses participate in determining the cause of HIV-associated fever. When a client with HIV is admitted with FUO, diagnostic evaluation often points to the possibility of infection, malignancy, or a fever that is related to one or more of the client's current medications. If the client is an injection drug user, persistent fever may be caused by infective endocarditis or osteomyelitis.

CD$_4$ Cell Counts

Knowing a client's CD$_4$ cell count is essential to assessing the etiology of fever, because different infections occur at different levels of immune function.

Febrile clients with CD$_4$ cell counts above 200 cells/mm³. Bacterial and viral respiratory infections and pulmonary and extrapulmonary TB are the most likely causes of fever when the client's CD$_4$ cell count is above 200 cells/mm³. Common opportunistic infections can have atypical presentations regardless of the client's CD$_4$ count (e.g., Pneumocystis of the ear, renal parenchymal disease caused by mycobacterium organisms or cytomegalovirus).

Febrile clients with CD$_4$ cell counts below 200 cells/mm^3. Opportunistic infections such as cryptococcal meningitis, histoplasmosis, *M. avium* complex, toxoplasmosis, and cytomegalovirus infection are common causes of fever in clients whose CD$_4$ cell counts are below 200 cells/mm^3. A client's risk for infection with particular organisms is based on the degree of immunosuppression. Refer to individual disorders in Chapters 13 to 17. As clients live longer with HIV, malignancies are emerging with more frequency than 10 years ago.

Evaluation of a Client with FUO
Careful review of history
- Recent travel history—Certain opportunistic infections are endemic in certain regions of the country (e.g., histoplasmosis is endemic in Ohio, the Mississippi River Valley, and Indianapolis). Travel to other countries can result in infections that are uncommon in the United States.
- Exposures to sick contacts—HIV-positive individuals may often be in the position of caring for others who are ill (e.g., an HIV-positive mother caring for a child with an upper respiratory infection).
- New sexual partners or recent sexual history—Even clients who report safer sexual practices may engage in sexual behaviors that have the ability to transmit organisms (e.g., oral-anal contact).
- Recent antiretroviral or other medication changes—Drug fever can result from therapy or prophylaxis with trimethoprim-sulfamethoxazole, dapsone, zidovudine, and didanosine, as well as medications such as interferon-α, which is one component of the treatment of hepatitis C infection.

Diagnostic Evaluation
1. Routine serum laboratory tests, such as routine chemistry panels and a complete blood count (CBC), are always included in the initial workup. Nurses should anticipate that the following additional serum laboratory specimens will be collected, depending on the suspected organism:
   - Liver enzymes—Abnormalities may be seen in clients with *M. avium* complex, especially when accompanied by hepatomegaly.
   - Lactic dehydrogenase—Marked increases in the lactic dehydrogenase (LDH) level can be seen in clients with PCP and non–Hodgkin's lymphoma.
   - Venereal Disease Research Laboratory (VDRL) or rapid plasma reagin (RPR) tests may be ordered to rule out primary or secondary syphilis as a cause of fever.
   - Serum cryptococcal antigen—If cryptococcal meningitis is suspected; a lumbar puncture is indicated if the client is cryptococcal antigen–positive.
2. Blood cultures—Clients with fever should have routine blood cultures. Routine cultures indicate the presence of any bacterial patho-

gens. The nurse should collect 2 to 4 sets of blood cultures, which consist of two bottles per set. Approximately 5 ml of blood should be instilled per bottle. Each set should be collected from a different culture site. Clients with indwelling catheters may have at least one set of blood cultures drawn from the indwelling line (controversy surrounds the benefit of this strategy). Removal of the line by a qualified health care provider is often indicated if the line is considered the cause of the client's fever. Viral and fungal culture tests can also be performed. The nurse should consult with the laboratory for proper collection and handling of these types of specimens.

3. Urine analysis and cultures—Urine should be collected for routine analysis and culture. The presence of leukocyte esterase and nitrite in the urine is indicative of urinary pathogens. A culture test will demonstrate the nature of the organism.

4. Radiographic studies—A routine chest x-ray study can rule out any pulmonary pathogen that may be involved in the etiology of the client's fever.

5. Other studies—If no source of fever can be determined, additional studies such as regional computed tomography (CT) scans, bone marrow biopsies, or lymph node biopsies may be indicated.

Nursing Considerations

1. The client's body temperature should be measured at least every 4 hours.

2. The client must maintain hydration. PO fluids are preferable. Intravenous replacement of fluid may be indicated with large losses. The client's laboratory data may indicate a state of dehydration (e.g., hypernatremia, increased specific gravity of urine, elevated hematocrit).

3. The client should be assessed for excessive insensible water loss (e.g., diaphoresis indicated by saturated bed sheets).

4. Antipyretics should be administered if ordered, and agency policy should be followed regarding other cooling measures.

DYSPNEA

A variety of pulmonary pathogens can invade the tracheobronchial tree of a person infected with HIV. *P. carinii*, a common opportunistic pathogen, affects persons with advanced immunosuppression (a CD_4 cell count less than 200 cells/mm^3) who are not receiving prophylaxis for this organism or are not compliant with prophylactic therapy. PCP is rare in clients with a CD_4 cell count greater than 250 cells/mm^3.

Bacterial pneumonia is also common in HIV-positive individuals; *Streptococcus pneumoniae* is the most common type of bacterial pneumonia seen in client with HIV infection. Clients who smoke cigarettes or illicit drugs are at increased risk for the development of bacterial pneumonia.

Diagnostic Evaluation

1. Pulse oximetry—Measuring the client's pulse oximetry (SpO_2) at rest and with activity is of value when determining whether or not a client has impaired gas exchange secondary to a pulmonary process. This measurement is often taken in the ambulatory setting when the index of suspicion for a pulmonary process is high.
2. Chest radiography—A chest x-ray study is the gold standard examination in the evaluation of chest abnormalities. A client with a bacterial pneumonia will demonstrate densities within a lung segment or lobe. A chest x-ray study of a client with PCP infection demonstrates diffuse interstitial infiltrates.
3. Sputum examination—The collection of sputum for culture may be necessary to determine the causative organism. Pneumocystis does not culture well. See Chapter 16 for other tests that may be used in the diagnosis of PCP.

Nursing Considerations

1. The client's respiratory status should be monitored at least every 4 hours and more frequently if indicated.
2. The client's SpO_2 should be evaluated continuously, and arterial blood gas measurements should be obtained if indicated.
3. Medication may be used to relieve the client's dyspnea (e.g., morphine sulfate, antitussives/expectorants).
4. Therapeutic modalities should be administered as needed, such as coughing and deep breathing exercises, postural drainage, suctioning, and oxygen.
5. Ambulation should generally be encouraged within the client's tolerance.

NUTRITIONAL AND FLUID ALTERATIONS

Diarrhea and subsequent fluid and electrolyte loss from the gastrointestinal tract can plague an HIV-positive client at any stage of illness. Infections and malignancies are most often contributing factors, however other factors such as medications, vitamin deficiencies, and lactose intolerance can lead to significant nutrient malabsorption or fluid and electrolyte losses. Clients with fever, abdominal pain, mental status changes, and cardiovascular instability are best treated in the acute care setting, because large fluid and electrolyte losses or an inability to tolerate food or fluid can be life-threatening.

Diagnostic Evaluation

1. Stool analysis—Evaluation of the client's stool is essential for determining whether the etiology of the client's diarrhea includes enteric pathogens. Special studies for cryptosporidium, microsporidia, and isospora may be indicated in clients infected with HIV. See Chapter 16 for discussion of these organisms and Figure 16-1 for diarrhea pathway information.

2. Invasive studies such as sigmoidoscopy, upper GI endoscopy, or colonoscopy may be indicated.

Nursing Considerations

1. The client should be weighed daily. Assessments for rehydration should occur at least every 8 hours. This includes but is not limited to the assessment of skin turgor, mucous membranes, mental status, and tissue perfusion.
2. The nurse should monitor the client for signs and symptoms of electrolyte imbalances (e.g., hypokalemia); the client may report weakness, constipation, paresthesias, and cramping. The nurse should monitor for orthostatic hypotension, arrhythmias, and ECG changes.
3. Clients with diarrhea should follow a diet that is high in protein and high in calories. The client should avoid substances that increase gastrointestinal motility (e.g., caffeine).
4. Containment of stool through a fecal collection device may be indicated to assist in maintenance of the client's skin integrity. The nurse should also monitor the characteristics of the stool. The appearance of frothy stool or an excessive amount of fat in the stool may indicate malabsorption.
5. Intravenous therapy may be indicated to replace lost fluids and electrolytes. The nurse should monitor fluid intake and losses.
6. Oral nutritional supplements may be indicated. The nurse should consult with a nutritionist to determine the most appropriate supplement.
7. Total parental nutrition (TPN) may be indicated for clients with severe electrolyte losses or malnutrition. Clients with TPN infusion must have regular electrolyte and glucose monitoring. Institutional protocol should be followed for managing a client receiving TPN.
8. Antimotility agents such as loperamide, Lomotil, or tincture of opium may be indicated. Antibiotics are indicated for diarrhea caused by susceptible organisms

NEUROLOGICAL ALTERATIONS

HIV-related neurological processes and nursing considerations are discussed in Chapter 22.

DISCHARGE PLANNING

Like clients with any chronic condition, clients with HIV often require support as they convalesce after acute illness. There are a wide range of services available to clients; the type and scope of a client's treatment is determined by client and caregiver preferences, community resources, and provisions of the client's health insurance plan. Discharge planning is a complex activity and requires a nurse to have special skills; the planner assesses the client's physical, financial, emotional, psychological, and spiritual needs in preparation for return to the community. Home care of clients with HIV is discussed in Chapter 12.

REFERENCES

1. Morrison C: HIV/AIDS units: is there still a need? *J Assoc Nurses AIDS Care* 9(6):16, 1998.
2. Torres R, Barr M: *Impact of potent new antiretroviral therapies on inpatient and outpatient hospital utilization by HIV-infected persons*, Fourth Conference on Retrovirus and Opportunistic Infections, p 113, 1997 (abstract, No. 264).
3. Parker DA, Barnes AJ, Mandal BK: Cause of hospitalization of HIV-seropositive individuals: regional AIDS unit, *International Conference on AIDS* 8(3):201, 1992 (abstract, No. PuD 9016).
4. Mars ME et al: *Protease inhibitors lead to a change of infectious disease unit activity*, Fourth Conference on Retrovirus and Opportunistic Infections, p 102, 1997 (abstract, No. 203).
5. Paul S et al: *Impact of HARRT on rates and types of hospitalization at a New York City hospital*, Fifth Conference on Retrovirus and Opportunistic Infections, p 117, 1998 (abstract, No. 205).
6. Durack DT, Street AC: Fever of unknown origin—reexamined and redefined, *Curr Clin Top Infect Dis* 11:35, 1991.

10 Tuberculosis Control

Dorothy Talotta

Tuberculosis (TB) is an airborne disease, and prevention of the spread of TB to other clients, visitors, and health care workers is essential. When considering isolation precautions to prevent transmission, it is important to remember that clients who are admitted to acute care facilities may not have a specific diagnosis of TB; they may be admitted for nonspecific complaints (e.g., fever of unknown origin) or for pneumonia. Although TB may not be included in the differential diagnoses, they may be infected. The most recent isolation precautions guideline, developed by the Centers for Disease Control and Prevention (CDC) and the Hospital Infection Control Practices Advisory Committee (HICPAC),[1] recognizes this problem and recommends the consideration of airborne precautions when clients present with certain clinical syndromes or conditions that might be manifestations of TB. In addition, hospitals must have systems in place to evaluate clients who are potentially infectious. The guideline suggests that airborne precautions be considered for HIV-negative clients or clients at low risk for HIV infection who present with a cough, a fever, and an upper lobe pulmonary infiltrate. Airborne precautions should also be considered for HIV-infected clients or clients at high risk for HIV infection who present with a cough, a fever, and a pulmonary infiltrate in any lung location.[1] If uncertain about the potential for transmission of the disease or the need to institute isolation precautions, the nurse should use the institution's infection control personnel as a resource to answer questions and provide appropriate guidance. When a client is known or suspected to have active TB, the public health department should be notified so that persons exposed to the client can be evaluated for infection and so that appropriate follow-up care for the client can be arranged.[2] (For additional information on TB infection control, see Chapter 7. For additional information on TB, see Chapters 7 and 13. For additional information on health care workers and TB, see Chapter 23.)

Airborne precautions are one type of what the isolation precautions guideline calls *transmission-based precautions.* (See Chapter 23 for a discussion of transmission-based and standard precautions.) Other transmission-based precautions are droplet and contact precautions. The purpose of airborne precautions is to decrease the risk of airborne transmission of infectious agents.[1] The organism that causes TB, *Mycobacterium*

167

tuberculosis (MTB), is carried by droplet nuclei which can remain suspended in the air for long periods and can be widely dispersed by air currents. The disease is spread when droplet nuclei are inhaled by a susceptible host. If a client is infected with an organism that is spread in this way, special air handling and ventilation systems are required, as well as other special precautions such as wearing respiratory protection.[1,2] If TB is suspected, to prevent transmission it is critical to institute airborne isolation precautions immediately and not wait for the diagnosis to be confirmed.[3] Clients with extrapulmonary TB are usually not infectious unless they have one of the following: (1) accompanying pulmonary disease, (2) nonpulmonary disease located in the oral cavity or respiratory tract, or (3) extrapulmonary disease that includes an open lesion or abscess in which there is a high concentration of organisms, particularly if there is extensive drainage.[2] (See Chapter 13 for a discussion of extrapulmonary TB.)

A TB infection control program in a health care facility is based on a hierarchy of control measures.[2] The first level in the hierarchy is the use of administrative measures; the second is the use of engineering controls; and the third is the use of personal protective respiratory equipment. Administrative measures are primarily intended to reduce the risk of exposure of uninfected persons to persons with infectious TB, including the development and implementation of effective written policies and protocols to ensure that persons likely to have TB are rapidly identified, isolated, diagnosed, and treated. They also include measures such as educating health care workers about TB, screening them for TB exposure and infection and implementing effective work practices—keeping doors to isolation rooms closed, for example. Engineering controls are measures to prevent the spread and reduce the concentration of droplet nuclei. They include the use of local exhaust ventilation, control of the direction of airflow, dilution and removal of contaminated air through general ventilation, and air cleaning by filtration or ultraviolet germicidal irradiation (UVGI).[2]

When a client is suspected of having or is known to have TB, the nurse should place the client in a TB isolation room.[2] These rooms are often called *negative pressure rooms;* when the door is opened, outside air is pulled into the room rather than allowing contaminated air to be released into the corridor. To maintain negative pressure, the door must be kept closed except when entering or leaving the room. The nurse should inspect the pressure meter (often located outside the door) to ensure that negative pressure is being maintained. If it is not, the problem should be reported promptly to the appropriate person, such as the nurse's supervisor or the facility's building maintenance department. In order to reduce the concentration of TB droplet nuclei within the isolation room, and for comfort as well as for odor control, there should be a minimum of six air changes per hour. New or renovated facilities should be designed to provide twelve air changes per hour.[2]

Some infection control systems are designed with high efficiency particulate air (HEPA) filters installed in the exhaust duct, which leads from the isolation room to the general ventilation system. Other infection control measures may include the use of UVGI lamps to kill or inactivate microorganisms. Potential hazards of exposure to ultraviolet irradiation need to be considered when these are used and there should be regular evaluation of the ultraviolet intensity to which health care workers, clients, and others are exposed.[2]

Clients placed in isolation for TB should be educated about the disease, the mode of transmission, and the reasons for isolation. The client should remain in the room and keep the door closed. The client should be transported as little as possible. If transport is necessary, the client should wear a surgical mask covering both nose and mouth during transport. Necessary procedures that require transportation should be scheduled at times when waiting areas are less crowded and when the procedure can be performed rapidly. The client should be returned promptly to the isolation room when the procedure is complete.[2]

PROVIDING DIRECT NURSING CARE TO A CLIENT WITH TB

The CDC suggests the use of administrative measures to minimize the number of health care workers exposed to TB while providing optimal care to TB clients.[2] Nursing care assignments should be structured so as to provide quality nursing care and meet the client's needs while minimizing the number of health care workers exposed to the disease. Nurses and all persons (including the client's visitors) entering a TB isolation room must wear respiratory protection.[2] The Occupational Safety and Health Administration (OSHA) mandates that health care facilities provide respiratory protective equipment to their employees who will be entering potentially hazardous areas and train them in its correct use.[4]

In addition, OSHA requires individual fit testing of each health care worker's personal respiratory protection to ensure that the face seal is tight enough to prevent the inhalation of droplet nuclei.[4] Face seal leakage testing can be done by determining whether a health care worker can identify a specific taste—saccharin, for example—while wearing the mask. It can also be done using an irritant fume to see whether or not the health care worker responds to it.[5] If the worker can taste the saccharin or responds to the fume, then the mask is not sealed properly. Nurses and other health care workers must be aware that factors such as a major weight change or beginning or ceasing to wear dentures can affect the fit of the mask and necessitate repeated fit testing. Beards may make it difficult to obtain an adequate face seal and OSHA requires that workers who use negative pressure respirators that depend on an adequate face seal for proper function be clean-shaven where the seal contacts the face. The wearer must perform a quick fit check each time the mask is used.[4]

All persons present must wear respiratory protection when cough-inducing or aerosol-generating procedures (e.g., diagnostic sputum induction, endotracheal intubation and suctioning, aerosol treatments such as pentamidine therapy or bronchoscopy, any other procedure that can generate aerosols) are performed on clients with known or suspected infectious TB. The CDC recommends that such procedures be performed only if absolutely necessary and with appropriate precautions.[2] They should be performed using local exhaust ventilation devices such as booths or special enclosures, or in a room that meets the ventilation requirements for TB isolation. The client should remain in the booth or room until coughing subsides and should be instructed to cover the mouth and nose with tissues when coughing. A sign should warn visitors against entry and warn staff that respiratory protection is required for entry. The booth or room should not be used again for another client until enough time has passed for airborne contaminants to be removed. The time necessary will vary according to the ventilation or filtration system in use.[2] The nurse should consult with the facility's infection control personnel as to the appropriate waiting time. A sign should indicate the time when it will be safe to enter without respiratory protection. Personal respiratory protection should also be worn by persons in certain other settings, such as while transporting clients with known or suspected TB in closed vehicles.[4]

Significant to the provision of nursing care is the knowledge that a client in isolation may experience adverse psychological effects. One such effect is sensory deprivation, which is a reduction in the intensity and variety of sensory input.[6] Clients subjected to airborne isolation may also feel neglected by health care providers and may experience feelings of loneliness and solitude as a result of having to remain alone in a room with the door closed. The fact that all who enter the room must wear respiratory protection can also be distressing for the client, who cannot see the complete faces of family members, friends, or caregivers. The nurse should make every effort to decrease the client's solitude and to promote quality care. Family members and friends who visit should be provided with respiratory protection and instructed in its use.[2] Telephone, television, and radio use can help decrease feelings of seclusion, but the nurse should monitor the client's wishes and reactions. Providing the client access to a window, if possible, can be helpful in decreasing sensory deprivation. A recreational or activity therapist, if available, may be helpful.[6] The nurse can also ensure that TB diagnostic procedures (e.g., sputum collection) are carried out promptly. (See Chapter 7 for a discussion of sputum collection.) This will enable a TB-negative client to return to the general client population as quickly as possible.

DISCONTINUING TB ISOLATION

For known or suspected cases of TB, isolation can be discontinued when the client is determined to be noninfectious. The amount of time required for a person to become noninfectious after being started on anti-TB therapy can vary significantly. Therefore, isolation should be discontinued only when the following criteria are met: (1) the client has had three consecutive negative sputum acid-fast bacillus (AFB) smears, collected on different days; (2) the client is on effective therapy; and (3) the client is improving clinically.[2] For clients with multidrug-resistant tuberculosis (MDR-TB), strong consideration should be given to continuing isolation throughout the hospitalization, because there is a tendency for treatment failure or relapse in such clients.[2] (See Chapter 13 for a discussion of MDR-TB.) The nurse should consult the facility's infection control nurse for guidance regarding discontinuing TB isolation. Hospitalized clients who have had active TB should have sputum AFB smears examined regularly to monitor for relapse.[2]

TRANSITIONING A CLIENT FROM ACUTE TO SUBACUTE OR HOME CARE

Before a client with TB is discharged from a health care facility, there must be collaboration between the staff of the facility and public health authorities to ensure continuation of therapy. Early notification that a client is known or suspected of having active TB facilitates the organization of follow-up care for the client. Before discharge, the client must have a confirmed appointment to see the provider who will be managing care until the client is cured. The client must have sufficient medication to last until the appointment and, in addition, must have been placed into case management or an outreach program of the health department.[2]

If the discharge of a client who may be infectious is being considered, he or she must be discharged either to the home or to a facility with isolation capability. If an infectious client is to be discharged home, the potential for transmission to other household members must be considered. If the household includes any uninfected members who are at very high risk for active TB if they become infected, arrangements must be made to prevent them from being exposed to the client until the client is noninfectious. Such household members include children under the age of 4 years and persons who are HIV-infected or severely immunocompromised.[2]

Other factors must be considered if an infectious client is to be discharged, such as the stability of the client's residence, the willingness and ability of the client to cover the mouth when coughing, and whether or not there is a need for social services that would require a provider (e.g., a home attendant) to see the client routinely for several hours at a time.[7] Any applicable state and local protocols must also be considered. In New York City, for example, the Bureau of Tuberculosis Control of the Department of Health indicates that a client suspected of having MDR-TB should remain hospitalized until three consecutive AFB smears, taken on three different days, are negative.[7]

According to the American Thoracic Society and the CDC, there should be consideration given to treating all TB clients with directly observed therapy (DOT).[8,9] DOT is the supervised observation of clients ingesting each dose of antituberculosis medication.[9] Observation may occur daily or less frequently, depending on the client's dosing regimen. DOT may take place in the client's home, school, or place of employment; in a clinic setting; or in another place agreed upon by the client and observer.[9] The effectiveness of DOT may be enhanced by offering incentives such as meals, subway tokens, and clothes.[10]

DOT is an important component of TB care and ensures that the client receives antituberculous treatment. Self-administration of the many required pills over the course of at least 6 months is difficult for many clients. If medications are missed or not taken consistently, drug resistance can develop. The Department of Health and Human Services (DHHS) recommends that, when possible, DOT programs be provided through already existing systems such as drug treatment centers, HIV clinics, or community-based agencies. DHHS also recommends that both the medications and services be available at low or no cost, easily accessible, and available at convenient times.[10] Depending on state law, a client with infectious TB who has not successfully engaged in or completed treatment, despite assistive interventions, may be detained involuntarily.[11]

REFERENCES

1. Garner JS, The Hospital Infection Control Practices Advisory Committee (HICPAC): Guideline for isolation precautions in hospitals, *Infect Control Hosp Epidemiol* 17(1):54, 1996.
2. Centers for Disease Control and Prevention: Guidelines for preventing the transmission of *Mycobacterium tuberculosis* in health-care facilities, 1994, *MMWR* 43(RR-13):1, October 28, 1994.
3. Boutotte J: TB: the second time around . . . and how you can help to control it, *Nursing 93* 23(5):42, 1993.
4. Decker MD: OSHA enforcement policy for occupational exposure to tuberculosis, *Infect Control Hosp Epidemiol* 14(12):689, 1993.
5. Clark RA: OSHA enforcement policy and procedures for occupational exposure to tuberculosis, *Infect Control Hosp Epidemiol* 14(12):694, 1993.
6. Ignatavicius DD, Workman ML, Mishler MA: *Medical-surgical nursing: a nursing process approach*, ed 2, Philadelphia, 1995, Saunders.
7. Fujiwara PI: *Clinical policies and protocols*, ed 3, New York, 1999, Bureau of Tuberculosis Control, New York City Department of Health.
8. American Thoracic Society: Treatment of tuberculosis and tuberculosis infection in adults and children, *Am J Resp Crit Care Med* 149:1359, 1994.
9. Simone PM: Essential components of a tuberculosis prevention and control program: recommendations of the Advisory Council for the Elimination of Tuberculosis, *MMWR* 44(RR-11):1, 1995.
10. United States Department of Health and Human Services: *Clinical practice guideline #7: evaluation and management of early HIV infection*, AHCPR Publication No. 94-0572, 1994, Agency for Health Care Policy and Research.
11. Anastasio CJ: HIV and tuberculosis: noncompliance revisited, *J Assoc Nurses AIDS Care* 6(2):11, 1995.

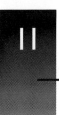

Palliative Care

Deborah Sherman

The World Health Organization has defined palliative care as the active, total care of clients whose disease is not responsive to curative treatment.[1] Palliative care is envisioned as life-affirming—neither hastening nor postponing death. Death is regarded as a natural process with profound individual and family meaning.[2,3] The aim of palliative care is therefore to address the physical, psychological, social, spiritual, and existential needs of clients with progressive, life-threatening illnesses, with the overall goal of improving the quality of life for individuals and families.[2] In palliative care, there is acknowledgment that, in advanced illness, a time comes for a change of goals from curing to caring. At that time, the emphasis must shift from the disease entity to the concerns, preferences, choices, and plans of the individual and family.[2] In the United States, hospice care has embodied the principles of palliative care, recognizing that, with death impending, the control of pain and symptoms and the emotional and spiritual preparation of the client and family must be given the highest priority.[4]

Although the term *palliative care* has been used in the past to describe care provided at the end of life, increasingly the term refers to the alleviation of suffering through pain and symptom management at any point in the illness trajectory.[5] Palliative care emphasizes the appropriate use of technology and treatment modalities for symptomatic benefit.[6] Radiotherapy, chemotherapy, and surgery have a place in palliative care, provided that the symptomatic benefits of treatment clearly outweigh the disadvantages.[7] The intensity and range of palliative interventions often increase as illness progresses, and the care needs of the client become more complex. Palliative care should, therefore, become increasingly important when there is a move away from attempts at cure to a concern for quality of life and quality of dying and death.[6]

PRECEPTS AND PRINCIPLES OF PALLIATIVE CARE

Current research has indicated that the care of dying persons in America has not met the needs or expectations of clients and families. A 2-year study[8] based in several institutions found that at the end of life there

173

continued to be aggressive medical interventions, a lack of communication between physicians and clients with regard to end-of-life preferences, and a high level of pain reported by seriously ill and dying clients. As a response, the Last Acts Palliative Care Task Force (1997) was convened to identify the precepts of palliative care, in an attempt to begin much needed reform in end-of-life care. The core precepts in palliative care include:

- Respecting the client's end-of-life goals, preferences, and choices about care settings, living situations, and services;
- Working toward the resolution of conflicts among clients, families, and providers;
- Comprehensive caring, which includes recognizing dying as a normal process; acknowledging the potential for personal growth; and providing physical, emotional, social, and spiritual comfort;
- Utilizing the strengths of members of various health professions and accessing a variety of institutional and community resources;
- Acknowledging the stress of fulfilling caregiving responsibilities and addressing caregiver concerns, risks, and needs for support; and
- Building systems and mechanisms of support by developing infrastructures supportive of the philosophy and practices of palliative care.

In addition, the principles of palliative care dictate that the individual has the right to be informed and to be autonomous in making end-of-life decisions; the client and family are to be respected with regard to information sharing (i.e., they have timely access to information and services in language that can be understood); palliative care services are to be available 24 hours a day, 7 days a week, without discrimination; confidentiality is to be assured; and an interdisciplinary team of caregivers are to be committed to the continuity of care, working collaboratively with the individual and family.[9] Furthermore, health care professionals are encouraged to make a diagnosis before treatment, be knowledgeable about the drugs being used, use medications that will accomplish more than one objective, and recognize that palliative care is aggressive care—with the belief that something can always be done to alleviate pain and suffering.[10]

PALLIATIVE CARE FOR CLIENTS WITH AIDS

AIDS, as defined by the Centers for Disease Control and Prevention (CDC), is a chronic illness characterized by opportunistic infections, specific cancers, and neurological manifestations.[11] It involves a multitude of symptoms that result from the related disease processes, as well as side effects from medications and other therapies. AIDS, characterized by bouts of severe illness and debilitation followed by periods of stabilization,[12] presents complex care issues, requiring extensive management of pain and symptoms to enhance the client's quality of life.

Although thousands of individuals have suffered and died from AIDS each year, the palliative care needs of HIV/AIDS clients have been largely neglected by organizations involved in medical care.[13] In the past, persons with AIDS have not fit into the traditional models of palliative care, which were developed in response to the needs of those with cancer.[14] The problem has been that the unique challenges of AIDS care, specifically the severity, complexity, and unpredictable trajectory of the disease,[15] have blurred the distinction between what was previously understood as curative care and what was considered supportive palliative care. It is now understood that clients with AIDS require not only the treatment of chronic debilitating conditions, but also the treatment of superimposed acute opportunistic infections and related symptoms. Intravenous therapy and blood transfusions, as well as preventive measures, such as ongoing intravenous therapy to prevent blindness from CMV retinitis, may be necessary if clients with AIDS are to maintain their quality of life.[6] In addition to the pain and suffering related to the various disease processes, new treatments may also give rise to symptoms and side effects. Palliative care may therefore be beneficial in ensuring tolerance of and compliance with difficult treatment regimens.

As a result, there has been increasing recognition of the importance of palliative care for clients with HIV/AIDS and the realization that as people live longer with the disease, the chance of their experiencing symptoms and needing palliation increases.[1] It is further understood that, although new treatments for AIDS hold promise, the quality of life for people with AIDS may still be compromised. In AIDS care, short-term aggressive curative therapy is often important in treating acute infections, while the overall goal may remain palliation.[16]

Palliative care may be administered throughout the disease continuum and may be concurrent with restorative and curative treatment.[12] The management decisions for clients with advanced AIDS revolves around the rate of progression of the disease, the ratio between the benefits and burdens of the various diagnostic and treatment modalities, and the client's expectations and goals, as well as future anticipated problems. Health care providers and clients together must determine the appropriate time to shift the balance and focus to a palliative rather than curative effort, particularly in the face of increasing debility, weight loss, and deteriorating cognitive function, which herald the onset of the terminal stage of AIDS.[17]

The complex needs of clients and families living with HIV/AIDS require a multidisciplinary team effort involving physicians, nurses, social workers, dieticians, physiotherapists, and clergy, particularly as the end of life approaches.[1,18] Given the belief that illness affects all family members, and that active participation of the family is beneficial, the "unit of care" is comprised of the client and family.[2] The palliative care team offers not only a support system to help clients live as actively as possible until death, but also a support system to help the family cope during the client's illness and in their own bereavement.[2]

An interdisciplinary approach also enables health care professionals to meet client's needs across a variety of health care settings. In the acute care setting, clients with advanced HIV disease may, at the request of their primary care provider, be seen by the palliative care consultation team or be admitted to the institution's inpatient palliative unit. Clients with advanced disease may also be admitted to a hospice care program, which may be an inpatient program or based in the community, a skilled nursing facility, or the client's home.

Today many acute care facilities are opening units dedicated to palliation. Nurses working in this emerging nursing specialty must be particularly skilled in the alleviation of suffering, pain and symptom management, and end-of-life care. What follows is a brief discussion of the practice of palliative care nursing.

PALLIATIVE CARE NURSING—NURSING ASSESSMENT AND MANAGEMENT

PAIN

Critical to the assessment and management of pain is the provider's acceptance of the definition of pain as what the client says it is and occurring when the client says it does. Like the pain experienced by clients with cancer, pain in advanced AIDS is more common and intense, with nearly two thirds of clients reporting pain.[19] The successful management of pain requires complete and continual reassessment of pain, and the following nursing interventions:

1. Pain assessment is comprised of the client's description of the pain, including its duration, location, intensity, and quality; the history of the pain (recent or ongoing); the associated physical and emotional symptoms; the history of successful and unsuccessful attempts at reducing or eliminating the pain; and the effect of pain on quality of life, including emotional, social, or economic aspects. It should also be realized that clients might suffer from pain at more than one site. In clients with AIDS, the common sites of pain include the lower extremities (e.g., peripheral neuropathy), abdomen, oral cavity, esophagus, skin, perirectal area, chest, joints, muscles, and head (i.e., headache).[15]
2. A complete physical examination should be conducted in order to determine the cause of pain and appropriate laboratory or radiological studies should be reviewed.
3. Pain should be quantified by using numeric or descriptive scales (Fig. 11-1) to assess the intensity of pain from the client's perspective.

Given the diversity of each client's characteristics and the uniqueness of each pain experience, the plan of care should be individualized using the World Health Organization's three-step guideline or "analgesic ladder" (Box 11-1). Management of pain must also be focused on treating the underlying cause, since pain often indicates treatable disease or injury. For clients with HIV/AIDS, pain arising from infection should be alleviated with treatment of the underlying infection, as in the case of candida, which can cause oral pain, or toxoplasmosis, which can cause headache.[20]

Simple Descriptive Pain Intensity Scale

No Pain	Mild Pain	Moderate Pain	Severe Pain	Very Severe Pain	Worst Possible Pain

0-10 Numeric Pain Intensity Scale[*]

0 No Pain	1	2	3	4	5 Moderate Pain	6	7	8	9	10 Worst Possible Pain

Visual Analog Scale (VAS)[*]

No Pain	Worst Possible Pain

[*]A 10 cm baseline is recommended.

Figure 11-1. Pain Intensity Scales. (*From Acute Pain Management Guideline Panel: Acute pain management: operative or medical procedures and trauma, clinical practice guideline, Rockville, Md, Agency for Health Care Policy and Research, Public Health Service, US Department of Health and Human Services, February, 1992 [Publication, No. 92-0032].*)

Clients with advanced HIV may experience painful peripheral neuropathy, which can be treated by tricyclic antidepressants (see Chapter 22). Tricyclic antidepressants are also useful in treating concurrent depression and pain-related sleep disturbances. With tricyclic antidepressants, the onset of analgesia is within 1 or 2 weeks of drug administration, with peak effects occurring in 4 to 6 weeks.[15] Within the context of a terminal illness, pain may also respond to the use of radiation. Radiation can serve a palliative function by lessening the size of a tumor, as well as the perception of pain.

The principles of pain medication administration in palliative care for clients with AIDS are the same as for clients with cancer and include regularity of dosing, individualization of dosing, and usage of drug combinations (Box 11-2).[15] The single most important rule in the management of all symptoms, including pain, is to anticipate the symptom and attempt to prevent it. If the symptom does occur, it should be treated with subsequent regular dosing of medication to prevent symptom recurrence.[13]

Client and provider concerns about addiction to pain medications can be a barrier to effective pain management. It should be emphasized that addiction is a compulsive craving for a drug for effects other than

BOX 11-1 WORLD HEALTH ORGANIZATION GUIDELINES FOR AN ANALGESIC LADDER

Step 1: For Mild Pain

Use a nonopioid analgesic such as nonsteroidal antiinflammatory drugs (NSAIDs), acetaminophen, or aspirin, with or without adjuvant medications such as anticonvulsants, corticosteroids, antidepressants, psychostimulants, or phenothiazine, which enhance analgesic efficacy or provide analgesic activity for distinct types of pain, such as neuropathic discomfort.

Step 2: If Mild Pain Persists or Increases or Client Presents with Mild to Moderate Pain

A weak opioid such as codeine, hydrocodone, oxycodone, or propoxyphene is added to the non-opioid analgesics and adjuvant therapy used in step 1.

Step 3: If Moderate Pain Persists or Increases or Client Presents with Moderate to Severe Pain

A strong opioid such as morphine, hydromorphone, methadone, levorphanol, fentanyl, or meperidine should be prescribed in place of the weak opioid and the nonopioid analgesics; adjuvant therapy can be continued or discontinued.

Note: NSAIDs have a ceiling effect, meaning that an increase in dosage above the recommended maximum dosage has no additional analgesic effect. In contrast, opioids do not have a ceiling effect, and therefore the dosage of opioids can be increased until clients state that pain has been relieved.

pain relief and is extremely uncommon in terminally ill clients. Addiction should not be confused with physical dependence, which is an expected physiological response to the use of opioids. Physical dependence will occur after 3 or 4 weeks of opioid administration, evidenced by withdrawal symptoms upon abrupt discontinuation. If a drug is to be discontinued, halving the daily dose every 1 to 2 days, until the dose is equivalent to 15 mg of morphine, can be effective in reducing withdrawal symptoms.[2] *Tolerance* of medication, defined as the need for increasing amounts of medication to achieve the same analgesic effect, is another expected physiological response. Increasing the dosage of the medication or adding adjuvant therapy to potentiate the action of the opioid is appropriate and of benefit in achieving pain relief. Client and family education should emphasize that physical dependence and tolerance to pain medications does not imply addiction, and therefore pain medications should not be withheld.

Health care providers in palliative care are often concerned with the administration of opioids to clients with a history of intravenous drug use. However, clients with substance abuse disorders must also receive effective pain management. Health care providers should openly discuss the substance-related problem with the client and family, and consultation should be obtained with specialists in the field. Because it limits the

BOX 11-2 PRINCIPLES OF PAIN MANAGEMENT

- Use medications that are appropriate to the severity and specific type of pain, based on the World Health Organization guidelines for the analgesia ladder (see Box 11-1).
- Give medications in amounts sufficient to control the pain and at intervals appropriate to the medication's duration.
- When changing medications, use equi-analgesic conversions (Table 11-1).
- Use oral medications when possible with controlled-release morphine, the drug of choice for clients with chronic pain, yet choose the route of drug administration most appropriate for the client and one that will maximize analgesic effect.
- Give medications around the clock at regular intervals (generally every 4 hours) so that a constant blood level concentration is maintained.
- Use rescue analgesic for breakthrough pain. The rescue dose is usually given every 4 hours by mouth and is 25% of the scheduled regular dose of opioid drug.
- Prevent, assess, and treat side effects and complications of medications (e.g., constipation from narcotics, nausea).
- Assess for tolerance, as manifested by shortened or diminished effects of analgesics. Give increased amounts of medications or decrease time interval between doses when tolerance is determined.

abuse potential, consistent use of a standard pain scale and regular monitoring of drug consumption by the nurse and the primary care provider can be helpful in ongoing assessment and pain management. Whenever possible, the oral route of medication is preferred, as it has a lower abuse potential than parenteral administration. As substance-abusing clients have a greater tolerance to morphine derivatives and benzodiazepines, increased doses may be necessary for effective pain management or it may be necessary to shorten the interval between doses. Given the possibility of hepatic failure in such clients, dosage of medications should be carefully monitored to avoid overdosing. Simultaneous use of agonists and antagonists are avoided in this population, as they may rapidly provoke withdrawal symptoms. Withdrawal symptoms can be treated effectively with benzodiazepine, clonidine, antispasmodics, or antiinflammatory agents.[9]

OTHER SYMPTOMS

Clients with HIV/AIDS also experience symptoms other than pain at all of the various stages of the illness that may be exacerbated as the disease progresses. In a study of 1128 HIV-infected, ambulatory clients, the most frequently reported symptoms other than pain were fatigue (65%), anorexia (34%), cough (32%), and fever (29%).[21] In a sample of 207 clients with AIDS, 50% of the participants experienced symptoms of shortness

Table 11-1	Equianalgesic Dosage of Weak and Strong Opioids		

Drug	Route	Equianalgesic Dose (mg)*	Recommended Schedule
Weak Opioids			
Codeine	Oral	200	q3-6h
	Intramuscular	130	q3-6h
Propoxyphene	Oral	65-130	q4-6h
Hydrocodone	Oral	N/A	q4-6h
Oxycodone	Oral	30	q3-6h
Strong Opioids			
Immediate-release oral morphine	Oral	30	q2-4h
Controlled-release morphine	Oral	30	q8-12h
Morphine	Intramuscular	10	q2-4h
Hydromorphone	Oral	7.5	q2-4h
	Intramuscular	1.5	q2-6h
Levorphanol	Oral	4	q4-8h
	Intramuscular	2	q4-8h
Methadone	Oral	20	q4-12h
	Intramuscular	10	q4-12h
Meperidine	Oral	300	q2-4h
	Intramuscular	75	q2-4h

*The equianalgesic dose is the amount that provides analgesia equivalent to 10 mg of intramuscular morphine. The equianalgesic dose should not be interpreted as the starting dose, but rather as a guide, particularly when switching drugs or changing the route of administration.

Adapted from Patt RB, Szalados JE, Wu CL: Appendix C: pharmacotherapeutic guidelines. In Patt RB, ed: *Cancer pain*, Philadelphia, 1993, Lippincott.

of breath, dry mouth, insomnia, weight loss, and headaches.[22] Understanding the causes of, presentations of, and nursing interventions for common symptoms (Table 11-2) is important in enhancing the quality of life of clients with AIDS. For effective symptom management, assessment of all body systems is necessary, and clients should be encouraged to report all symptoms, as well as changes in the quality of symptoms as the illness progresses. The relief of physical suffering by the management of various symptoms often affords clients and families the energy they need to deal with many other end-of-life issues.

END-OF-LIFE CARE

Advanced planning is an important issue related to end-of-life care for clients with HIV/AIDS. Nurses, as members of the palliative care team, can assist clients and families with end-of-life issues by:

1. Ensuring that the client understands the benefits of health care and other social support programs, such as unemployment insurance,

Table 11-2	Selected Symptoms Associated with HIV/AIDS		
Symptoms	**Causes**	**Presentation**	**Nursing Interventions**
Fatigue (asthenia)	• HIV infection • Opportunistic infections • AIDS medications • Prolonged immobility • Anemia • Sleep disorders • Hypothyroidism • Medications	• Weakness • Lack of energy	• Pace activities according to client's tolerance • Schedule rest periods or naps • Ensure adequate nutrition • Use relaxation exercises • Encourage meditation • Suggest warm (rather than hot) showers or baths • Keep room temperatures cool • Administer dextroamphetamine 10 mg PO daily as ordered
Anorexia (loss of appetite) and cachexia (wasting)	• Metabolic alterations caused by cytokines and interleukin 1 • Opportunistic infections • Intestinal nutrient malabsorption • Chronic diarrhea • Depression • Taste disorders	• Diminished food intake • Profound weight loss	• Consult with dietitian about food choices • Make food appealing in color and texture • Avoid noxious odors at mealtime • Avoid fatty, fried, and strong-smelling foods • Offer small frequent meals and nutritious snacks • Encourage clients to eat whatever is appealing • Provide high-energy, high-protein liquid supplements • Use appetite stimulants as ordered, such as megestrol acetate 800 mg/day PO qd or bid • Administer testosterone as ordered by 5 mg transdermal patch to increase weight and muscle mass • Administer dronabinol 2.5 mg PO qd or bid

Continued

Note: The nurse should ensure that an appropriate diagnostic workup is implemented for symptoms as indicated.
Adapted from Ferris F et al: *Palliative care: a comprehensive guide for the care of persons with HIV disease*, Ontario, Canada, 1995, Mount Sinai Hospital/Casey House Hospice.

Table 11-2 Selected Symptoms Associated with HIV/AIDS—cont'd

Symptoms	Causes	Presentation	Nursing Interventions
Fever (elevated body temperature)	• Bacterial toxins • Viruses • Yeast • Antigen-antibody reactions • Drugs • Tumor products • Exogenous pyrogens	• Body temperature greater than 99.5° F (oral), 100.5° F (rectal), or 98.5° F (axillary) • Chills, rigor • Sweating, night sweats • Delirium • Dizziness • Dehydration	• Maintain fluid intake • Provide loose clothing and sheets with frequent changing • Avoid plastic bed coverings • Exceptionally high temperature may require ice packs or cooling blankets • Administer around-the-clock antipyretics as ordered, such as acetaminophen or aspirin 325-650 mg PO q6-8h
Dyspnea (shortness of breath) and cough	• Bronchospasm • Embolism • Effusions • Pulmonary edema • Pneumothorax • Kaposi's sarcoma • Obstruction	• Productive or non-productive cough • Crackles • Stridor • Hemoptysis • Inability to clear secretions	• Elevate bed to Fowler's or high Fowler's position • Provide abdominal splints • Administer humidified oxygen therapy to treat dyspnea • Use fans or open windows to keep air moving for dyspnea • Remove irritants or allergens, such as smoke • Teach pursed-lip breathing for clients with chronic obstructive pulmonary disease

	• Opportunistic infections • Anxiety • Allergy • Mechanical or chemical irritants • Anemia	• Wheezing • Tachypnea • Gagging • Intercostal retractions • Areas of pulmonary dullness • Anxiety	• Encourage frequent mouth care to decrease discomfort from dry mouth • Treat bronchospasm • Suppress cough as ordered with dextromethorphan hydrobromide 15-45 mg PO q4h prn; or with opioids, such as codeine 15-60 mg PO q4h, even if taking other opioids for pain, or hydrocodone 5-10 mg PO q4-6h prn, or morphine 5-20 mg PO q4h prn (may be increased) to relieve dyspnea, cough, and associated anxiety • For hyperactive gag reflex use nebulized lidocaine as ordered 5 ml of 2% solution (100 mg) q3-4h prn
Diarrhea	• Idiopathic HIV enteropathy • Diet • Bowel infections (e.g., bacteria, parasites, protozoa) • Chronic bowel inflammation • Medications • Obstruction with overflow incontinence • Stress • Malabsorption	• Flatulence • Multiple bowel movements per day • Cramps or colic • Hemorrhoids	• Maintain adequate hydration • Replace electrolytes with Gatorade or Pedialyte. • Offer rice, bananas, or apple juice to reduce diarrhea • Increase protein and calories • Avoid dairy products, alcohol, caffeine, extremely hot or cold foods, and spicy or fatty foods • Provide an atmosphere in which dignity is maintained while toileting • Provide ready access to bathroom or commode • Maintain good perianal care • Administer medications as ordered such as Lomotil 2.5-5 mg q4-6h; Kapectalin 60-120 ml q4-6h (not to exceed 20 mg/day); Immodium 2-4 mg q6h (not to exceed 16 mg/day); or paregoric (tincture of opium) 5-10 ml q4-6h

Note: The nurse should ensure that an appropriate diagnostic workup is implemented for symptoms as indicated. Adapted from Ferris F et al: *Palliative care: a comprehensive guide for the care of persons with HIV disease*, Ontario, Canada, 1995, Mount Sinai Hospital/Casey House Hospice.

Continued

Table 11-2 Selected Symptoms Associated with HIV/AIDS—cont'd

Symptoms	Causes	Presentation	Nursing Interventions
Insomnia (inability to fall asleep or stay asleep)	• Anxiety • Depression • Pain • Medications • Delirium • Sleep disorders such as sleep apnea • Excessive alcohol intake • Caffeine	• Early morning awakening • Nighttime restlessness • Fear • Nightmares	• Establish a bedtime routine • Reduce daytime napping • Avoid caffeinated beverages and alcohol • Have client take a warm bath 2 hours before bedtime • Use relaxation techniques • Provide an environment conducive to sleep (e.g., dark, quiet, at a comfortable temperature) • Administer anxiolytics as ordered such as benzodiazepines (use for less than 2 weeks because of dependency), antidepressants (helpful over long term), or other sedatives (e.g., Benadryl)
Headache	• Infections such as encephalitis, herpes zoster, meningitis, toxoplasmosis • Sinusitis	• Pain in one or more areas of the head or over sinuses	• Suggest chiropractic manipulation • Provide massage therapy • Use relaxation therapy • Apply transcutaneous electrical nerve stimulation (TENS) if ordered • Use stepwise analgesia as ordered • Administer corticosteroids as ordered to reduce swellings around space-occupying lesions

Note: The nurse should ensure that an appropriate diagnostic workup is implemented for symptoms as indicated. Adapted from Ferris F et al: *Palliative care: a comprehensive guide for the care of persons with HIV disease*, Ontario, Canada, 1995, Mount Sinai Hospital/Casey House Hospice.

worker's compensation, pension plans, insurance, and union or association benefit packages. The nurse should ensure that the client and family members are able to access appropriate documents and information.

2. Ensuring that financial matters are in order, such as powers of attorney on bank accounts, credit cards, property, legal claims, and income tax preparation.

3. Discussing advance directives or power of attorney for care and treatment (see Box 11-3).

4. Discussing decisions related to the setting and manner of death, including who the client wants at the bedside, what rituals are important, whether an autopsy should be performed, what arrangements the client wants regarding funeral services and burial, and where donations in remembrance should be sent. It is important to realize that these issues should be discussed at appropriate stages in the person's illness, respecting the client's ability and wish to do so, in a way that promotes the client's sense of control over his or her life and death.

5. Clients and families may also express concern about writing the diagnosis of AIDS on the death certificate for fear of stigmatization in their communities. Physicians may write a nonspecific diagnosis on the main death certificate and sign section B on the reverse side to signify to the registrar general that further information will be available at a later date.

HOPE AND SPIRITUAL WELL-BEING

Maintaining a sense of hope is important for clients who are terminally ill. However, hope may shift away from the hope for cure toward the hope that the client will live for at least a particular amount of time (e.g., for an important family event). Hope for cure may also shift to the hope for a peaceful, dignified death—without physical pain or suffering, in the company of supportive and significant others, in the setting or context of the client's choice, and with the knowledge that the client's end-of-life wishes will be honored.

The spiritual care of the client may present unique opportunities for personal growth and transcendence. The assessment of client and family spiritual values and needs should occur before the progression of illness and the approach of death. Spiritual assessment includes an assessment of the client's beliefs about the meaning and purpose in life and connection with self, others, and God. This knowledge may inform interventions that promote spiritual well-being. The nurse can assist the client to maintain hope and spiritual growth through the following interventions:

1. The client should be assisted with life review. Life review helps individuals to find meaning in their lives and to face death with dignity. Clients and families should be encouraged to tell their life stories and reflect on the mistakes and accomplishments of the past. This provides opportunities for growth even at the end of life and a sense of integrity versus despair.

2. Clients and families should be assisted in finding meaning in the face of adversity. This begins with encouraging the client and family to discuss feelings, issues, and concerns and to recognize past successful ways of coping and their unique internal strengths.

3. Open communication between client and family should be encouraged. This can help resolve old issues and be an opportunity to express feelings of love and support.

4. In the face of life-threatening illness, clients may express anger at God if they view their illness as a punishment or believe that God is not answering their prayers for cure and recovery. The expression of feelings, while exploring the perception of suffering in accordance with their religious affiliation, may offer a new perspective and be a source of spiritual comfort. Clergy serve as valuable members of the palliative care team in offering spiritual support to clients and families and alleviating spiritual distress.

5. For individuals who have no religious affiliation but who express spiritual needs or concerns, the use of imagery, meditation, or spiritual readings can promote a sense of harmony and peace. Very often the greatest spiritual comfort that can be offered to any individual is active listening and meaningful presence. Simply sitting with a client or family member and holding their hand can convey a deep level of caring and commitment, and the promise that they will not be abandoned and left to suffer alone. Often this relationship is of mutual benefit, as persons with AIDS teach their families and health care providers how to transcend suffering and how to die with grace and dignity.

THROUGH THE DYING TRAJECTORY

The unpredictable course of HIV infection imposes a great deal of uncertainty regarding the illness and dying trajectory. Death is usually due to multiple causes, including chronic infections, malignancies, neurological disease, malnutrition, and multisystem failure.[23] However, even for clients with HIV/AIDS in whom death appears to be imminent, spontaneous recovery with survival of several more weeks or months is possible. The terminal stage is often marked by a period of increasing weight loss and deteriorating physical and cognitive functioning.[17] The general rule related to mortality is that the greater the cumulative number of opportunistic infections or illnesses, complications, or deviance of serologic or immunologic markers, the less the survival time.[15] Survival time is also decreased by psychosocial factors such as a decrease in physical and emotional support because of increased demands on the caregivers, feelings of hopelessness, and older age (greater than 39 years).[24] Decisions related to diagnosis, treatment, and prevention thus pose ethical and clinical issues for both clients and their health care providers in the terminal stage of infection—specifically, decisions related to the frequency of laboratory monitoring, use of invasive procedures, use of antiretroviral and prophylactic measures, and participation in clinical trails.[15]

For clients in the terminal stage of HIV/AIDS, as for persons with other terminal illnesses, palliative care ideally facilitates a personal acceptance of death. The end of life is an important time for individuals to accept their own shortcomings and limitations and differences with significant others so that death may be accepted without physical, psychosocial, or spiritual anguish.[2] This can be facilitated by reducing internal conflicts, such as fears about loss of control; promoting a sense of identity; supporting the client in maintaining important interpersonal relationships; and encouraging clients to identify and attempt to reach meaningful, though limited, goals.[10] Encouraging clients and families to express feelings through such statements as "I love you," "I forgive you," "Forgive me—I am sorry," "Thank you," and "Goodbye," is important to the completion of relationships.[25] Peaceful death can occur as families give the client "permission" to die, and assure them that they will be remembered.[1]

RESPONSES TO LOSS AND BEREAVEMENT IN HIV/AIDS

The close and continual contact with clients and families during the progression of illness enables nurses to identify their fears and concerns. Although many of the acute illnesses experienced by clients may be treated, clients and families must come to terms with continued decline in health and multiple losses. Such losses include the loss of identity, as they perceive their status changing to that of an "AIDS victim"; loss of control over their health; loss of sexual expression because of changes related to safer sexual behavior; loss of body image due to weight loss, wasting, and the lesions of Kaposi's sarcoma; loss of relationships due to the death of others from the disease or rejection by friends or family; and loss of a lifestyle, often due to changes in financial status.[26]

In addition, each occurrence of illness reinforces the eventuality of death and associated fears. Occurrences of illness can be opportunities for nurses to approach the subject of dying and death and to recognize cues sent by clients and families indicating their concerns and feelings. Upon the death of a client, bereavement counseling should be available to friends and family to help them recognize normal responses to grief (Box 11-4).[27] The support of health care professionals and family is important in assisting the bereaved through the tasks of grieving, which are identified by Worden[28] as: (1) accepting the reality of the death; (2) experiencing the pain of grief; (3) adjusting to a changed physical, emotional, and social environment in which the deceased is missing; and (4) finding an appropriate emotional place for the deceased person in the emotional life of the bereaved. Alan Wolfelt[29] describes the tasks of mourning as: (1) experiencing and expressing outside oneself the reality of the death; (2) tolerating the emotional suffering that is inherent in the work of grief, while nurturing oneself both physically and emotionally; (3) converting the relationship with the deceased from one of presence to one of memory;

BOX 11-3 ADVANCE DIRECTIVES

If an individual is competent and anticipates the future loss of competency, he or she may initiate an *advance directive*, which refers to a living will or designation of a health care proxy who is to carry out the client's health care wishes and decisions in the event that the client becomes incompetent. The client may also give an individual the power of attorney with regard to financial matters and care or treatment issues. Advance directives include the client's wishes regarding the use of life-sustaining treatments such as cardiopulmonary resuscitation, vasoactive medications to sustain blood pressure or heart rate, dialysis, artificial nutrition and hydration, and ventilatory support.

Initiation of an advance directive is often done in consultation with the client's primary care provider. The signing of advance directives must be witnessed by at least two individuals who are not related to the client or involved in his or her treatment. Individuals who are mentally competent can revoke their advance directives at any time. If a client is deemed mentally incompetent, state statutes may allow the court to designate a surrogate decision-maker for the client. Advance directives should be placed in the client's medical record or in an area that all health care providers can access. Nursing personnel should review their institution's policy on the review and renewal of advance directives.

(4) developing a new self-identity based on life without the deceased; and (5) relating the experience of loss to a context of meaning.

Given the stigma attached to AIDS and to death in general, clients with AIDS and their close family and friends are often isolated in their grief and may have difficulty in accomplishing the tasks of mourning. The complications of AIDS-related grief often come from secrecy that results from the social stigma associated with the disease.[30] Reluctance to contact family and friends can restrict the normal support systems available for the bereaved. Families and partners of clients with AIDS may experience *disenfranchised grief*, defined as the grief that persons experience when they incur a loss that is not openly acknowledged, publicly mourned, or socially supported.[31] Through clear, truthful, and sensitive communication, nurses can offer families support in their grief and promote trust that their needs are understood and validated. Cultural differences related to loss and grief must also be acknowledged to enhance a sense of dignity in the lives of all who are touched by the illness.

Clients with AIDS need both active and palliative care. In some clients, the focus of care shifts from the management of a single treatable infection to the suppression of multiple chronic infections and malignancies. If appropriate, the goal of treatment changes from cure to the relief of physical, emotional, social, and spiritual suffering and, ultimately, a dignified death. Health care providers have a responsibility to be knowledgeable about the various treatment options and resources available for

BOX 11-4 NORMAL RESPONSES TO GRIEF

- Emotional release (e.g., crying, screaming, constant tearfulness)
- Sense of losing one's mind
- Feelings of depression, irritability, numbness, shock, isolation, yearning, and longing
- Restlessness or aimless wandering
- Sense of frustration with others
- Panic, self-doubt, and confusion
- Guilt feelings
- Hostility, anger, or rage
- Physical symptoms of distress (e.g., sighing, trouble catching breath, heaviness in the chest, loss of appetite, tightness in the throat, weight loss, insomnia, exhaustion)
- Reexperiencing feelings related to previous deaths
- Telling and retelling stories about the loved one and death experience
- Assuming traits of the deceased
- Expecting the deceased to appear, or having a sense of their presence
- Increased dreaming about the deceased
- Questioning purpose and meaning in life
- Reevaluating goals and values
- Gradually overcoming grief feelings
- Restitution—readjustment to life with and without the deceased

pain and symptom management and should encourage clients to be active partners in developing and implementing the plan of care. The control of pain and many other symptoms related to HIV/AIDS enables both client and family to expend their energies on spiritual and emotional healing, with the opportunity for personal growth and transcendence. Palliative care thus preserves a person's quality of life by protecting his or her integrity, reducing perceived helplessness, and lessening the threat of exhausting coping resources.[5] Overall, palliative care seeks to alleviate all aspects of personal suffering for the client and family by comprehensive care and respect of client and family goals and end-of-life wishes. Ira Byock believes that through competent and compassionate end-of-life care, clients can achieve a sense of inner well-being, and that for families the death of a loved one may be as precious as it is painful: "When the human dimension of dying is nurtured, for many the transition from life can become as profound, intimate and precious as the miracle of birth."[28]

REFERENCES

1. O'Neill J, Alexander C: Palliative medicine and HIV/AIDS, *HIV/AIDS Management in Office Practice* 24(3):607, 1997.
2. Bone R: Hospice and palliative care, *Dis Mon* 61(12):773, 1995.

3. *Palliative care core precepts,* 1997, Last Acts Palliative Care Task Force. http://www.lastacts.org

4. George RJ: Palliation in AIDS: where do we draw the line? *Genitourinary Medicine* 67(1):85, 1991.

5. Bayes R: A way to screen for suffering in palliative care. *J Palliat Care* 13(2):22, 1997.

6. Higginson I: Palliative care: a review of past changes and future trends, *J Public Health Med* 15(1):3, 1993.

7. Storey, P: *Primer of palliative care,* Gainsville, Fla, 1994, The Academy of Hospice Physicians.

8. Knaus W et al: A controlled trial to improve care for seriously ill hospitalized patients, *JAMA* 274(20):1591, 1995.

9. Ferris F et al: *Palliative care: a comprehensive guide for the care of persons with HIV disease,* Ontario, Canada, 1995, Mount Sinai Hospital/Casey House Hospice.

10. Breitbart W, Jaramillo, Chochinov H: Psychooncology research: the road less traveled, the road ahead, *J Psychosom Res* 45(3):185, 1998.

11. Goldstone I: Trends in hospital utilization in AIDS care 1987-1991: implications for palliative care, *J Palliat Care* 8(4):22, 1992.

12. Bloomer S: Palliative care, *J Assoc Nurses AIDS Care* 9(2):45, 1998.

13. Walsh TD: An overview of palliative care in cancer and AIDS, *Oncology* 3:7, 1991.

14. Foley FJ et al: AIDS palliative care: challenging the palliative paradigm, *J Palliat Care* 11(2):19, 1995.

15. Kemp C, Stepp L: Palliative care for patients with acquired immunodeficiency syndrome, *Am J Hospice Palliat Care* 12(6):14, 1995.

16. Fraser J: Sharing the challenge: the integration of cancer and AIDS, *J Palliat Care* 11(2):23, 1995.

17. Glare PA: Palliative care in acquired immunodeficiency syndrome (AIDS): problems and practicalities, *Ann Acad Med Singapore* 23(2):235, 1994.

18. Post L, Dubler N: Palliative care: a bioethical definition, principles, and clinical guidelines, *Bioethics Forum* 13(3):17, 1997.

19. Singer EJ et al: Painful symptoms reported in ambulant HIV-infected men in a longitudinal study, *Pain* 54:15, 1993.

20. American Pain Society: *Principles of analgesic use in the treatment of acute pain and cancer pain,* ed 3, Skokie, Ill, 1992, American Pain Society.

21. Fantoni et al: Multicenter study on the prevalence of symptoms and somatic treatment in HIV infection, Central Italy PRESINT Group, *J Palliat Care* 13(2):9, 1997.

22. Holzemer W, Henry S, Reilly C: Assessing and managing pain in AIDS care: the patient perspective, *J Assoc Nurses AIDS Care* 9(1):22, 1998.

23. Wood C, Whittet S, Bradbeer C: ABCs of palliative care, *BMJ* 315(7120):1433, 1997.

24. Goldstone et al: Patterns of care in advanced HIV disease in a tertiary treatment center, *AIDS Care* 7(Suppl 10):47, 1995.

25. Byock I: *Dying well: the prospect for growth at the end of life,* New York, 1997, Riverhead Books.

26. Welsby P, Richardson A, Brettle R: AIDS: aspects in adults. In Doyle D, Hanks G, MacDonald N, eds: *Oxford textbook of palliative medicine,* ed 2, New York, 1998, Oxford University Press.

27. Klein SJ: *Heavenly hurts: surviving AIDS-related deaths and losses,* New York, 1998, Baywood.
28. Worden J: *Grief counseling and grief therapy: a handbook for the mental health practitoner,* New York, 1991, Springer Publications.
29. Wolfelt A: Reconciliation needs of the mourner: reworking a critical concept in caring for the bereaved, *Thanatos,* Spring 1998 (newsletter).
30. Maxwell N: Responses to loss and bereavement in HIV, *Professional Nurse* 12(1):21, 1996.
31. Doka K: *Disenfranchised grief: recognizing hidden sorrow,* Lexington, Mass, 1989, Lexington Books.

Unit III   Frequently Asked Questions

I have just learned that I have TB. Is it possible that my family or friends have caught TB from me?

Yes, it is possible that someone may have caught TB from you, and this is why all cases of TB are reported to the health department. Health department workers will contact people who might possibly have caught the TB germ so they can be tested and receive treatment if they need it. Most people who come into contact with TB will not get sick even if the TB germ gets into their body. However, if this happens, they will have to take medicine to prevent the germ from causing infection.

How long will everyone who comes in to my hospital room have to wear a special mask?

People coming into your room will have to wear the masks until it is sure that your TB cannot be transmitted to anyone else. After you have been taking TB medications for a certain period of time, other people won't be able to catch TB from you because your sputum (i.e., phlegm that you cough up) will no longer have the TB germ in it. However, the period of time it takes for this to happen is different for each individual and is determined by checking your sputum regularly to see if it contains the germ that causes TB. When three consecutive sputum specimens do not contain the germ and your health is improving, then it is sure that no one can catch TB from you. Then people can stop wearing the masks. However, your sputum will be rechecked several times to make sure that it still does not contain the germ.

Can I have my viral load measured while I am in the hospital?

It is neither common nor advisable to measure viral load or CD_4 cell counts while you are in the hospital. Illness often raises the viral load and decreases the CD_4 cell count, particularly if you have an infection. When you are discharged from the hospital, your physician may want to see you within 1 to 2 weeks. If you are completely well your physician will then obtain a specimen for viral load and CD_4 cell count determination.

Will I have to take care of this intravenous line in my arm after I go home from the hospital? How long will it have to stay in?

You have a special intravenous (IV) line in your arm called a peripherally inserted central catheter (PICC). This is a special catheter that is similar to a regular IV but is placed near your heart so that you can receive infusions in the home. It will need to remain in place for as long as you need to receive this medication. You should be taught how to care for your catheter at home while you are in the hospital, beginning with how to flush (rinse) the catheter, which must be done daily. When you are discharged a visiting nurse should come to your home and continue the teaching that was started in the hospital. The visiting nurse will meet with you as many times as necessary to ensure that you or your family members can care for this catheter adequately; it is the goal of the home care nurse to ensure that you or your family can care for your catheter with minimum assistance from the nurse.

I have heard the term the "Lazarus Effect"—what does this mean?

The "Lazarus Effect" is sometimes used to describe clients with AIDS who, as a result of HAART therapy, have returned from a debilitated and dying state to a relatively healthy and productive life. Although HAART therapy has given many people a chance for a new and productive life, it can also cause a series of problems.[1] It may cause feelings of guilt, because these drugs are not available to everyone who needs them (e.g., the poor, the uninsured, those in underdeveloped countries); or, simply, because they have survived while others they know have died. Second, it may create difficulties in reestablishing relationships. Old friends may have stopped coming by if you were very ill and you may have become isolated. Finally, it can cause problems related to work. Now that people with AIDS are no longer expected simply to die, there is pressure to go back to work. This may create feelings of excitement, fear, or confusion. It may cause anxiety about the possible prospect of losing disability payments. Also, your job skills may have deteriorated. Or, after having come so close to death, you may no longer find your old jobs fulfilling. You may also feel that if HAART begins to fail you, you may lose your jobs again.

How does one distinguish between sadness, grief, and depression?

Sadness and grief are well correlated with changes in life circumstances. Major depression, on the other hand, produces changes that are out of proportion to changes in life circumstances. People who have major depression are likely to exhibit the following: sadness, anxiety, irritability, apathy, low energy with a decreased sense of vitality, insomnia (especially with middle of the night or early morning awakening), decreased appetite, decreased interest in sex, inappropriate feelings of self-blame, guilt, worthlessness, loss of interest or pleasure in usual activities, tendency toward social isolation, and hopelessness, sometimes with thoughts of suicide. In very severe cases, major depression may occur with delusions or hallucinations.[2] Rates of major depression are significantly higher among HIV-positive clients than in the general population. This is thought to be because of preexisting lifetime rates among at-risk populations. As HIV disease progresses, major depression may become more common. Major depression is very responsive to treatment with antidepressant drugs. No one single medication seems to be more effective than any other. There is no way of predicting in advance which drug will be most effective in an individual.

REFERENCES

1. Stine G: *Acquired immune deficiency syndrome: biological, medical, social, and legal issues,* ed 3, Upper Saddle River, New Jersey, 1998, Prentice Hall.
2. Fishman M, Treisman G: A guide to the use of antidepressants in HIV, *The Hopkins HIV Report,* May, 1997. http://www.ama-assn.org/special/hiv/treatmnt/hopkins/depress.htm#toc

Unit IV

Home Care Nursing of Clients with HIV/AIDS

12

Home Care Visitation: Nursing Assessment and Interventions

*Gail Kropf**

Clients in all stages of HIV illness are cared for in a variety of settings. Care in the community setting is an important option for clients with end-stage disease, and even clients with chronic stable disease often require the support of nursing services in the community through nursing case management. Nursing case management and the provision of home care services have been integral parts of AIDS care from the very beginning of the epidemic, and these continue today. The purpose of HIV/AIDS home care is to maintain the client in his or her home by providing services to meet health care needs identified by both the client and caregiver. The client may require various levels of services in the home. The levels range from housekeeping—carrying out household chores while the client recovers from illness—to skilled nursing services of various complexities. Other services provided to clients include mental health care, social and financial services, nutritional support, rehabilitation services, and referrals to community resources.

Home care services may be initiated through the process of discharge planning done while the client is hospitalized. Discharge planning is the process of preparing the client to return to the community. A plan for home care services may also be initiated in the primary care setting (e.g., physician's office or clinic). It is important for the nurse to understand the services provided by home health agencies to ensure that clients receive appropriate care in the home.

TYPES OF HOME CARE AGENCIES

There are basically two types of home care agencies: Certified Home Health Agencies (CHHAs) and Licensed Home Care Agencies (LHCAs). CHHAs are monitored by both their respective State's Department of Health and an accrediting agency such as the Joint Commission for Accreditation of Health Care Organizations. To be eligible to bill the federal government for the services they provide, CHHAs must meet strict governmental regula-

*The author and editors would like to acknowledge the contributions that Michele Crespo-Fierro and Carol Wetherbee made in the preparation of this manuscript.

197

tions. CHHAs may be affiliated with a hospital or be an independent (free-standing) organization. Hospital-affiliated agencies generally have a nurse or discharge planner on site that can review clients' needs for possible home care. Freestanding agencies usually receive referrals from hospitals, physicians, community-based organizations, and, in some cases, other home care agencies. CHHAs provide skilled nursing services, rehabilitative services, nutritional assessments, social work interventions, and home health aide (HHA) services. They can bill directly to Medicare, Medicaid, third-party payers, and clients for the services they provide. LHCAs provide the care permitted by their state license, which can include skilled nursing, HHA, rehabilitative, and social work services. Licensed agencies bill the client, and some third-party payers, directly but must bill through the CHHA for clients with Medicare, Medicaid, and other third-party payers. A major distinction among home care agencies is whether they are not-for-profit or for-profit. Not-for-profit agencies provide some services free of charge for indigent clients who are ineligible for insurance coverage.

REFERRAL TO AND PAYMENT FOR HOME CARE

To initiate a request for home care services, the discharge planner, primary care provider, or case manager notifies the home care agency of the intent to request services and then provides the agency with medical and nursing orders indicating the scope of service. The next step before home care services are provided is verifying the client's insurance coverage, which must be reviewed carefully so that the services provided will be within the insurance guidelines. (The staff of the home care agency often does this assessment.) Private insurance carriers, including managed care corporations, often require prior approval before any care can be initiated. These carriers often define the exact number and types of home care visits that are covered, the supplies and services that can be provided, and the expected discharge date of the client from service. Government-funded third-party payers (e.g., Medicare, Medicaid) provide standardized guidelines to CHHAs regarding the type and scope of services that can be provided. These guidelines are strictly enforced. Sometimes a client who has been accepted by Medicare or Medicaid may be provided with home care while the paperwork is still pending. Once the insurance carrier finalizes the paperwork, the billing may be retroactive to the start of care.

Clients without insurance or who do not qualify for Medicare or a public assistance program may be eligible for coverage via the Ryan White Care Act. The Ryan White Care Act represents the United States Federal Government's largest financial allocation specifically for HIV-related health and support services. Since fiscal year 1991, close to $6.4 billion in federal funds have been appropriated under the Ryan White Care Act to help people with little or no insurance pay their health care expenses.*

---

*Information courtesy of http://www.hrsa.gov/hab/.

Under Title II of the Ryan White Care Act, grants are awarded to states and other eligible areas (e.g., localities, territories) to improve the quality, availability, and organization of HIV health care and support services. In addition to other specific service programs, Title II also funds the AIDS Drug Assistance Program (ADAP). ADAP provides funds to pay for medications in all 50 States, the District of Columbia, Puerto Rico, the Virgin Islands, and Guam to low-income individuals with HIV infection who have limited or no coverage from private insurance or Medicaid. The administration of these funds, as well as whether additional funds are provided, varies from state to state. Obtaining these services often requires the expertise of a social worker. Most home care agencies employ social workers that can assist with these tasks.

THE HOME CARE VISIT: PREVISIT NURSING ACTIVITIES

Prior to visiting the client in the home, the nurse reviews the client referral form, which should indicate the client's needs based on the referring person's assessment. This form is a preliminary plan of care and may need to be modified based on a complete home nursing assessment. Prior to the visit, the client is called by the home care nurse, who arranges a time for the initial home evaluation, gets directions to the home, and determines if an HHA (i.e., a specialized paraprofessional) is needed at once, and, if so, arranges for one within the limits of the insurance coverage. The HHA may meet the nurse at the home during the initial evaluation. If supplies or equipment are needed, arrangements are made for their delivery to the home either before or during the initial visit.

An essential tool for the home care nurse is the nursing bag, which contains supplies for use in assessing and caring for the client. These include liquid soap, paper towels, nonsterile and sterile gloves, a stethoscope, a sphygmomanometer with different size cuffs (i.e., pediatric, adult, and large), sterile gauze and cotton swabs, paper tape, thermometers, alcohol swabs, syringes, disposable measuring tape, epinephrine, a glucometer and strips to assess blood glucose, and paper and plastic bags for trash disposal. Along with these items, the nurse should have the client's chart, the appropriate agency forms necessary for admission to home care, progress notes, and other forms that facilitate the provision of care in the home. If education regarding a specific topic is needed, then client education handouts are always advised. Some home care agencies use laptop computers for documentation of the nursing assessment. The client's chart is transferred to the computer before the visit and reviewed by the nurse. Once the assessment is completed and documented on the laptop, the client information is uploaded to the main computer for printout the following day. On the following day, the nurse reviews and signs the hard copy that is placed in the client's chart. Many home care agencies are participating in the Outcomes Assessment and Information Set

(OASIS) study, a federally supported initiative designed to assess and standardize home care needs. Agencies that participate in this study are required to document client-related care on a specially designed form called the Outcome Based Quality Improvement (OBQI) form. Some agencies have incorporated the OBQI into their documentation system.

The transport of medical equipment and supplies used in home care can be difficult. Many home care nurses travel by car and secure their equipment in the trunk of the car. Other nurses, particularly in large cities, must travel by public transportation and find that it is easier and safer if backpacks (not black medical bags) are used to carry supplies.

HOME ASSESSMENT

THE INITIAL NURSING VISIT

The assessment and care of clients with HIV/AIDS in their homes is extremely complex and involves physical, psychological, social, financial, and spiritual evaluations. The nursing process guides nursing care in the home. The five components of the nursing process are:

- Assessment—The collection of subjective and objective data.
- Nursing Diagnosis—The identification of the problem, based on data from the assessment, as the nurse and client understand it.
- Planning—Setting goals from the perspectives of the nurse, the client, the primary care provider, and significant others.
- Implementation—Interventions and treatments following nursing and primary care provider orders.
- Evaluation—Analysis of the effects of the nursing interventions and modification of the nursing plan as needed.

The trust and confidence of the client is needed if care given at home is to be effective. Therefore the nurse must maintain strict confidentiality regarding the client's diagnosis and must respect the client's choices regarding disclosure of his or her HIV status. Because confidentiality is absolutely imperative, the initial interview with the client should be private if at all possible. Discussions about the disease process are important, as are the client's personal feelings about the diagnosis and whom the client has told or would feel comfortable telling about the diagnosis. The nurse must explore with the client who knows about the diagnosis and whether the responsible caregiver, significant others, and family members know. The lack of disclosure cannot affect the provision of care; however, the nurse may need to modify the care plan based on the client's response to these questions. The nurse must also explore with the client and possibly the family how to reduce the potential for transmission of HIV to others in the home. A discussion of infection control should include safer sex practices and other measures to protect household members from transmission, as well as measures to protect the client from infection (Box 12-1). Clients and caregivers should be taught how to handle blood and body fluid spills (Box 12-2). Some clients' family members may want to be

BOX 12-1 INFECTION CONTROL IN THE HOME

Food Preparation/Eating*

- All foods should be fully cooked, properly stored, and used by the expiration date.
- Raw eggs, fish, or foods containing raw fish or eggs should not be eaten.
- Shellfish should be avoided.
- Use of bottled water is preferred over tap water for drinking and making ice cubes.
- Kitchen counters should be kept clean and washed thoroughly, especially after contact with raw meat.

Personal Care*

- Toothbrushes, razors, enema equipment, and sexual devices should never be shared with others.
- Towels and washcloths should not be shared with others without laundering.
- Razor blades should be discarded carefully in a metal puncture-resistant container.

Accidental Cuts/Bleeding*

- Caregivers should wear gloves (disposable or yellow kitchen gloves are okay) when the client receives an accidental cut or bleeds. The client or caregiver should apply pressure to the affected site, apply a bandage or Band-Aid to the site once the client has stopped bleeding, examine the area for any spills, and treat the area accordingly.

General Housekeeping*

- Sinks and toilets should be cleaned daily with a freshly-made bleach solution (see Box 12-2).
- Bathtubs should be cleaned before and after use by the client.
- Sponges used to clean in the kitchen where food is prepared should *never* be used in the bathroom.
- Dirty sponges should not be used in food preparation areas or to wash dishes.
- Sponges and dishcloths should be bleached periodically.
- The inside of the refrigerator should be cleaned with soap and water to control mold.
- Kitchen and bathroom floors should be mopped at least weekly using a solution of soap and a disinfectant.
- Spills should be cleaned up as soon as they occur.
- In the bathroom, bleach solution should be used in the shower stall to kill the fungus that causes athletes foot.
- Body fluids should first be cleaned with soap and water (gloves should be worn) followed by a 10% bleach solution. A little full-strength bleach can be poured into the toilet for disinfection.

* Handwashing should precede and conclude any infection control activity.

Continued

BOX 12-1 INFECTION CONTROL IN THE HOME—CONT'D

Pet Care*

- Cleaning of litter boxes, birdcages, fish tanks, reptile cages, or dog excrement should be performed while wearing gloves or by someone other than the client.
- A mask should be worn when cleaning birdcages.

Linens*

- If not contaminated with blood or body fluids, linens can be handled as usual with regular laundry.
- If linens are splashed or soaked with body fluids, they should be cleaned as soon as possible or stored in a plastic bag.
- Gloves should be used only if linens are soiled with body fluids.
- If a washing machine is not available, soiled items should be soaked in the bathroom sink in cold soapy water then in the bleach solution for about 10 minutes (see Box 12-2). Soiled water should be rinsed down the drain and item(s) rewashed using hot soapy water. Gloves should be used when hand washing soiled linens.
- Commercial or home dryers are preferred; hanging in the sun is also acceptable; or, if necessary, hanging indoors.
- No special treatment is necessary for the washing machine or dryer after use.
- If clothing or linens cannot be bleached, then they should be soaked in a household disinfectant such as Lysol, followed by washing with a detergent. They should be rinsed extremely well after use of a Lysol-type of disinfectant.

Needle Disposal*

- Used needles and syringes should be placed in a puncture-resistant metal or opaque plastic container with a cover; for example, a liquid laundry detergent container or heavy milk quart container. Used hypodermic needles *must not* be recapped or thrown into the garbage—someone could get stuck. The container must be stored safely, away from children. When the container is three-quarters full, some bleach should be poured in and the top should be replaced and taped securely in place. This container should be placed into a plastic bag, tied shut, and then placed inside another plastic bag and tied shut. Finally, the container may be discarded into the trash.

Household Waste Disposal*

- A waste container should be lined with two plastic bags for the disposal of bandages, pads, or tissues containing urine, feces, or blood. Bags should be tied securely and disposed of in the garbage. Feces, urine, and vomitus should be disposed of in the toilet and flushed away.
- Items containing blood, urine, or feces (e.g., bandages, diapers) must never be placed directly into the household garbage and body waste should never go directly into the garbage or sink.
- Hands must be washed after the disposal of any waste.

_____
* Handwashing should precede and conclude any infection control activity.

BOX 12-2 CLEANING BLOOD AND BODY FLUID SPILLS

Preparing a 10% Bleach Solution
- This should be made daily (it will lose its potency if made too far in advance) and kept in a closed, well-marked container with a lid. A 10% bleach solution can be made by mixing ¼ cup bleach with 2½ cups water. This solution must not be mixed with any other cleaning agent.

Cleaning a Spill
- Disposable latex gloves or yellow household cleaning gloves should be worn before any cleaning proceeds.
- The area should be cleaned with soap and water.
- The area should be cleaned with freshly made 10% bleach solution.

involved in the care of the client; others may remain aloof and provide minimal care. The nurse must respect the level of family involvement in client care. Many people fear "catching" HIV/AIDS from living with or caring for an infected person. Any misconceptions need to be explored with the client and the family so that basic knowledge about the disease is known. For example, the family and client need to know how HIV is spread, how to protect themselves from HIV, and how to deal with the emotional "roller coaster" that many clients and their caregivers experience on an ongoing basis.

If family members or significant others want to be involved in the care of the client, the nurse should teach basic client care, including proper handwashing technique, food preparation, medication administration, wound care, and other necessary types of treatment. When providing client and family education, care must always be taken not to overload the client or family with too much information. The nurse may need to provide education over many sessions. The nursing plan of care should clearly reflect realistic goals and time frames within which to achieve the desired outcomes of education. This plan should also include how goal attainment will be evaluated.

THE CLIENT ASSESSMENT

Physical Assessment

After an introduction to the client , the nurse should prepare for the assessment by asking permission to wash hands with soap and water. Sometimes clients prefer that the nurse use the kitchen sink and other times, the bathroom. It is wise for the nurse to use soap and paper towels from the nursing bag. If possible, the client should be interviewed in a quiet place (e.g., without the television) and privately. After assessing the client's comfort level and readiness for the interview, the nurse can begin by reviewing the reason for the home care referral and reviewing the home care mission and paperwork. After the initial paperwork is completed, the nurse should begin the examination by reviewing all of the client's body systems. The nurse should do a "head-to-toe" assessment, much like those done in the hospital. Vital signs should be recorded along with height and weight (the nurse may need to bring a scale). During the complete physical assessment, if it is apparent that wound care is needed, the client's supplies should be checked for adequacy. An inventory of necessary equipment and supplies should be made at the time of the visit. It is the nurse's responsibility to order supplies and equipment in a timely manner. *All soiled supplies should be put in plastic bags and disposed of in the client's home before leaving.* See Box 12-1 for a description of how to discard soiled supplies and needles in the home.

Psychological Assessment

The nurse should also assess the client's psychological state. Topics such as self-concept; body image; current social supports or social isolation; feelings of depression, anxiety, grief, loss, guilt, or hopelessness; drug and alcohol use or dependency; violence in the home; suicidal ideations; and any desire to harm others should be explored with the client. Many of these feelings can be assessed by listening to clients as they answer other questions, as well as by direct questions related to their mental status. Some clients may have a history of sexual or physical abuse that may also need to be explored. The nurse should evaluate whether clients are currently using drugs or alcohol in an abusive or addictive manner. If they are, the nurse should determine whether they want to seek treatment, are already in treatment, or have no current plans to deal with the addiction. The safety of the home care staff is of great importance if the client is an active user of recreational drugs or alcohol. Many home care agencies have policies regarding how such cases are handled to ensure the safety of all.

If the client is participating in a methadone maintenance program, arrangements can be made to ensure that clients continue to obtain the methadone daily or three times a week at a specific site. Methadone maintenance programs are not allowed to dispense methadone to anyone but the client, and so the social worker and nurse will need to work with personnel at the site to make appropriate plans for the client to pick up this vital medication.

Economic Assessment

When clients are discharged from the hospital with home care services they are often worried about the household bills. Other concerns often include who will care for them and their children, who will pick up or cash checks, and when and if they will be able to return to work. Clients' abilities to provide for basic needs such as food and shelter are important issues in home care. Home care agencies often employ a social worker that is an expert in helping clients obtain financial assistance. Nurses should also be familiar with community resources that may be able to assist clients until economic entitlements are available. See p. 210 for a discussion of community resources.

Spiritual Assessment

Spirituality is an area that may be overlooked by the nurse but that can be a great source of strength, peace, and hope for clients with HIV/AIDS. The spiritual assessment can begin by asking clients if they want to discuss this topic. If they do, questions can be asked related to how they express their spirituality, whether or not they attend a place of worship, and if they would like to see a spiritual provider. The nurse needs to be open to this subject and allow the client the freedom to express ideas that may differ from his or her own. Members of a spiritual group will often come to the aid of a sick member; if the client belongs to such a group, other members may be willing to assist him or her. The nurse can encourage clients to call their place of worship or the nurse can call with the client's permission, remembering to protect confidentiality. The nurse should explore with clients how they intend to respond to those who ask about their health.

HOME SAFETY ASSESSMENT

Along with the complete assessment of the client, the home or apartment must be assessed for safety. This includes noting the presence of scatter rugs, overused electrical outlets, inadequate refrigeration, and any sanitation problems (e.g., roaches, lack of garbage pick-up, problems with general cleanliness). The nurse should also note the availability of running water, and the adequacy of bathroom facilities, heating, and air conditioning. The exterior of the dwelling should also be evaluated. Unsafe stairs or stairwells, hallways, and elevators should be reported to building management. Outside safety (especially regarding the neighborhood and security of the home or apartment) should be evaluated as well. In collaboration with the client, family, and other paraprofessionals, the nurse creates a plan for making the home as safe as possible for the client.

GENERAL ASSESSMENT

A comprehensive nursing assessment includes evaluating the client's ability to manage the treatment regimen for the illness. The following are some questions that need to be answered when assessing a client in the home:

- Can the client ingest his or her own medications? Can he or she open the containers?
- Does the client know the names and doses of the medications, and the times to take them?
- Does the client know how to take the medications properly (e.g., with or without food)?
- Does the client know the medications' side effects and which side effects to report to the provider?

- Who will get the prescriptions and where will the prescriptions be filled?
- Where will the client sleep? Does he or she need assistance to get into the sleeping area?
- Where is the bathroom in relation to the client's living areas?
- Can the client get into a bath? Shower?
- Where will the client eat? In the kitchen? In the dining area?
- Who will prepare meals? Do shopping? Laundry? Housekeeping? Care for the children? Care for pets?
- How will the client manage to attend medical appointments? Public transportation? Taxi? Private automobile?
- Are the home and neighborhood safe?
- Does the client have a support system? Is someone willing to assist in the client's care? How much? How often?

This list represents some of the questions that must be answered during the initial home assessment; however, it is not all-inclusive.

Other vital information important in the care of the client includes a sexual history, an obstetric history, and data about the HIV status of any children. Further questions include:

- Does the client have custody of the children?
- If the client is hospitalized, are there plans to provide care for the children?
- Has guardianship been set up for the children if the client dies?
- Are others in the home also HIV-positive?

Assessment Of Legal Issues

The client may be an undocumented immigrant and face difficult legal problems with his or her residency status. The nurse may refer the client to the social worker or to a community agency that assists immigrants in obtaining residency status. The nurse should also explore and discuss advanced directives (e.g., health care proxy and durable power of attorney) with the client. For a discussion of the health care proxy and durable power of attorney see Chapter 11.

NURSING INTERVENTIONS IN HOME CARE

Once the assessments of the client and home are completed, the nurse makes the appropriate nursing diagnoses and goals are outlined. A plan of care is then designed that includes the medical plan, the nursing plan, plans for meeting the other needs of the client, and the agency's responsibilities. The nurse acts as the case manager and makes referrals for all other services to be carried out in the home. These may include a nutritional evaluation; home health aide services; homemaker services; a social work assessment; home-delivered meals; medical equipment and supplies; and physical, occupational, speech, or language therapy. If the client requires highly technical intravenous (IV) therapy, then a special IV team from the home care agency should be notified or another agency should be subcontracted to perform this service.

Medication management for clients with HIV/AIDS is crucial in home care. All medications must be reviewed, including the purpose, name, dose, frequency, and time of administration, as well as side effects. The client may have "old" medications at home that are no longer needed and could even be dangerous if taken with the new regimen. The nurse should ask to discard these in the toilet to protect others and the client as well. It is useful to use a medication box with individual compartments marked with the appropriate day and time of administration so that medications can be prepared for a period of up to a week at a time. The need for medications to be refrigerated necessitates other methods for remembering to take them, such as notes. The medication box can assist the nurse in evaluating the client's adherence to medication regimens. It may be helpful to provide the client with written sheets containing information about each medication. Occasionally home care nurses are inventive and create their own teaching devices for clients; for instance, making a list of the medications and taping one pill of each kind on pieces of paper so the client can identify medication properly. The refrigerator is usually a good place to hang information or educational tools but medications must be kept out of the reach of children. The family should also receive education if they are assisting with the medication regimen.

USE OF PARAPROFESSIONALS

After completing an evaluation of the client, family, home, and environment, the nurse may determine that the services of a specialized paraprofessional are needed. The use of paraprofessionals is a vital component of providing care to clients with HIV/AIDS in the home. Box 12-3 lists the types of paraprofessionals and their general duties. The availability of the type of paraprofessional is dependent upon the insurance coverage, special program enrollment, and the geographical area. The scope of activities varies from area to area.

All paraprofessionals are provided with specialized training and observed before they are certified. The agency may provide regular inservice classes on standards of care. When a paraprofessional is placed in the home of a client, state requirements dictate the frequency of supervision by the registered nurse (e.g., every 2 weeks). While it is important that paraprofessionals be informed of a client's diagnosis, state laws regarding confidentiality and HIV may not permit this disclosure. All paraprofessionals' training programs should include a component on the specialized needs of an HIV-positive client. Standard precautions are to be included in the general training.

HHAs and PCAs

HHAs and PCAs are specifically trained to assist with the personal care needs of the client. If the client needs assistance with personal care (e.g.,

BOX 12-3 PARAPROFESSIONALS USED IN THE HOME

Paraprofessional	Duties
Home Health Aid (HHA)	Provides personal care (assistance with activities of daily living [ADLs]), including checking vital signs, performing special exercises, assisting with oxygen therapy, and performing chore services (for the client only).
Homemaker	Provides chore services and childcare services; may act as a surrogate parent, staying 24 hours/day when a parent is hospitalized or bedbound.
Personal care assistant (PCA); also called a "home attendant" or "personal care attendant"	Provides chore services such as shopping, cleaning, laundry and meal preparation, and assistance with ADLs; may travel with the client to and from appointments
Housekeeper	Provides chore services such as shopping, cleaning, laundry, and meal preparation, but provides no personal care.

activities of daily living [ADLs]) then an HHA is "placed and oriented" at the time of the initial visit or at a subsequent visit. (See Box 12-3 for the duties for HHAs and PCAs.) These paraprofessionals are supervised by the registered nurse on a regular basis depending on the state, local, and agency guidelines.

When a paraprofessional enters a client's home, a care plan is developed based on the individual needs of the client. The paraprofessional is instructed about the exact care that he or she is expected to provide. The duties and responsibilities of the HHA are written down by the nurse and reviewed by both the client and the HHA. The care plan is reviewed and updated regularly with the client and the paraprofessional and is placed in the client's home (usually on the refrigerator) where it can be easily consulted by the paraprofessional or the nurse. A copy is kept with the client's chart. The paraprofessional should also keep a copy. After the nurse completes the evaluation of the client and the home and family situation, the HHA or other paraprofessional performs specific tasks that are written out by the nurse. It is important for the nurse to remind the paraprofessional that he or she is not able to dispense medications personally, but can remind the client to take medication. The nurse should carefully assess the relationship between the HHA, the client, the family, and significant others.

HOUSEKEEPERS

Housekeepers can perform chores in the home such as light housekeeping, laundry, grocery shopping, and food preparation. They also must receive training on household cleaning (i.e., the use of bleach solutions) and on the proper selection, storage, and preparation of food.

HOMEMAKERS

Homemakers can care for the client's minor children who are well and who live in the home. If an HIV-positive child is in the home and is ailing, he or she should be referred for home personal care. Homemakers provide meal preparation, clean the home, and feed and play with children. If the children are school-aged, homemakers may also assist with homework. Generally they assist with meal planning for the client and children but not the entire family. Any other family members should be responsible for meeting their own housekeeping needs. Again, confidentiality is vital in this situation, as the children and other family members may not be aware of the client's HIV status.

NURSING DOCUMENTATION IN HOME CARE

The nurse must complete several forms to meet regulatory requirements of insurers that are billed by the home care agencies and to provide a record of the planned and provided nursing care. Table 12-1 lists some of the most common forms used. The nurse providing coordination of home care services is responsible for preparing the "485" (and, if necessary, the "487") form, which includes physician's orders and a nursing plan of care (Figures 12-1 and 12-2). It is signed by the physician every 62 days and sent to the insurance company for reimbursement. The plan of care for a client is based on the combined assessments of the nurse, the physician, and other care providers and the designated benefits of the health care insurance policy. In addition to the forms listed in Table 12-1, the agency usually requires appropriate notes for each visit made by the nurse, therapist, or paraprofessional. The nurse is generally the coordinator of services and is responsible for appropriate and timely documentation.

ENDING THE VISIT

When the visit is complete, the nurse should have documented all appropriate information. The nurse should wash his or her hands, thank the client, and schedule the next nursing appointment.

CASE MANAGEMENT

Case management has become a necessity in the United States because there are multiple health care plans and the average consumer has difficulty in understanding and negotiating the complexities of entitlements offered through private insurance policies, Medicaid, and Medicare. The role of the nurse case manager is to provide an assessment, plan care, obtain services, set goals and objectives, and monitor and evaluate the client's care so that his or her needs are met. In the home care setting, nurses often act as case managers, interacting with all of the care providers. They review cases along with physicians and other care providers

	Forms Used in Nursing Documentation of Home Health Care

Table 12-1

Form	Comments
"485" Home Health Certification and Plan of Care; for Medicaid, Medicare, and private health insurance companies (see Figure 12-1).	Standardized HCFA form, due every 62 days (physician's orders). Completed by the nurse; includes diagnosis, mental status, allergies, activities and functional limitations, orders for supplies, medications, treatments, goals, and discharge plans. Must be signed and dated by physician and placed with the client's chart in a timely manner.
"487" Addendum to Plan of Treatment or Medical Update (see Figure 12-2).	Standardized HCFA form, used if more space is needed on "485." Completed by the nurse; must be signed and dated by the physician and placed in client's record in a timely manner.
Interim Order Sheet	Not standardized—Created by each agency to provide interim orders until the next "485" is due.
60 Day/Discharge Summary	Not standardized—Created by each agency; required every 60 days and upon discharge. Copies are sent to the physician and placed with the client's chart. Includes all services and therapies that were provided, vital signs, and a summary of outcomes. Signature required by only the nurse.
Interim Summary	Not standardized—Created by each agency; required every 30 days by some agencies. Copies are sent to the physician and placed with the client's chart. Includes summary of problems and interventions for all disciplines. Signature required by only the nurse.
Team Conference Form	Not standardized—Created by each agency; used for summarizing a team conference. Original copy goes with the client's chart.

(e.g., physical therapists, occupational therapists, social workers) and decide on the plan of care.

COMMUNITY-BASED RESOURCES FOR HIV-POSITIVE CLIENTS

A community-based organization (CBO) is a service organization that provides social services at the local level. CBOs that are exclusively devoted to the needs of people living with AIDS (PLWA) are called AIDS service organizations (ASO). These agencies provide advocacy, education, internet resources, medical and dental services, social and religious support, and access to specialized support groups. ASOs can also provide insurance and

Text continued on p. 217

Department of Health and Human Services
Health Care Financing Administration

Form Approved
OMB No. 0938-0357

HOME HEALTH CERTIFICATION AND PLAN OF CARE

1. Patient's HI Claim No.	2. Start of Care Date	3. Certification Period	4. Medical Record No.	5. Provider No.
		From: To:		

6. Patient's Name and Address

7. Providers Name, Address and Telephone Number

8. Date of Birth		9. Sex ☐ M ☐ F

10. Medications: Dose/Frequency/Route (N)ew (C)hanged

11. ICD-9-CM	Principal Diagnosis	Date
12. ICD-9-CM	Surgical Procedure	Date
13. ICD-9-CM	Other Pertinent Diagnoses	Date

14. DME and Supplies

15. Safety Measures:

16. Nutritional Req.

17. Allergies:

18. A. Functional Limitations

1 ☐ Amputation   5 ☐ Paralysis   9 ☐ Legally Blind
2 ☐ Bowel/Bladder (Incontinence)   6 ☐ Endurance   A ☐ Dyspnea With Minimal Exertion
3 ☐ Contracture   7 ☐ Ambulation   B ☐ Other (Specify)
4 ☐ Hearing   8 ☐ Speech

18. B. Activities Permitted

1 ☐ Complete Bedrest   6 ☐ Partial Weight Bearing   A ☐ Wheelchair
2 ☐ Bedrest BRP   7 ☐ Independent At Home   B ☐ Walker
3 ☐ Up As Tolerated   8 ☐ Crutches   C ☐ No Restrictions
4 ☐ Transfer Bed/Chair   9 ☐ Cane   D ☐ Other (Specify)
5 ☐ Exercise Prescribed

19. Mental Status:

1 ☐ Oriented   3 ☐ Forgetful   5 ☐ Disoriented   7 ☐ Agitated
2 ☐ Comatose   4 ☐ Depressed   6 ☐ Lethargic   8 ☐ Other

20. Prognosis:

1 ☐ Poor   2 ☐ Guarded   3 ☐ Fair   4 ☐ Good   5 ☐ Excellent

Figure 12-1. Form HCFA-485.

Continued

21. Orders for Discipline and Treatments (Specify Amount/Frequency/Duration) Finite and predictable end date to daily visits _____

SN ORDERS FREQUENCY & DURATION

☐ Assess Vital Signs
☐ Assess & Instr. Pt/Caregiver: health status maintenance, activities permitted, safety measures, reporting significant changes to M.D. symptom management.
☐ Report to following M.D.: _____
☐ Lab. _____

☐ Assess & Instr. Pt/Caregiver on medication action & S/E.
☐ Assess & Instr. on prescribed diet/fluids
☐ Instr. Pt./Caregiver/aide on universal precautions, incl. safe disposal of medical waste.
☐ Skilled Mgmt and evaluation of Care Plan.
☐ Supv. Aide q 2wks. & prn
☐ Assess mental status & judgement.

☐ Instr. use of equip.
☐ Instr. Pt/Caregiver to access emergency services and home safety precautions.
☐ Provide Rehab nursing for _____

☐ Teach _____

☐ CONTINUATION OF ORDERS _____

SN Order: _____

22. Goals/Rehabilitation Potential/Discharge Plans

Goals:

Rehab Potential: ☐ Good ☐ Fair ☐ Poor ☐ Unclear At This Time

Discharge Plan:

23. Nurse's Signature and Date of Verbal SOC Where Applicable:

25. Date HHA Received Signed POT

24. Physician's Name and Address

26. I certify/recertify that this patient is confined to his/her home and needs intermittent skilled nursing care, physical therapy and/or speech therapy or continues to need occupational therapy. The patient is under my care, and I have authorized the services on this plan of care and will periodically review the plan.

27. Attending Physician's Signature and Date Signed

28. Anyone who misrepresents, falsifies, or conceals essential information required for payment of Federal funds may be subject to fine, imprisonment, or civil penalty under applicable Federal laws.

Form HCFA-485 (C-4) (02-94)

PAGE _____ OF _____

PROVIDER

Figure 12-1, cont'd.   Form HCFA-485.

Department of Health and Human Services
Health Care Financing Administration

Form Approved
OMB No. 0938-0357

ADDENDUM TO: ☐ **PLAN OF TREATMENT** ☐ **MEDICAL UPDATE**

1. Patient's HI Claim No.	2. SOC Date	3. Certification Period	4. Medical Record No.	5. Provider No.
		From: To:		

6. Patient's Name	7. Provider Name

8. Item No.

CARDIO/VASCULAR/PULMONARY CARE

☐ Assess C/P, C/V status incl. Lung Fields, peripheral circulation and edema.
☐ Instr. pursed lip breathing/deep breathing/coughing.
☐ Instr. use of O₂ at _____ l/min.
   continuous/prn (circle one) via _____
☐ Other _____

☐ Instr. O₂ Safety Precaution
☐ Instr. Trach care, incl. suctioning with
   (size) _____ cath at (freq) _____ using (Sol) _____
☐ Change Trach. Tube Size _____ (freq.)
   instr. _____

☐ Trach. care: cleanse with _____
   Apply DSD, change neck tape, qD & prn.
☐ Instr. on removal of inner cannula, cleanse
   _____, using brush; Rinse thoroughly
   & replace qD & prn.
☐ Instr. proper use of humidifier via trach
   mask as follows: _____ (freq.)

PSYCH/NEURO/CARE

☐ Assess Neuro/Muscular Status/Symptom management.
☐ Assess S/S depression, anxiety, psychosis, ineffective coping.
☐ Other _____

☐ Instr. Caregiver to S/O Pt. behavior, reducing stress level and improving coping mechanisms.
☐ Instr. Pt./Caregiver seizure precautions.

☐ Instr. Pt./Caregiver gait, balance motor coordination.
☐ Assess & Instr. on pain management.
☐ Assess risk of falls, teach safety measures.

GASTROINTESTINAL/GENITOURINARY CARE

☐ Assess & Instr. Pt./Caregiver on GI/GU status.
☐ Instr. on Abdomen & elimination patterns.
☐ Assess/Instr. weight gain/loss: I&O
☐ Assess/Instr. perineal care.
☐ Change foley cath (size) _____
   balloon _____ (freq) q _____ & prn x2
☐ Other _____

☐ Teach on foley care
☐ Assess & Instr. Colostomy/Ileostomy care. (Size/Type) _____
☐ Instr. Stoma Care: S/S Obstruction, S/S Infection
☐ Instr. appliance change (freq)

☐ Instr. on _____ irrigation(s)
   Using (Sol) _____ every _____
   (freq) _____, Irrigate – prn
   X _____ for _____
☐ Instr. bladder training.
☐ Assess & Instr. on S/S UTI

Figure 12-2. Form HCFA–487.

Continued

WOUND/SKIN CARE

☐ Assess/Instr. on skin care. S/S Skin breakdown/rash.

☐ Instr. on measures to ↓ pressure over bony prominences.

☐ Instr. _____ on wound care, S/S Infection & approp. actions.

☐ Other _____

☐ Assess & Provide Wound Care to (loc) _____ as follows: _____ _____

☐ Remove staples from _____ suture line on _____ (date).

DIABETIC CARE

☐ Instr./Supv. Pt./Caregiver on Diabetic regime including _____

☐ Administer Insulin as ordered.

☐ Teach Insulin prep. & admin.

☐ Other _____

☐ Prefill Insulin Syringes q WK as ordered by M.D. Instr. _____ to prefill syringes.

☐ S/O response to diabetic meds & diet. Assess compliance.

☐ Teach diet & emergency measures

☐ Assess/Instr. on DM blood glucose monitoring via _____ (freq.)

☐ Report _____ to M.D.

HOME HEALTH AIDE ORDERS FREQ: _____ DAYS _____ HRS _____ WKS _____

☐ ADL ASSIST
☐ PERSONAL CARE
☐ ASSIST HOME EXER. PROG.
☐ ASSIST AMBULATION

☐ PREPARE MEALS
☐ ERRANDS/SHOP
☐ WASH CLOTHES
☐ HOUSEKEEPING

☐ MAINTAIN SAFE ENVIRONMENT
☐ REMIND TO TAKE MEDICATIONS

OTHER _____
_____
_____

9. Signature of Physician

10. Date

11. Optional Name/Signature of Nurse/Therapist

12. Date

Form HCFA-487 (C4) (4-87)

PAGE _____ OF _____ **PROVIDER**

Department of Health and Human Services
Health Care Financing Administration

Form Approved
OMB No. 0938-0357

ADDENDUM TO: ☐ **PLAN OF TREATMENT** ☐ **MEDICAL UPDATE**

1. Patient's HI Claim No.	2. SOC Date	3. Certification Period	4. Medical Record No.	5. Provider No.
		From: To:		

6. Patient's Name	7. Provider Name

8. Item No.

PHYSICAL THERAPY ORDERS FREQUENCY & DURATION:

☐ EVALUATION
☐ AROM, PROM, EXER. TO ____ UE ____ LE
☐ AMB. TRAINING W/APPROP. ASSIST DEVICE
☐ GAIT TRAINING & BAL. EXER.
☐ TRANSFER TRAINING
☐ ESTABLISH H.E.P.

☐ STRENGTHENING EXER. TO ____ UE ____ LE
☐ COORDINATION / BALANCE PROGRAM
☐ PRE- AND POST-PROSTHETIC TRAINING
☐ ENERGY CONSERVATION TRAINING
☐ PAIN OR EDEMA MANAGEMENT
☐ ADL TRAINING   WEIGHT BEARING STATUS ☐ FWB ☐ PWB ☐ NWB

☐ EQUIP. EVAL & TRAINING
☐ HOME EXERCISE PROGRAM
PT. ORDER ____

PRECAUTIONS

PHYSICAL THERAPY GOALS:

☐ INCREASE STRENGTH & MOBILITY BY ____ VISIT/WEEK
☐ IND. AMB. W/APPROP. ASSIST. DEVICE BY ____ VISIT/WEEK
☐ AMB. PROSTHESIS/ASSIST DEVICE BY ____ VISIT/WEEK

☐ DISPLAY IMPROVED GAIT & BAL. BY ____ VISIT/WEEK
☐ DISPLAY IMPROVED TRANSFER TECHNIQUE BY ____ VISIT/WEEK
☐ DECREASE PAIN/EDEMA BY ____
☐ IMPROVE ENERGY CONSERVATION

☐ PT./CAREGIVER DEMONSTRATE CORRECT USE OF EQUIPMENT
PT GOALS: ____

OCCUPATIONAL THERAPY ORDERS FREQUENCY & DURATION:

☐ EVALUATION
☐ ADL TRAINING
☐ MUSCLE RE-EDUCATION
☐ FINE MOTOR TRAINING
☐ WHEELCHAIR EVAL/TRAINING

☐ ADAPTIVE EQUIP. EVAL/TRAINING
☐ AROM/PROM EXERCISE TO ____ UE
☐ STRENGTHENING EXER. TO ____ UE
☐ SPLINT EVAL/TRAINING
☐ ENERGY CONSERVATION TRAINING

OT ORDER: ____

INSTR: ____

OCCUPATIONAL THERAPY GOALS:

☐ INCREASED IND. W/ADL BY ____ VISIT/WEEK
☐ INCREASE MUSCLE FUNCTION BY ____ VISIT/WEEK
☐ INCREASE FINE MOTOR COORD. BY ____ VISIT/WEEK
☐ IMPROVED IN ENERGY CONSERVATION

☐ INCREASED ABILITY TO USE ADAPT. EQUIP. BY ____ VISIT/WEEK
☐ PT. WILL PERFORM ROM EXER. BY ____ VISIT/WEEK
☐ PT. WILL HAVE INCREASED STRENGTH TO UE BY ____ VISIT/WEEK

OT GOALS: ____

Continued

Figure 12-2, cont'd. Form HCFA–487.

BY _____
☐ SET UP SYSTEM OF CUES TO FACILITATE
  COGNITIVE PROCESSING BY _____

☐ PT./CAREGIVER DEMONSTR. KNOWLEDGE OF
  CORRECT USE OF ADAPTIVE DEVICES BY _____

SPEECH THERAPY ORDERS FREQUENCY & DURATION:

☐ EVALUATION
☐ SPEECH ARTICULATION DISORDER Rx
☐ COGNITIVE TRAINING

☐ VOICE DISORDER Rx
☐ APHASIA RX
☐ LANGUAGE DISORDER RX

ST ORDER: _____

INSTR: _____

SPEECH THERAPY GOALS:

☐ INCREASED ARTICULATION
  ABILITY BY _____ VISIT/WEEK
☐ VOICE CONTR. BY _____ VISIT/WEEK
☐ SET UP SYSTEMS OF CUES TO FACILITATE
  COGNITIVE PROCESSING BY _____

☐ EFFECTIVE COMMUNICATION
  BY _____ VISIT/WEEK
☐ INDEP. IN USE OF ELECTRONIC DEVICE
  BY _____
☐ INDEP. IN ESOPHAGEAL SPEECH BY _____

ST GOALS: _____
_____
_____

MEDICAL SOCIAL WORKER ORDERS FREQUENCY & DURATION:

☐ EVALUATION
☐ ASSESS OF SOCIAL & EMOTIONAL FACTORS
☐ COUNSEL FOR LONG RANGE PLANNING

☐ SHORT TERM THERAPY FOR MGMT. OF
  ILLNESS
☐ COUNSEL RE: UNSAFE ENVIRONMENT
☐ COUNSEL RE: FINANCIAL PROBLEMS
  WHICH INHIBITS PROPER CARE TO PT.

MSW ORDER _____
_____
_____

MEDICAL SOCIAL WORKER GOALS:

☐ ABILITY TO MAKE LONG RANGE PLANS

☐ DECREASE STRESS & ANXIETY
  BY _____ VISIT/WEEK

☐ PT. WILL IMPROVE IN
  THROUGH BENEFIT OF COUNSELING
  BY _____ VISIT/WEEK

MSW GOALS: _____
_____
_____

9. Signature of Physician

10. Date

11. Optional Name/Signature of Nurse/Therapist

12. Date

Form HCFA-487 (C4) (4-87)

PAGE _____ OF _____

PROVIDER

Figure 12-2, cont'd. Form HCFA-487.

legal information and social work services. While services are provided to anyone affected by or infected with HIV, some ASOs target specific groups such as adolescents, people of various sexual orientations, people of color, people living with hemophilia, people belonging to particular ethnic groups, people with low literacy, or inmates. Some ASOs provide education to other ASOs. For example, the Southeast AIDS Training and Education Center provides education to health departments and other AIDS organizations.

As client advocates, nurses who work in the community should be aware of CBOs and ASOs that can provide services to their clients. A physician's order is not required to make a referral to one of these agencies; however, the referral should be incorporated into the client's plan of care. Many communities publish a booklet of local agencies that may be helpful to clients.

CONTINUING CARE

Continuing home care for persons with HIV/AIDS is based on ongoing evaluation and planning by the nurse. The client's care plan is based on the original nursing assessment of the client and the home and family situation and is implemented continuously with each visit. These visits are made daily (if IV therapy or daily dressing changes are needed), weekly, or as needed. The plan of care is reassessed regularly to ensure that the services provided by the nurse are necessary for the well-being of the client and continue to meet guidelines provided by the health insurance company. Other services the client may be receiving need to be coordinated, and thus a weekly or monthly review of the entire case with all providers is very valuable. This can be accomplished with phone calls, summaries, or e-mail. These case reviews also provide the opportunity for the nurse and others involved in the client's care to reassess the client's physical progress, social situation, and psychosocial status. Revisions to the plan of care are made based on these team conferences. Care must be provided so as not to make the client or family unnecessarily dependent on the services, because self-care and independence are the goals of home care.

Clients are monitored closely for the development of new or recurrent opportunistic infections (OIs) or syndromes. An HHA may note that a client has decreased appetite, which may be a sign of oral or esophageal candidiasis; weakness in performing ADLs, which may indicate *Mycobacterium avium-intracellulare;* or shortness of breath when walking about the house, which may indicate *Pneumocystis carinii* pneumonia (PCP). An HHA is often with a client for 4 to 8 hours per day and often plays a key role in identifying subtle differences in the client's behavior and any new symptoms. The nurse must teach HHAs to record any of these findings on the HHA worksheet and to notify the nurse by phone if there is any sudden change. A copy of a typical HHA worksheet may be found in Figure 12-3. Each organization that trains and supervises HHAs has its own form that must be completed in duplicate with one copy for the client's home and one for the visiting nurse.

PARAPROFESSIONAL PLAN OF CARE

Client Name _____ Age _____   Primary Nurse _____

Address _____ Apt. _____   Coordinator _____

_____ Zip _____   HHA _____ PCA _____ HM _____

Directions _____   Days/Wk _____

_____   Hours/Day _____ AM _____ PM _____

Phone (___) _____   _____ PM _____ PM _____ AM _____

Lives With _____   Start Date _____

Emergency Contact _____   Is Replacement Essential? Yes _____ No _____

Phone (H) _____ (W) _____   Pets(s) in Home _____ Dog _____ Cat _____ Bird _____

Language Spoken _____   Other _____

Client Status

Oriented _____ Disoriented _____ Forgetful _____ Hearing Impaired _____ Visually Impaired _____

Ambulation

Independent _____ Needs Assistance _____ Cane _____ Walker _____ W/C _____ Bedbound _____

FIRE/POLICE/AMBULBANCE – CALL 911
Notify Primary Nurse of any change in condition or unusual occurrences.
Use universal precautions at all times.

PERSONAL CARE (circle all that apply)	ACTIVITIES/AMBULATION (circle all that apply)	SPECIFY CARE:
Bed bath	Ambulation (specify below)	
Sponge bath	Transfers	
Tub bath	Turning and positioning	
Shower	Exercise (as per instruction of nurse or therapist)	
Mouth care	Reinforce safety measures	
Foot care	Accompany to MD Visits	
Hair care		
Skin care (specify below)	NUTRITION (circle all that apply)	
Nail care	Meal preparation	
Toileting:	Breakfast	
Bed pan/urinal/bathroom/commode	Lunch	
Incontinent care (specify below)	Dinner	
Dressing/grooming	Snack (specify)	
Reinforce/change simple dressing (specify below)	Diet (specify)	
Catheter care (specify below)	Feed client	
Ostomy care (specify below)	Assist with feeding	
Temperature:	Record Intake/output	
Oral/rectal/axillary		
Pulse/respirations	HOME MAINTENANCE	
Weigh client	Clean client's room/bathroom/kitchen/pt. care equipment	
Medications (remind)	Laundry	
	Shopping	

Registered Nurse: _____ Home Health Aide: _____

I have read, understand and agree with this plan of care:

Client: _____ Date: _____

Figure 12-3. Paraprofessional Plan of Care Worksheet.

The social worker is also an important team member and provides ongoing assessments of the client and family's ability to cope with the client's condition. The social worker can assist in providing referrals to CBOs that may be able to fill gaps in care.

LONG-TERM CARE PROGRAMS

While the goal of home care is to assist the client and family to become independent in meeting their needs, long-term care sometimes becomes necessary. Long-term care programs that were previously devoted to meeting the needs of older adults who did not desire nursing home placement are revamping their programs so that they can serve the needs of the population living with HIV. In some cases, with the availability of appropriate reimbursement sources, up to 24 hours of in-home care may be provided, usually on a short-term basis. If care is complicated or there is no caregiver willing to accept responsibility for working with the nurse to manage these services, then placement in a long-term care facility may be necessary. At this printing there are several long-term care programs available for HIV/AIDS clients when they can no longer be maintained in their homes with intermittent home care services. One such program, Nursing Homes Without Walls, provides HHA services 24 hours a day, but the scope of services provided ultimately depends on the client's type of insurance coverage. Often, maintaining a client in the home with 24-hour care is less expensive than nursing home care. However, if this is not an option, several long-term care facilities are available in larger metropolitan areas. They resemble hospitals or upscale nursing homes. Clients are in 1- or 2-bed rooms and can receive high-tech therapy (e.g., IV therapy) and other nursing care, as well as nutritional and social work services and physical, occupational, and speech therapy. In this setting clients are a part of the team and help form the plan of care. Meals can be served individually but a common dining room is available to encourage socialization while eating. Family and friends can visit for most of the day (unlike hospitals with specific visiting hours), and the client is encouraged to go home for weekend overnight stays, if possible. The number of available beds in this type of facility varies from state to state and city to city; larger metropolitan areas tend to have more of these types of facilities.

Trying to place clients with HIV/AIDS in traditional long-term care facilities (e.g., nursing homes) may be difficult because of the lack of education regarding AIDS care, activities that are more appropriate for older adults, meals that are specific for older adults, schedules that may not match those of younger AIDS clients, and the lack of high-tech equipment. The reactions of uninfected residents and their families to HIV/AIDS can make clients with HIV/AIDS feel isolated; in addition, the age of HIV/AIDS clients is generally much younger than that of the typical nursing home client. Dementia is seen in many clients with advanced AIDS and can result in bizarre behavior, violent "acting out," a decline in self-care skills, and delusional thinking. Both staff and residents should be informed of the etiology of these behaviors and taught how to respond appropriately.

RESIDENTIAL CARE FACILITIES

Residential care facilities for persons living with AIDS were initially started in July 1993 in San Francisco, and since then several other programs have been started across the country. Residential care facilities meet the needs of clients when there is no caregiver or no domicile for the client. There are several models for this type of care, but basically all clients have their own rooms with a bathroom, some type of cooking facility (e.g., toaster oven, microwave), and a small refrigerator. The clients are encouraged to eat together in a main dining room and there are activities in which they may choose to participate. There is generally a nurse on staff who is available to assist with medications. If the client becomes too ill for self-care, then home care services are used until health can be restored.

DISCHARGE FROM HOME CARE

Discharge from home care is the long-term goal of every admission and involves all of the caregivers involved in the client's care, including the nurse, paraprofessional, and significant others and care partners. Before discharge the nurse must assess the client's clinical, social, and physical needs. The client may be discharged to self-care, to the care of significant others, or to a facility. Clients who are to remain in the home should be engaged with community-based programs that can help them maintain the achieved level of independence. Community outreach resources include "buddy" systems, in which a volunteer visits clients usually 1 to 2 times each week. The buddy is there primarily to visit with the client for an hour or so or do errands but is, in general, there to be a friend. Other community resources that have developed in the HIV age are day care programs. These provide the client with a home-like setting, one to two meals (e.g., breakfast and/or lunch), and group activities like painting, sewing, group therapy, and field trips. Public assistance programs often assist with the payment for this particular service. If a client needs meals delivered to the home, there are meals-on-wheels programs designed particularly for people with HIV/AIDS.

END-OF-LIFE CARE IN THE COMMUNITY

Many dying clients want to remain at home until they die. The process can certainly be managed in the home setting so as to maintain dignity and meet the spiritual and emotional needs of the client and significant others. Hospice and palliative care is an option for those clients who wish to remain at home and receive palliation for their signs and symptoms. A

Health Care Proxy

(1)   I, _____

hereby appoint _____

(name, home address and telephone number)

_____

as my health care agent to make any and all health care decisions for
me, except to the extent that I state otherwise. This proxy shall take effect
when and if I become unable to make my own health care decisions.

(2)   Optional instructions: I direct my agent to make health care decisions in
accord with my wishes and limitations as stated below, or as he or she
otherwise knows. (Attach additional pages if necessary.)

_____

_____

_____

(Unless your agent knows your wishes about artificial nutrition and hydration [feeding tubes], your agent will not be allowed to make decisions
about artificial nutrition and hydration. See instructions on reverse for
samples of language you could use.)

(3)   Name of substitute or fill-in agent if the person I appoint above is unable, unwilling, or unavailable to act as my health care agent.

_____

(name, home address and telephone number)

_____

(4)   Unless I revoke it, this proxy shall remain in effect indefinitely, or until
the date or conditions stated below. This proxy shall expire (specific date
or conditions, if desired):

_____

(5)   Signature _____

Address _____

Date _____

Statement by Witnesses (must be 18 or older)

I declare that the person who signed this document is personally known
to me and appears to be of sound mind and acting of his or her own free
will. He or she signed (or asked another to sign for him or her) this document in my presence.

Witness 1 _____

Address _____

Witness 2 _____

Address _____

Figure 12-4.   Health Care Proxy Form.

complete discussion of palliative care can be found in Chapter 11. Hospice care can be initiated if the client, family, and physician agree that this is the best choice for the client and family. The physician must determine, to the best of his or her knowledge, that the client has 6 months or less to live. The concept of home hospice care is to allow the client to die at home with dignity and in as little pain as possible. No further curative treatment can be pursued except what is necessary to reduce pain or suffering.

The nurses involved in this end-of-life cycle should encourage the client and family together to compose a living will and designate a health care proxy (Figure 12-4). The *living will* provides dying clients with choices for what happens when they are no longer competent to make decisions for themselves. Such decisions may include medical decisions, such as whether to have a feeding tube placed if the client can no longer eat or whether to start oxygen if breathing becomes labored. These and other issues are discussed with the client and documented on a specially designed state form. The *health care proxy* is a person designated to act as the client's spokesperson if he or she is no longer able to make health care decisions. This person needs to understand the living will and must follow it to the best of his or her abilities. If the client, physician, and family agree, the client may consider a "Do not resuscitate" (DNR) order, which requires the physician to complete a special form. This will allow the client to die without any extraordinary interventions to prolong life. It is vital that the forms meet department of health (DOH) standards to be honored by emergency medical staff. Copies are kept with the client's chart at the home care agency, in the physician's records, and in the client's home in a safe, easy-to-find place. Generally it is kept on the wall by the phone or on the refrigerator. Other information that is helpful to have in advance includes a list of the names and phone numbers of the private medical doctor (PMD), the funeral home of choice, and those who are to be notified of the death. The nurse should guide the client and family in performing the necessary tasks.

Home care is often the preferred option for clients, family and insurance payers. The comfort of the home and the support of the community can be beneficial to the client and may be more economical for payers. It is a way to maintain independence and dignity throughout the HIV disease trajectory.

BIBLIOGRAPHY

Bartlett JA: *Care and management of patients with HIV infection*, 1996, Glaxo-Wellcome.

Casey-Mahon K, Hughes A, Cohen F: *The Association of Nurses in AIDS Care—core curriculum for HIV/AIDS nursing*, Philadelphia, 1996, Nursecom.

Southeast AIDS Training and Education Center: *Metro Atlanta/Georgia resources for HIV/AIDS*, ed 11, Atlanta, 1999, The Association.

Ungvarski PJ, Flaskerud JH: *HIV/AIDS: a guide to nursing care,* ed 4, Philadelphia, 1999, Saunders.

Dunn S: Providing care in a county nursing home AIDS unit. In Fransen VE, ed: *Proceedings: AIDS prevention and service workshop,* Princeton, NJ, 1990, Robert Wood Johnson Foundation.

Unit IV   Frequently Asked Questions

My home attendant only comes 4 hours a day and I feel like I need her for more hours. Who decides how many hours she can stay and what would I have to do to get her to stay for the whole day?

There are a number of factors that help determine how long you may have a home health aide in your home. First and foremost is the number of hours your insurance carrier will approve; second is the number of hours your provider approves based on your condition; and finally the number of hours your home care nurse determines are needed after making a home assessment. If all three agree that more hours are needed, then the home care nurse will increase the hours and/or days necessary to assist with your care. If any one of the three disagrees, then there may be resources available to fill in the gaps, like a "Buddy" or friend, day care, or other community resources. Your case manager can assist you with determining the scope of coverage that your insurance carrier provides.

If I get sick at night or over the weekend, whom should I call?

If you become ill during the night or over the weekend, it is best to call your primary care provider. He or she should have an emergency contact number for nights and weekends. If you cannot reach him or her, then you could certainly call the nurse, who might be able to assess you over the phone and make appropriate decisions about your care.

My physician won't fill out these forms because he says that I don't need home care services anymore. What should I do?

According to federal law, a physician must order home care services. If your physician will not fill out the required paperwork to continue home care services, the nurse will try to intervene on your behalf, if appropriate. The nurse's home assessment may uncover factors that affect your health and well-being that are not apparent during the provider's office assessment. This communication between provider and nurse should be sufficient to reinstate your home care services. However, if your primary physician does not think you need home care services then you cannot receive them unless you are willing to pay for them privately.

I've been told that I don't need a home health aide anymore and that I'll be getting a home attendant instead. I like my home health aide, and I don't want to have a stranger come into my home. Why is this change being made, and is there anything I can do to keep my current home health aide?

The type of paraprofessional in your home is determined by the type of services that you need based on the nursing assessment. To receive the services of a home health aide there must be "skilled nursing needs"; for example, transfer from bed to chair, provision of simple skin care, or assistance with nutrition. When a client's level of care changes or the insurance presents obstacles, then a change in service type may be warranted. The nurse will continue to visit and make assessments of the care that the home attendant provides. Any concerns that you have should be brought to the attention of the nurse immediately.

When I go home, I have to keep changing my dressing and it usually has blood on it. How should I get rid of the soiled dressing?

Soiled dressings should be placed in a plastic leakproof bag, tied, and then placed in a second bag and tied closed and disposed of along with the regular trash. Soiled dressings handled in this manner pose very little threat to those in the immediate area or to sanitation workers. The dressings should not be burned or destroyed in any other way.

Suppose when I go home I cut myself shaving and get blood in the bathroom. How can I clean it up so that my family won't catch HIV from me?

Your concern for others in your home is valid and shows that you understand the risk of transmission. If you happen to spill or splash blood during shaving or when you get a cut, you can initially rinse the sink with water to remove the blood and then follow this by rinsing the sink with a 10% bleach solution. You can purchase this solution at a surgical supply store but it may be costly. You can also make this solution by diluting household bleach with water in a 1:10 ratio.

I don't want my home health aide to know that I have HIV. Does she have to be told?

Your aide does not need to know your diagnosis because he or she will use universal precautions with all clients, including you. That means that home health aides treat all clients as if they are HIV positive.

Unit V

Opportunistic
Infections in
HIV/AIDS

13

Bacterial Infections

- Bacillary angiomatosis
- *Mycobacterium avium* complex
- *Mycobacterium tuberculosis*
- *Rhodococcus equi*

Kenneth Zwolski and Dorothy Talotta

Bacillary Angiomatosis

■ DEFINITION AND ETIOLOGY

A small, gram-negative bacillus, *Bartonella henselae* (also sometimes referred to as *Rochalimaea henselae*) and a closely related species, *B. quintana*, are responsible for causing bacillary angiomatosis, a Category B condition. Bacillary angiomatosis frequently produces skin lesions, although it may also involve other systems of the body such as the viscera, bone, and brain. It is thought that arthropods may serve as a vector of transmission, as well as ticks; but the most common reservoir for the bacillus is the domestic cat and the cat flea.

■ CLINICAL OVERVIEW

The most common presentation is the appearance of papules, nodules, or plaques that occur anywhere on the body. The nodules are tender to the touch. The skin lesions may resemble those associated with Kaposi's sarcoma. Visceral disease is common; involvement of the liver produces a syndrome called peliosis hepatitis, which is associated with fever, abdominal pain, weight loss, hepatomegaly and splenomegaly, and increases in liver enzymes (alkaline phosphatases tend to be more elevated then the hepatic transaminases). Bacteremia may develop, with or without endocarditis. About one half of clients with liver involvement also have skin lesions and one half have lymphadenopathy.

In rare cases Bartonella may infect bones, causing painful osteolytic bone lesions, or the brain, resulting in focal brain lesions and associated neurological symptoms. In the case of brain involvement, skin or liver lesions are always present. Approximately two thirds of those infected with Bartonella have a history of either a cat bite or cat scratch.

■ DIAGNOSIS

Diagnosis is made by biopsy of suspected tissue. Biopsy results show vascular proliferation with edema and polymorphonuclear (PMN) infiltrates. A Warthin Starry stain shows the presence of *B. henselae*.

▓ MEDICAL MANAGEMENT

Medical management is focused on correct diagnosis and then instituting and monitoring response to antibiotic therapy. Erythromycin often gives a good response within 1 to 3 days, but therapy must be continued for up to 2 months to normalize laboratory parameters.

▓ NURSING CONSIDERATIONS

1. Because of the high risk of being infected with *Bartonella* from cats, nurses should educate clients with AIDS about cat ownership. It is recommended that those who are severely immune suppressed should consider the risks of cat ownership. Clients with AIDS should avoid rough play with cats and situations in which scratches from cats are likely to occur. If a scratch or wound develops from interaction with a cat, then the wound should be washed promptly. Cats should not be allowed to lick open wounds or cuts. All cats should be treated for fleas, and flea control measures should be followed.
2. For medical regimens see Table 13-1.

Mycobaterium Avium Complex

▓ DEFINITION AND ETIOLOGY

M. avium complex (MAC) is composed of *M. avium* and *M. intracellulare*, which are closely related species. *M. avium* is more commonly associated with disease in clients with AIDS. Before the AIDS epidemic, MAC was a rare cause of pneumonia. MAC is usually limited to the lungs in immunocompetent individuals. In clients with AIDS, however, MAC can cause infection that is widely disseminated.[1] Prior to the availability of highly active antiretroviral therapy (HAART) and prophylactic medications, it was estimated that as many as one third to one half of clients with AIDS might develop disseminated MAC (DMAC). However, the incidence of MAC has decreased markedly with the widespread use of MAC prophylaxis and the advent of HAART.[2] DMAC infections occur frequently when CD_4 cell counts are below 50 cells/mm^3.

MAC is not considered to be a contagious disease, and organisms of MAC are known as ubiquitous (i.e., occurring everywhere or in many places). MAC can be found in food, water, soil, and animal sources.[3] Because MAC is common in environmental sources, there are currently no specific recommendations to avoid exposure.[4]

▓ CLINICAL OVERVIEW

MAC may enter the body via the gastrointestinal or respiratory tracts. Data suggest that disseminated disease results from newly acquired organisms rather than from reactivation (as immunosuppression becomes severe) of quiescent mycobacteria already present.[2] Localized infection in the gastrointestinal or respiratory tract eventually causes bacteremia and

Table 13-1	Medical Regimens

Bacillary Angiomatosis	Regimens
Prevention	None recommended
Treatment	Erythromycin 500 mg PO or IV qid × 2-4 months
	Or
	Doxycycline 100 mg PO bid
	Or
	Clarithromycin 500 mg PO bid
	Or
	Ciprofloxacin 500-700 mg PO bid
	Or
	Azithromycin 250 mg PO qd
Maintenance	Erythromycin 250-500 mg PO bid
	Or
	Clarithromycin 500 mg PO bid
	Or
	Ciprofloxacin 500-750 mg PO bid

systemic dissemination that is frequently widespread. The liver, lymph nodes, bone marrow, and spleen are common sites of dissemination.[1]

Signs and symptoms of DMAC include fever, fatigue, weight loss, night sweats, abdominal pain, and diarrhea. Lymphadenopathy and organomegaly can also occur. Laboratory data abnormalities include anemia and elevations in alkaline phosphatase and lactic dehydrogenase. It can be difficult to distinguish these signs and symptoms from those of advanced HIV infection and from those of other opportunistic infections and malignancies.[5]

◼ DIAGNOSIS

When disseminated MAC is suspected, mycobacterial blood cultures should be done. If a single blood culture is positive for MAC, this is considered diagnostic for DMAC. When bacteremia is very low, cultures may fluctuate between positive and negative. A positive culture from certain other sites that are normally sterile (e.g., the liver, bone marrow) is also considered by many experts to be diagnostic.[6] An advantage of obtaining biopsy specimens from such sites is that staining may indicate the presence of acid-fast bacteria well before blood cultures become positive.[2]

The significance of finding MAC in sputum or stool is controversial.[2] MAC found in sputum is typically colonization.[1] The presence of MAC organisms in sputum or stool may be predictive of the development of DMAC, but no data are available regarding the effectiveness of prophylaxis in such situations when the client's blood culture result is negative. Therefore, currently, routine screening of stool or sputum to identify clients likely to develop MAC bacteremia is not recommended.[4]

Advances in microbiology have shortened the time needed to detect and identify mycobacteria. Depending on the system used, MAC can be detected in from five to nineteen days. If DNA probes are used, MAC can be identified within a few hours.[1]

It should be noted that both *M. tuberculosis* and *M. avium* are acid-fast bacilli (AFB), and in HIV-positive clients it may be difficult to distinguish MAC disease from tuberculosis (TB).[2] Therefore a sputum smear that is positive for AFB should be treated as tuberculosis until the organism has definitely been identified as nontuberculous.[1]

■ MEDICAL MANAGEMENT

Historically, MAC was very difficult to treat because the organism was inherently resistant to most standard antimicrobial drugs. However, newer drugs, including the advanced generation macrolides (azithromycin and clarithromycin), can now be used to prevent DMAC, and combinations of these macrolides with standard agents can be used for its treatment. Three drugs—rifabutin, azithromycin, and clarithromycin—are approved for single-agent prophylaxis against MAC.[7]

The United States Public Health Service and the Infectious Diseases Society of America recommend that HIV-positive clients receive prophylaxis against DMAC if their CD_4 cell counts are below 50 cells/mm^3. Clarithromycin or azithromycin are the preferred agents for this prophylaxis. Rifabutin can be used as an alternative if the preferred agents cannot be tolerated.[4] In some individuals receiving prophylaxis, macrolide resistance has developed; drug combinations for prophylaxis are being studied in an attempt to delay the development of resistance in future clients.[7]

Before prophylaxis is instituted, the possibility that MAC has already disseminated must be ruled out by clinical assessment, which must include a negative blood culture.[1,4] If DMAC is present, a treatment regimen must be instituted that is different from a prophylactic regimen. In addition, if rifabutin is used alone for prophylaxis and DMAC is already present, MAC organisms resistant to rifabutin can develop.[8]

Also to be ruled out before initiating MAC prophylaxis with rifabutin is active TB. If a client has active TB and receives rifabutin as a single agent, he or she can develop a cross-resistance to rifampin.[4] This would eliminate a mainstay of TB therapy and might contribute to the development of multidrug-resistant TB (MDR TB) (see later in this chapter). Skin testing and chest x-ray studies may be done to check for TB, but the skin test may not be reliable due to anergy (see Chapter 7). Sputum testing for AFB is another means of ruling out TB and may be done especially in areas of high TB prevalence. Some providers may choose not to use rifabutin for prophylaxis in clients at high risk for TB.[8]

In selecting prophylactic agents for MAC disease, the provider should consider cost, the client's tolerance of the drug, and possible drug interactions. Consideration of potential drug interactions is particularly important; for example, there are a number of drug interactions between rifabutin and protease inhibitors (PIs) and nonnucleoside reverse transcriptase inhibitors (NNRTIs).[4]

With the advent of HAART, the CD_4 cell counts of some clients have increased so that the question of discontinuing primary prophylaxis for MAC has arisen. According to current guidelines, the optimal criteria for discontinuation are still not known. However, the guidelines state that a reasonable option is to discontinue the prophylaxis if a client's CD_4 cell count remains above 100 cells/mm[3] for longer than 3 to 6 months and there is sustained suppression of HIV plasma RNA for a similar period.[4]

In treating MAC, there is general agreement that multiple drugs should be used. Treatment should include at least two drugs, one of which should be either clarithromycin or azithromycin.[7] Drugs that may be used in addition include ethambutol, rifabutin, ciprofloxacin, ofloxacin, and, in some cases, amikacin[6,9] (see Table 13-2). A number of experts select ethambutol as the second drug and might add a third or a fourth drug.[6] Some providers may choose a three- or four-drug regimen if the client is very ill.[1] When clarithromycin is used to treat MAC in HIV-positive individuals, the dose should not exceed 1000 mg/day (given as 500 mg bid) because larger doses are associated with increased mortality.[2] According to present recommendations, once a client has been treated for DMAC, secondary prophylaxis (i.e., chronic maintenance therapy) with full therapeutic doses of antimycobacterial drugs should be continued for life.[4]

During initial therapy, symptoms such as fever, weight loss, and night sweats should be monitored. Blood cultures are usually done about every 4 weeks to determine the effectiveness of treatment. Clients will usually experience substantial improvement during the first 4 to 6 weeks of therapy if they are going to improve. If there is no response to therapy then the client should be reevaluated.[6]

■ NURSING CONSIDERATIONS

1. The nurse should be aware that constitutional symptoms, such as those noted above, can be signs of DMAC, especially in clients with low CD_4 cell counts. The nurse should report symptoms to the primary care provider so that appropriate diagnostic tests can be performed. Screening for DMAC by blood culture testing should be done for clients with constitutional symptoms and CD_4 cell counts below 50 cells/mm[3].

2. If a client is receiving rifabutin prophylaxis and does not adhere to the prophylactic regimen, there is potential for the development of rifabutin-resistant MAC. The nurse should encourage adherence, explaining its importance to clients. Some providers may not prescribe rifabutin prophylaxis for clients who have a habit of skipping or stopping medications.[8]

3. While there are more extensive data supporting the use of clarithromycin against MAC, when issues of compliance and cost are considered, the use of azithromycin for MAC prophylaxis has the

advantages of once a week dosing, lower cost, and possibly, fewer drug interactions.[7]

4. If a client receiving rifabutin develops TB, the possibility of TB resistant to both rifabutin and rifampin must be considered.[6]

5. As more drugs are added to the client's medication regimen, the number of possible drug interactions increases. There are many possible drug interactions when drugs for MAC prophylaxis or treatment are used and are added to other medications the client may be taking. The following are some of the Rifabutin interactions that the nurse should be aware of:

- The use of rifabutin in doses greater than 300 mg/day in combination with a macrolide for treatment of MAC disease has been associated with the development of uveitis (i.e., intraocular inflammation). The risk is much less in those taking 300 mg/day.[10] The client with uveitis may complain of eye redness, pain, blurred vision, and photophobia.

- The use of rifabutin with hard-gel saquinavir has been considered contraindicated and data regarding the use of rifabutin with soft-gel saquinivir have been considered insufficient to make a recommendation.[4] However, new guidelines regarding tuberculosis (TB) provide updated information regarding concurrent use of these drugs in TB prevention and treatment.[11] See TB nursing considerations later in this chapter.

- The rifabutin dose should be decreased by 50% (i.e., from 300 mg daily to 150 mg daily) when it is given with indinavir, nelfinavir, or amprenavir.[4]

- According to the CDC's 1999 guidelines for the prevention of opportunistic infections, the dose of rifabutin should be decreased to ¼ of the usual dose (i.e., 150 mg every other day or 3 times weekly) if used with ritonavir.[4]

- Rifabutin should not be used with delavirdine.[4]

- The 1999 guidelines state that if used with efavirenz, the rifabutin dose should be increased to 450 mg daily.[4] The new TB guidelines recommend that the dose of rifabutin be increased to 450 or 600 mg daily when it is used with efavirenz.[11]

- For additional information on rifabutin see the nursing considerations for TB later in this chapter.

6. The following are some clarithromycin interactions that the nurse should be aware of[4,12]:

- Clarithromycin can decrease effects of zidovudine. The nurse should teach the client that these drugs must be taken at least 4 hours apart.

- PIs may increase clarithromycin levels. However, at this time, there is not sufficient data for a recommendation to be made about dosage adjustment.

- Ritonavir increases clarithromycin levels. Dosage adjustment is needed if creatinine clearance is below 30 mL/minute.

Table 13-2	Medical Regimens

Mycobacterium Avium Complex	Regimens
Prophylaxis	**First Choice**
	Clarithromycin 500 mg PO bid
	Or
	Azithromycin 1200 mg PO weekly
	Alternative Regimens
	Rifabutin 300 mg PO qd
	Or
	Azithromycin 1200 mg PO weekly **plus** rifabutin 300 mg PO qd
Treatment	Optimal treatment regimen still not clear.
	One drug should be either:
	Clarithromycin 500 mg PO bid
	Or
	Azithromycin 500-600 mg PO qd
	Plus
	Ethambutol 15 mg/kg PO qd
	And/or
	Rifabutin*
	And/or
	Ciprofloxacin, ofloxacin, amikacin, others
Maintenance	**First Choice**
	Clarithromycin 500 mg PO bid **plus** ethambutol 15 mg/kg PO qd
	With or without
	Rifabutin* 300 mg PO qd
	Alternative Regimen
	Azithromycin 500 mg PO qd **plus** ethambutol 15 mg/kg PO qd
	With or without
	Rifabutin* 300 mg PO qd

*See text in this chapter for interactions and dose changes when rifabutin is used with PIs and NNRTIs. From Centers for Disease Control and Prevention: 1999 USPHS/IDSA guidelines for the prevention of opportunistic infections in persons infected with human immunodeficiency virus, *MMWR* 48(RR-10):1, Aug 20, 1999; Framm SR, Soave R: Agents of diarrhea, *Med Clin North Am* 81(2):427, 1997; Jacobson MA: *Mycobacterium avium* complex. In Cohen PT, Safrin S, eds: *The AIDS knowledge base*, 1997—http://hivinsite.ucsf.edu/akb/1997/section6.html; Masur H et al: US Public Health Service Task Force on Prophylaxis and Therapy for *M. avium* complex, recommendations on prophylaxis and therapy for disseminated *M. avium* complex disease in patients infected with the HIV, *New Engl J Med* 329(12):898, 1993.

- Nevirapine can decrease clarithromycin levels, which can result in decreased effectiveness of prophylaxis. If clients receive this combination, they must be monitored closely.
7. Prophylactic medication for MAC is underprescribed. In 1997, 56% of clients with CD_4 cell counts less than 50 cells/mm³ had not had such medication prescribed.[13] The nurse should ensure that the client receives prophylaxis if appropriate.

BOX 13-1 PEDIATRIC CONSIDERATIONS
Mycobacterium avium complex

Prophylaxis

For children aged >6 years, CD$_4$ cell count <50 cells/mm^3; aged 2-6 years, CD$_4$
 cell count of 75 cells/mm^3; aged 1-2 years, CD$_4$ cell count <500 cells/mm^3; aged
 <1 year, CD$_4$ cell count <750 cells/mm^3:
Clarithromycin 7.5 mg/kg (not to exceed 500 mg) PO bid
Or
Azithromycin 20 mg/kg (not to exceed 1200 mg) PO weekly

Alternative Regimens

Rifabutin 300 mg PO qd (for children ≥ 6 years)
Or
Azithromycin 5 mg/kg (not to exceed 250 mg) PO qd

Treatment*

Clarithromycin 30 mg/kg (not to exceed 2 g) qd in divided doses PO q12h
Or
Ethambutol 15-25 mg/kg qd
Or
Rifabutin 10-20 mg/kg qd
Or
Ciprofloxacin 500-750 mg PO bid
Or
Amikacin 15-22.5 mg/kg IV qd in divided doses q8h

Maintenance
First Choice
Clarithromycin 7.5 mg/kg (not to exceed 500 mg) PO bid
Plus
Ethambutol 15 mg/kg (not to exceed 900 mg) PO qd
With or without
Rifabutin† 5 mg/kg (not to exceed 300 mg) PO qd

---

* A combination of drugs is generally used.
† See text for interactions of rifabutin with PIs and NNRTIs.

8. For medical regimens see Table 13-2. For pediatric regimens see
 Box 13-1.

Mycobacterium Tuberculosis

■ DEFINITION AND ETIOLOGY

Individuals who are HIV-positive are at increased risk of contracting TB.[14]
When a person with more advanced HIV disease, for example, a CD$_4$ cell
count less than 200/mm^3, is newly infected by the organism that causes TB,
there is likely to be a much more rapid progression of the infection which
may be fatal if not treated.[15] Data also suggest that active TB may accelerate

the progression of HIV infection, perhaps by acting as a potent stimulus for replication of HIV at the cellular level.[16] TB is caused by *M. tuberculosis* (MTB), which is an aerobic AFB. It is a communicable disease that is almost always spread via the airborne route. The organism, present in infected particles called droplet nuclei, is emitted into the air by an infected person during activities such as coughing, sneezing, talking, and laughing.[3,17] The microscopic droplet nuclei are inhaled by another person. TB cannot be spread by contact with items such as food, eating utensils, clothing, or bedding.[18]

When mycobacteria are inhaled, the body's first line of defense is the upper airway, which prevents most of the inhaled organisms from reaching the lungs. In order for pulmonary TB to occur, the organisms must penetrate lung tissue, resisting the lung's defense mechanisms. The first time a person is infected with TB is known as primary infection.[17] After entering the lungs, the bacilli are transported to hilar lymph nodes by alveolar macrophages and then spread via the blood. They eventually lodge in oxygen-rich areas such as the apex of the lung.[19] During this process, the body's cell-mediated immunity is activated; this immune response can be detected by a tuberculin skin test (i.e., a PPD test). Infection can usually be detected within 2 to 10 weeks after exposure.[18] Spread of the organism can be contained by an effective cell-mediated immune response. However, once a person has been infected with *M. tuberculosis,* PPD results may continue to be positive for life.[19]

Most people who become infected, however, do not progress to a stage of active disease.[18] Alveolar macrophages surround the organisms and wall them off inside solid tubercles, known as Ghon tubercles, where they lie dormant but remain viable indefinitely. This asymptomatic condition is called latent tuberculosis and is not harmful or contagious.[19]

When the bacilli multiply, however, active disease occurs. Active disease is primary if it occurs when the bacilli first enter the lungs. Active disease can also result from reactivation of TB, which occurs when the solid tubercles break down and bacilli multiply. About 85% of all TB cases are a result of reactivation TB.[18]

In individuals who are HIV-positive, the risk of rapid progression of primary infection is much greater because the ability to contain the infection is impaired. The likelihood of reactivation of a latent infection is also greater due to immune defects.[15] TB can occur relatively early in the course of HIV infection, probably because of the virulence of the organism.[20] It is the only HIV-related opportunistic infection that is also a threat to the general public.[21]

■ CLINICAL OVERVIEW

In HIV-positive clients, the clinical presentation of TB varies somewhat depending on the degree of immunosuppression.[22] Clients with CD_4 cell counts above 300 cells/mm^3 commonly present in a manner similar to that of immunocompetent individuals.[15] Symptoms of TB can be insidious and this may hinder the clinician in diagnosis.[23] Constitutional symptoms such as fever, chills, weight loss, fatigue, and night sweats are character-istic of early reactivation TB. When respiratory symptoms develop, they may include a productive cough and hemoptysis if there has been ulcer-ation of a blood vessel.[24] Clients may report shortness of breath as a result of pleural effusion or, less frequently, pleuritic chest pain as a result of pleural inflammation.

When CD_4 cell counts are below 200 cells/mm^3, there is greater like-lihood of atypical presentations and extrapulmonary TB.[3] Extrapul-monary TB is TB anywhere in the body outside the lungs. Extrapulmo-nary TB can occur in the renal cortex, lymph nodes, bone, meninges, genitourinary tract, abdomen, pericardium, or lymph nodes, for example. Assessment findings in extrapulmonary TB are often indistinct and symp-toms such as fever, weight loss, fatigue, and night sweats may or may not occur. There can be widespread dissemination of TB throughout the body, involving the lungs and many other organs.[17] Disseminated TB is more common in clients with advanced HIV disease.[20]

Clinicians should be acutely aware of the possibility of TB in clients infected with HIV. The presence of other risk factors for TB, such as alco-holism, homelessness, advanced age, and a history of communal living (e.g., in a shelter, prison, or nursing home), should increase the clinician's suspicion of TB.[23]

▮ DIAGNOSTIC TESTING

The PPD test using the Mantoux method is the cornerstone of identifica-tion of individuals infected with TB.[19] The test determines whether or not infection has occurred; however, it does not determine whether infection is active or not. A client receiving a PPD test receives an intradermal injection of a protein derived from the organism. The accuracy of the test result de-pends on the ability of the client's immune system to mobilize the delayed-type hypersensitivity (DTH) response to previous infection.[25] This re-sponse causes a skin reaction at the site of the intradermal injection if the client has been infected. Tuberculin skin testing is described in Chapter 7.

If TB is suspected, a chest x-ray study is an important part of the di-agnostic work-up. In latent TB, most clients will have normal chest x-ray study results, although Ghon lesions are sometimes present. In immuno-compromised anergic clients (see Chapter 7 for a discussion of anergy) who are in danger of reactivation TB, a chest x-ray study may take the place of a nonreactive PPD result in determining if the client has been in-fected with TB. However, in most anergic persons with latent TB, the x-ray study results may still be normal.[19] Chest x-ray study findings in HIV-positive clients with active TB vary.[26] In clients with CD_4 cell counts above 300/mm^3, findings are likely to be typical for reactivation TB with cavities involving the upper lobes of the lungs and focal infiltrates. In clients with CD_4 cell counts less than 200/mm^3, atypical findings such as lympha-denopathy and diffuse, interstitial, or lower lobe infiltrates are more likely, or the findings may be normal.[15]

Sputum studies are also used in the diagnosis of TB. If a client cannot produce an adequate amount of sputum spontaneously, sputum may be obtained by other methods such as bronchoalveolar lavage (BAL).[19] When obtaining sputum specimens from a client suspected of having TB, precautions to prevent transmission of the organism must be taken (see Chapter 7 for sputum specimen collection procedure; and Chapters 7 and 10 for infection control procedures during specimen collection). Examination of sputum can confirm a diagnosis of TB.

An AFB smear is a rapid way of identifying infections caused by mycobacteria, as well as some other organisms. The presence of AFB in a smear is suggestive of the diagnosis of TB, but is not proof of TB disease[27]; positive smears have traditionally detected the presence of mycobacteria, but have not determined the type of mycobacteria present. (Clients with AIDS may have pulmonary infection with MAC or other mycobacteria.) Newer tests, however, are quite sensitive and can identify TB in sputum smears, but these tests are still not as sensitive as cultures.[15] Cultures are essential in determining the type of mycobacteria infecting the client, but require a longer time for results to be obtained.[19]

■ MEDICAL MANAGEMENT

Drug therapy is the primary form of treatment for TB. Drug therapy may be given for prophylaxis (prevention) of TB when indicated or for treatment of the disease.

Considerations for Treatment with Antituberculous and Antiretroviral Therapy

The decision about an appropriate antituberculosis regimen (whether for prophylaxis or treatment) for an HIV-positive person must take into account the antiretroviral treatment that the client may already be receiving. The use of rifampin with protease inhibitors (PIs) or with nonnucleoside reverse transcriptase inhibitors (NNRTIs) has been considered contraindicated.[16] However, recently published guidelines indicate that there are three situations in which rifampin can be used with certain PI and efavirenz drug regimens to treat active TB.[11] (See "Nursing Considerations.")

When rifabutin is used, dosage adjustments of both the rifabutin and some of the antiretrovirals may be necessary and the use of rifabutin with delavirdine is contraindicated. There are also many other medications commonly used in individuals with HIV infection that have drug interactions with both rifampin and rifabutin. These interactions require dose adjustments, use of alternative therapies, or other interventions.[16] (See "Nursing Considerations" later in this chapter.) There are no contraindications to the use of isoniazid (INH), pyrazinamide, ethambutol, or streptomycin with nucleoside reverse transcriptase inhibitors (NRTIs), NNRTIs, or PIs.[16] There are also no contraindications for the concurrent use of NRTIs and rifamycins.[11] Because of the many complex drug interactions that can occur, recommended antituberculosis regimens for both prophylaxis and treatment of TB differ depending on the antiretrovirals being used.

Prophylaxis—Indications and Considerations

In prophylaxis, the goal is to prevent clients from developing active disease. HIV-positive clients with positive PPD skin test results (i.e., greater than or equal to 5 mm of induration), no evidence of active TB, and no history of TB treatment or prophylaxis should receive prophylactic therapy. HIV-positive clients who are close contacts of individuals with infectious TB should also receive prophylactic therapy (after active TB has been ruled out), regardless of their PPD skin test results or prior courses of chemoprophylaxis.[4] HIV-positive clients who have a history of prior untreated or inadequately treated past TB that healed and no history of adequate TB treatment should also receive prophylactic therapy regardless of their PPD skin test results. Some experts recommend consideration of primary TB prophylaxis for HIV-positive clients whose PPD skin test results are negative but who are at ongoing high risk for exposure to TB, such as residents of homeless shelters or prisons with a high prevalence of TB. Such prophylaxis should continue for the duration of the exposure time.[16] Prophylaxis has also been recommended for clients with positive PPD skin test results, and risk factors for HIV infection, whose HIV status is unknown but who are suspected of being HIV-positive.[28]

Prior to beginning prophylactic therapy, active disease must be ruled out. If INH, for example, is used alone and the client has active disease, there is a risk of inducing INH resistance. Therefore, if there is doubt as to whether or not the TB is active, treatment (as opposed to prophylactic) regimens may be used until the client's TB status is clarified. Also, before prophylaxis is begun, clients must be questioned about their history of TB therapy and any adverse reactions, as well as any contraindications or necessary special precautions.[28] Baseline laboratory tests include a CBC and, if the client is to receive a rifamycin, a platelet count; a chemistry panel, including liver enzymes and total bilirubin; and a uric acid level if the client is to receive pyrazinamide. A chest X-ray study is indicated to rule out active TB. If a client has symptoms that indicate active TB or has chest X-ray findings indicating past healed TB and a history of no or inadequate TB treatment, three consecutive sputum samples should be tested to rule out active disease.[16]

Prophylaxis—medical regimens. For prophylaxis against TB for HIV-positive adults, whether or not they are receiving PIs or NNRTIs, the CDC recommends a 9-month regimen of INH daily or twice a week. (Available data, according to the CDC, suggest that the same protection should be obtained from INH prophylaxis whether administered daily or twice a week.) An alternative regimen for HIV-positive adults who are *not* receiving PIs or NNRTIs is a 2-month regimen of rifampin and pyrazinamide administered daily. An alternative prophylactic regimen for HIV-positive adults who *are* receiving PIs or NNRTIs is a 2-month regimen of rifabutin and pyrazinamide administered daily.[16] However, as previously noted, when rifabutin is used with PIs or NNRTIs, there are some contraindications and there is frequently the need for dosage adjustments.[4,11] (See "Nursing Considerations" later in this chapter.)

While receiving prophylaxis against TB, the client should be monitored monthly. During these visits, signs and symptoms of active disease and of drug reactions should be assessed and reviewed with the client. The client should be taught the signs and symptoms of hepatotoxicity and reminded to stop therapy and promptly report such signs and symptoms if they occur (see "Nursing Considerations"). All medications that the client is taking should be reviewed with an assessment of the potential for drug interactions. Appropriate laboratory tests should be performed.[16]

Prophylaxis—duration of regimens.   Completion of a prophylactic regimen should be based on the total number of medication doses administered rather than the duration of therapy only. Daily INH regimens should consist of a minimum of 270 doses administered for 9 months or, if interruption in therapy occurs, for up to 12 months. INH regimens administered twice weekly should consist of a minimum of 76 doses administered for 9 months or, if interruption in therapy occurs, for up to 12 months. Regimens of either rifampin or rifabutin and pyrazinamide should consist of a minimum of 60 doses administered for 2 months. The duration may be extended to 3 months if therapy is interrupted. When therapy is interrupted for 2 months or more, it is essential to rule out active TB disease and perform drug-susceptibility testing. Interruption in therapy may necessitate renewal of the entire regimen.[16]

Treatment

Treatment of TB focuses on elimination of the organism. Current recommendations for the treatment of TB in HIV-positive adults include several options. Note that the client's response to treatment is a critical consideration in determining the duration of treatment for any antituberculous regimen.[16]

Treatment—medical regimens for clients not receiving antiretroviral therapy.   The preferred option for individuals who are not receiving antiretroviral therapy is a 6-month regimen of treatment. INH, rifampin, pyrazinamide, and ethambutol (or streptomycin) are administered for the first 2 months of therapy. (As previously noted, new guidelines indicate three situations in which rifampin can be used with certain PI and efavirenz regimens. (See "Nursing Considerations.") The drugs may be administered daily for the 2-month phase of induction, or daily for at least the first 2 weeks and then 2 or 3 times a week for 6 weeks until the 2-month phase of induction is completed. (Ethambutol may be discontinued if susceptibility tests indicate that the organism is susceptible to both INH and rifampin.) INH and rifampin are then continued for at least an additional 4 months so that the client is treated for at least 6 months. INH and rifampin may be administered daily or two or three times a week during this 4-month period. Alternatively, INH, rifampin, pyrazinamide, and ethambutol (or streptomycin) can be administered three times per week for 6 months.[16]

When a regimen that contains rifampin is used, the minimum duration of treatment is 6 months. The number of doses required depends on whether administration is daily or 2 or 3 times a week. At least 180 daily doses are required or 14 daily induction doses followed by 12 to 18 induction doses administered 2 to 3 times a week for 6 weeks, followed by 36 to 54 continuation doses administered 2 to 3 times a week for 18 weeks. If a regimen containing rifampin is administered on a three times a week schedule, at least 78 doses administered over 26 weeks are required.[16]

Treatment—medical regimens for clients receiving antiretroviral therapy. The recommended initial treatment regimen for individuals who are receiving PIs or NNRTIs is a 2-month induction phase of INH, rifabutin, pyrazinamide, and ethambutol. The drugs may be given daily for the 2-month period, or daily for at least the first 2 weeks followed by twice a week dosing for 6 weeks until the 2-month phase of induction is completed. Then, INH and rifabutin, administered either daily or twice a week, are continued for the next 4 months.[16] As previously noted, the use of rifabutin is contraindicated with some antiretrovirals and dosage adjustment is required with others. Rifampin may be used with efavirenz and certain PIs in three specific situations[11] (see "Nursing Considerations").

When a regimen that contains rifabutin is used, the minimum duration of treatment is 6 months. The number of doses required depends on whether administration is daily or twice a week. At least 180 daily doses are required or 14 daily induction doses followed by 12 induction doses administered twice a week for 6 weeks, followed by 36 doses administered twice a week for 18 weeks.[16]

Non–rifamycin-containing regimens. If a client is intolerant to rifamycin, a decision is made not to combine rifabutin with antiretroviral therapy or, for some other reason, a regimen is used that does not contain a rifamycin, 9 months of treatment is necessary. The initial 2-month phase consists of INH, streptomycin, pyrazinamide, and ethambutol. The drugs may be administered daily for the 2-month period or daily for at least the first 2 weeks and then 2 or 3 times per week for the next 6 weeks. For the next 7 months, the client is treated with INH, streptomycin, and pyrazinamide administered 2 or 3 times per week.[16]

When this regimen is used, at least 60 daily induction doses are required or 14 daily induction doses followed by 12 to 18 induction doses administered 2 or 3 times per week for 6 weeks. The next phase of treatment consists of either 60 doses (when a twice a week schedule is used) or 90 doses (when a three times a week schedule is used) over a period of 30 weeks. For clients who experience a delayed response to this treatment, the duration of therapy should be prolonged from 9 to 12 months or to 6 months after documented conversion of sputum culture.[16]

Clients receiving treatment for TB should be monitored monthly and may need more frequent monitoring during the early stages of treatment. They should be assessed for signs and symptoms of TB and response to treatment. Sputum specimens for smear and culture should be obtained until results are negative. Delayed response to treatment or persistence of positive cultures should be evaluated and appropriate action taken. The potential for drug interactions should be reviewed. The client should be reminded about signs and symptoms of hepatotoxicity (see Nursing Considerations) and the need to discontinue TB medications and notify the provider immediately if these occur. Appropriate laboratory tests should be performed as necessary (e.g., CBC, tests of liver and kidney function).[16]

Paradoxical Reactions

When an individual begins antituberculous therapy, there is a possibility of a paradoxical reaction although these are rare. Paradoxical reactions are temporary exacerbations of TB lesions and symptoms after the therapy is begun. They can occur whether or not the client is HIV-positive but are more common when antiretroviral and antituberculous therapies are being taken concurrently. Paradoxical reactions can cause lymphadenopathy, hectic fevers, worsening of chest x-ray manifestations of TB, and worsening of TB lesions.[16]

It is critical that the clinician rule out other possible causes of these signs and symptoms prior to diagnosing a paradoxical reaction. Paradoxical reactions frequently do not necessitate a change in antituberculous or antiretroviral therapy. If symptoms are severe or life threatening, short-term treatment with steroids is a possible option; hospitalization may be required.[16]

Directly Observed Therapy

Directly observed therapy (DOT) is the observation of the client ingesting antituberculous medications by either a health care provider or another responsible person.[28] The CDC states that DOT and other strategies that increase adherence to therapy should be used for all persons with HIV-related TB.[16] DOT can be used with daily, twice a week, or three times a week medication regimens. The setting for the observation can be an office or other clinical setting; the client's home, school, or place of employment; or another place agreed upon by the client and observer. The observer may be a staff member at a facility, a home health worker, a family member, or a responsible member of the community.[28] DOT greatly increases the likelihood of cure[29] and has been recommended to ensure compliance with therapy.[30]

Multidrug-Resistant TB (MDR-TB)

Multidrug-resistant TB (MDR-TB) is defined by the CDC as active TB that is caused by "organisms that are resistant to more than one antituberculous drug."[31] MDR-TB includes organisms that are resistant to both INH and rifampin,[16] and INH and rifampin are the two drugs most effective for treating TB.[32] In the 1990s, reports of outbreaks of MDR-TB occurred with increasing frequency[33]; organisms have even been found that were resistant to seven antituberculosis drugs.[32] A major cause of the development of drug-resistant organisms is not completing a course of curative therapy.[29] Difficult treatment problems are presented by MDR-TB, and it is recommended that an expert in MDR-TB be consulted in such cases.[16] MDR-TB should be suspected when a client does not respond to therapy.[28] Drug regimens that may be used to treat MDR-TB usually include an aminoglycoside (e.g., streptomycin, kanamycin, amikacin) or capreomycin and a fluoroquinolone. In HIV-positive individuals, treatment of MDR-TB should be continued for 24 months after sputum culture conversion. DOT should always be used for clients with MDR-TB because of serious risks to both the client's and the public's health. Adherence to therapy must be ensured.[16]

If the TB strain is not MDR-TB but is resistant to INH only, it should generally be treated with either rifampin or rifabutin plus pyrazinamide and ethambutol for the duration of therapy (6 to 9 months or for 4 months after sputum culture conversion). If TB is resistant to rifampin only, it should be treated with a 9-month regimen, beginning with 2 months of INH, streptomycin, pyrazinamide, and ethambutol, followed by 7 months of INH, streptomycin, and pyrazinamide.[16]

■ NURSING CONSIDERATIONS

1. The nurse must be aware of factors that facilitate the spread of TB and should maintain a high index of suspicion for the disease.
2. Although cough, fever, and night sweats are among the characteristic symptoms of pulmonary TB, the nurse should keep in mind that atypical presentations can occur.
3. Accurate skin testing and sputum collection are important in establishing the diagnosis of TB. (See Chapter 7 for discussions of Mantoux test administration and sputum collection procedure.)
4. Because of the long duration of therapy for TB, adherence to TB treatment can be difficult for clients. (Approximately 20% of TB clients do not complete a course of therapy within 12 months.[29]) The nurse-client relationship can have an important influence on adherence. It is critical that there be mutual trust and respect for cultural values, health care beliefs, and lifestyle choices.[34] To facilitate adherence, interventions such as DOT are needed. In addition, community outreach workers, particularly those who are of the client's culture and who speak the client's language, can help encourage adherence. Incentives such as food, carfare, or babysitting can be helpful in encouraging clients to continue therapy.[18,28] Also, newer combinations of antituberculosis drugs are available, which may make the regimen easier for the client; for example, INH is now available in combination with rifampin and in combination with both rifampin and pyrazinamide (PZA). Depending on state law, infectious TB clients who have not successfully engaged in or completed treatment despite assistive interventions may be detained involuntarily.[34]

5. HIV-positive individuals who are receiving INH should also receive 25 to 50 mg of vitamin B_6 (pyridoxine) daily or 50 to 100 mg twice a week to reduce the occurrence of side effects in the peripheral and central nervous systems.[16] INH can cause hepatotoxicity. Elevated hepatic enzymes; bilirubinemia; jaundice; and, rarely, severe hepatitis can occur. The risk of hepatitis is greater in older clients and in alcoholics. The nurse should instruct clients to report any fatigue, anorexia, or vomiting, which may be early signs of hepatitis.[35] The client should avoid alcohol use and also report any dark urine, jaundice, or abdominal tenderness.

6. There are interactions between rifampin and PIs and between rifampin and NNRTIs. Rifampin markedly lowers the blood levels of PIs and NNRTIs and has been considered contraindicated when the client is taking these drugs. However, new guidelines suggest that rifampin can be used to treat clients with active TB in three situations: (1) a client's antiretroviral regimen includes the NNRTI, efavirenz, and two NRTIs; (2) a client's antiretroviral regimen includes the PI, ritonavir, and one or more NRTIs; and (3) a client's antiretroviral regimen includes the combination of two PIs (i.e., ritonavir and either hard-gel or soft-gel saquinavir). If efavirenz is used with rifampin, some experts recommend increasing the efavirenz dose from 600 mg to 800 mg daily.[11] In clients receiving other regimens, it is recommended that there be at least a 2-week period between the last dose of rifampin and the first dose of PI or NNRTI.[16]

7. The nurse needs to be aware of a number of factors when the client is receiving rifampin or rifabutin. These include the following:
   - The client should be informed that the medication causes saliva, sputum, sweat, tears, urine, and feces to become red-orange to red-brown in color and that permanent discoloration of soft contact lenses may occur.
   - These drugs can cause hepatitis and the client should be taught to report any warning signs and to avoid alcohol, as it may increase the potential for hepatotoxicity.
   - These drugs can also cause thrombocytopenia and the client should be taught to report signs such as unusual bleeding or bruising.[12]
   - Rifampin and rifabutin cause an increase in the metabolism of methadone and oral contraceptives (as well as a number of other drugs).[12,36] Clients receiving rifampin and methadone will require incremental increases in their dose of methadone in order to avoid withdrawal symptoms. The effect of rifabutin on methadone, however, is milder and withdrawal symptoms are less frequent. The client should be monitored for withdrawal symptoms and the methadone dose increased if necessary.[36] When rifampin or rifabutin is used, there may be a decrease in the effectiveness of oral contraceptives and, in addition, these drugs have teratogenic properties. Therefore, the client should be advised to use another, nonhormonal form of contraception during therapy.[12] When the

client is receiving rifampin or rifabutin, there are drug interactions with many medications that an HIV-positive client may be receiving. Some of these include: anticoagulants, anticonvulsants, beta-blockers, cardiac glycosides, corticosteroids, dapsone, diazepam, fluconazole, ketoconazole, itraconazole, hormonal contraceptives, hypoglycemics (sulfonylureas), narcotics (including methadone as mentioned above), and theophylline. Concomitant use of these drugs with a rifamycin requires interventions such as adjustments in dosage or use of alternative therapies.[16]

8. The nurse needs to be aware of a number of factors when the client is receiving rifabutin. These include the following:

- Rifabutin should not be used with delavirdine.[4] Recent guidelines indicate that rifabutin can possibly be used with hard-gel saquinavir if ritonavir is also included in the drug regimen. Rifabutin in the ususal dose can possibly be used with soft-gel saquinavir.[11]

- When rifabutin is used, dosage adjustments of it and some of the antiretrovirals are recommended as follows[4,11,16]:
  - Combinations of rifabutin with saquinavir and ritonavir are possibilities, with the dose of rifabutin decreased to 150 mg two or three times per week. There is limited data and clinical experience with these combinations.
  - When rifabutin is used in a daily regimen with indinavir, nelfinavir, or amprenavir, the daily dose should be decreased from 300 to 150 mg. The recommended dose of rifabutin for twice weekly administration is 300 mg if indinavir, nelfinavir, or amprenavir are being used concurrently.
  - If used with ritonavir, the rifabutin dose should be decreased to 150 mg two or three times per week.
  - When used with efavirenz, the dose of rifabutin should be increased. One recommendation is to increase the dose from 300 mg to 450 mg regardless of whether it is administered daily or twice weekly.[16] A more recent recommendation is to increase the dose to 450 mg or 600 mg daily or to 600 mg two or three times per week.[11]
  - There are no published clinical experiences for the concurrent use of rifabutin and nevirapine. However, new guidelines suggest that this combination is a possibility with the dose of rifabutin remaining at the usual dose of 300 mg daily or 2 or 3 times per week.
  - When rifabutin is used concurrently with PIs or NNRTIs, the client should be monitored carefully for signs of rifabutin drug toxicity, such as arthralgia, uveitis, and leukopenia, as well as for decreased antiretroviral activity.
  - When indinavir is used with rifabutin, some experts recommend that the indinavir dose be increased from 800 mg every 8 hours to 1000 mg every 8 hours.[11]

- When nelfinavir is used with rifabutin, some experts suggest that the dose of nelfinavir be increased from 750 mg three times a day to 1000 mg three times a day.

9. Clients receiving PZA should be monitored for both hepatotoxicity and hyperuricemia. Clients may also experience arthralgia and photosensitivity. PZA may decrease the effectiveness of antigout agents. The client should be taught to notify the provider if any signs of hepatotoxicity occur or if any pain or swelling of the joints occurs. In addition, the client should be advised to wear protective clothing and use sunscreen to prevent photosensitivity reactions. Evaluation of hepatic function prior to and every 2 to 4 weeks during therapy has been recommended.[12] PZA can also make glucose control more difficult in clients with diabetes.[16]

10. Clients receiving ethambutol are at risk for the development of optic neuritis, which may be bilateral or unilateral. All clients who are to receive ethambutol should have a baseline visual acuity examination and a test for red-green color perception. These should be repeated monthly.[16] The client should be taught to report any blurred vision, constriction of the visual fields, or changed color perception immediately. If not identified early, visual impairment can lead to permanent impairment of sight.

11. Aminoglycosides such as streptomycin, amikacin, or kanamycin can cause ototoxicity and nephrotoxicity. To monitor for ototoxicity, audiometry should be done prior to and throughout the course of therapy. The client should be taught to report any tinnitus, vertigo, dizziness, or hearing loss. To monitor for nephrotoxicity, renal function tests should be done periodically. The client should be taught to drink plenty of fluids.[12]

12. For complete drug information, the reader is referred to a nursing drug reference.

13. There should be consultation with an expert in the field when the client has MDR-TB.[28]

14. When receiving a two or three times weekly drug regimen, there is increased risk that the client will forget doses, which can lead to the emergence of drug-resistant organisms. This type of therapy should only be used when the client is receiving supervised therapy (DOT).[16,28]

15. Clients whose sputum was positive for TB prior to treatment should have sputum examinations at least monthly (weekly smears are encouraged) until the sputum becomes negative. More than 85% of clients whose sputum was positive prior to treatment should have negative sputum after 2 months of treatment with regimens containing both INH and rifampin. If this does not occur, careful reevaluation is needed with repeated drug susceptibility studies and the use of DOT. If resistant organisms are found, the drug regimen must be modified.[28]

16. Screening for TB in HIV-positive individuals includes an annual chest x-ray study and Mantoux test.[25]

Table 13-3	Medical Regimens

Tuberculosis	Regimen
Prophylaxis	Isoniazid (INH) 300 mg PO **plus** pyridoxine 50 mg PO qd *Or* INH 900 mg PO **plus** pyridoxine 100 mg PO twice weekly Duration: Usually 9 months. **Short-course regimens:** ***Not Receiving PIs or NNRTIs*** Rifampin 600 mg **plus** pyrazinamide 20 mg/kg PO qd Duration: Usually 2 months. ***Receiving PIs* or NNRTIs**** Rifampin is contraindicated except in certain situations (see "Nursing Considerations"). Clients receiving some PIs or NNRTIs can receive rifabutin plus pyrazinamide 20 mg/kg PO qd. However, the dose of rifabutin depends on the PIs or NNRTIs administered concurrently (see "Nursing Considerations"). Duration: Usually 2 months. **For MDR-TB:** Consultation with expert in MDR-TB.
First-Line Treatment	***Not Receiving Antiretroviral Therapy*** Induction phase: (Dosage should be daily for at least the first 2 weeks) INH 5 mg/kg (not to exceed 300 mg) qd **or** 15 mg/kg (not to exceed 900 mg) 2 or 3 times per week *Plus* Rifampin 10 mg/kg (not to exceed 600 mg) qd **or** 2-3 times per week

*For dose changes of antiretrovirals, see the appropriate section on nursing considerations.
From American Thoracic Society: Treatment of tuberculosis and tuberculosis infection in adults and children, *Am J Respir Crit Care Med* 149:1359, 1994; Centers for Disease Control and Prevention: Updated guidelines for the use of rifabutin or rifampin for the treatment and prevention of tuberculosis among HIV-infected patients taking protease inhibitors or nonnucleoside reverse transcriptase inhibitors, *MMWR* 49(9):185, 2000; Centers for Disease Control and Prevention: Prevention and treatment of tuberculosis among patients infected with human immunodeficiency virus: principles of therapy and revised recommendations, *MMWR* 47(RR20):1, 1998.

17. For medical regimens see Table 13-3. For pediatric regimens see Box 13-2.

ADDITIONAL RESOURCES

Division of Tuberculosis Elimination:
http://www.cdc.gov/nchstp/tb
Francis J. Curry National Tuberculosis Center:
http://www.nationaltbcenter.edu/ics.html

Table 13-3	Medical Regimens—cont'd

Tuberculosis	Regimen

	Plus
	Pyrazinamide 15-30 mg/kg (not to exceed 2 g) qd **or**
	  50-70 mg/kg (not to exceed 3.5 g) 2 times per week **or**
	  50-70 mg/kg (not to exceed 2.5 g) 3 times per week
	Plus
	Ethambutol or streptomycin at the following doses:
	  Ethambutol 15-25 mg/kg (not to exceed 1600 mg) qd **or**
	    50 mg/kg (not to exceed 4000 mg) 2 times per week
	    or 25-30 mg/kg (not to exceed 2000 mg) 3 times per week
	  Or
	  Streptomycin 15 mg/kg (not to exceed 1 g) qd **or** 25-30 mg/kg
	    (not to exceed 1.5 g) 2-3 times per week (not to exceed 1 g for
	    those aged 60 years and over)
	Duration: Usually 2 months, followed by:
	  Continuation phase:
	  INH **plus** rifampin qd or 2-3 per week
	  Duration: Usually 4 months.
	  Minimum duration for total regimen: 6 months. See text for
	    specifics of duration.
	
	Receiving PIs* or NNRTIs*
	Rifampin is contraindicated except in certain situations. Clients
	  receiving some PIs and NNRTIs can receive rifabutin. However,
	  the dose of rifabutin depends on the PIs or NNRTIs adminis-
	  tered concurrently (see "Nursing Considerations").
	Induction phase:
	  (Dosage should be daily for at least the first 2 weeks)
	  INH **plus** Pyrazinamide **plus** Ethambutol qd **or** 2 times per
	    week at above doses **plus** rifabutin qd or 2 times per week
	Duration: Usually 2 months, followed by (continuation phase):
	  INH **plus** Rifabutin qd **or** 2 times per week
	  Duration: Usually 4 months.
	  Minimum duration of total regimen: 6 months. See text for
	    specifics of duration and regimens for when the use of a
	    rifamycin is limited or contraindicated.

Second-Line
Treatment
	Second-line drugs with daily doses (note that some may require
	  divided dosing) include:
	• Capreomycin 15-30 mg/kg (not to exceed 1 g) IM (not to ex-
	  ceed 750 mg in older adults)
	• Kanamycin 15-30 mg/kg (not to exceed 1 g) IM
	• Ethionamide 15-20 mg/kg (not to exceed 1 g) PO
	• Paraaminosalicylic acid 150 mg/kg (not to exceed 12 g) PO
	• Cycloserine 15-20 mg/kg (not to exceed 1 g) PO
	Second-line drugs should be used only when necessary and by a
	  provider experienced in their use.

Maintenance	**For MDR-TB:** Consultation with expert in MDR-TB. Not indicated.

 ## BOX 13-2 PEDIATRIC CONSIDERATIONS
Mycobacterium avium complex

M. *avium* complex	Regimens
Prophylaxis	Isoniazid 10-15 mg/kg (not to exceed 300 mg) PO qd × 9 months *Or* Isoniazid 20-30 mg/kg (not to exceed 900 mg) PO twice weekly × 9 months (Most experts recommend that pyridoxine be given to HIV-infected children treated with isoniazid) **Alternative Regimen** Rifampin 10-20 mg/kg (not to exceed 600 mg) PO qd × 4-6 months (Note that the use of rifampin with protease inhibitors [PIs] or nonnucleoside reverse transcriptase inhibitors [NNRTIs] is generally contraindicated.)
Treatment	If drug-susceptibility results are not available, a four-drug regimen (e.g., isoniazid, a rifamycin, pyrazinamide, and ethambutol*) for 2 months, followed by isoniazid and a rifamycin administered intermittently for 4 months, is recommended. (If a child is receiving PIs or NNRTIs, drug interactions and contraindications for use with rifamycins must be considered.)

---

* For HIV-positive children (even those who are too young to have visual acuity and red-green color perception monitored), ethambutol at a dose of 15 mg/kg should be included in the initial regimen unless the *M. tuberculosis* (MTB) strain is known or suspected to be susceptible to isoniazid and rifampin.
From Centers for Disease Control and Prevention: 1999 USPHS/IDSA guidelines for the prevention of opportunistic infections in persons infected with human immunodeficiency virus, *MMWR* 48(RR-1):1, 1999; Centers for Disease Control and Prevention: Prevention and treatment of tuberculosis among patients infected with human immunodeficiency virus: principles of therapy and revised recommendations, *MMWR* 47(RR20):1, 1998.

Rhodococcus Equi

■ DEFINITION AND ETIOLOGY

R. equi is a gram-positive, non–spore-forming, aerobic coccobacillus that is found in the soil of all continents except Antarctica. It is especially prevalent in horse ranches. It has a long history of being a veterinary pathogen. In 1967, however, it was recognized as a human pathogen as well, causing mostly respiratory-related complications in severely immunosuppressed clients. It is transmitted by exposure to soil (through either inhalation or ingestion) that is contaminated with the manure of infected animals.

■ CLINICAL OVERVIEW

A client infected with *R. equi* presents with chest pain, a productive cough, hemoptysis, dyspnea, and fever. Often clients are symptomatic for weeks

Table 13-4	Medical Regimen	

Rhodococcus equi	**Regimen**
Prevention	None recommended.
Treatment	Vancomycin 2.0 gm IV qd
	With or without
	Rifampin 600 mg PO qd **plus** imipenem 0.5 g IV q6h **plus** ciprofloxacin 750 mg PO bid × 2-4 weeks
	Or
	Erythromycin 2-4 g IV qd
Maintenance	Ciprofloxacin 750 mg PO bid (resistance is likely to develop)

to months before diagnosis. Anorexia, fatigue, and weight loss may be present. Bacteremia develops in 53% of clients. Rarely, brain abscesses may develop. X-ray studies of the chest in HIV-positive clients show pulmonary infiltrates, empyema, pleural effusion, and cavitary lung disease, particularly in the upper lobes.

■ DIAGNOSIS

Diagnosis is made by isolation of the organism from sputum or bronchoalveolar lavage fluid, or from normally sterile sites such as blood, pleural fluid, or biopsy tissue.

■ MEDICAL MANAGEMENT

R. equi infection is treated with antibiotics, usually erythromycin, rifampin, vancomycin, ciprofloxacin, or imipenem. Antimicrobial susceptibility testing on initial isolates is done to direct antimicrobial therapy. Follow-up cultures need to be done because resistance can easily develop to antibiotics. Often treatment with more than one drug is needed and treatment can last as long as 2 to 6 months. Lifelong suppressive therapy is often necessary.

■ NURSING CONSIDERATIONS

1. Most clients with HIV who become infected with *R. equi* do not have a well-defined exposure. However, it is wise to counsel severely immunosuppressed clients to avoid any situation that may potentially put them into contact with infected soil. They should avoid visiting or working on a horse farm or working as a groom, for instance.

2. Infection with *R. equi* produces a cavitary lung disease, similar in many respects to TB. However, TB, as compared to *R. equi*, tends to occur in clients with higher CD_4 cell counts. Therefore any client with a low CD_4 cell count, no history of tuberculosis, and a cavitary lung disease should be suspected of *R. equi* infection (Table 13-4).

REFERENCES

1. French AL, Benator DA, Gordin FM: Nontuberculous mycobacterial infections, *Med Clin N Am* 81(2):361, 1997.
2. Jacobson MA: Disseminated mycobacterium avium complex and other atypical mycobacterial infections. In Sande MA, Volberding PA, eds: *The medical management of AIDS,* ed 6, Philadelphia, 1999, Saunders.
3. Casey KM, Cohen F, Hughes A: *ANAC's core curriculum for HIV/AIDS nursing,* Philadelphia, Nursecom, 1996.
4. Centers for Disease Control and Prevention: 1999 USPHS/IDSA guidelines for the prevention of opportunistic infections in persons infected with human immunodeficiency virus, *MMWR* 48(RR-10):1, August 20, 1999.
5. Gordin FM et al: Early manifestations of disseminated *M. avium* complex disease: A prospective evaluation, *J Infect Dis* 176:126, 1997.
6. Masur H et al: US Public Health Service Task Force on Prophylaxis and Therapy for *M. Avium* Complex: recommendations on prophylaxis and therapy for disseminated *M. avium* complex disease in patients infected with the HIV, *N Engl J Med* 329(12):898, 1993.
7. Amsden GW, Peloquin CA, Berning SE: The role of advanced generation macrolides in the prophylaxis and treatment of *Mycobacterium avium* complex (MAC) infections, *Drugs* 54(1):69, 1997.
8. Klaus B D, Prophylaxis of *Mycobacterium avium* complex infections in AIDS, *Nurse Pract* 20(6):80, 1995.
9. Framm SR, Soave R: Agents of diarrhea, *Med Clin North Am* 81(2):427, 1997.
10. Shafran SD et al, for the Canadian HIV Trials Network Protocol 010 Study Group: A comparison of two regimens for the treatment of *Mycobacterium avium* complex bacteremia in AIDS: rifabutin, ethambutol, and clarithromycin versus rifampin, ethambutol, clofazimine, and ciprofloxacin, *N Engl J Med* 335(6):377, 1996.
11. Centers for Disease Control and Prevention: Updated guidelines for the use of rifabutin or rifampin for the treatment and prevention of tuberculosis among HIV-infected patients taking protease inhibitors or nonnucleoside reverse transcriptase inhibitors, *MMWR* 49(9):185, March 10, 2000.
12. Deglin JH, Vallerand AH: *Davis' drug guide for nurses,* ed 5, Philadelphia, 1997, FA Davis.
13. Centers for Disease Control and Prevention: Surveillance for AIDS-defining opportunistic illnesses, 1992-1997, *MMWR* 48(SS-2):1, 1999.
14. Coker R, Miller R: HIV-associated tuberculosis, *BMJ* 314(7098):1847, June 28, 1997.
15. Chambers HF: Tuberculosis in the HIV-infected patient. In Sande MA, Volberding PA, eds: *The medical management of AIDS,* ed 6, Philadelphia, 1999, Saunders.
16. Centers for Disease Control and Prevention: Prevention and treatment of tuberculosis among patients infected with human immunodeficiency virus: principles of therapy and revised recommendations, *MMWR* 47(RR20):1, October 30, 1998.
17. Cronin SN: Nursing care of clients with disorders of the lung parenchyma and pleura. In Black JM, Matassarin-Jacobs E, eds: *Medical-surgical nursing: clinical management for continuity of care,* ed 5, Philadelphia, 1997, Saunders.
18. Boutotte J: TB: the second time around . . . and how you can help to control it, *Nursing 93* 23(5):42, 1993.

19. Leiner S, Mays M: Diagnosing latent and active pulmonary tuberculosis: a review for clinicians, *Nurse Pract* 21(2):86, 1996.

20. Hopewell PC: Tuberculosis in persons with human immunodeficiency virus infection. In Sande MA, Volberding PA, eds: *The medical management of AIDS,* ed 5, Philadelphia, 1997, Saunders.

21. Gordin FM et al: A controlled trial of isoniazid in persons with anergy and HIV infection who are at risk for tuberculosis, *N Engl J Med* 337:315, 1997.

22. Schecter GF: *Mycobacterium tuberculosis* infection. In Cohen PT, Sande MA, Volberding PA, eds: *The AIDS knowledge base,* ed 2, Boston, 1994, Little, Brown & Co.

23. Waxman S, Gang M, Goldfrank L: Tuberculosis in the HIV-infected patient, *Emerg Med Clin North Am* 13(1):179, 1995.

24. Rakel RE: *Textbook of family practice,* ed 5, Philadelphia, 1995, Saunders.

25. Jo HS: Assessment and management of persons coinfected with tuberculosis and human immunodeficiency virus, *Nurse Pract* 18(11):42, 1993.

26. Miller WT: Tuberculosis in the 1990s, *Radiol Clin North Am* 32:(4):649, 1994.

27. Scharer LL, McAdam JM: *Tuberculosis and AIDS: the epidemiology of tuberculosis and human immunodeficiency virus,* New York, 1995, Springer.

28. American Thoracic Society: Treatment of tuberculosis and tuberculosis infection in adults and children, *Am J Respir Crit Care Med* 149:1359, 1994.

29. Centers for Disease Control and Prevention: Meeting the challenge of multidrug-resistant tuberculosis: summary of a conference, *MMWR* 41(RR-11):51, June 19, 1992.

30. Advisory Committee for the Elimination of Tuberculosis: A strategic plan for the elimination of tuberculosis in the United States, *MMWR* 38(Suppl 3), 1989.

31. Centers for Disease Control and Prevention: Guidelines for preventing the transmission of *M. tuberculosis* in health-care facilities, *MMWR* 43(RR-13):1, October 28, 1994.

32. Centers for Disease Control and Prevention: National action plan to combat multidrug-resistant tuberculosis, *MMWR* 41(RR-11):7, June 19, 1992.

33. Serkey JM: Multidrug-resistant tuberculosis: a new era in prevention and control, *Dim Crit Care Nurs* 14(5):236, 1995.

34. Anastasio CJ: HIV and tuberculosis: noncompliance revisited, *J Assoc Nurses AIDS Care* 6(2):11, 1995.

35. Anastasi JK, Rivers J: Understanding prophylactic therapy for HIV infections, *Am J Nurs* 94(2):36, 1994.

36. Friedland G: HIV disease in substance abusers: treatment issues. In Sande MA, Volberding PA, eds: *The medical management of AIDS,* ed 6, Philadelphia, 1999, Saunders.

14

Fungal Infections

- Aspergillosis
- Candidiasis
- Coccidioidomycosis
- Cryptococcosis
- Histoplasmosis

Kenneth Zwolski

Aspergillosis

■ DEFINITION AND ETIOLOGY

Three species of the fungus *Aspergillus* (i.e., *A. fumigatus, A. flavus,* and *A. terreus*) can cause aspergillosis. These species live in soil, water, and air and are ubiquitous in geographical distribution. Spores of Aspergillus are inhaled into the lungs. Once in the lung they can cause a serious, life-threatening pulmonary infection in immunosuppressed clients. Rarely does Aspergillus disseminate to other sites in the body.

About 4% of clients with AIDS with CD_4 cell counts of less than 50 cells/mm^3 develop aspergillosis. Two predisposing factors are severe neutropenia (an absolute neutrophil count [ANC] of less than 500/mm^3) and the use of corticosteroids.

■ CLINICAL OVERVIEW

Most clients who develop aspergillosis had an episode of pneumonia in the year preceding diagnosis of aspergillosis and before their CD_4 cell counts dropped to less than 50 cells/mm^3. Symptoms are mostly pulmonary in nature and include fever, cough, dyspnea, chest pain, and hemoptysis. Occasionally, central nervous system (CNS) signs occur. Chest x-ray studies typically show bilateral interstitial infiltrates, although focal or reticulonodular infiltrates can also be present. Despite treatment, the mean time to death after diagnosis of aspergillosis is about 8 weeks.

■ DIAGNOSIS

The most reliable tests are positive stains of respiratory secretions or biopsy evidence of tissue invasion. False-positive and false-negative cultures are common.

■ MEDICAL MANAGEMENT

Amphotericin B is most commonly used to treat aspergillosis. If the client responds, then chronic suppressive therapy is required indefinitely. Be-

Table 14-1	Medical Regimens	

Aspergillosis	Regimen
Prophylaxis	None recommended.
Treatment	Amphotericin B 1.0-1.4 mg/kg qd
	Or
	Itraconazole 200 mg PO bid
	Or
	Amphotec 3-6 mg/kg/d IV
	Or
	Abelcet 5 mg/kg IV qd
Maintenance	Usually not necessary.

cause corticosteroids are a predisposing factor for infection, they should be stopped or decreased as necessary. Granulocyte colony-stimulating factor (G-CSF) can treat neutropenia.

■ NURSING CONSIDERATIONS

1. Clients who are severely immunosuppressed should be taught how to take precautions against infection with *Aspergillus*. *Aspergillus* can be found in basements, crawlways, bedding, humidifiers, ventilation ducts, potted plants, wicker or straw material, condiments, pasta, and household dust. To the extent possible, the client should avoid or eliminate these sources of *Aspergillus* in his or her living space.
2. *Aspergillus* is also associated with decaying matter and may be found in marijuana.
3. The nurse needs to provide intense monitoring of any client receiving antifungal agents and be aware of the possible drug-drug interactions between antifungal agents and other medications.
4. For medical regimens see Table 14-1.

Candidiasis

■ DEFINITION AND ETIOLOGY

Candida albicans is a unicellular yeast that is found on soil, food, and inanimate objects. In humans it can inhabit the teeth, gingiva, skin, oropharynx, vagina, and large intestine. It can be transmitted from mother to child during vaginal delivery, it can be passed from one person to another through sexual intercourse, or it can be acquired nosocomially in a health care setting. Ordinarily, unless the immune system is suppressed or the normal flora or fauna on the skin or mucous membranes is disrupted, *C. albicans* does not cause a candidiasis infection. Treatment with antibiotics or the presence of indwelling catheters or IV devices increases the risk for infection. Anywhere from 75% to 90% of clients who are HIV-positive will develop candidiasis at some time during the course of their illness.

In clients who are HIV-positive, oral and vaginal forms of candidiasis are often seen in the early stages of the disease and many times this may be the initial indicator of infection with HIV. Thrush, which is a pseudomembranous form of candidiasis, is the most common form of oral candidiasis. Both oral candidiasis and vulvovaginal candidiasis, which is recurrent, persistent or poorly responsive to therapy, represent Category B conditions. *C. albicans* may cause intertrigo, especially in genital areas, upper thighs, and under the breasts, and occasionally it may produce an infection of the nails or surrounding tissues.

In AIDS clients, candidiasis may progress to infection of the esophagus and, more rarely, infection of the bronchi, trachea, or lungs. These forms of candidiasis are classified as AIDS indicator conditions. Esophageal candidiasis actually accounts for 10% to 17% of AIDS-defining diagnoses. Overall, clients with AIDS have a lifetime risk of 20% to 30% of developing esophageal candidiasis. Candidiasis of bronchi, trachea, or lungs can also develop and accounts for 1% to 2% of initial AIDS-defining diagnoses.

■ CLINICAL OVERVIEW

Oral candidiasis can occur in either a pseudomembranous form (thrush) or in an erythematous form. In thrush, presentation is whitish to creamy colored patches, about 1 to 2 mm, surrounded by an erythematous base. These patches are found mostly on buccal mucosa and tongue surfaces. Often they can be wiped off, leaving an erythematous or even bleeding mucosal surface. Occasionally, they cannot be wiped off. If this is the case, then it can easily be confused with oral hairy leukoplakia. The erythematous form is seen as red patches on the hard or soft palate, buccal mucosa, or dorsal surface of the tongue. These lesions can appear insignificant and can easily be missed. Even though erythematous oral candidiasis is much less frequent then the pseudomembranous form, it can be just as serious as a prognostic indicator for the progression to AIDS. Angular cheilitis caused by *C. albicans* may occur with or without oral candidiasis. Angular cheilitis presents as cracks, fissures, and erythema at the corner of the mouth.

Vaginitis associated with *C. albicans* can cause erythema, pruritus, and swelling of external genitalia. Physical examination shows whitish to yellowish cottage cheese–like discharges that adhere to the vaginal walls, producing a musty odor. Recurrent or resistant cases of fungal vaginitis may be due to infection with *Torulopsis glabrata,* another species of yeast that is more resistant to treatment with imidazoles. Esophageal candidiasis typically presents with a complaint of dysphagia, a sensation that food is sticking. Other symptoms include pain on swallowing (odynophagia) and retrosternal esophageal pain (esophagospasm). Occasionally, a client with esophageal candidiasis is asymptomatic. Clients with esophageal candidiasis often have thrush at the same time. Esophageal candidiasis tends to occur when the CD_4 count is below 200 cells/mm^3. Antibiotic therapy can easily result in the overgrowth of *C. albicans* and increases the risk of occurrence of esophageal candidiasis. A deficiency of hydrogen chloride (HCL) in gastric juice (hypochlorhydria) has been associated with an increased risk for Candida esophagitis. Hypochlorhydria can happen in clients who are being treated for gastric ulcers or clients who have had gastric surgery or AIDS-associated gastropathies.

■ DIAGNOSIS

The diagnosis of oral and vaginal candidiasis is made by potassium hydroxide preparation of a smear from the lesion. A culture provides information concerning the species involved and can be very useful. The differential diagnosis of oral candidiasis includes oral hairy leukoplakia. *C. albicans* can be identified in the vagina even in the absence of symptoms, so a diagnosis of fungal vaginitis must include clinical symptoms in addition to a positive culture.

Endoscopy is used to make the diagnosis of esophageal candidiasis. Large white to yellow plaques are usually noted throughout the esophagus. A biopsy or direct cytology should be done. Radiography is not useful in establishing the diagnosis of esophageal candidiasis but may be useful to assess esophageal motility; demonstrate complications such as ulcerations, perforations, or fistulas; and identify obstructions.

Dysphagia, odynophagia, and retrosternal pain can be associated not only with esophageal candidiasis but also cytomegalovirus (CMV) esophagitis and herpes esophagitis. To make the differential diagnosis a histopathological examination of the lesions needs to be done. Generally speaking, though, the pattern of symptoms may be useful in making a differential diagnosis. In esophageal candidiasis, dysphagia is most severe and odynophagia and esophagospasm are rare, whereas in CMV and herpes esophagitis, dysphagia is moderate and odynophagia and esophagospasm are more severe.

■ MEDICAL MANAGEMENT

Oral candidiasis usually responds to antifungal agents, including nystatin, clotrimazole, and fluconazole (Diflucan). More potent antifungals, such as Itraconazole or amphotericin B oral solution can be used as alternatives in clients who fail the usual oral regimen. Generally clients are treated until symptoms resolve, about 10 to 14 days in most cases. Many clients will relapse within 3 months after therapy. Clients can be treated for each episode as it occurs, or they can be put on a maintenance schedule to prevent further incidences. Prophylaxis is not recommended. Angular cheilitis usually responds to topical antifungal creams.

Vaginal candidiasis responds well to antifungal creams such as clotrimazole or miconazole. It can also be treated with oral fluconazole. Certain conditions may require continuous treatment in order to prevent relapse. Other forms not related to candida (e.g., glabrata) may respond to boric acid suppositories.

Clients presenting with symptoms suggestive of esophagitis need to be evaluated. There may be noninfectious causes of esophagitis. For instance, HIV itself has been implicated in causing esophageal ulcerations during acute HIV infection and during the development of AIDS. If an infectious origin is suspected, a differential diagnosis needs to be established. The most common organisms causing esophagitis are *C. albicans,* herpes simplex, and CMV. Rarely, other organisms such as *M. tuberculosis, M. avium-intracellulare, P. carinii,* cryptosporidium, *Aspergillus,* or Epstein-Barr virus (EBV) may be causing esophagitis.

Most cases of *Candida* esophagitis can be treated with oral ketoconazole, itraconazole, or fluconazole. In clients who have difficulty swallowing, fluconazole or low-dose amphotericin B can be given intravenously. For severe cases, the drug of choice is amphotericin B. The relapse rate is 84% within 1 year with the absence of maintenance therapy. Prolonged antifungal therapy increases the risk of resistant organisms.

■ NURSING CONSIDERATIONS

1. Any adult presenting with oral candidiasis should be tested for HIV. To decrease the incidence of *Candida* infections, clients with HIV should be encouraged to practice good oral hygiene and skin care routinely, while being cautioned not to do anything that might be traumatic to mucosal surfaces. Skin surfaces should be kept dry and exposed to air.

2. Women should be advised that vaginal candidiasis that occurs in the absence of antibiotic treatment or that is refractory to standard treatment warrants testing for HIV. Women with HIV can be taught to reduce or prevent the occurrences of vaginal candidiasis by:
   - Avoiding clothing that is too tight.
   - Changing menstrual pads frequently.
   - Avoiding panty hose and all tight-fitting synthetic underwear.
   - Avoiding douching and feminine hygiene products.
   - Avoiding spreading anal secretions to the vaginal area during sex or after a bowel movement.
   - Boiling, bleaching, ironing, or microwaving underpants to kill yeast.
   - Minimizing sugar, sweets, and refined foods in the diet.
   - Eating 8 ounces of yogurt that contains *Lactobacillus acidophilus* each day.

Table 14-2	Medical Regimens

Oral Candidiasis	Regimen
Prophylaxis	None recommended.
Treatment	Nystatin 500,000 units gargled five times daily
	Or
	Clotrimazole oral troche 10 mg five times daily
	Or
	Fluconazole 100 mg PO
Maintenance*	Nystatin 500,000 units gargled five times daily
	Or
	Fluconazole 100 mg PO qd **or** 200 mg PO three times weekly

*Optional.

3. In clients with HIV, *Candida* infections tend to recur, so the nurse needs to monitor clients continually for signs and symptoms and teach clients how to recognize the early signs themselves. Clients with esophageal candidiasis usually have difficulty in swallowing and adequate caloric intake may become a problem. A good nutritional assessment with possible referral to a nutritionist may be required.

4. If a client is receiving amphotericin B, the nurse needs to be aware of the potential nephrotoxicity of this drug and monitor renal function carefully.

5. For clients receiving ketoconazole, fluconazole, or flucytosine, liver function needs to be assessed routinely and the client instructed to notify the provider if signs and symptoms of liver dysfunction occur such as unusual fatigue, anorexia, nausea, vomiting, dark urine, pale stools, or jaundice. Alcohol should be avoided.

6. Ketoconazole absorption from the gastrointestinal tract is dependent on the gastric pH. Increasing pH decreases absorption. Clients with AIDS may have decreased absorption of ketoconazole because of gastric hypochlorhydria. In such cases the drug may be administered in an acidic fluid or juice.

7. The safety of fluconazole during pregnancy and lactation has not been established. Ketoconazole is contraindicated during pregnancy and lactation

8. Ketoconazole may be administered with meals or snacks to decrease nausea and vomiting.

9. For medical regimens for oral candidiasis see Table 14-2 and Box 14-1; for vaginitis see Table 14-3; and for esophagitis see Table 14-4 and Box 14-2.

BOX 14-1   PEDIATRIC CONSIDERATIONS
Oral candidiasis

Prophylaxis for oral candidiasis is not recommended for children; however, maintenance therapy is recommended for frequent or severe recurrences:
Fluconazole 3-6 mg/kg PO qd

Table 14-3   Medical Regimens

Vaginitis	Regimen
Prophylaxis	None recommended.
Treatment	Intravaginal miconazole suppository 200 mg **or** cream (2%) × 7 days
	Or
	Clotrimazole cream (1%) **or** 100 mg troche qd × 7 days **or** 100 mg bid × 3 days **or** 500 mg × 1
	Or
	Fluconazole 150 mg PO × 1
Maintenance*	Ketoconazole 100 mg/day PO
	Or
	Fluconazole 50-100 mg PO qd

*Optional

Table 14-4   Medical Regimens

Esophagitis	Regimen
Prophylaxis	None recommended.
Treatment	Fluconazole 200 mg (not to exceed 400 mg) PO qd × 2-3 weeks
	Or
	Ketoconazole 200-400 mg PO bid × 2-3 weeks
	Or
	Itraconazole 100-200 mg PO bid or 100 mg oral suspension qd
	Or
	Amphotericin B 0.3-0.5 mg/kg IV qd
Maintenance*	Fluconazole 100-200 mg PO qd

*Optional

BOX 14-2 PEDIATRIC CONSIDERATIONS
Esophagitis

Prophylaxis for esophageal candidiasis is not recommended for children; however, maintenance therapy is recommended for frequent or severe recurrences:
Fluconazole 3-6 mg/kg PO qd
Or
Itraconazole 5-10 mg/kg PO q24h
Or
Ketoconazole 5-10 mg/kg PO q12-14h

Coccidioidomycosis

◼ DEFINITION AND ETIOLOGY

Coccidioidomycosis is caused by infection with the *Coccidioides immitis* fungus, which is endemic to southwestern United States, northern Mexico, and portions of Central and South America. In Arizona, coccidioidomycosis is the third most frequently reported opportunistic infection in clients with AIDS and the incidence is increasing in central California valley regions. About 15% of those with coccidioidomycosis also are infected with *Pneumocystis carinii*. Extrapulmonary coccidioidomycosis is an AIDS indicator condition.

C. *immitis* lives in the soil in the mycelial phase. When the soil is disturbed, aerosolized particles are breathed into the lung. *C. immitis* multiplies in the alveolar spaces of the lung, resulting in giant spherules. Macrophages may ingest these, but they are unable to kill them. As in infection with histoplasmosis, *C. immitis* can become disseminated after infecting the lung. Intact cellular immune mechanisms can halt the infection, but if impaired, the infection can either progress or become reactivated.

◼ CLINICAL OVERVIEW

Coccidioidomycosis can produce life-threatening pneumonia or meningitis. It occurs when the CD_4 count is less than 250 cells/mm^3. Initial symptoms often include fever, weight loss, fatigue, dry cough, or pleuritic chest pain. The clinical course often mimics that of infection with other respiratory pathogens. Clients with pulmonary involvement may have cutaneous lesions. These lesions are nonpruritic and maculopapular in nature. Arthralgia without associated joint effusion is a frequent finding. Chest x-ray studies show diffuse pulmonary disease that may be indistinguishable from that seen with *P. carinii*.

Infections of the meninges may occur, producing signs and symptoms of meningitis. Unlike clients with cryptococcal meningitis, clients with coccidioidal meningitis have high cerebral spinal fluid (CSF) cell counts. CSF glucose is usually suppressed and CSF protein is elevated.

Table 14-5	Medical Regimens	

Coccidioidomycosis	Regimen
Prophylaxis	Recommended only for clients who have CD_4 counts less than 50 cells/mm³ and live in endemic regions: Itraconazole 200 mg PO qd *Or* Fluconazole 200 mg qd
Treatment	Amphotericin B 0.5 mg/kg IV qd × 8 weeks, for a total dose of 2.0-2.5 g *Or* Fluconazole 400 mg PO qd *Or* Itraconazole 200 mg PO bid
Maintenance	Fluconazole 200 mg PO qd *Or* Amphotericin B 1 mg/kg/wk *Or* Itraconazole 200 mg PO bid

■ DIAGNOSIS

Diagnosis is made by culturing the organism from clinical specimens or by demonstrating the presence of the organism in tissue via histopathological stains. Blood cultures are positive in less than 30% of clients with coccidioidomycosis. The majority of clients, though, will have positive serological titers for *C. immitis* at the time of diagnosis.

■ MEDICAL MANAGEMENT

Amphotericin B is the principal treatment for coccidioidomycosis. Fluconazole and itraconazole may be used in the treatment of coccidioidomycosis, especially in maintenance therapy. Once a person has had coccidioidomycosis, lifetime suppressive therapy is needed. Ketoconazole does not work well.

■ NURSING CONSIDERATIONS

1. Clients who are severely immunosuppressed should be advised to avoid unnecessary exposure to *C. immitis* when traveling in endemic areas. These measures, for example, would include staying away from disturbed soil, avoiding building excavation sites, or seeking shelter during dust storms. The incidence of exposure increases in dry months that follow a rainy season.
2. Routine skin testing with coccidioidin is not predictive of disease and should not be done.
3. For medical regimens see Table 14-5 and Box 14-3.

BOX 14-3 PEDIATRIC CONSIDERATIONS
Coccidioidomycosis

Coccidioidomycosis infection in children has not been established. Consultation with a pediatric HIV specialist is warranted for treatment of primary infection. For prophylaxis after initial infection:
Fluconazole 6 mg/kg qd PO
Or
Amphotericin B 1.0 mg/kg IV weekly
Or
Itraconazole 2-5 mg/kg PO q12-48h

Cryptococcosis

■ DEFINITION AND ETIOLOGY

Cryptococcus neoformans is a round to oval shaped yeast, approximately 4 to 6 μm in diameter enclosed in a capsule that can be up to 30 μm thick. It lives in soil and can be inhaled into the lungs in the nonencapsulated form, becoming deposited in the small airways of the lung. Based on analysis of DNA base sequences and the antigenic differentiation of its capsule, four serotypes can be identified: A, B, C, and D. Serotypes A and D, both of which occur in clients with AIDS, are identified as *C. neoformans* var. *neoformans*. Serotypes B and C, which are not known to infect clients with HIV/AIDS, are identified as *C. neoformans* var. *gattii*.

   Cryptococcosis (i.e., infection with *C. neoformans* var. *neoformans*) is the most common systemic fungal infection in clients with AIDS, and it is the fourth most common cause of opportunistic infection in clients with HIV/AIDS. Of those who develop cryptococcosis it is the initial AIDS-defining diagnosis 40% to 45% of the time. About 6% to 10% of all clients with HIV become infected with *C. neoformans* var. *neoformans*.

   Infection with *C. neoformans* var. *neoformans* typically occurs when the CD_4 count is less then 200 cells/mm³. Although it gains access to the body through inhalation, pulmonary manifestations are present in only about 15% to 20% of cases. The most common complication (in 80% to 85% of cases) is the development of cryptococcal-induced meningitis. Actually, cryptococcosis is the third most common CNS disorder in clients with HIV/AIDS, after toxoplasmosis and CNS lymphoma in frequency. Occasionally, infection with *C. neoformans* may involve the skin, bone, and genitourinary (GU) tract.

■ CLINICAL OVERVIEW

The onset of symptoms is slow, sometimes not appearing until 30 days after infection. In addition, symptoms are nonspecific and may follow a waxing and waning course, often making diagnosis difficult. A prolonged febrile prodrome (indistinguishable from many other opportunistic infections), as well as headache and malaise are the most frequent symptoms. Other neurological symptoms may include nausea and vomiting, altered mental status, stiff neck, visual disturbances, cranial nerve palsies, papilledema, ataxia, seizures, aphasia, and photophobias. In about 20% to 60% of AIDS-infected clients, extraneural cryptococcal disease may present with involvement of joints, oral cavity, pericardium, myocardium, GU tract, and skin. If the lungs become involved, pneumonia may develop. X-ray studies show a variable pattern with single or multiple well-defined nodules, with or without cavitation.

C. neoformans invades primarily the CNS, resulting in meningitis, but nuchal rigidity is present in only one third of those infected. Increased intracranial pressure (presenting as a pressure greater than 200 mm H_2O) develops in about two thirds of those with CNS involvement. Altered mental status, which is present in 20% to 30% of cases, is the most important predictor of a poor outcome. Involvement of the skin can result in umbilicated, round lesions, which resemble those of molluscum contagiosum; occasionally, they can also resemble the lesions of Kaposi's sarcoma.

■ DIAGNOSIS

A positive CSF culture for *C. neoformans* is the standard for diagnosis. Other diagnostic tests include cryptococcal antigen (CRAG) testing of blood and CSF, analysis of CSF fluid, and brain imaging studies.

For clients with headache and fever, CRAG is a good screening test. A negative CRAG makes cryptococcal meningitis unlikely. In the event of a positive CRAG, however, further work-up would be indicated, including a CSF fungal culture. Regarding CSF analysis, in 50% of those clients with AIDS and infected with *C. neoformans,* the opening pressure obtained on lumbar puncture is elevated and an India ink preparation of CSF is positive. These are the most significant findings of CSF analysis. Elevated CSF white blood cell count, hypoglycorrhachia, and elevated CSF protein—findings typical of infection with *C. neoformans* in non–AIDS-infected clients—are not reliable indicators in clients with AIDS.

Brain imaging studies, if done, are likely to show cerebral atrophy, ventricular enlargement, and some evidence of generalized cerebral edema. Computed tomography (CT) or magnetic resonance imaging (MRI) scans can be useful in distinguishing cryptococcosis from CNS toxoplasmosis and CNS lymphoma. In these latter cases, space-occupying lesions would be present.

■ MEDICAL MANAGEMENT

All clients suspected of cryptococcosis generally have a screening CRAG performed. In those clients with a positive CRAG, a lumbar puncture is often done to determine the possibility of cryptococcal meningitis. If cryptococcal meningitis is present then initial treatment is with IV amphotericin, oral flucytosine, and oral fluconazole, followed by life-long maintenance therapy with PO fluconazole (50% to 70% of clients will experience recurrent disease after successful treatment if no maintenance therapy is initiated). In cases in which there are no changes in mental status, initial treatment with fluconazole alone may be acceptable. Since cryptococcal antigen is almost always found in CSF, the measurement of CRAG in CSF is useful in monitoring response to treatment. Clients with symptomatic increased intracranial pressure (with headache, nausea, and vomiting) often find relief by undergoing serial lumbar punctures, provided there is no contraindication to this procedure (e.g., obstructive hydrocephalus). Usually 10 to 20 cc of spinal fluid are removed with each tap.

In clients with cryptococcosis without meningitis, initial therapy consists of oral fluconazole. Prophylaxis for cryptococcosis is generally not recommended, although it may be considered in clients whose CD_4 count is less than 50 cells/mm^3.

■ NURSING CONSIDERATIONS

1. If a client has been diagnosed with cryptococcal meningitis, it is important to make the client aware that, if left untreated, the condition is fatal.
2. The administration of intravenous amphotericin is very toxic, often causing fever, rigors, headache, and thrombophlebitis during administration; to reduce the toxicity associated with administration, the nurse can ensure that the following steps are taken:
   - The medication is delivered over a 4- to 6-hour period. Because of pain and phlebitis at the infusion site, heparin 1000 units per 500 ml of infusate may be added.
   - The client should be premedicated with antipyretics (e.g., acetaminophen, diphenhydramine).
   - In clients who have experienced severe rigor in the past, Demerol can be used for premedication.
   - Electrolytes must be monitored and replaced aggressively as needed; amphotericin may also cause renal failure, so renal status must be scrutinized and monitored carefully.
3. *C. neoformans* is a soil saprophyte with worldwide distribution. It seems to occur with a higher frequency in soil contaminated with pigeon droppings. Therefore, clients with low CD_4 counts should be advised to avoid these areas as much as possible.
4. For medical regimens for cryptococcal meningitis see Table 14-6 and for cryptococcosis without meningitis see Table 14-7 and Box 14-4.

Histoplasmosis

■ DEFINITION AND ETIOLOGY

Histoplasmosis is caused by infection with the fungal organism, *Histoplasma capsulatum*. This organism is endemic in the central and south central regions of the United States and along river basins into Canada,

Table 14-6	Medical Regimens

Cryptococcal Meningitis	Regimen
Prophylaxis	None recommended.*
Treatment	Amphotericin B 0.7 mg/kg/day IV × 10-14 days **plus** flucytosine 100 mg/kg PO qd **then** fluconazole 400 mg PO bid × 2 days **then** 400 mg qd × 8-10 weeks *Or* (if no mental status change) Fluconazole 400 mg PO qd × 6-10 weeks
Maintenance	Fluconazole 200 mg (not to exceed 400 mg) PO qd *Or* Amphotericin B 0.6-1.0 mg/kg once to thrice weekly *Or* Itraconazole 400 mg PO **or** 200 mg oral suspension qd (suspension is preferred due to better bioavailability)

*Except in some cases when CD_4 cell count is less than 50 cells/mm^3.

Table 14-7	Medical Regimens

Cryptococcosis Without Meningitis	Regimen
Prophylaxis	None recommended.
Treatment	Fluconazole 200 mg PO bid × 6-10 weeks *Or* Itraconazole 200 mg PO bid **or** 100 mg oral suspension qd × 6-10 weeks
Maintenance	Fluconazole 200 mg PO qd *Or* Itraconazole 200 mg PO qd **or** 100 mg oral suspension qd *Or* Amphotericin B 0.6-1.0 mg/kg IV once or twice weekly

BOX 14-4 PEDIATRIC CONSIDERATIONS
Cryptococcosis Without Meningitis

For treatment of *Cryptococcus neoformans* infection in children see Table 14-7; however, consultation with a pediatric HIV specialist is warranted for treatment of primary infection. Infants and children with severe immunosuppression should be offered prophylaxis against infection. Maintenance therapy after initial infection is warranted as follows:
Fluconazole 3-6 mg/kg PO qd
Or
Itraconazole 2-5 mg/kg PO q12-24h
Or
Alternative therapy after initial infection:
Amphotericin B 0.5-1.0 mg/kg IV thrice weekly

southern Mexico, Central America, and South America. Indianapolis and Kansas City are two American cities with very high incidences of infection with *H. capsulatum*. In these cities, histoplasmosis is the second or third most common opportunistic infection. Overall, the rate of infection with *H. capsulatum* in endemic regions represents 5% of all opportunistic infections in clients with AIDS. Extrapulmonary histoplasmosis is an AIDS-indicator condition.

Initially infection begins in the lungs, after inhalation of the spore form of *H. capsulatum*. Once in the lung, because of the warm temperatures, the spores are rapidly converted into the yeast phase of the histoplasma life cycle. While in the yeast phase, they are phagocytized by reticuloendothelial cells. They continue to multiply within these cells. Once the infection is established in the lung, then histoplasma disseminates to the lymph nodes, and then to target organs. In an immunocompetent person, mechanisms of cell-mediated immunity are sufficient to control the infection within 2 to 3 weeks. In an immune suppressed individual, cell-mediated mechanisms are not sufficient, and either the initial infection progresses or an old infection becomes reactivated.

■ CLINICAL OVERVIEW

Histoplasmosis generally does not occur until the CD_4 count is less than 50 cells/mm^3. Fever, weight loss, and night sweats are present in over 95% of cases. Respiratory complaints, such as shortness of breath, occur in 50% to 60% of cases. Other symptoms include lymphadenopathy (20%), and skin and mucosal involvement (2% to 5%). Typically histoplasmosis causes slightly pink, cutaneous papules (about 2 to 6 mm); larger, reddish plaques; and multiple, shallow crusted ulcerations.

In 18% to 20% of cases there is neurological involvement. Septicemia, characterized by high fever, hypotension, and sometimes acute respiratory distress syndrome (ARDS), occurs in about 10% of cases. In rare cases, retinitis, pericarditis, prostatitis, pancreatitis, pleuritis, or colitis develops. Routine laboratory tests are generally nonspecific, although in cases of liver involvement, alkaline phosphatase and gamma glutamyl transferase are elevated. Chest x-ray studies are abnormal in about 60% of cases with the most common finding being diffuse infiltration.

■ DIAGNOSIS

A positive culture of the organism from peripheral blood or tissue specimens is considered the standard for diagnosis. However, culture of the organism can take 2 to 3 weeks. Histopathological evaluation of tissues obtained by biopsy specimen testing may identify the organism. The bone marrow is the tissue most accessible for biopsy samples. However, the presence of antibodies to *H. capsulatum* does not distinguish between active and previous infection, so it is not a good indicator for active infection. A better indicator for active infection is the measurement of *H. capsulatum* antigen in the urine. *H. capsulatum* antigen in the urine is positive in 95% of clients with AIDS and disseminated histoplasmosis.

■ MEDICAL MANAGEMENT

Treatment with amphotericin B often provides good results and rapid defervescence within days. Itraconazole may also be used for induction and subsequently for maintenance. Ketoconazole does not work well. Measurements of *H. capsulatum* antigen in the urine are useful for determining response to treatment and relapse.

■ NURSING CONSIDERATIONS

1. It is important to teach immunosuppressed clients to avoid activities that may bring them into direct contact with *H. capsulatum.* These include cleaning chicken coops, disturbing the soil beneath bird roosting sites (e.g., those of pigeons, starlings, and blackbirds) and exploring caves. Routine skin testing with histoplasmin is not predictive of disease and should not be done.

2. Treatment with amphotericin requires intensive monitoring. Amphotericin is nephrotoxic and so the nurse needs to assess blood urea nitrogen (BUN) and creatinine (CR) levels. A BUN greater than 40 mg/dl and CR greater than 3 mg/dl warrants discontinuation or reduction of the dose. Clients should be encouraged to drink adequate fluids and other nephrotoxic drugs should be avoided. When administered IV, amphotericin B can cause chills. Chills frequently develop 1 to 3 hours after infusion, and can last up to 4 hours. Chills can be reduced by adding hydrocortisone (10 to 15 mg) to the infusion. Alternatively, meperidine or ibuprofen can be given prior to infusion. Hypotension, nausea, and vomiting may occur 1 to 3 hours after infusion of amphotericin B, but these can be reduced by administering Compazine. An initial test dose of amphotericin B should be given. During

Table 14-8	Medical Regimens

Histoplasmosis	Regimen
Prophylaxis	Only for clients with CD_4 cell counts less than 50 cells/mm³ and from endemic areas: Itraconazole 200 mg PO qd *Or* Fluconazole 200 mg PO qd
Treatment	Amphotericin B 0.5-1.0 mg/kg IV qd × 7-14 days *Or* Itraconazole 300 mg PO bid × 3 days **then** 200 mg PO bid **or** 100 mg oral suspension qd
Maintenance	Itraconazole 200 mg PO bid *Or* Amphotericin B 1.0 mg/kg once to twice weekly *Or* Fluconazole 400 mg PO qd

the first 4 hours of amphotericin B infusion, vital signs should be monitored every 30 minutes. Hypokalemia, hypomagnesia, and hypocalcemia may all occur secondary to amphotericin B therapy. Deficiencies need to be corrected with supplemental K^+, Ca^{++}, and Mg^{++}. Phlebitis and pain at the infusion site are common. About 1200 to 1600 units of heparin added to the infusate can help reduce this complication.

3. When amphotericin B is given in the oral form, side effects include rash, gastrointestinal intolerance, and allergic reactions. Other antifungal drugs may be used in the treatment of histoplasmosis. Some of these drugs, such as itraconazole, may cause liver dysfunction. Clients with prior liver disease should be screened and monitored carefully. Gastrointestinal intolerance is a common side effect of most antifungals. Itraconazole and fluconazole are both category C medications, so their use in pregnant women should be approached with the greatest caution (see Chapter 20 for explanation of category C). Before administering antifungals, the nurse should determine what other medications the client is using and check to see if there are any drug-drug interactions that might warrant attention. In some cases, the dosage of one of the drugs may need to be adjusted to ameliorate drug-drug interactions.

4. Clients for whom itraconazole capsules are prescribed should be instructed to take these capsules with acidic food or beverages, such as cola or orange juice. Itraconazole solution is better absorbed and does not require an acidic environment to enhance absorption.

5. For medical regimens see Table 14-8 and Box 14-5.

BOX 14-5 PEDIATRIC CONSIDERATIONS
Histoplasmosis

Prophylaxis for histoplasmosis is generally not recommended for children, but should be considered in children with CD_4 counts less than 50 cells/mm^3 and those that reside in endemic areas:
Itraconazole 2-5 mg/kg PO q12-24h
Treatment
Amphotericin B 0.5-1.0 mg/kg/day IV × 7 days, *then* 0.8 mg/kg qod (or thrice weekly)
Maintenance
Itraconazole 2-5 mg/kg PO q12-48h
Or
Amphotericin B 1.0 mg/kg/day IV × 1 week

BIBLIOGRAPHY

Bartlett J: *Medical management of HIV infection,* Baltimore, 1997, Port City Press.

Centers for Disease Control and Prevention: USPHS/IDSA guidelines for the prevention of opportunistic infections in persons infected with human immunodeficiency virus, MMWR 46(RR-12):18, June 27, 1997.

Libman H, Witzberg R: *HIV infection: a primary care manual,* ed 3, Boston, 1996, Little, Brown & Co.

Sande M, Volberding P: *The medical management of AIDS,* Philadelphia, 1997, Saunders.

15

Oncologic Conditions

- Kaposi's Sarcoma
- Lymphomas

Carl A. Kirton

Kaposi's Sarcoma

▐ DEFINITION AND ETIOLOGY

Kaposi's Sarcoma (KS) is one of the most common types of neoplasm that develops in clients with AIDS. Men who have sex with men (MSM) have the highest incidence of KS among all groups with HIV infection. KS is infrequently seen in heterosexual men, women, and children. KS is thought to be caused by the sexual transmission of the human herpes virus 8 (HHV8) or KS-associated herpes virus (KSHV).[1] Because of the decrease in the incidence of sexually transmitted diseases (STDs) in MSM, the overall incidence of KS has declined. It is thought that the pathogenesis of KS is caused by the activation of certain circulating inflammatory cytokines (see Chapter 2 for explanation of cytokines). When these cellular elements come in contact with vascular cells, they alter the physiology of these cells. Several cytokines have been implicated in the proliferation of KS, including basic fibroblast growth factor (bFGF), oncostation-M, vascular endothelial growth factor (VEGF), and interleukin-6 (IL-6).

▐ CLINICAL OVERVIEW

KS most commonly affects the skin first, but it can affect almost any organ in the body. It has been found that when KS occurs on the skin, it also frequently occurs in the gastrointestinal tract.[2] KS first appears as a macular, painless, nonpruritic, nonblanchable lesion confined to the reticular dermis. Early lesions can vary in color—pink, red, purple, or brown. Sometimes KS presents initially on the face, mouth, gums, palate, or penis. Macular lesions can progress to a palpable vascular lesion, infiltrating the dermis. The most severe form of KS is the nodular type, which consists of large palpable lesions within a network of extensive vascular spaces.[3] This often leads to edema of the surrounding areas. The nodules are painless. In lightly pigmented individuals, the lesions are typically a deep violet color. In darkly pigmented individuals, the nodules are often are black in color.

When confined to the skin, KS does not cause any symptoms. However, tumors may grow in the lungs and the gastrointestinal system. If the lungs are involved, the client may have a cough and dyspnea. If the gastrointestinal tract is involved, the client may experience gastrointestinal bleeding.

■ DIAGNOSTIC TESTING

KS is often diagnosed by clinical appearance; however, the lesions of bacillary angiomatosis (BA) can mimic those of KS. BA is a bacterial infection that is easily treated and should be ruled out (see Chapter 13). The most definitive test for the diagnosis of KS is a biopsy. A specimen of tissue for biopsy can be obtained by the punch method or by surgical excision of the lesion. A *punch biopsy* is the process of obtaining a full-thickness skin specimen for histological evaluation. The nurse may assist the health care provider in preparing the client for the procedure and obtaining the specimen. The site is prepared by cleansing it with a solution for sterilization, such as povidone-iodine. A 1% lidocaine solution is injected into the area for analgesia. The health care provider uses a punch knife (i.e., a 2 to 10 mm tubular knife) to obtain the specimen. When the specimen has been obtained, it is placed in a bottle of formalin (often supplied by the laboratory) and shipped according to laboratory specifications.

■ MEDICAL MANAGEMENT

Because there is no cure for KS, treatment is considered palliative. Treatment options vary, including simple observation, highly active antiretroviral therapy (HAART), surgical removal, cryotherapy, radiotherapy, and chemotherapy. A very important component of the management of KS is maximal suppression of the viral burden. When viral burden is suppressed, tumors may regress completely or become smaller in size or lighter in color. A client with a few small lesions may not need to be treated beyond this but may desire treatment because of concern about the appearance of the lesions.* Cosmetic treatment for KS-related lesions can be done with cryotherapy, radiotherapy, or intralesional injection of chemotherapeutic agents. In cryotherapy, the lesions are frozen with liquid nitrogen; in radiotherapy, varied doses of radiation are aimed at tumors to suppress their growth; and in intralesional injection of chemotherapeutic agents, lesions that are less than 1 cm in diameter are treated with an injection of vinblastine (Velban) directly into the lesion.

Systemic chemotherapeutic agents are generally reserved for KS lesions that alter the function of organs, such as the lungs, liver, or spleen, or for those that alter the function of the gastrointestinal system. Systemic therapies for KS include liposomal daunorubicin (DaunoXome) and

---

*Some clinicians have begun to question the practice of delaying treatment of small lesions. This violates one of the principles of cancer therapy, that of chemotherapy being more effective with a lower tumor burden (written communication, Kathy Handy, 1998).

generic doxorubicin HCL (Doxil), both approved by the FDA as first-line and second-line agents, respectively, for treatment of AIDS-related KS. Other systemic therapies that may be used in the treatment of KS are: α-interferon, Bleomycin, and paclitaxel (Taxol).

■ NURSING CONSIDERATIONS

1. Because KS is caused by the sexual transmission of the HHV8, protected sexual intercourse is the only known means of prevention.
2. Teach clients that tumor growth varies from person to person. One factor that may influence the growth of lesions is the client's viral load. Tumor regression correlates with drops in viral load. This may be due to the fact that when the virus is suppressed, there is some restoration of immune functioning that may suppress the spread of KSHV.
3. Teach clients that regardless of the therapy chosen, KS tends to reoccur. Even with systemic therapies tumors may reappear in as little as 6 months.
4. Teach clients that cryotherapy has residual cosmetic effects. There is often some mild scarring at the site of treatment and hypopigmentation may occur where lesions have been treated.
5. Teach clients receiving radiotherapy that several doses (or treatments) will be required to deliver the full dose of radiation. Low-dose radiation (1000 to 1500 rads) is generally given in divided doses over a period of 7 to 10 days. Moderate-dose radiation (1800 to 2100 rads) may be given over a period of 2 weeks. Teach clients that side effects of this therapy depend on the treatment site. Treatment to the face may result in mouth ulcers that may alter the client's ability to eat. There is often skin irritation at the site of treatment.
6. Teach clients receiving treatment by intralesional injections with chemotherapy that side effects are common with this type of therapy. Injections of chemotherapeutic agents are painful and there may be some localized residual pain. Some chemotherapeutic agents may cause hyperpigmentation at the injection site.
7. Teach clients receiving intravenous infusions of agents such as liposomal daunorubicin (DaunoXome) and doxorubicin HCL (Doxil) that although the liposomal formulation reduces traditional chemotherapeutic side effects, such as hair loss and bone marrow suppression, they can still occur. Severe side effects such as cardiomyopathies (rarely), myelosuppression, and palmar-plantar erythrodysesthesia (rubor appearance to the palms of the hand and the soles of the feet) can occur with systemic therapies. The nurse should refer to a more comprehensive text of cancer chemotherapies when caring for a client receiving these therapies.
8. Important side effects of liposomal agents are a first-dose reaction consisting of back pain, chest tightness, and shortness of breath. This is managed by stopping the infusion and notifying the prescribing

provider or oncology clinical nurse specialist. This type of reaction is often managed with diphenhydramine or dexamethasone. The offending drug can almost always be reinstituted without a recurrence of this effect.

9. Ulceration and bacterial cellulitis are common complications associated with nodular KS lesions. The nurse should examine clients for ulcerated lesions and edema, particularly of the lower extremities. Ulcerated lesions can cause the client pain and place the client at increased risk for infection.

10. Clients with cutaneous KS should be questioned routinely about blood in the stool or abdominal pain. Gastrointestinal KS often accompanies cutaneous lesions. Hematochezia is one manifestation of gastrointestinal KS.

11. Clients with pulmonary KS may have a dry, nonproductive cough, shortness of breath, hemoptysis, or chest pain. Chest x-ray study results are not specific for KS lesions but may show a pulmonary infiltrate or nodular density. A bronchoscopy with biopsy is the definitive test in detecting pulmonary KS.

12. To diagnose suspected pulmonary KS, clients may undergo gallium scanning. The nurse prepares clients for this procedure by informing them that they will receive an IV injection of gallium. The scan usually requires two visits to the nuclear medicine department. On the first day, the client will receive an injection of gallium and be scheduled for imaging. The initial scan is the longest part of the procedure and may take up to 2 hours. The client may be asked to return on another day for more imaging.

13. For medical regimens see Table 15-1.

Lymphomas

■ Definition and Etiology

Lymphomas are malignant neoplasms that originate in lymphoid tissue, such as the bone marrow, spleen, thymus gland, or intestinal lymphatic tissues. Immunodeficient clients have a fourteen times greater risk than the general population for the development of lymphomas.[4]

There are two classes of lymphomas—Hodgkin's and non-Hodgkin's. Non-Hodgkin's lymphoma (NHL) is the second most common malignancy found in clients with AIDS. The majority of malignant cells in non-Hodgkin's lymphomas originate from B cells. These neoplastic cells seem to develop as a result of the arresting of the maturation process of lymphocytes. The cause of this process in HIV-positive persons is thought to be multifactorial, including (but not limited to) the presence of the Epstein-Barr virus (EBV), loss of immune surveillance, destruction of dendritic cells of the lymph nodes, dysregulation of cytokines, and elevated IL-6 levels.

Table 15-1	Medical Regimens

Kaposi's Sarcoma	Regimens
Prophylaxis	No known therapy.
Treatment	**Local Therapies** Reserved for small, localized lesions: Cryotherapy—Liquid nitrogen is applied to site for 30 seconds. Reserved for single lesions or intraoral/pharyngeal lesions (can be used to shrink bulky tumors): Radiotherapy—Tumor is exposed to a single dose of 150 rad. Reserved for lesions of the face or other exposed parts of the body: Intralesional injection—Vincristine (Velban) as a 0.2 mg/cc dilution[5] **or** vinblastine 0.01 mg mixed with 0.1 ml of sterile water in an insulin syringe. Interferon alpha—10 million units SQ OD are administered to clients receiving antiretroviral therapy. Higher doses (36 million units) are administered to clients not receiving antiretroviral therapy. Treatment is continued indefinitely. **Systemic Chemotherapy** (Should only be prescribed by a medical oncologist) Reserved for advanced systemic KS (i.e., >25 lesions, internal KS, severe edema): First-line therapy—Daunorubicin HCL liposome injection (DaunoXome) 40 mg in D_5W infused over 30 minutes, once every 2-3 weeks for as long as client responds satisfactorily and can tolerate treatment. Second-line therapy—Doxorubicin HCL liposome injection (Doxil) 20 mg in D_5W infused over 30 minutes, once every 3 weeks for as long as client responds satisfactorily and can tolerate treatment.
Maintenance	No known therapy.

Unfortunately, the incidence of lymphomas is rising, because clients with HIV are living longer as a result of better therapies for HIV and opportunistic infections. In general, the prognosis of a client with NHL is poor, because by the time NHL is diagnosed, the disease is often widely disseminated. With chemotherapy, the median survival of clients with NHL is 4.5 months in those with CD_4 cell counts of less than 100 cells/mm^3 and 24 months in those with CD_4 cell counts higher than 100 cells/mm^3.[6]

■ CLINICAL OVERVIEW

Generally, the condition originates in the lymph nodes and begins with a single painless enlarged lymph node. NHL can occur in extranodal sites, such as the mediastinum, gastrointestinal tract, bones, and the testes. Almost all HIV-positive clients with lymphoma eventually develop the disease in extranodal sites. Symptoms vary according to the site involved, making diagnosis difficult because they are often vague, constitutional, or "B" symptoms such as chills, fever, night sweats, and weight loss, which can be attributed to other HIV-related diseases such as tuberculosis (TB). However, fever that has been present for over 2 weeks is a strong indicator of lymphoma.

In HIV, NHL can involve almost any site of the body and is seen primarily when the CD_4 cell count has fallen below 200 cells/mm^3. In the face of severe immunosuppression (i.e., CD_4 cell count of less than 50 cells/mm^3) the most common site of involvement is the central nervous system (CNS). When CNS lymphomas occur, focal neurological signs and symptoms are present. For clients who have CNS lymphoma, the prognosis, in general, is very poor with a median survival of approximately 2 months.

■ DIAGNOSTIC TESTING

Diagnosis often begins with an evaluation of the complete blood count (CBC), which in the early stages of the disease often reveals anemia or thrombocytopenia. The clinician will usually then implement other diagnostic examinations to determine the cause of abnormalities in the CBC, abnormal physical examination results, and constitutional symptoms. These examinations may include, but are not limited to, chest x-ray studies; computed tomography (CT) scans of the chest, abdomen, and pelvis; bone marrow smear and biopsies; and lumbar puncture. These diagnostic tests and procedures are important in the determination of the stage of the disease.

Biopsies of lymph nodes or extranodal sites and subsequent classification of any tumors are important in the determination of prognosis and response to treatment. There are several classification systems used with NHL—*The Working Formulation of Non-Hodgkin's Lymphoma*[7] is the most common. In brief, according to this classification system, tumors are classified as being low-grade, intermediate-grade, or high-grade. A lower grade corresponds to slower growth of the tumor, with survival extended for years. However, low-grade tumors are less responsive to chemotherapeutics than high-grade tumors.

CT scans or magnetic resonance imaging (MRI) of the head are important tools in the diagnosis of NHL. When CNS lymphoma is present, it often appears as a ring-enhanced lesion on the film, although other CNS infections such as toxoplasmosis yield a similar picture. Differential diagnosis is essential. One criterion that distinguishes the lesions of toxoplasmosis from the lesions seen in lymphomas is the size of the ring-enhanced lesions. Toxoplasmosis lesions are typically smaller, approximately 1 to 3 cm in diameter, whereas lesions of lymphomas are usually greater than 3 cm in diameter. In MRI results, toxoplasmosis lesions are multiple, whereas lymphomas are singular.

▓ MEDICAL MANAGEMENT

Because of its insidious nature, it is rare that lymphomas are detected in a single node or two contiguous nodal areas. When detected in these early stages, however, radiation is the treatment of choice. Stage III and stage IV lymphatic involvement or involvement of the CNS requires the administration of a combination of chemotherapeutic agents. Complete response to chemotherapy occurs in a little over 50% of clients with stage III and stage IV NHL. A favorable response to chemotherapy is more likely in clients with a CD_4 cell count greater than 200 cells/mm^3 and when the disease is confined to a single node or organ. Decreased survival is seen in clients with elevated lactic dehydrogenase (LDH) levels (greater than 1000 u/dl), with Stage III or IV disease and low CD_4 cell counts, who are over 35 years of age, who have a history of injection drug use, or who have a history of AIDS-defining illness prior to lymphoma.[8]

▓ NURSING CONSIDERATIONS

1. Clients who are older than 40 years, have a history of IV drug use, have a CD_4 cell count less than 100 cells/mm^3, or have an LDH level greater than 1000 u/dl have a very poor prognosis. Median survival is approximately 18 months.[9] The nurse should provide care, support, and referrals as indicated to assist clients, families, and significant others in coping with the diagnosis and its implications.

2. If none of the aforementioned conditions are present, there is an 80% chance of complete remission with chemotherapy. Even with remission, however, relapses tend to occur within 2 years. Some relapses will present as a higher stage.

3. Clients receiving chemotherapies for lymphomas are often hospitalized. With systemic therapies there is the possibility of the occurrence of tumor lysis syndrome (TLS), which results in hyperkalemia, hyperphosphatemia, hypocalcemia, hyperuricemia, and renal failure. Clients receiving systemic chemotherapy have nursing care considerations beyond those that can be discussed in this text. The reader is referred to a more comprehensive review of chemotherapeutic agents. General considerations for selected chemotherapeutic agents are listed in Table 15-2.

4. See Table 15-3 for medical regimens.

Table 15-2	Chemotherapy Used for Lymphomas

Drug	General Nursing Considerations
Cyclophosphamide	Bone marrow depression occurs.
	Leukopenia occurs in 7-14 days.
	Thrombocytopenia and anemia occur.
	Clients receiving this drug are at high risk for hemorrhagic cystitis. Clients must be hydrated before and after infusion to avoid hemorrhagic cystitis. The client should be encouraged to void at regular intervals. Nausea and vomiting 2-4 hours after infusion may last for 24 hours. Antiemetics may be indicated.
	Syndrome of inappropriate secretion of antidiuretic hormone (SIADH) may occur.
	Cardiotoxicity may occur 1-6 months after initiation of therapy. Clients are at risk for cardiomyopathy, hemorrhagic cardiac necrosis, transmural hemorrhage, and coronary artery vasculitis—especially if they are receiving high doses or concurrent Doxorubicin.
Doxorubicin	Although rare, interstitial pneumonitis can occur.
	Alopecia is a common side effect.
	This drug is a potent vesicant and preferably should be infused via central line.
	When given with cyclophosphamide, there is increased risk of hemorrhage and cardiac dysfunction.
	Nausea and vomiting begin 1-3 hours after administration; premedication may be warranted.
	Contains dye that causes red urine.
	Drug can cause bone marrow suppression (WBC and platelet nadir occurs around day 10-14 and recovery occurs around day 15-21).
	Drug causes irreversible cardiomyopathy at cumulative doses >550 mg/m².
Vincristine	Alopecia may occur.
	This drug is a vesicant and preferably should be infused via central line.
	Drug may cause mild bone marrow depression within 4-10 days.
	Drug is toxic to nerve fibers. May cause peripheral neuropathy, weakness, myalgia, cramping, or severe motor difficulty. Discontinuation of drug considered if these conditions occur.
	Autonomic dysfunction may occur. The client should be monitored for ileus and hypotension.
Bleomycin	SIADH may occur.
	Anaphylactoid reaction can occur in clients with lymphoma. The client should be monitored for signs and symptoms suggestive of a reaction, such as wheezing, urticaria, tachycardia, and fever. A test dose or premedication should be considered.
	May cause chemical fevers. Temperatures up to 103-105° F may occur. Fevers generally occur 4-10 hours after drug administration. Fevers are treated with acetaminophen.

Table 15-2	Chemotherapy Used for Lymphomas—cont'd

Drug	General Nursing Considerations
Bleomycin—cont'd	Drug can cause pneumonitis. High concentrations of oxygen are contraindicated in clients who have received bleomycin. Skin reactions can occur. These include rash, erythema, striae, hyperpigmentation, hyperkeratosis, and peeling of the hands.
Methotrexate	Can crystallize in the kidneys. The client should be hydrated both before and after receiving the drug. Urine should be alkalinized with bicarbonate. The pH of urine must be maintained >7.0. Leucovorin rescue must be given to prevent excess toxicity. Multiple gastrointestinal problems can occur, including stomatitis, diarrhea, enteritis, intestinal perforations, melena, hematemesis. Sometimes back pain can occur with infusion. Slowing the infusion rate may help.
Leucovorin	This drug is administered 24 hours after the first methotrexate dose. It must be given on time to avoid methotrexate toxicity, which can be fatal.

Table 15-3	Medical Regimens

Lymphomas	Regimen
Prophylaxis	No known therapy.
Treatment	**CHOP Regimen** 4-6 cycles of the following drugs are given at 28-day intervals: • Cyclophosphamide (Cytoxan) 750 mg/m^2 • Doxorubicin hydrochloride (Adriamycin) 50 mg/m^2 • Vincristine (Oncovin) 1.4 mg/m^2 • Prednisone 50 mg/m^2 **mBA-COD Regimen** • Methotrexate 200 mg/m^2 • Bleomycin 4 mg/m^2 • Doxorubicin 25 mg/m^2 • Cyclophosphamide 300 mg/m^2 • Vincristine 1.4 mg/m^2 • Dexamethasone 3 mg/m^2 • Leucovorin 25 mg q6h × 6 doses (24 hours after methotrexate)
Maintenance	No known therapy.

REFERENCES

1. Chang Y et al: Identification of herpesvirus-like DNA sequence in AIDS-related Kaposi's Sarcoma, *Science* 266:1865, 1994.
2. Bartnof HS: Kaposi's Sarcoma, *BETA* 52:14, 1996.
3. Tappero JW et al: Kaposi's Sarcoma: epidemiology, pathogenesis, histology, clinical spectrum, staging criteria, and therapy, *J Am Acad Dermatol* 28:371, 1993.
4. Penn I: De novo malignancy in pediatric organ transplant recipients, *J Pediatr Surg* 29:221, 1994.
5. Fathering C: Dermatological procedure in primary HIV care, *PRN Notebook* 2(4):11, 1997.
6. Kaplan LD et al: AIDS-associated non-Hodgkin's lymphoma in San Francisco, *JAMA* 261:719, 1989.
7. Gorell AH, May LA, Mulley AG: *Primary care medicine: office evaluation and management of the adult patient,* ed 3, Philadelphia, 1995, Lippincott.
8. Kaplan L: Lymphomas. In Powderly W, ed: *Manual of medical therapeutics,* Philadelphia, 1997, Lippincott-Raven.
9. Vaccher E et al: Age and serum lactate dehydrogenase level are independent prognostic factors in human immunodeficiency virus–related non-Hodgkin's lymphomas, *J Clin Oncol* 14(8):2217, 1996.

HIV / AIDS
MEDICATIONS

Color photos courtesy Mosby's GenR$_x$, St Louis, MO, Mosby, 2000 and
Abbott Laboratories, Agouron Pharmaceuticals, Bristol-Myers Squibb,
DuPont Pharmaceutical, Glaxo Wellcome, Merck and Co, Inc., Roche
Laboratories, Roxanne Laboratories, and Pharmacia & Upjohn.

HIV/AIDS MEDICATIONS*

Nucleoside Reverse Transcriptase Inhibitors (NRTI)

Brand/Generic Name	Usual Regimen	Common Side Effects	Important Nursing Consideration
  ZIDOVUDINE (Retrovir, AZT, ZDV) *FDA approval: 3/87* Supplied as: *Capsules*—100 mg *Tablets*—300 mg *Combivir Tablet*—300 mg ZDV + 150 mg 3TC *Solution*—50 mg/5 ml (bottle contains 240 ml) *Injection*—200 mg/20 ml	600 mg daily—200 mg q8h **or** 300 mg q12h *Prevention of vertical transmission*—Start treatment at 14 wks gestation: 100 mg five times daily until labor. *Intrapartum*—Load with 2 mg/kg over first hr, followed by a maintenance dose of 1 mg/kg/hr until umbilical cord is clamped. *Neonates*—Syrup 2 mg/kg PO q6h × 6 wks. Start 8-12 hrs after birth. If unable to use oral route, deliver IV dose of 1.5 mg/kg q6h. *Pediatric dosing, for ages 3 mos-2 yrs*—90-180 mg/m² q6-8h. Usual pediatric dose is approximately 160 mg/m² q8h. *Continuous IV infusion*—20 mg/m²/hr *Intermittent IV infusion*—120 mg/m² q6h.	Fever, rash, anorexia, headache, weakness	This drug should always be used in combination with other medications to treat HIV infection. (AZT can be used as monotherapy in cases to prevent vertical transmission.) **DRUG-FOOD INTERACTIONS** • Food and milk do not appear to affect GI absorption substantially. **ADVERSE EFFECTS** • Anemia may be seen in clients taking AZT, usually occurring after 2-12 wks of therapy. • Other cytopenias may occur, such as leukopenia or thrombocytopenia. • Prolonged use (i.e., >1 year) may result in myopathies. **DOSAGE ADJUSTMENTS** • AZT is metabolized by the liver. Dosage may need alteration in severe liver disease. • AZT is eliminated by the kidneys. For clients with renal failure receiving dialysis, the recommended dosage is 100 mg q6-8h. The IV dose is 1 mg/kg. **MONITORING AND EDUCATION** • Because anemia is common to this medication, the nurse should monitor the Hgb and reticulocyte count. Significant anemia may require discontinuation of drug (with a switch to another agent) or dose adjustment. If severe anemia occurs, serum erythropoietin (EPO) levels should be checked;

			if <500, epoetin alpha (ProCrit) is indicated, and if >500, blood transfusion is indicated. • A complete blood count (CBC) with a differential should be performed every 2-3 wks for the first 1-2 mos to monitor for cytopenia. • The creatine kinase (CK) level must be monitored. An increased level, with clinical findings of extremity weakness or muscle tenderness, may indicate myopathy. These findings necessitate switching to another medication. • This medication may cause lengthening of eyelashes and hyperpigmentation of nails (this is more prevalent in dark-skinned individuals).
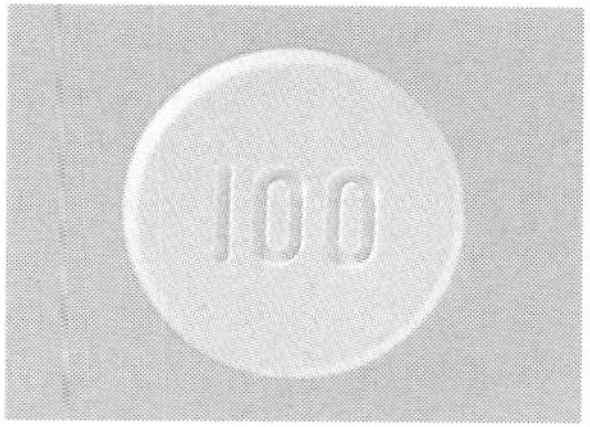 **DIDANOSINE** (Videx, ddI) *FDA approval:* 10/91 Supplied as: *Tablets*—25, 50, 100, and 150 mg	400 mg daily—200 mg q12h **or** 400 mg qd Buffered tablets: *For <60 kg*—125 mg q12h *For >60 kg*—200 mg q12h Buffered powder (25% less bioavailable than buffered tablets): *For <60 kg*—167 mg PO q12h *For >60 kg*—250 mg PO q12h *Neonatal (infants aged >90 days) dosage*—50 mg/m² q12h.	Parethesias, diarrhea, anxiety, headache, irritability, insomnia, abdominal pain, nausea	This drug should always be used in combination with other medications to treat HIV infection. **DRUG-FOOD INTERACTIONS** • Must be taken on empty stomach ½ hr before meals or 2 hrs after meals. Tablets are chewable. • Acid rapidly degrades drug. Contains a buffering agent to prevent degradation. When ddI dosage requires more than one pill, the pills must be taken together to achieve benefit from buffers. Doses are ineffective if done otherwise. • Powder must not be placed in acidic liquids, such as orange juice. • Alcohol should be taken with caution. **ADVERSE EFFECTS** • Neuropathy with pain can occur 2-6 mos after drug administration.

*See Appendix D for important drug-drug interaction information.

Continued

HIV/AIDS MEDICATIONS—cont'd

Brand/Generic Name	Usual Regimen	Common Side Effects	Important Nursing Consideration
Powder Packets—100, 167, and 250 mg single-dose packets *Solution*—4 oz bottles containing 2 g of drug and 8 oz bottles containing 4 g of drug	*Pediatric dosage*—90-150 mg/m² q12h. The usual dosage in combination with other antiretrovirals is 90 mg/m² q12h.		• Pancreatitis has been reported and in some cases has been fatal. This finding increases in those who drink alcohol or take other medications that can cause pancreatitis. **DOSAGE ADJUSTMENTS** • ddI is eliminated by the kidney. In clients with renal failure receiving dialysis, it is recommended that ¼ of the total daily dose be administered once daily. • No specific dose has been listed, but it is recommended that the dose be reduced for severe hepatic impairment. **MONITORING AND EDUCATION** • The client should chew, crush, or disperse tablets in water (i.e., not swallow tablets whole). • Any numbness and tingling in the client's hands and feet should be assessed and reported to the primary health care provider. The client may need to be switched to another NRTI. The use of ddI with ddC or d4T should be avoided because all of these drugs have peripheral neuropathy as a major adverse effect. • The client should be assessed for signs of pancreatitis (i.e., nausea, vomiting, abdominal pain). Serum amylase or lipase should be evaluated. Elevations may indicate acute pancreatitis, in which case the drug must be switched to another NRTI. • Changes in vision have been reported in adult and pediatric clients receiving ddI because of optic neuritis and retinal depigmentation. Retinal examinations q6mo are recommended for individuals receiving therapy.

Continued

ZALCITABINE
(HIVID, ddC)
FDA approval: 6/92

Supplied as:
Tablets: 0.375 and 0.75 mg

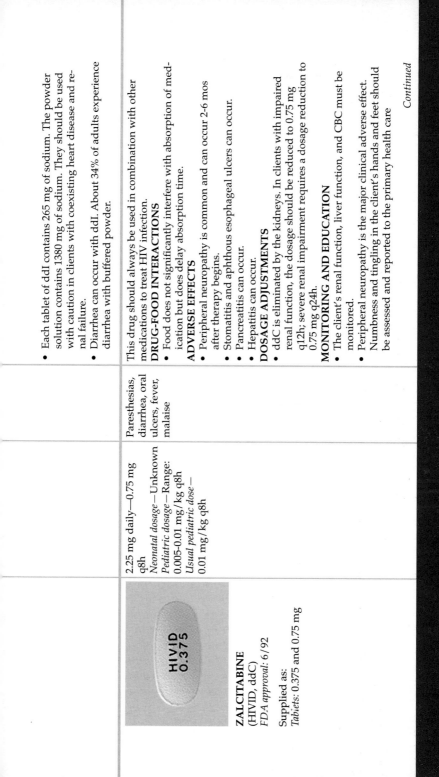

2.25 mg daily—0.75 mg q8h
Neonatal dosage—Unknown
Pediatric dosage—Range: 0.005-0.01 mg/kg q8h
Usual pediatric dose—0.01 mg/kg q8h

Paresthesias, diarrhea, oral ulcers, fever, malaise

- Each tablet of ddI contains 265 mg of sodium. The powder solution contains 1380 mg of sodium. They should be used with caution in clients with coexisting heart disease and renal failure.
- Diarrhea can occur with ddI. About 34% of adults experience diarrhea with buffered powder.

This drug should always be used in combination with other medications to treat HIV infection.

DRUG-FOOD INTERACTIONS

- Food does not significantly interfere with absorption of medication but does delay absorption time.

ADVERSE EFFECTS

- Peripheral neuropathy is common and can occur 2-6 mos after therapy begins.
- Stomatitis and aphthous esophageal ulcers can occur.
- Pancreatitis can occur.
- Hepatitis can occur.

DOSAGE ADJUSTMENTS

- ddC is eliminated by the kidneys. In clients with impaired renal function, the dosage should be reduced to 0.75 mg q12h; severe renal impairment requires a dosage reduction to 0.75 mg q24h.

MONITORING AND EDUCATION

- The client's renal function, liver function, and CBC must be monitored.
- Peripheral neuropathy is the major clinical adverse effect. Numbness and tingling in the client's hands and feet should be assessed and reported to the primary health care

Brand/Generic Name	Usual Regimen	Common Side Effects	Important Nursing Consideration
			provider; medication may need to be switched to another NRTI. The use of ddC with ddI or d4T should be avoided because all of these drugs have peripheral neuropathy as a major adverse effect.
			• The client should be assessed for signs of pancreatitis (i.e., nausea, vomiting, abdominal pain). Serum amylase or lipase should be evaluated. Elevations may indicate acute pancreatitis, in which case the drug must be switched to another NRTI.
			• Liver function tests (AST, ALT, and GGT) must be monitored. Hepatitis can occur, in which case the client must be switched to another medication.
BMS 1965 20 **STAVUDINE** (Zerit, d4T) *FDA approval: 6/94*	80 mg daily—40 mg q12h *For <60 kg*—30 mg q12h *Neonatal dosage*—Unknown *Pediatric dosage*—For <30 kg; 1 mg/kg/day q12h (in two divided doses)	Paresthesias, headache, insomnia, malaise, fatigue, agranulocytopenia	This drug should always be used in combination with other medications to treat HIV infection. **DRUG-FOOD INTERACTIONS** • Stavudine should be taken on an empty stomach. **ADVERSE EFFECTS** • Peripheral neuropathy is common and can occur 2-6 mos after therapy begins. **DOSAGE ADJUSTMENTS** • d4T is partially eliminated by the kidney. Dosage adjustment varies by severity of renal function impairment and body weight. With severe renal impairment (creatinine clearance between 10-25 ml/min) dosage may be adjusted to 20 mg

q24h. For those with severe renal impairment weighing <60 kg, the dosage should be reduced to 15 mg q24h.

MONITORING AND EDUCATION
- Peripheral neuropathy is the major clinical adverse effect. Numbness and tingling in the client's hands and feet should be assessed and reported to the primary health care provider. The use of d4T with ddI or ddC must be avoided because all of these drugs have peripheral neuropathy as a major adverse effect. In some cases, symptoms of peripheral neuropathy may worsen temporarily following discontinuation of therapy.
- Mild to moderate increases in AST and ALT can be seen with therapy and tend to resolve following discontinuation of therapy.

Supplied as:
Capsules—15, 20, 30, and 40 mg

LAMIVUDINE
(Epivir, 3TC)
FDA approval: 11/95

300 mg daily
For >50 kg—150 mg bid
For <50 kg—2mg/kg PO bid
Neonatal (infants aged <30 days) dosage—2 mg/kg bid
Pediatric dosage, for ages 3 mos-12 yrs—4 mg/kg (not to exceed 150 mg) bid

Well tolerated in adults; infrequent nausea, diarrhea, abdominal pain, insomnia

This drug should always be used in combination with other medications to treat HIV infection.

DRUG-FOOD INTERACTIONS
- Epivir tablets and solution may be taken with or without food.

ADVERSE EFFECTS
- Generally well tolerated.

DOSAGE ADJUSTMENTS
- 3TC is eliminated by the kidneys. Dosage adjustment varies with the severity of renal function. In severe renal function, the dosage should be reduced to 25 mg daily.

MONITORING AND EDUCATION
- This medication has activity against the hepatitis B virus.
- Insomnia and nausea may occur.

Continued

HIV/AIDS MEDICATIONS—cont'd

Brand/Generic Name	Usual Regimen	Common Side Effects	Important Nursing Consideration
Supplied as: *Tablets*—150 mg *Solution*—10 mg/ml (bottle contains 240 ml)			This drug should always be used in combination with other medications to treat HIV infection. **DRUG-FOOD INTERACTIONS** • There are no known dietary restrictions for this drug. **ADVERSE EFFECTS** • May cause hypersensitivity reaction consisting of fever, nausea, vomiting, malaise, and rash, in which case the medication should be stopped permanently. Rechallenging can be life-threatening. Hypersensitivity reaction should be reported to the *ABC Hypersensitivity Registry* (1-800-270-0425).
ABACAVIR (Ziagen, 1592, ABC) *FDA approval:* 12/98 Supplied as: *Tablets*—300 mg *Solution*—20 mg/ml (bottle contains 240 ml)	600 mg daily—300 mg q12h *Neonatal dosage*—Unknown *Pediatric dosage, for ages 3 mos-16 yrs*—8 mg/kg (not to exceed 300 mg) q12h	Rash	**DOSAGE ADJUSTMENTS** • No renal or hepatic dosage adjustment necessary. **MONITORING AND EDUCATION** • Mild to moderate increases in AST and ALT may be seen and tend to resolve if therapy is changed. • Abacavir may not be efficacious in persons already resistant to other nucleoside analogues. • The client should avoid alcohol, which increases the blood levels of abacavir.

Nonnucleoside Reverse Transcriptase Inhibitors (NNRTI)

Brand/Generic Name	Usual Regimen	Common Side Effects	Important Nursing Consideration
NEVIRAPINE (Viramune) *FDA approval:* 6/96 Supplied as: *Tablets*—200 mg *Solution*—50 mg/ml (solution contains 240 ml)	400 mg daily—200 mg qd × 14 days, then 200 mg bid *Neonatal dosage*— **Under study:** 5 mg/kg PO qd × 14 days, followed by 120 mg/m² PO q12h × 14 days, followed by 200 mg/m² PO q12h *Pediatric dosage, for ages 2 mos–8 yrs*—4 mg/kg PO qd × 14 days; if no rash develops, can be increased to 7 mg/kg PO bid *For >8 yrs*—4 mg/kg PO qd × 14 days; if no rash develops, can be increased to 4 mg/kg PO bid (not to exceed 400 mg/day)	Rash, head- ache, fever, diarrhea	This drug should always be used in combination with other medications to treat HIV infection. **DRUG-FOOD INTERACTIONS** • The drug may be administered with food, antacids, or ddI. • Has good oral bioavailability with or without food. **ADVERSE EFFECTS** • Drug is metabolized in the liver by the cytochrome P450 system. There are many drug-drug interactions. See Appendix D. • Rash is common early in treatment. If severe rash occurs, especially if accompanied by fever, blistering, lesion, swelling, or general malaise, discontinue medication. • Stevens-Johnson syndrome can occur. • Clinical hepatitis can occur. **DOSAGE ADJUSTMENTS** • The drug is partially eliminated by the kidney. Dosage adjustments for clients with renal failure have not been studied. **MONITORING AND EDUCATION** • If client is noncompliant, full daily dosage can be given once per day. • Because clinical hepatitis has been reported with the use of this drug, monitoring of the AST, ALT, and GGT is recom- mended, especially during the first 6 mos of use. The drug should be discontinued if hepatitis occurs.

Continued

Brand/Generic Name	Usual Regimen	Common Side Effects	Important Nursing Consideration
  DELAVIRDINE (Rescriptor) *FDA approval: 4/97* Supplied as: *Tablets*—100 and 200 mg	1200 mg daily—400 mg tid **or** 600 mg bid *Pediatric and neonatal dosages are unknown. Dosage is for clients 16 yrs and older.*	Rash, headache	This drug should always be used in combination with other medications to treat HIV infection. **DRUG-FOOD INTERACTIONS** • The drug can be taken with or without food but should not be taken with a fatty meal. • Clients taking antacids and ddI should take these at least 1 hr apart from delavirdine (Rescriptor). • The drug can be dispersed in water for consumption. A dispersion consists of four tablets placed or mixed in at least 3 ounces of water, allowed to stand for a few minutes, and then stirred. The dispersion should be consumed promptly. **ADVERSE EFFECTS** • Rash is a common side effect. The drug can be continued or restarted in most cases. • The drug is metabolized in the liver by the cytochrome P450 system, which may alter the activity of other drugs. See Appendix D. **DOSAGE ADJUSTMENTS** • The drug is partially eliminated by the kidneys. Dosage adjustments for clients with renal failure have not been studied. • Severe hepatic insufficiency may warrant decreased dosage. **MONITORING AND EDUCATION** • Clients who are achlorhydric should take this medication with an acidic beverage to increase its absorption.

This drug should always be used in combination with other medications to treat HIV infection.

DRUG-FOOD INTERACTIONS

- The drug can be taken with or without food. A high fat meal should be avoided. Foods high in fat may increase the bioavailability of efavirenz by 50%.
- Capsules may be opened and added to liquids or foods but efavirenz has a peppery taste; grape jelly has been used to disguise the taste.

ADVERSE EFFECTS

- The most common type of rash seen in studies of this drug was a diffuse maculopapular type. The rash often appeared within the first 2 wks of initiating therapy and resolved within 1 mo when therapy was continued.

DOSAGE ADJUSTMENTS

- No renal or hepatic dosage adjustment necessary.

MONITORING AND EDUCATION

- The drug is metabolized in the liver. Liver function tests LFT, AST, ALT, and GGT should be monitored.
- The drug may cause central nervous system (CNS) side effects. To minimize these effects, the client should take this drug at night.
- Nightmares have been reported.
- If a client develops resistance to this drug, the client may not be able to use drugs in this same class because of cross-resistance.
- The drug may cause hyperlipemia. Cholesterol and triglyceride levels should be monitored.

Continued

CNS side effects such as dizziness, vivid dreams, nightmares, difficulty concentrating; rash.

---

600 mg daily—600 mg qd HS

Tablets can be placed in water to form slurry.
Neonatal dosage—Unknown
Pediatric dosage, for children >3 yrs (administered once daily)—Body weight: 10 to <15 kg—200 mg; 15 to <20 kg—250 mg; 20 to <25 kg—300 mg; 25 to <32.5 kg—350 mg; 32.5 to <40 kg—400 mg; >40 kg—600 mg.

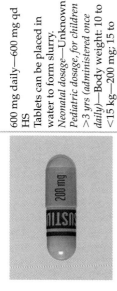

EFAVIRENZ
(DMP-266, Sustiva)
FDA approval: 12/98

Supplied as:
Capsules—50, 100, and 200 mg

Protease Inhibitors (PIs)

Brand/Generic Name	Usual Regimen	Common Side Effects	Important Nursing Consideration
  SAQUINAVIR (Invirase, "hard gel capsule") *FDA approval:* 12/95 Supplied as: *Capsules*—200 mg	1800 mg daily—600 mg q8h *Neonatal and pediatric dosages are unknown.*	Nausea, vomiting, diarrhea, rash, paresthesias, weakness	This drug should always be used in combination with other medications to treat HIV infection. **DRUG-FOOD INTERACTIONS** • The drug should be taken with a meal that is high in fat. • Saquinavir absorption may be enhanced with ingestion of grapefruit juice. **ADVERSE EFFECTS** • There are many drug interactions. See Appendix D. **DOSAGE ADJUSTMENTS** • No dosage adjustment for renal impairment necessary. Severe hepatic insufficiency may warrant decreased dosage. **MONITORING AND EDUCATION** • The client should avoid direct exposure to sunlight and use sunscreen. • Gastrointestinal (GI) side effects are common—diarrhea, abdominal discomforts, and gas. These may improve within 4-8 wks after starting the drug. • The drug is principally metabolized by the liver. Liver function tests (AST, ALT, and GGT) should be monitored periodically. • Elevated nonfasting triglyceride levels have been reported. The client's lipid panel (e.g., cholesterol and triglyceride levels) should be monitored.

SAQUINAVIR
(Fortovase, "soft gel capsule")
FDA approval: 11/97

Supplied as:
Capsules—200 mg | 3600 mg daily—1200 mg q8h
Neonatal and pediatric dosages are unknown.
Under study: 50 mg/kg PO tid | Nausea | • New onset type II diabetes mellitus has been reported with this and all PIs. The client's glucose levels should be monitored periodically.

This drug should always be used in combination with other medications to treat HIV infection.
DRUG-FOOD INTERACTIONS
• The drug should be taken with a meal that is high in fat.
• The drug can be kept out of the refrigerator but not for longer than 3 mos.
ADVERSE EFFECTS
• There are many drug interactions. See Appendix D.
DOSAGE ADJUSTMENTS
• No dosage adjustment for renal impairment necessary. Severe hepatic insufficiency may warrant decreased dosage.
MONITORING AND EDUCATION
• The client should avoid direct exposure to sunlight and use sunscreen.
• GI side effects are common—diarrhea, abdominal discomforts, and gas. These may improve within 4-8 wks after starting the drug.
• The drug is principally metabolized by the liver. Liver function tests (AST, ALT, and GGT) should be monitored periodically.
• Elevated nonfasting triglyceride levels have been reported. The client's lipid panel (e.g., cholesterol and triglyceride levels) should be monitored. |

Continued

HIV/AIDS MEDICATIONS—cont'd

Brand/Generic Name	Usual Regimen	Common Side Effects	Important Nursing Consideration
			• New onset type II diabetes mellitus has been reported with this and all PIs. The client's glucose levels should be monitored periodically.
RITONAVIR (Norvir, "soft-gel capsule") *FDA approval: 3/96* (*Semisolid capsules no longer available after 7/98. Soft-gel capsules approved by FDA: 6/99.*) Supplied as: *Capsules*—100 mg *Solution*—80 mg/ml (bottle contains 240 ml)	1200 mg daily—600 mg PO bid To minimize side effects Ritonavir can be administered in escalating doses: Day 1—300 mg q12h; day 2-3—400 mg q12h; day 4-13—500 mg q12h; then 600 mg q12h. *Neonatal dosage*—Unknown *Pediatric dosage*—400 mg/m² q12h; maximum daily dose is 1200 mg daily (600 mg bid). To minimize nausea/vomiting, start at 250 mg/m² q12h and add 50 mg/m² daily.	Nausea, GI distress	This drug should always be used in combination with other medications to treat HIV infection. **DRUG-FOOD INTERACTIONS** • Soft-gel capsule refrigeration is recommended but not required if the drug is used within 30 days and stored below 77° F. • Drug must be taken with meals. There may be a bitter aftertaste. To decrease the aftertaste, the drug can be mixed in chocolate milk or Ensure or another nutritional supplement. **ADVERSE EFFECTS** • The client may report circumoral paresthesias (i.e., numbness around the mouth). This diminishes after several weeks of therapy. • This drug is metabolized through the cytochrome P450 system. There are several drugs that should not be taken with ritonavir (see Appendix D). **DOSAGE ADJUSTMENTS** • There are no adjustments for renal insufficiency. Ritonavir has not been studied in hepatic insufficiency. **MONITORING AND EDUCATION** • This drug *often* causes GI upset—nausea and vomiting (use dose escalation). However, the effect may disappear after 4

| INDINAVIR (Crixivan) FDA approval: 3/96 | 2400 mg daily—800 mg q8h
Neonatal dosing: Not recommended
Pediatric dosage—
Under study: 500 mg/m² q8h | Flank pain, hematuria (suggests a kidney stone), nausea, headache, asthenia, rash, dizziness, metallic taste | wks of continued administration. An anticipatory management plan, in collaboration with the health care provider, may prevent the client from discontinuing this medication.
• The drug may cause hypertriglyceridemia. The lipid panel, including triglycerides, should be monitored.
• This drug is metabolized by the liver. Levels of AST, ALT, CPK, and uric acid should be monitored regularly.
• When using Ritonavir solution, the following table indicates the correct dosage:
    300 mg → 3.5 ml
    400 mg → 5.0 ml
    500 mg → 6.25 ml
    600 mg → 7.5 ml
• New onset type II diabetes mellitus has been reported with this and all PIs. The client's glucose levels should be monitored periodically. |

This drug should always be used in combination with other medications to treat HIV infection.

DRUG-FOOD INTERACTIONS

• Drug must be taken on an empty stomach or with a light meal—with skim milk, juice, or coffee.
• Clients must drink at least six 8-ounce glasses of water daily to prevent the formation of kidney stones.

ADVERSE EFFECTS

• Nephrolithiasis can occur.
• Hemolytic anemia has been reported.
• Hepatitis, although rare, can occur.
• Thrombocytopenia, although rare, can occur.

Continued

HIV/AIDS MEDICATIONS—cont'd

Brand/Generic Name	Usual Regimen	Common Side Effects	Important Nursing Consideration
Supplied as: *Capsules*—200 and 400 mg			**DOSAGE ADJUSTMENTS** • No adjustment for renal failure necessary. If there is mild to moderate hepatic insufficiency, dosage should be decreased to 600 mg q8h **MONITORING AND EDUCATION** • Since hemolytic anemia can occur with this drug, the client's complete blood count should be monitored. • If indinavir is administered with ddI, the drugs should be given at least 1 hr apart. • Clients may develop dry skin. • Clients may develop ingrown toenails. • The drug may cause GI upset. • To ensure adequate hydration, it is recommended that the client drink at least 1.5 liters (approximately 48 ounces) of liquid during the course of 24 hrs. • New onset type II diabetes mellitus has been reported with this and all PIs. The client's glucose levels should be monitored periodically.

This drug should always be used in combination with other medications to treat HIV infection.

DRUG-FOOD INTERACTIONS

• The drug must be taken with food.

ADVERSE EFFECTS

• This drug is metabolized through the cytochrome P450 system; several medications are contraindicated for concurrent use (see Appendix D).

DOSAGE ADJUSTMENTS

• No adjustments for hepatic or renal insufficiency are necessary.

MONITORING AND EDUCATION

• The current formulation of the pill disintegrates quickly on contact with moisture. This can cause the client to choke when swallowing the tablet. The company recommends crushing the pills with the back of a spoon and mixing with food. The client can also dissolve the pills in water, juice, or milk. If the pill gets stuck in the throat, drinking a large volume of water can help dissolve the pill.

• This drug often causes diarrhea. An anticipatory management plan, in collaboration with the health care provider, may prevent the client from discontinuing this medication.

• For children unable to take tablets, Viracept oral powder may be administered. It can be mixed with water, milk, formula, soy formula, and soymilk. When mixed, it should be used within 6 hrs. The powder should not be mixed in an acidic beverage.

Mild to moderate diarrhea

2250-2500 mg daily—1250 mg bid **or** 750 mg tid
Neonatal dosage—
Under study: 10 mg/kg PO bid
Pediatric dosage, for ages
2-13 yrs—20-30 mg/kg tid (not to exceed 750 mg tid).

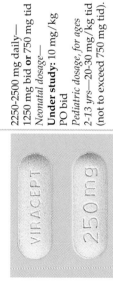

NELFINAVIR
(Viracept)
FDA approval: 3/97

Supplied as:
Tablets—250 mg
Powder—Bottle containing 144 g of powder; one level scoop (1 g) equals 50 mg of drug.

Continued

HIV/AIDS MEDICATIONS—cont'd

Brand/Generic Name	Usual Regimen	Common Side Effects	Important Nursing Consideration
			• New onset type II diabetes mellitus has been reported with this and all PIs. The client's glucose levels should be monitored periodically.
AMPRENAVIR (Agenerase, 141W94) *FDA approval:* 4/99 Supplied as: *Tablets*—50 and 150 mg *Solution*—15 mg/ml (bottle contains 240 ml) *Note:* Agenerase capsules and Agenerase oral solution are not interchangeable on a milligram per milligram basis.	2400 mg daily—1200 mg bid *Neonatal dosage*—Under study *Pediatric dosage, for ages 4-12 yrs or <50 kg*—Capsules: 20 mg/kg bid **or** 15 mg/kg tid (not to exceed 2400 mg daily). Solution: 22.5 mg/kg (1.5 ml/kg) bid **or** 17 mg/kg (1.1 ml/kg) tid (not to exceed 2800 mg daily).	Nausea, vomiting, diarrhea, rash, paresthesia, altered mood	This drug should always be used in combination with other medications to treat HIV infection. **DRUG-FOOD INTERACTIONS** • The drug may be taken with or without food; however, a high fat meal decreases absorption of amprenavir. • Vitamin E supplements should not be taken with amprenavir, which already contains vitamin E. • Clients taking ddI or antacids should take these at least 1 hr before or after Agenerase. **ADVERSE EFFECTS** • This drug is a sulfonamide. It should be used with caution in clients with allergies to sulfonamides. • This drug is metabolized through the cytochrome P450 system; several medications are contraindicated for concurrent use (see Appendix D). • Stevens-Johnson syndrome has been reported. Clients should notify provider if skin changes occur. • Acute hemolytic anemia may occur. • Because of the potential risk of toxicity from the large amount of the excipient propylene glycol, Agenerase oral solution is contraindicated in infants and children below the age of 4 yrs,

pregnant women, clients with hepatic or renal failure, and clients treated with disulfiram or metronidazole.

DOSAGE ADJUSTMENTS

• Decrease dosage for liver impairment.

MONITORING AND EDUCATION

• The client should be made aware that he or she may experience some perioral paresthesia.

• Since hemolytic anemia is associated with this drug, CBC should be monitored.

16

Parasitic Infections

- Cryptosporidiosis
- Isosporiasis
- Microsporidiosis
- *Pneumocystis carinii* pneumonia
- Toxoplasmosis

Glenda Winson
Carl A. Kirton
Kenneth Zwolski

Cryptosporidiosis

■ DEFINITION AND ETIOLOGY

Cryptosporidium parvum is a member of the coccidia family, which also includes *Pneumocystis carinii* and *Toxoplasma gondii*. The cryptosporidium parasite typically affects the small intestines, but can infect the colon; the biliary tract; and, less commonly, the respiratory tract and sinuses. While well known in veterinary medicine, it has only been recognized as a cause of diarrhea in humans since 1980.[1]

Cryptosporidium is found throughout the world, but the incidence is higher in developing countries. Infection with this organism is an AIDS-defining illness, and in the past it has accounted for 5% to 10% of AIDS cases reported to the Centers for Disease Control and Prevention. The organism is ubiquitous in nature and affects a wide variety of different species. It is transmitted by ingestion of oocysts (spores enclosed in a thick membrane), which are excreted in the feces of infected humans and most farm animals, rodents, puppies, and kittens. It is very infectious and only one oocyst may cause infection. The most common route of transmission is the fecal-oral route. The organism can be ingested by consuming contaminated water (oocysts are resistant to chemical disinfectants commonly used to treat water) and food or as a result of sexual contact involving exposure to fecal material. Nosocomial infection of health care workers can occur from handling contaminated feces. Oocysts can remain infective for 2 to 6 months after leaving the body. The risk of infection increases with degree of immunosuppression and is seen most often in clients with CD_4 cell counts below 200 cells/mm^3.

■ CLINICAL OVERVIEW

After ingestion of the oocysts, the sporozoite commonly infects the small intestines where it damages the epithelial cells. The organism is small, round, 2 to 4 μm in diameter, and appears to stick to the surface of infected cells. On average it is 7 to 10 days after ingestion of the oocysts before the client notes the onset of the most common manifestation of disease, severe watery diarrhea. In immunocompetent clients, this diarrhea resolves in a few days. In immunocompromised clients (CD_4 lymphocyte counts less than 200 cells/mm³) it can lead to unrelenting, voluminous, watery diarrhea and dehydration. The severity of symptoms may vary and on occasion the infection resolves spontaneously, especially in the face of immune system reconstitution (CD_4 cell counts above 200 cells/mm³).

While diarrhea resulting from intestinal infection is the most common manifestation of cryptosporidiosis, biliary infections do occur. Biliary infections include sclerosing cholangitis or calculous cholecystitis. It has been suggested that the difficulty in eradicating cryptosporidium from the gastrointestinal (GI) tract may be due to its presence in the gallbladder. Clients infected with cryptosporidium rarely have fever unless the organism has infected the gallbladder. Sinus and respiratory infections with cryptosporidium are rare, but when present the client may complain of a cough, sinus trouble, or a postnasal drip.

Since highly active antiretroviral therapy (HAART) was introduced in 1996, the incidence of cryptosporidiosis has fallen. This may be explained, in part, by the fact that as the immune system begins to recover (as evidenced by a rising CD_4 count), there is more likelihood of spontaneous remission.

■ DIAGNOSTIC TESTING

Examination of the client's stool for oocysts is the cornerstone of diagnosis. In clients with HIV, diarrhea can be caused by a variety of organisms. Therefore, when examining the stool for sources of diarrhea, specimens are collected for examination for ova and parasites, enteric pathogens, and *Clostridium difficile* toxin. Tests for cryptosporidia, microsporidia, and *Isospora* sp. may not be done routinely in clinical laboratories and should be specifically requested in the stool analysis.

When cryptosporidiosis is suspected, it is advised to collect three separate stool samples due to variability in shedding of the oocysts, although in 80% of cases oocysts are found in the first sample. If the stool sample contains cryptosporidium oocysts, an acid-fast stain reveals unevenly colored red or pink spheres 2 to 4 microns in diameter. In cases where stool analysis does not yield any organism, yet diarrhea persists, intestinal biopsy by esophagogastroduodenoscopy (EGD) or a colonoscopy may be needed to rule out other infections and to localize the site of infection.

■ MEDICAL MANAGEMENT

Management of a client with diarrhea begins with a thorough, detailed history about the frequency and volume of bowel movements, any presence of blood, and urgency felt by the client. It may be possible to determine that the cause of diarrhea is either colitis or mucosal malabsorption by a detailed history. Clients with colitis have large numbers of bowel movements that are small in volume. Clients with malabsorption often

Table 16-1	Clinical Differences in Stools of Malabsorption and Colitis	

Symptom	Malabsorption	Colitis
Frequency	3-4	4-30
Stool Volume per day	750-10,000 ml	250-1000 ml
Interval of bowel movements	Variable	Regular
Occult blood	No	Yes
Urgency	Yes	Yes
Tenesmus	No	Variable

Table 16-2	Medical Regimens

Cryptosporidiosis	Regimens
Prophylaxis	No known therapy.
Treatment	No curative treatments.
	The following drugs are used and are sometimes helpful in reducing diarrhea (maximum daily dosages):
	Paromomycin sulphate (Humatin) 2000 mg (in 4 divided doses)
	Azithromycin (Zithromax) 2000 mg qd in divided doses (to be taken with empty stomach)
	Thalidomide* 100 mg hs
	Nitazoxanide* (NTZ) 3000 mg qd (in 2 divided doses)
Maintenance	No known therapy.

*Not FDA approved; available on compassionate use basis.

have moderately elevated numbers of bowel movements that are large in volume (Table 16-1). The D-xylose absorption test can be used to establish whether there is diffuse small bowel disease. (See p. 355 for a description of this test.)

Therapy with the drugs listed in Table 16-2 is sometimes helpful in reducing diarrhea, but is not effective in eradicating the organism. Management focuses on identifying the organism and controlling the symptoms. Clients with diarrhea should be given medications to slow GI motility. Common antidiarrheal medications are as follows:

- Lomotil 5 mg PO qid, initially, then titrated according to response
- Deodorized tincture of opium (DTO) 0.3 to 1 ml qid (not to exceed 6 ml daily)
- Paregoric 5 to 10 ml qid

Prolonged diarrhea caused by cryptosporidiosis may lead to weight loss, abdominal cramps, flatulence, general malaise, electrolyte imbalances, weakness due to potassium depletion, and dehydration. Clients who are volume depleted may require parenteral infusions. Figure 16-1 outlines the evaluation of a client who has diarrhea for longer than 2 weeks.

■ NURSING CONSIDERATIONS

1. The client should be taught that the best way to prevent transmission of infection is to wash hands before and after touching food and after using the bathroom.
2. The client should be taught to use a latex barrier condom for oral-anal sex and to wash hands well after sexual contact.
3. The client should wear gloves when cleaning pet litter.
4. Clients with CD_4 cell counts below 100 cells/mm^3:
   - ■ Should boil water for 1 minute or use a water filter that screens out particles down to 1 micron. Brita brand filters are *not* able to filter out cryptosporidia. Purplus brand filters are guaranteed to filter out cryptosporidiosis. Clients should be informed that bottled water must come from underground wells or springs to be safe. Poland Springs and Deer Park brands make that claim. Commercially bottled soft drinks and seltzers are safe. Bottled juices are safe if they have been pasteurized.
   - ■ Should be taught to use safe water (i.e., filtered, boiled, or bottled as previously noted) to make ice cubes and to wash fruits and vegetables.
   - ■ Should avoid swimming in pools or bodies of water that may be contaminated. It is estimated that 65% to 96% of rivers, lakes, and streams in the United States may be contaminated with cryptosporidia.
   - ■ Should not drink raw, untreated milk. Pasteurized milk is safe.
   - ■ Should be instructed to use weak ammonia to clean laundry and to clean kitchen countertops to kill organisms. Chlorine bleach is ineffective against cryptosporidia.
5. Clients should be informed that dishes, silverware, pots, and pans can be washed in tap water as long as they are dried before use.
6. Infection with cryptosporidium produces enough diarrhea to cause dehydration and electrolyte abnormalities. When diarrhea is present, the nurse should instruct the client to consume a diet low in fat and residue and high in protein and calories. The client should increase fluid intake to approximately 3 liters per day and avoid milk and milk products. The client should also be instructed to ingest food that is high in potassium.
7. The client's weight and body composition should be monitored. Several indirect measures of body composition are available. Lean body mass, body fat, and body water can be monitored by bioelectrical impedance analysis (BIA). BIA should be done at least monthly in clients

A. Assess clinical history, past gastrointestinal history, current medications, disease stage, CD_4 cell count, travel history, dietary history, behavioral risk factors, reports of fever, weight loss, and signs of dehydration.

B. Stool examination for ova and parasites (send 3 samples), *Giardia* spp., ameba, *Isospora* spp., *Cyclospora* spp., microsporidia, and cryptosporidia*; stool culture for enteric pathogens, salmonella, shigella, and campylobacter; assay for *Clostridium difficile* toxin[†]; stool for acid-fast bacillus (AFB)[‡]; urinalysis.[§]

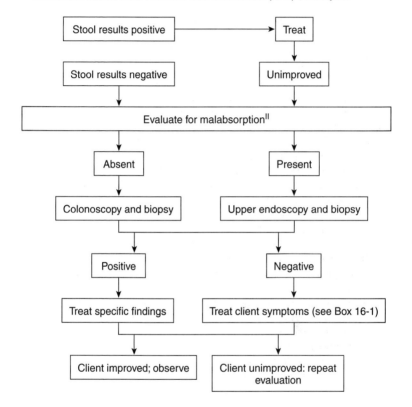

*If CD_4 cell count <100 cells/mm^3.
[†]With concurrent or recent antibiotic use or hospitalization.
[‡]If CD_4 cell count <100 cells/mm^3.
[§]For microsporidiosis, encephalitozoon intestinalis.
[II]D-xylose absorption test, fecal fat, serum carotene, breath test.

Figure 16-1. Evaluation of chronic diarrhea.

with chronic diarrhea. If BIA is not available, the nurse can assess skinfold measurements at each visit. Skinfold measurements provide an estimate of the size of subcutaneous fat stores, which can be used to estimate total body fat.[2] (See p. 351 for a discussion of BIA.)

8. Nutritional considerations for clients with diarrhea due to small bowel disease are listed in Box 16-1.
9. For medical regimens see Table 16-2.

Isosporiasis

■ DEFINITION AND ETIOLOGY

Isosporiasis is caused by infection with a coccidian protozoa, *I. belli*, which is similar to the protozoa that cause cryptosporidiosis. Isosporiasis has a frequency of 1% to 3% and typically does not occur until the CD_4 cell count is less than 100 cells/mm^3. Isosporiasis is more likely to occur in foreign born clients, especially those from El Salvador and Mexico and, generally, has a higher incidence in persons of Hispanic ethnicity than in those of non-Hispanic ethnicity. Clients who have been treated previously for *P. carinii* pneumonia (PCP) have a decreased risk of getting isosporiasis, probably because Bactrim, which is used to treat PCP, is effective in killing *I. belli* as well. *I. belli* is transmitted by the fecal-oral route.

■ CLINICAL OVERVIEW

Clients typically present with watery diarrhea—often more than 2 to 3 bowel movements per day—which can persist for more than 21 days. Symptoms of enteritis may be present, fever is not present, and weight loss and symptoms of malabsorption are common.

■ DIAGNOSIS

Isosporiasis is detected by an acid-fast bacillus (AFB) smear of stools, in which red-stained oocysts can be found. There are no white blood cells present in fecal samples. See Figure 16-1 for a description of the complete work-up of a client with diarrhea.

■ MEDICAL MANAGEMENT

Isosporiasis is treated with trimethoprim sulfamethoxazole or pyrimethamine plus folinic acid. Antidiarrheal agents such as Lomotil, loperamide, or paregoric are often prescribed to relieve symptoms.

■ NURSING CONSIDERATIONS

1. The best advice to give clients to reduce their risk of being infected with *Isospora* spp. is to practice good handwashing techniques and personal hygiene and to avoid ingestion of fecally contaminated food or water.
2. Nutritional supplements often have to be provided to clients because of the chronic nature of diarrhea and malabsorption. Careful

BOX 16-1 NUTRITIONAL CONSIDERATIONS FOR CLIENTS WITH SMALL BOWEL DISEASE

1. Diets should be low in fat, lactose free, and contain no caffeine or alcohol. Oil should not be used in cooking for clients with malabsorption because they cannot digest or absorb fat. To enhance the flavor of foods, clients should be instructed to substitute broth stocks for oils. Medium-chain triglycerides (obtained from health food stores) can be used for cooking.
2. Clients should be advised to eat foods that help to bind stools (e.g., rice, bananas, applesauce). Pectin, which is found in apples, for example, helps bind stools and should be recommended.
3. Undernourished clients should be offered chemically defined, nutritionally sound diets in the form of an enteral formula. Elemental diets, in the form of enteral formulas, are low in long-chain triglycerides and lactose free. Elemental diets require little digestion and thus are maximally absorbed. The enteral product, not food, should be the main source of calories. Food needs to be broken down and digested before it can be absorbed. Clients should be advised to consume 6 to 8 packets or cans a day of the enteral product. Examples of such products include Vivonex and Peptamin. Elemental products are not palatable to clients. Fruit flavor can be added to improve the taste of the formula. Clients should be advised not to eat food concurrently with formula because food decreases transit time in the small bowel and decreases absorption. Eating less food and taking an elemental formula also reduces diarrhea. Enteral feeding with elemental formula of clients with malabsorption is effective in preserving lean body mass and body weight. In a study to compare the effects of such enteral feeding with the effects of total parenteral nutrition (TPN), little difference was found between the study groups. Enteral feeding is preferable, however, because it is cheaper and because there is a high risk of infection with TPN. It is also better that the gut be used; intestinal mucosa quickly becomes atrophied if not used. Some medical insurance companies will not cover enteral formula. For some insurers a letter is needed explaining the reasons for use, including that the alternative of TPN is much more expensive and carries a high risk of infection.
4. TPN should be used when enteral feeding is not possible or effective. TPN has been shown to increase weight and lean body mass in malnourished clients with AIDS. Standard- or high-nitrogen parenteral fluids can be administered by either peripheral or central vein infusion. Intravenous (IV) lipids are usually administered at least twice a week. The serum triglycerides of clients receiving IV lipids should be monitored routinely because hypertriglyceridemia can occur. Strict aseptic technique must be followed when administering TPN. It is recommended that a family member or friend and a skilled nurse assist in the management of the parenteral feeding program. Clients receiving long-term parenteral support should receive supplements of trace minerals, such as zinc and selenium. Additional potassium and magnesium are often necessary in clients with diarrhea. Nutritional assessment should be conducted regularly to assess the adequacy of the feeding program, as well as the client's tolerance of TPN. Vitamins and minerals can be adjusted to individual needs.

From Kotler DP et al: Enteral alimentation and repletion of body cell mass in malnourished patients with AIDS, *Am J Clin Nutr* 53:149, 1991; Kotler DP, Tierney A, Fogleman L: *Comparison of TPN and semi-elemental diet in AIDS patients with malabsorption*, presentation at the International AIDS Conference in Vancouver, 1996; Kotler DP et al: Effects of home TPN upon body composition in patients with AIDS, *Am J Clin Nutr*, 14:454, 1990.

Table 16-3	Medical Regimens

Isosporiasis	Regimens
Prophylaxis	No known therapy, but PCP prophylaxis with Bactrim may prevent occurrence.
Treatment	Trimethoprim sulfamethoxazole PO qid × 10 days **then** bid × 3 weeks. *Or* Pyrimethamine 75 mg PO qd **plus** folinic acid 10 mg qd × 14 days then maintenance therapy
Maintenance	Recommended—Bactrim therapy.

attention should be paid to the potential for fluid and electrolyte disturbances.

3. Because of the prevalence of *I. belli* in Latin America, nurses should have a high index of suspicion for isosporiasis in clients with AIDS who have diarrhea and who have immigrated from or traveled to Latin America, in clients who were born in the United States but are of Hispanic ethnicity, and in clients who are not receiving PCP prophylaxis.
4. For medical regimens see Table 16-3.

Microsporidiosis

■ DEFINITION AND ETIOLOGY

Microsporidia are intracellular spore-forming parasites, approximately 3 to 6 μm in diameter. In humans, microsporidia affect not only the small intestines but also the kidneys, eyes, and sinuses. Cells infected with microsporidia may contain a single parasite or several different species. *Enterocytozoon bieneusi* is the most common species to infect humans and was first described in 1985. *Encephalitozoon intestinalis* (formerly Septata) is also seen but only occurs in about 10% of cases.[1] Microsporidia are found in many other species (e.g. fish, insects, many mammals). Infection is thought to occur by ingestion of contaminated spores, which can live outside of the body for up to 4 months. However, the actual source of human infections is not known. The distribution of microsporidiosis is also not known; however, the incidence is higher in clients who have traveled to tropical areas.

Since HAART was introduced in 1996, the incidence of microsporidiosis has declined. This may be explained, in part, by the fact that as the immune system begins to recover (as evidenced by a rising CD_4 cell count), there is more likelihood of spontaneous clearance.

■ CLINICAL OVERVIEW

The major symptom of microsporidiosis is profuse, watery diarrhea. Other accompanying symptoms may include malabsorption and weight loss, flatulence and abdominal cramps, and symptoms of electrolyte imbalances. Microsporidia usually affect the small intestines by causing fusing of the villi (see Figures 19-1 and 19-2). As a result, there is partial atrophy of villi in the duodenum, jejunum, and ileum. This change in morphology decreases the surface area for absorption and curtails the production of digestive enzymes, resulting in malabsorption of fats and disaccharides. Undigested food in the small intestine is hyperosmotic, pulling more fluid into the small intestines. In the colon, the bacteria in undigested food ferments, producing gas and further increasing osmolality, pulling in yet more fluid and leading to profuse, watery diarrhea.

■ DIAGNOSTIC TESTING

When microsporidiosis is suspected, stool samples are collected for examination. However, microsporidia are difficult to isolate from stools because of their small size. Urine should also be examined for microsporidia (*E. intestinalis* to rule out extraintestinal disease. See Figure 16-1 for complete work-up of the client with diarrhea. To confirm the diagnosis, a small bowel biopsy may be necessary.

■ MEDICAL MANAGEMENT

Management focuses on identifying the organism and controlling the symptoms caused by the disease and is similar to that of the client with cryptosporidiosis.

■ NURSING CONSIDERATIONS

1. The client should be informed that there is no known curative or even effective therapy available. Clients who are treated with albendazole who have *E. bieneusi* tend to have a limited response, whereas clients with *E. intestinalis* have a good response to albendazole and other experimental therapies.
2. The nurse should be aware that albendazole is a hepatotoxic drug. The nurse should monitor the client's liver enzyme levels—lactic dehydrogenase (LDH), alanine aminotransferase (ALT), aspartate aminotransferase (AST), and gamma glutamyl transpeptidase (GGTP).
3. Thalidomide is being used with some success in clients with microsporidiosis. This drug is not FDA approved for this indication; however, it is available on a compassionate use basis. The nurse should instruct both male and female clients receiving thalidomide about the importance of very strict birth control. This involves using at least two methods of birth control. Clients should be instructed to use a barrier method as well as another form of birth control because

Table 16-4	Medical Regimens	

Microsporidiosis	Regimens
Prophylaxis	No known therapy.
Treatment	No curative treatments. For palliative treatment (maximum daily doses—not to exceed):
	Paromomycin (Humatin) 150 mg/kg PO qid in divided doses
	Azithromycin (Zithromax) 2000 mg PO (to be taken with empty stomach)
	Nitazoxanide (NTZ) 3000 mg/day PO bid
	Albendazole 800 mg PO bid in divided doses*
	Thalidomide 100 mg PO in divided doses*
Maintenance	No known therapy.

*Not FDA-approved; available on compassionate use basis.

thalidomide is known to cause birth defects—including, but not limited to, the absence of limbs in the newborn. The nurse should ensure that clients understand that thalidomide should be kept in a place that is not accessible to other family members to prevent inadvertent administration.

4. For medical regimens see Table 16-4.

Pneumocystis carinii Pneumonia

■ DEFINITION AND ETIOLOGY

P. carinii is a fungal organism that is acquired by inhalation. Most children are exposed to it by the age of two and demonstrate serological evidence of *P. carinii* antibodies in their serum. These antibodies, however, are not long-lasting; adults rarely demonstrate these antibodies.

PCP in HIV-positive clients is caused almost exclusively by the reactivation of latent organisms. PCP as a result of primary infection is thought to be rare. Early in the AIDS epidemic, PCP was the most common opportunistic infection to affect those with AIDS and was one of the most common causes of death in clients with AIDS. Today, PCP is the second leading cause of death in clients with AIDS, second to pneumonia due to unspecified organisms. This decline in PCP-related deaths is due to effective PCP prophylaxis regimens and potent antiretroviral therapy.

■ CLINICAL OVERVIEW

When *P. carinii* activates, its cysts lodge in the interstitial spaces of the pulmonary parenchyma, creating a mechanical barrier to ventilation and perfusion of respiratory gases. This process causes dyspnea on exertion, which is typical in clients with PCP. Other symptoms that often occur are fever and a nonproductive cough. Clients with PCP typically have normal lung examination findings but may also present with adventitious breath sounds. PCP rarely occurs in extrapulmonary sites, but when it does it can affect almost any organ.

■ DIAGNOSIS

Because the organism cannot be cultured, the diagnosis of PCP is often made on the presence of the classical triad of symptoms—fever, dyspnea, and a nonproductive cough—in a person with immunosuppression (i.e., a CD_4 cell count less than 200 or CD_4 percentage less than 14). However, these classical symptoms may be absent in clients with advanced HIV disease, individuals receiving PCP prophylaxis (especially with aerosolized pentamidine), and clients with chronic obstructive pulmonary disease (COPD).[3] There is no single test that can diagnose a client with PCP. A variety of tests are often used to support the diagnosis. The chest x-ray study, when abnormal, demonstrates diffuse bilateral interstitial infiltrates. Approximately 10% of clients may have normal chest x-ray study results. Pulse oximetry (i.e., measuring oxygen saturation) can be useful in supporting a working diagnosis. Arterial blood gas (ABG) measurements often reveal hypoxemia (reduced Po_2). ABG measurements can also be used to calculate the alveolar-arterial (A-a) gradient, which is a measure of intrapulmonary shunting. The A-a gradient, breathing room air, of a client with PCP will be increased (normal is 0 to 20 mm Hg). Box 16-2 shows the formula used to calculate the A-a gradient.

Serum LDH measurement (normal is 118 to 273 IU/L) may also be useful in supporting the diagnosis. A rise in LDH is usually seen in clients with PCP, although this finding does not always indicate PCP because many other conditions (e.g., myocardial infarction, hepatic failure) can also increase LDH.

Gallium scanning may be useful in ruling out PCP infection. When clients undergo gallium scanning, they are injected with a radionuclide that is "taken up" by or concentrated in areas of inflammation. Special gallium scanners reveal these areas. Clients with any inflammation or

BOX 16-2   MEASURING THE A-A GRADIENT

1. The client must be breathing room air.
2. Draw the client's arterial blood and measure arterial blood gases.
3. Using the PCO_2 and the PO_2 in the following equation:
$$\text{A-a gradient} = 150 - Po_2 - (Pco_2/0.8)$$

abscesses demonstrate increased uptake of gallium in these areas. The presence of *P. carinii* causes an uptake of gallium in the lungs. However, many other pulmonary conditions also yield the same results. Thus a positive test does not prove the presence of *P. carinii,* although a negative test reduces the likelihood that *P. carinii* or any other inflammation is present.

The diagnosis of PCP is often confirmed by the detection of the organisms in an induced sputum specimen or, if necessary, by the detection of the organism in a specimen obtained through bronchoalveolar lavage (BAL).

■ NURSING CONSIDERATIONS

1. Prophylaxis is considered for clients with a CD_4 cell count less than 200 cells/mm^3 or a CD_4 percentage of less than 14% of total lymphocytes, clients with unexplained persistent fevers and thrush, clients with hematological malignancies requiring chemotherapy, splenectomized clients, and clients receiving high-dose steroids.

2. Sputum induction is often necessary to confirm diagnosis of PCP. Clients inhale a hypertonic solution of nebulized saline. The mist is irritating to the respiratory mucosa and causes the client to cough forcibly, producing a specimen sufficient to diagnose PCP. In most facilities, sputum induction is carried out in negative pressure rooms. This is done because clients may be coinfected with *Mycobacterium tuberculosis* (MTB), which can be spread if aerosolized. (See Chapters 10 and 13 regarding MTB.) The nurse ensures that collection is done according to laboratory standards to ensure the highest yield of cyst in the specimen.

3. One double-strength (160 mg/800 mg) tablet of trimethoprim/sulfamethoxazole (Bactrim) is the drug of choice for prevention and treatment of PCP. Regimens with Bactrim may include daily dosage or three times weekly dosage. A recent clinical trial examined whether it was more advantageous for clients to take Bactrim once daily or thrice weekly. The researchers found that there was no difference in the development of PCP in clients who took Bactrim once a day compared to those who took Bactrim three times a week. However, they did find that survival was significantly prolonged in those who took Bactrim daily. Clients who took Bactrim daily also had significantly lower rates of bacterial pneumonia. Results from this trial seem to indicate that it is more advantageous for clients to take Bactrim on a daily basis.[4]

4. Up to 40% of clients receiving Bactrim experience fever and rash as side effects. These side effects can be managed by switching to a single-strength dosage; to a three times weekly schedule of administration; or to another drug, such as dapsone. Because of the superiority of Bactrim over other drugs, clients who experience mild adverse reactions should be encouraged to "work through" the effects. When

the adverse reactions are severe, Bactrim desensitization can be carried out. Desensitization therapies vary among institutions. Because of the potential for severe cardiopulmonary or dermatological reactions, this procedure is carried out in a monitored setting. The nurse is referred to the institution's protocol when participating in desensitization procedures.

5. Clients who are being treated for PCP should have ABGs measured. Clients with severe hypoxia (i.e., PO_2 less than 70 mm Hg or an A-a gradient greater than 35 mm Hg) must receive concomitant therapy with oral corticosteroids. Treatment with steroids is as follows:

    Prednisone $\times$ 21 days:

    40 mg PO bid $\times$ 5 days

    Then

    40 mg PO qd $\times$ 5 days

    Then

    20 mg PO qd $\times$ 11 days

6. Clients taking Bactrim should have their complete blood count (CBC) monitored every 4 to 6 months because the sulfa component of the drug often causes thrombocytopenia and neutropenia.

7. Clients being considered for dapsone therapy must have blood drawn for glucose-6-phosphate dehydrogenase (G6PD) testing. Clients who are deficient in G6PD and take dapsone are prone to hemolytic anemia. Dapsone may also cause abnormalities in liver function tests (LFTs).

8. Clients receiving IV infusions of pentamidine should be monitored for pancreatitis. The nurse should monitor the serum amylase and lipase. Hypoglycemia can occur as a side effect of IV infusion, so it is necessary to check blood capillary glucose by fingersticks 1 hour after infusion. Since pentamidine is nephrotoxic, the client's blood urea nitrogen (BUN) and creatinine should be monitored. Diluted solution is infused over a period of 60 minutes.

9. Clients may develop sudden, severe hypotension after a single dose of pentamidine isethionate, whether given IM or IV. Clients should receive the medications while lying down and blood pressure should be monitored closely during and after the period of administration.

10. Clients who have had PCP must be maintained on lifelong therapy regardless of the amount of immune reconstitution that occurs. It is safe to discontinue therapy in clients who are receiving *P. carinii* primary prophylaxis (i.e., never having had PCP infection) after having a sustained CD_4 cell count greater than 200 cells/mm^3 and a sustained reduction in viral load for at least 3 to 6 months.[5]

11. Bactrim therapy for *P. carinii* prophylaxis simultaneously provides prophylaxis against *T. gondii,* since Bactrim can also be used to prevent infection with *T. gondii.*

12. For medical regimens see Table 16-5 and Box 16-3.

Table 16-5	**Medical Regimens**

Pneumocystis Carinii Pneumonia	Regimens

Prophylaxis	Trimethroprim/sulfamethoxazole (Bactrim, Septra) double-strength (160/800 mg) PO qd
	For those intolerant to Bactrim:
	  Dapsone 100 mg PO qd
	  Or
	  Atovaquone (Mepron) 1500 mg PO qd
	  Or
	  Dapsone 200 mg PO weekly **plus** pyrimethamine 75 mg PO weekly **plus** folinic acid 25 mg PO weekly
	  Or (rarely)
	  Aerosolized pentamidine (Pentam) 300 mg in 6 ml of sterile water via aerosolization once monthly
	  Or
	  Pentamidine 4 mg/kg IM monthly
	  Or
	  Pentamidine 4 mg/kg IV monthly

Treatment	Trimethoprim/sulfamethoxazole 5 mg/kg/day (trimethoprim component) PO qid × 21 days
	(For the average adult this is the equivalent to 2 double-strength tablets daily.)
	  Or
	For clients unable to take oral medication:
	  Trimethoprim/sulfamethoxazole 5 mg/kg/day (trimethoprim component) IV q8h × 21 days
	  Or
	  Dapsone 100 mg PO qd **plus** trimethoprim 5 mg/kg PO tid × 21 days
	  Or
	  Clindamycin 600 mg (900 mg if very ill) IV **or** 300-450 mg PO q8h **plus** primaquine 15 mg PO qd × 21 days
	  Or
	  Atovaquone suspension 750 mg PO tid × 21 days
	  Or
	  Pentamidine isethionate 4 mg/kg IV qd × 21

Maintenance	Same as prophylaxis.

BOX 16-3 PEDIATRIC CONSIDERATIONS
Pneumocystis carinii *pneumonia*

Initiating PCP Prophylaxis in an HIV-Exposed Infant

PCP prophylaxis should be initiated at 4-6 weeks of life in all infants born to HIV-positive mothers, regardless of their CD_4 cell counts. PCP prophylaxis is not administered under 4 weeks of age because the risk of PCP is low and because the use of sulfa drugs in infants under 4 weeks of age is not advised because of the potential for adverse drug effects resulting from immature bilirubin metabolism. PCP prophylaxis can be discontinued once infection has been excluded.

Initiating PCP Prophylaxis in an HIV-Infected Infant or Child

All infants with confirmed HIV infection must receive PCP prophylaxis regardless of CD_4 cell count and T-lymphocyte count until 12 months of age. HIV-infected children aged 1-5 years must receive PCP prophylaxis if CD_4 cell count <500 cells/mm³ or CD_4 percentage <15%. HIV-infected children aged 6-12 years must receive PCP prophylaxis if CD_4 cell count <200 cells/mm³ or CD_4 percentage <15%. Initiation or continuation of PCP prophylaxis should also be considered on a case by case basis in consultation with an HIV expert for HIV-infected children aged 12 months or older who might otherwise be at risk for PCP (e.g., children with severely symptomatic disease or rapidly declining CD_4 cell counts or percentages).

PCP Prophylaxis in Children

Any child with a history of PCP should receive lifelong PCP prophylaxis to prevent recurrence, regardless of CD_4 cell counts or clinical status.

PCP Prophylaxis Regimens for Children Aged 4 Weeks or Older

Recommended regimen:
Trimethoprim 150 mg/M²/day **plus** sulfamethoxazole 750 mg/M²/day PO in 2 divided doses 3 times per week on consecutive days (e.g., Monday, Tuesday, and Wednesday).
Alternative regimens, if trimethoprim/sulfamethoxazole is not tolerated*:
- Dapsone 2 mg/kg (not to exceed 100 mg) administered once daily
- Aerosolized pentamidine 300 mg administered via Respirgard II inhaler monthly (for children ≥5 years of age)

Treatment of PCP in Infants and Children

The preferred regimen is:
Trimethoprim/sulfamethoxazole 5 mg/kg/day (trimethoprim component) PO or IV q6h × 21 days

---

* If neither Dapsone nor aerosolized pentamidine is tolerated, some clinicians use intravenous pentamidine 4 mg/kg administered every 2 or 4 weeks. From Centers for Disease Control and Prevention: 1995 revised guidelines for prophylaxis against *Pneumocystis carinii* pneumonia for children with or perinatally exposed to human immunodeficiency virus infection, *MMWR* 44(RR-4):1, 1995; Centers for Disease Control and Prevention: Revised classification system for human immunodeficiency virus infection in children less than 13 years of age, *MMWR* 43(RR-12):1, 1994.

Toxoplasmosis

■ DEFINITION AND ETIOLOGY

T. gondii is a protozoan organism that has a worldwide distribution. Infection with *T. gondii* is more prevalent in Europe and tropical climates than in the United States. Cats, mammals, and birds can serve as hosts of the organism. The form of the protozoan varies between cats, mammals, and birds. All forms of the protozoan are considered infectious to humans. People become infected with *T. gondii* by ingesting contaminated, undercooked meat or vegetables, or through the inappropriate handling of contaminated cat feces. Cat feces contain oocysts that are broken down by digestive enzymes, which results in the release of *T. gondii* protozoan. Once infection occurs, the organisms spread throughout the body via the lymphatic system. In immunocompetent clients, the majority of the organisms are killed, though a small number of organisms survive immune system surveillance and develop cysts within the host's tissues. These tissue cysts can remain there for many years without causing any disease or tissue reaction. Immunodeficiency is the most common cause of reactivation of a latent infection. In HIV-positive clients, primary infection is rarely seen; more than 95% of cases of infection are caused by reactivation of a latent infection.

A fetus may also become infected in utero if the mother either acquires the protozoan during pregnancy or experiences reactivation of a latent infection.

■ CLINICAL OVERVIEW

Nurses must be aware that *T. gondii* can infect any tissue of the body and therefore can cause altered functioning in any system. The most common sites of involvement, however, are the brain, lung, and eyes. Primary infection with toxoplasmosis in immunocompetent clients often presents as cervical adenopathy and "flulike" symptoms, such as fever, myalgia, arthralgia, fatigue, headache, and sore throat. In immunodeficient clients, toxoplasmic encephalitis is the most common form of the disease and occurs when a client's CD_4 cell counts are less than 100 cells/mm^3. When disease is reactivated in cerebral tissue, clients often present with neurological complaints such as dull, constant headache, weakness in the extremities, and seizures. Other neurological signs that may be present are altered level of consciousness, hemiparesis, cerebellar tremor, visual field defects, and cranial nerve palsy.

Pulmonary infection with *T. gondii* results in a febrile illness with a nonproductive cough and dyspnea. Toxoplasmosis pneumonia has a clinical profile that mimics PCP. Therefore, in the presence of symptoms, both organisms must be suspected. After CMV infection, *T. gondii* infection is the most common cause of retinitis in clients with AIDS. Clients that report photophobia and loss of visual acuity should have *T. gondii* infection as one of their differential diagnoses.

■ DIAGNOSIS

About 10% to 40% of all adults in the United States have been infected with *T. gondii* and demonstrate serological evidence of past infection. At the time of HIV diagnosis, the client should be tested for antibodies to *T. gondii*, which indicate previous exposure to the organism. When severe immunosuppression occurs, clients are at high risk for reactivation of the organism, resulting in disease. As previously stated, the central nervous system is the system most affected by this protozoan (resulting in toxoplasmosis encephalitis). The most common indicators of a diagnosis of toxoplasmosis encephalitis are clinical symptoms and serological and radiological evidence of disease. Toxoplasmosis encephalitis must be detected early and treated to prevent significant mortality; if not treated, it is fatal.

Factors that favor a diagnosis of toxoplasmosis encephalitis are the presence of IgG *Toxoplasma* sp. antibodies and two or more focal cerebral lesions detected by computed tomography (CT) scan or magnetic resonance imaging (MRI). A single cerebral lesion favors the diagnosis of lymphoma. In the absence of a positive antibody test, the diagnosis of *T. gondii* is unlikely. Clients with positive antibodies at the time of HIV diagnosis should receive preventative therapy if their CD_4 cell counts fall to less than 100 cells/mm^3.

■ NURSING CONSIDERATIONS

1. At the time of HIV diagnosis, clients should have titers for *T. gondii* done. Clients who are seronegative for antibodies should be taught how to prevent primary infection. During the HIV work-up, the nurse takes a dietary history. Any client that reports a history of favoring raw or undercooked meats or fish is at risk for developing infection with *T. gondii*. Nurses should work with clients in modifying dietary habits to prevent infection if they are not already infected. Clients should be taught to avoid undercooked meats and to always order meats well done.

2. Because infection can be transmitted from undercooked meats, the client should be taught to wash hands and utensils immediately after touching raw meats. Fruits and vegetables should also be washed before being consumed.

3. Clients who are seronegative should have yearly tests for antibodies to *T. gondii* when their CD_4 cell counts fall below 100 cells/mm^3. Any client who seroconverts should begin prophylaxis therapy.

4. Cat ownership for clients who are seronegative does not increase risk for seroconversion. If the client owns a cat, the client should avoid contact with materials that are potentially contaminated with cat feces (e.g., litter boxes). Activities such as daily emptying of litter boxes (while wearing gloves or by someone other than the client) with prompt handwashing can protect the client from infection.[6] The client should avoid inhalation of cat feces. Dry feces can sporulate; inhaled

Table 16-6 Medical Regimens

Toxoplasmosis	Regimens
Prophylaxis	Trimethoprim/sulfamethoxazole (Bactrim, Septra) 1 DS tab PO OD *Or* Pyrimethamine 50 mg once per week **plus** dapsone 50 mg OD **plus** leucovorin 25 mg once per week
Treatment	Pyrimethamine 100-200 mg load then 50-100 mg PO OD **plus** sulfadiazine 1-1.5 g PO q6h **plus** leucovorin 10-20 mg OD × 6 weeks *Or* (for clients allergic to sulfa) Pyrimethamine 100-200 mg load then 50-75 mg PO OD **plus** clindamycin 600 mg PO q6h **plus** 10-20 mg leucovorin OD × 6 weeks **Alternative regimens** Pyrimethamine 100-200 mg load **then** 50-100 mg PO qd **plus** leu- covorin 10-20 mg qd × 6 weeks **plus** one of the following: Azithromycin 1200 mg-1500 mg OD *Or* Clarithromycin 1 g PO bid *Or* Atovaquone 750 mg PO qid (with food)
Maintenance	Pyrimethamine 25-50 mg PO OD **plus** sulfadiazide 1 g PO q12h **plus** leucovorin 10 mg OD

BOX 16-4 PEDIATRIC CONSIDERATIONS
Toxoplasmosis

Treatment

Pyrimethamine 2 mg/kg/day (not to exceed 50 mg) PO × 2-3 days, then mainte-
nance therapy with 1 mg/kg/day PO (in two divided doses)
Plus
Sulfadiazine 100 mg/kg PO bid (not to exceed 6 g/day)
Plus
Folinic acid (leucovorin) 5-10 mg PO three times weekly

Alternative Regimens

Clindamycin 20-40 mg/kg PO q8h **plus** Pyrimethamine 2 mg/kg/day PO (not to
 exceed 50 mg) × 2-3 days
Or
Clarithromycin 30 mg/kg/day PO (in two divided doses)

spores can cause infection. To reduce the cat's potential for exposure to the organism, the client should consider keeping the cat indoors. The client should be taught to refrain from feeding cats raw meats, which may be a potential source of exposure.

5. Clients that are antibody positive generally have low levels of circulating IgG antibodies (i.e., approximately 1:16 to 1:64). A fourfold increase in IgG antibodies or the appearance of IgM antibodies indicates active infection.[7]

6. Clients who are treated for *T. gondii* should show radiological evidence of diminution or disappearance of the lesions by 3 to 5 weeks of treatment.[8] If there is no change in the lesions, a diagnosis other than *T. gondii* must be considered. In such a case, brain biopsy may be indicated but often is not done.

7. Bactrim, used to treat *P. carinii,* can be used to prevent disease. See p. 292 for nursing considerations related to the administration of Bactrim.

8. Pyrimethamine, a drug used to treat toxoplasmosis encephalitis, has myelosuppressive effects. The client's CBC should be monitored during therapy.

9. For medical regimens see Table 16-6 and Box 16-4.

REFERENCES

1. Kolter DP et al: Small intestine and parasitic disease in AIDS, *Ann Intern Med* 113(6):444, 1990.
2. Gibson R: *Principles of nutritional measurement,* New York, 1990, Oxford University Press.
3. Hardy WD: Options for prophylaxis of *Pneumocystis carinii* pneumonia, *HIV: Adv Res Ther* 6(1), 1996.
4. El-Sadr W et al for the Terry Beirn Community Programs for Clinical Research on AIDS (CPCRA): A randomized trial of daily and thrice-weekly trimethoprim-sulfamethoxazole for the prevention of *Pneumocystis carinii* pneumonia in human immunodeficiency virus–infected persons, *Clin Infect Dis* 29:775, 1999.
5. Furrer H et al: Discontinuation of primary prophylaxis against *Pneumocystis carinii* pneumonia in HIV-1–infected adults treated with combination antiretroviral therapy, *N Engl J Med* 340(17):1301, 1999.
6. Wallace MR, Rossetti RJ, Olson PE: Cats and toxoplasmosis risk in HIV-infected adults, *JAMA* 269(1):76, 1993.
7. Bakerman S, Bakerman P, Strausbauch P: *ABC's of interpretive laboratory data,* ed 3, Myrtle Beach, South Carolina, 1994, Interpretive Laboratory Data.
8. Sande ME, Volberding PA: *Medical management of AIDS,* ed 6, Philadelphia, 1999, Saunders.

17

Viral Infections

- Cytomegalovirus
- Herpes Simplex and Zoster
- Oral Hairy Leukoplakia
- Progressive Multifocal Leukoencephalopathy

Kenneth Zwolski

Cytomegalovirus

■ DEFINITION AND ETIOLOGY

Cytomegalovirus (CMV) is a herpes virus that circulates widely in the human population. It is a linear double-stranded DNA virus that can encode over 200 different proteins. CMV can be found in semen, cervical secretions, saliva, urine, blood, and organs. Transmission from an infected to a noninfected person can occur in several ways: perinatally (intrauterine transmission, during vaginal delivery through an infected cervix or as a result of breastfeeding), from child to child or child to adult (especially in crowded conditions; transmission from adult to adult in this way is rare), through sexual contact, through blood, and through transplantation of infected organs or tissues.

In undeveloped countries, the seroprevalence of CMV can approach 100%. In the United States, seroprevalence is greater than 90% in lower socioeconomic groups and 50% in higher socioeconomic groups. Among men who have sex with men and intravenous drug users (IVDU), seroprevalence approaches 100%. In an immunocompetent host, infection with CMV rarely results in any clinical manifestations. However, in clients with AIDS, infection with CMV can be a major cause of morbidity and mortality. The most common complications of infection with CMV in a person with AIDS include: chorioretinitis, radiculopathy, subacute encephalitis, colitis, esophagitis, and pneumonia.

■ CLINICAL OVERVIEW

CMV chorioretinitis (CMV retinitis) accounts for 90% of all infectious retinopathies in HIV clients. It occurs mostly in clients with severe immunodeficiency (i.e., a CD_4 count of less than 50 cells/mm^3). As a result of routine prophylaxis against PCP, CMV retinitis is often a presenting AIDS diagnosis. The symptoms of CMV retinitis include: decreased visual acuity, presence of floaters, unilateral visual field loss, which can progress to bilateral visual field loss, and other visceral organ involvement. Often, unilateral visual field loss is the presenting symptom. If left untreated,

CMV retinitis is progressive and can result in blindness. Even in those treated, visual field defects present at the beginning of therapy do not reverse. However, decreased visual acuity caused by edema of the macula may improve.

The most common neurological complication of infection with CMV is radiculopathy. This presents as a spinal cord syndrome. The client is likely to complain of lower extremity weakness. Spasticity, areflexia, and urinary retention may also be present. CMV may also cause subacute encephalitis, presenting as personality changes, difficulty in concentrating, headaches, or somnolence.

CMV may produce either colitis or esophagitis. The symptoms of colitis include diarrhea, weight loss, anorexia, and fever. Since many other pathogens can cause colitis in clients with HIV/AIDS, it is necessary to differentiate between infection with cryptosporidia, *Giardia* spp., *Entamoeba* spp., mycobacteria, *Shigella* spp., *Campylobacter* spp., and *Strongyloides stercoralis.* Involvement of the large intestine in lymphoma or Kaposi's sarcoma must also be ruled out. Most cases of esophagitis in clients with HIV/AIDS are due to infection with *Candida albicans.* However, CMV infection may also cause esophagitis. The main symptom of esophagitis is painful swallowing.

Pneumonia may develop as a result of infection with CMV, especially in those clients who have a concomitant infection with another pathogen; for example, infection with *Pneumocystis carinii.* Symptoms include: gradually worsening shortness of breath, dyspnea on exertion, dry nonproductive cough, and increased respiratory and cardiac rates. Auscultation reveals minimal findings and little evidence of consolidation.

▪ Diagnosis

It is important to keep in mind that there is a difference between infection with CMV and CMV-caused disease. Those infected with CMV will have a positive serological test for CMV, and CMV can often be shed in urine, semen, or saliva in the absence of disease. If CMV is suspected of causing a client's disease, more specific measures are necessary to confirm the diagnosis. Table 17-1 summarizes the diagnostic findings typical in the most common CMV diseases.

The characteristic funduscopic lesions associated with CMV retinitis need to be distinguished from cotton wool spots. Cotton wool spots appear as small, fluffy, white lesions with indistinct margins. They are not associated with exudates or hemorrhages and are common in asymptomatic AIDS clients. They represent focal areas of ischemia. They do not progress and many times will spontaneously regress.

▪ Medical Management

The medical management of CMV includes prevention, treatment (once disease has manifested) and prevention of recurrence (through the use of maintenance therapy). Three drugs are available for use: ganciclovir

Table 17-1	Common CMV Diseases

CMV Disease	Diagnostic Findings
Chorioretinitis	Funduscopic examination reveals large, creamy to yellowish-white granular areas with perivascular exudates and hemorrhages (described as cottage cheese and catsup). Initially found at periphery of fundus, but if not treated will progress within 2-3 weeks.
Radiculopathy	Culture results of cerebrospinal fluid may be negative, but antigen to DNA assays are usually positive.
Subacute encephalopathy	Can only be confirmed by brain biopsy.
Colitis	Endoscopic examination reveals ulceration and diffuse submucosal hemorrhages. Biopsy reveals vasculitis, neutrophilic inflammation, characteristic CMV inclusion bodies, CMV antigen, CMV DNA, or absence of other pathogens.
Esophagitis	Endoscopic examination reveals large, yellow-white plaques throughout the esophagus, and biopsy shows tissue-invasive pseudomycelia.
Pneumonia	X-ray studies show diffuse infiltrates, similar to those with PCP. Histologic findings confirm the presence of CMV in lung tissue. No other pathogens are identified with bronchoscopy.

(Cytovene), foscarnet (Foscavir), and cidofovir (Vistide). Recommended drug dosages for medical management are outlined in Table 17-2. If CMV occurs, prompt initiation of therapy is indicated.

Ganciclovir has both oral and parenteral formulations. Intravenous ganciclovir is used for initial therapy. The oral form can be used for maintenance and prevention. Ganciclovir is excreted through the kidneys, hence the dosage needs to be adjusted for clients with renal impairment (this is true for both IV and oral administrations). The toxicity of ganciclovir can limit its therapeutic benefit. Ganciclovir can affect hematopoiesis. Leukopenia, thrombocytopenia, and anemia can occur in response to ganciclovir therapy, especially when using IV formulations; incidence is lower when using oral formulations. Neutropenia is usually reversible with the administration of granulocyte colony-stimulating factor (G-CSF). If the absolute neutrophil count (ANC) is less than 500 cells/mm^3 a ganciclovir dose interruption is recommended until there is evidence of marrow recovery. Ganciclovir can also cause gastrointestinal (GI) side effects, such as diarrhea, nausea, vomiting, and anorexia. Neuropathy and paresthesia are also possible.

Foscarnet is available only as an IV medication. It is often used to treat ganciclovir-resistant CMV retinitis. The side effects of foscarnet in-

Table 17-2	Medical Regimens

Cytomegalovirus	Regimens
Prophylaxis **Treatment**	Ganciclovir 1 g PO tid with meals
	Ganciclovir 5 mg/kg IV q12h × 14-21 days
	Or
	Foscarnet 60 mg/kg IV q8h × 14-21 days
	Or
	Foscarnet 90 mg/kg IV q12h × 14-21 days
	Or
	Cidofovir 5 mg/kg IV every week × 2 **then** 5 mg/kg every 2 weeks **plus** Probenecid 2 g PO 3 hours before each dose, 1 g PO 2 and 8 hours after each dose
	Or
	Intraocular ganciclovir release device every 6 months **plus** Ganciclovir 1 g PO tid with meals
Maintenance	Ganciclovir 5 mg/kg/day IV 5-7 days per week
	Or
	Foscarnet 90-120 mg/kg IV daily
	Or
	Ganciclovir 1 g PO tid with meals

clude renal impairment, anemia, hypocalcemia, hypomagnesemia, and hypophosphatemia. Any client receiving foscarnet needs to have renal function assessed frequently, and the dosage of foscarnet needs to be adjusted accordingly. A daily infusion of 1 liter of saline before drug administration may reduce nephrotoxicity.

The newest drug available for CMV therapy is cidofovir (Vistide). It is used in the treatment of CMV retinitis and can only be given by IV infusion. The biggest advantage of cidofovir is that it only has to be administered once a week for the first 2 weeks of therapy and then once every other week for maintenance. However, it can be very toxic to the kidneys. Hence renal function needs to be assessed carefully and continuously—blood and urine tests of renal function should be monitored frequently, and the client should be observed for early warning signs of renal problems, such as decreased urination, increased thirst, and lightheadedness. It is recommended that cidofovir be given with probenecid and plenty of fluids to reduce its nephrotoxicity. Since probenecid contains sulfa, it should be used with caution in clients with sulfa allergies.

Treatment of CMV retinitis may include the use of an intravitreal injection of ganciclovir. This is done by the surgical placement of an implant into the eye. Implants typically last from 6 to 9 months and then need to be replaced. The advantage of the implant is that it eliminates the need for intravenous or oral administration of ganciclovir. Some disadvantages are possible trauma to the eye secondary to the implant procedure and the lack of systemic protection against CMV disease.

Whether or not to treat someone prophylactically for the prevention of CMV disease is an important issue in the care of HIV/AIDS clients. The side effects of treatment with ganciclovir, conflicting studies regarding the efficacy of the practice, and the cost of therapy are all factors that need to be considered. The U.S. Public Health Services (USPHS) have recommended that for some clients in unusual circumstances (e.g., clients who have CD_4 cell counts less than 50 cells/mm^3 and are CMV positive), prophylaxis should be initiated.

■ NURSING CONSIDERATIONS

1. The majority of clients with HIV/AIDS are likely to be already infected with CMV. A simple blood test, however, can determine seropositivity or negativity. Clients who are seronegative should be counseled as to how best to avoid infection. Any HIV-positive adults who are care providers for children or parents of children in childcare facilities should be made aware of their increased risk of acquiring CMV. This risk can be decreased by good hygienic measures, including handwashing.

2. If a client who is seronegative for CMV needs a blood transfusion, CMV-negative or leukocyte-reduced cellular blood should be requested.

3. Prophylaxis for CMV may be considered for some clients who are CMV positive. Acyclovir is not effective in preventing CMV-related disease. The most important method of preventing complications of CMV retinitis is to teach clients early warning signs. These include the presence of "floaters" in the eye or decreased visual acuity as might be noticed through such simple techniques as reading the fine print in newspapers. Regular funduscopic examinations should be encouraged. Anyone with a CD_4 cell count less than 100 cells/mm^3 should have a dilated ophthalmological examination and those with less than 50 cells/mm^3 should have such examinations routinely.

4. CMV disease cannot be cured. Once a client has experienced an episode of CMV disease, he or she will need to be maintained on a regimen of either parenteral or oral ganciclovir, parenteral foscarnet, combined parenteral ganciclovir and foscarnet, parenteral Cidofovir, or (for retinitis only) ganciclovir intraocular implant. Any client with an implant needs to be made aware of the fact that the implant does not provide protection to the contralateral eye or to other organ systems. Also, clients receiving maintenance therapy for CMV retinitis may experience a recurrence and need the reinstitution of high-dose induction therapy or the replacement of the implant.

5. Clients should be aware of the toxicity and side effects of the anti-CMV medications and should be assessed, screened, taught, and treated appropriately. Because of the nephrotoxicity associated with

BOX 17-1 PEDIATRIC CONSIDERATIONS
Cytomegalovirus

Prophylaxis against CMV infection is indicated for children with CMV antibody positivity and CD_4 cell counts less than 50 cells/mm³. Ganciclovir 30 mg/kg PO tid is currently recommended.

Treatment

Ganciclovir 10 mg/kg IV daily in two divided doses × 14-21 days
Or
Foscarnet: 180 mg/kg IV daily in three divided doses × 14-21 days

Maintenance

Ganciclovir 5 mg/kg/day IV 5 days/week
Or
Intraocular ganciclovir release device every 6 months **plus** ganciclovir 30 mg/kg PO tid
Or
Foscarnet 90-120 mg/kg IV daily

foscarnet and Cidofovir, it is important to determine if other drugs with nephrotoxic potential are being used, such as amphotericin B, aminoglycoside antibiotics, nonsteroidal antiinflammatory drugs, or IV pentamidine.

6. Induction doses of IV drugs should be administered in the clinical setting to allow for the observation of any potential reactions and provide an opportunity to teach clients about possible side effects. Follow-up home care needs to be provided. It is recommended that blood work should be done twice weekly during induction and then once weekly for maintenance therapy.

7. Because of the decreased visual acuity and threat of blindness that face a client with CMV retinitis, the nurse needs to recognize the physical and psychological stresses inherent in the situation. Referral to organizations for the visually impaired may be warranted. Such organizations can provide assistance to clients in dealing with disability.

8. For medical regimens see Table 17-2 and Box 17-1.

Herpes Simplex and Herpes Zoster

■ DEFINITION AND ETIOLOGY

Both herpes simplex and herpes zoster are members of the herpes virus group. In general, infection with either of these viruses follows a similar pattern: primary outbreak, latency, and then possible reactivation at some later point in the host's life. There are two herpes simplex viruses: herpes simplex, type 1 (HSV-1) and herpes simplex, type 2 (HSV-2).

Initial infection with HSV-1 most often occurs in childhood as a result of contact with infected droplets from orolabial or nasal secretions. Usually initial infection is subclinical. The risk of infection with HSV-1 increases with crowded living conditions. Infection with HSV-2 is acquired as a result of sexual activity. Although initial infection with HSV-2 can be asymptomatic, it often produces a clinically noticeable syndrome characterized by the presence of fluid-filled vesicles and, occasionally, systemic symptoms such as fever, headache, and malaise. The risk for acquiring HSV-2 begins at puberty and increases with the number of different sexual partners.

HSV can infect the mouth and lips (orolabia), the genitals, and anorectal area. It remains latent in the sacral ganglia. Serologic studies show that over 70% of HIV-positive clients have been previously infected with HSV, either HSV-1 or HSV-2 or both types. When this virus is reactivated in these clients, it can cause significant disease and extensive tissue destruction.

Herpes zoster or the varicella zoster virus (VZV) infects over 90% of all children. This initial infection with VZV is commonly called "chicken pox." In immunocompetent children, this primary infection is generally benign, but if a person with AIDS gets a primary infection with VZV, it can be life threatening. Transmission of VZV occurs as a result of cutaneous exposure to the serum contained within vesicles of an infected person, or as a result of inhalation of aerosolized droplets. After primary infection, VZV remains latent primarily in the dorsal root ganglion, though on occasion it can remain latent in the trigeminal nerve.

Because over 90% of all children become infected with VZV, nearly all adult clients with AIDS carry the virus—the reactivation of which is a major problem. In immunosuppressed clients, reactivation of VZV can cause pneumonia, encephalitis, and, most frequently, painful mucocutaneous outbreaks (often referred to as "shingles").

■ CLINICAL OVERVIEW

Herpes Simplex

Most clients with HIV have already been infected with HSV, and therefore the major concern is recurrence of infection. Primary infections are not uncommon, however. The severity of the illness depends upon the anatomic site of the initial infection and the degree of immunosuppression; HSV can involve orolabial, genital, anorectal, esophageal, brain, and retinal tissue.

Primary infection of orolabial tissue in clients with immunosuppression is much more severe than in healthy HIV-positive clients. For immunocompetent clients, primary orolabial infection is typically asymptomatic. In immunosuppressed clients, primary infection is usually characterized by painful vesicular eruptions along the lip, tongue, pharynx, or buccal mucosa. These vesicles rapidly coalesce, forming large ulcers covered with a whitish/yellowish necrotic film. Ulcers may be accompanied by fever, pharyngitis, and cervical lymphadenopathy. In infants, poor feeding and drooling is often apparent.

Recurrences of orolabial infections in clients with HIV tend to increase in severity and frequency with increasing immunosuppression. Prodromal symptoms begin about 12 to 24 hours before the appearance of fluid-filled vesicles (commonly referred to as "fever blisters"). Prodromal symptoms include tingling or numbness at the site of impending recurrence. Compared with HIV-negative clients, there is delayed healing of lesions. If left untreated, the lesions ulcerate. There is persistent viral shedding and prolonged contagiousness.

In primary genital herpes there is normally a 2- to 12-day incubation period after which symptoms appear. Small papules arise, which rapidly evolve into fluid-filled vesicles that are painful and tender to touch. These vesicles ulcerate rapidly and heal in 3 to 4 weeks by crusting. Inguinal adenopathy is common and dysuria may be present. Once in a while systemic symptoms, such as fever, headache, myalgias, malaise, and meningismus (i.e., vomiting, constipation, and fever) may be present.

Recurrent genital herpes in HIV-negative clients is less severe than primary genital herpes. It results in fewer lesions, a shorter duration of illness, and, generally, no systemic symptoms. In clients with HIV/AIDS, the severity and duration of recurrent genital herpes are greater. There is prolonged lesion formation with persistent shedding and often severe localized pain. Symptoms can last for several weeks, and there is a prolonged period of asymptomatic shedding of the virus.

Anorectal infection with HSV is a special problem for HIV-positive men who have sex with men. HSV is the most common cause of nongonococcal proctitis in sexually active men who have sex with men. It is usually the result of infection with HSV-2, but it may be from HSV-1 as well. The symptoms include severe anorectal pain, perianal ulcerations, constipation, tenesmus (i.e., straining in attempt to produce stool; usually ineffectual), and neurological symptoms related to infection of the sacral plexus. These neurological symptoms are sacral radiculopathy, impotence, and neurogenesis of the bladder. Physical examination may reveal shallow ulcers, which often coalesce and extend along the gluteal crease to involve the overlying sacrum.

Should infection with HSV involve the esophagus, the presentation is often one of acute onset odynophagia and dysphagia. This may be accompanied by retrosternal pain, nausea, and vomiting. It can easily be confused with *C. albicans* or CMV esophagitis. HSV encephalitis occurs rarely, but when it does it can be life threatening. Both HSV-1 and HSV-2 have been identified in brain tissue. Encephalitis is usually a result of primary or reactivated orolabial HSV infection. The presentation is highly atypical—a subacute illness with subtle neurological abnormalities. Headache, meningismus, and personality changes may develop gradually. In a few instances, the presentation may consist of an abrupt onset of fever, headache, nausea, confusion, and focal seizures. HSV can cause a rapidly progressing retinitis (i.e., acute retinal necrosis syndrome). Complete visual loss in the affected eye is the usual outcome.

Herpes Zoster

Recurrent herpes zoster is common in clients with AIDS. It usually begins with radicular pain and is followed by localized or segmental erythematous rash of maculopapules, covering one to three dermatomes. The maculopapules become fluid-filled vesicles that are contagious. The vesicles can enlarge to form bullae. Mostly the lesions remain confined in a dermatomal distribution and heal by crusting. Sometimes dissemination may occur to skin and visceral organs. If dissemination is to the skin, it may appear identical to primary VZV. If dissemination is to the viscera, it can involve the lungs, liver, or central nervous system (CNS) and can be life threatening. Dissemination to these organs is associated with a mortality of 6% to 17%.

Varicella pneumonia (due to dissemination to the lungs) may occur during primary or recurrent infection. The symptoms are variable, ranging from mild respiratory symptoms to severe hypoxemia and death. Dissemination to brain tissue is rare, but can occur, causing encephalitis. This begins typically with headache, vomiting, lethargy, and cerebellar symptoms (e.g., ataxia, tremor, dizziness). Other complications can include postherpetic neuralgia and acute retinal necrosis syndrome (similar to that caused by infection of the retina with HSV). In postherpetic neuralgia, there is a prolonged and disabling pain that develops and persists after resolution of the cutaneous lesions of zoster.

■ DIAGNOSIS

Herpes Simplex

Culture, Tzanck preparation, or endoscopy, when indicated, makes the diagnosis of HSV. In the presence of genital ulceration, the differential diagnoses are syphilis, chancroid, scabies, mucocutaneous candidiasis, or venereal warts. For suspected anorectal infection with HSV, a sigmoidoscopic examination may be done. An indicative examination would show a friable mucosa with diffuse ulcerations and occasional intact vesicular or pustular lesions.

For suspected esophagitis secondary to infection with HSV, the definitive diagnosis requires endoscopic visualization with positive viral studies. The diagnosis of HSV-induced encephalitis is difficult to make, since it resembles many other CNS infections. Viral cerebrospinal fluid cultures are usually negative, although it may be possible to demonstrate the presence of HSV DNA in cerebrospinal fluid. The definitive diagnosis requires brain biopsy and the recovery of the virus or demonstration of the presence of viral antigen in tissue specimens.

Herpes Zoster

The diagnosis of infection with herpes zoster is done through culture, Tzanck smear, or immunofluorescent assay (IFA). In suspected cases of VZV-induced encephalitis, VZV antibody can be found in cerebrospinal fluid (CSF).

■ MEDICAL MANAGEMENT

Herpes Simplex

Any client presenting with perianal ulcerations or anal fissures should be examined for the presence of HSV. Generally, HSV infection is treated with either acyclovir or foscarnet. Two newer drugs, famciclovir and valacyclovir have recently been approved for use in the treatment of recurrent HSV infection. The treatment of choice is usually acyclovir. IV acyclovir is reserved mostly for clients with severe or extensive mucocutaneous ulcerations or who have viral dissemination to visceral organs or neurological involvement.

Clients who either suffer from frequently recurring HSV infections or develop a new HSV infection shortly after treatment is discontinued can be treated for each separate episode or they can be given maintenance (suppressive) therapy with acyclovir. If a new outbreak occurs while the client is receiving maintenance therapy, the dosage is increased. However, two problems have to be addressed. First, the dosage tolerated by any one client may be limited by side effects, especially those that are gastrointestinal. Second, the new outbreak may represent the development of acyclovir-resistant organisms. Acyclovir resistance is an increasing problem. It is estimated that incidence is about 4% to 5%. In cases of acyclovir resistance, management requires switching to foscarnet or initiating a continuous infusion of acyclovir for up to 6 weeks. Clients who demonstrate a good response to suppressive therapy may have their daily dosages decreased.

Herpes Zoster

The treatment is similar to that of HSV infection. Acyclovir and foscarnet are the two preferred antivirals. Generally speaking, larger doses of these drugs are needed than in the management of HSV infection. Valacyclovir may be used. Also, as in the case of HSV infection, acyclovir-resistant strains of VZV can occur. In these cases, foscarnet is useful.

In those few clients with HIV who have not had a primary infection with VZV as children, varicella zoster immune globulin can be effective in preventing primary disease should they become exposed to VZV. The globulin, however, has to be administered within 96 hours of exposure.

■ NURSING MANAGEMENT

1. The nurse should educate the client regarding the care of mucocutaneous lesions common in both HSV and VZV infection. Clients should be instructed to:
   - Maintain good hygiene without drying out the skin.
   - Avoid deodorant astringent soaps.
   - Use tepid water when cleansing and pat skin dry without rubbing.

Table 17-3	Medical Regimens

Herpes Simplex	Regimens

Prophylaxis	For clients with previous infection or HSV antibodies:
	    Acyclovir 400 mg PO bid **or** 800 mg OD
	    Or
	    Famciclovir 500 mg PO bid
	    Or
	    Valacyclovir 500 mg PO bid

Treatment	For mild cases:
	    Acyclovir 400 mg PO tid × at least 10 days or until lesions crust
	    Or
	    Famciclovir 250 mg PO tid × 5-10 days
	    Or
	    Valacyclovir 1 g PO bid × 5-10 days
	For severe or refractory cases:
	    Acyclovir 5 mg/kg IV q8h **or** 800 mg PO five times daily × at least 7 days
	    Or
	    Foscarnet 40 mg/kg IV q8h **or** 60 mg/kg q12h × 3 weeks
	For visceral infection:
	    Acyclovir 30 mg/kg IV daily × at least 10 days
	    Or
	    Foscarnet 40 mg/kg IV q8h × at least 10 days

Maintenance	Acyclovir 400 mg PO bid **or** 200 mg PO tid
	    Or
	    Famciclovir 250 mg PO bid
	    Or
	    Valacyclovir 500 mg PO OD

- Apply moisturizing cream after bathing and at bedtime.
- Maintain environmental humidification.
- Avoid scratching.
- Use a separate cloth for cleansing affected areas in order to avoid autoinoculation and dissemination.

2. Some wounds need special care. A saline wet-to-dry dressing compress can be applied to debride necrotic tissue and should be followed with antibiotic ointment. Clients with HIV should avoid contact with any open lesions, which can occur readily during sexual relations.

3. Clients who have never had chicken pox should avoid exposure. If exposure occurs, they can be given varicella zoster immune globulin if less than 96 hours have elapsed since the exposure.

4. The management of postherpetic neuralgia in clients with VZV infection can be a challenge. Touching may exacerbate the pain, but some-

Table 17-4	Medical Regimens	

Herpes Zoster	Regimens
Prophylaxis	None indicated.
Treatment	Acyclovir 800 mg PO five times daily × 7 days
	Or
	Famciclovir 500 mg PO tid*
	Or
	Valacyclovir 1 gm PO tid*
	For severe dermatomal infection (>1 dermatone, trigeminal nerve, or disseminated):
	Acyclovir 10-20 mg/kg IV q8h × 7-14 days (until lesions crust)
	Or
	Foscarnet 40 mg/kg IV q8h **or** 60 mg/kg IV q12h × 14-26 days
	For visceral infection:
	Acyclovir 30-36 mg/kg IV daily × at least 7 days
	Or
	Foscarnet 40 mg/kg IV q8h **or** 60 mg/kg q12h
	Or
	Famciclovir 250 mg PO bid*
	Or
	Valacyclovir 500 mg PO OD*
Maintenance	Acyclovir 800 mg PO five times daily

*Not FDA-approved; use in immunocompromised host.

times vigorous stimulation of the affected area may actually reduce the pain. This can be achieved through brisk rubbing with a terrycloth towel. Pharmacological treatment for postherpetic neuralgia can include treatment with topical lidocaine, capsaicin ointment, tricyclic antidepressants, and neuroleptics. Often a combination of physical therapy, psychological support, and pharmacological treatment is required.

5. Acyclovir can cause bone marrow suppression, renal and hepatic damage, and seizures. The nurse needs to be aware of these side effects and monitor the client appropriately.

6. The nurse also needs to be aware that there is risk of nosocomial transmission of HSV-1 and HSV-2 from infected clients to health care workers, so barrier precautions should be used when examining oral, genital, or anal lesions and when performing any procedure that may involve exposure to body fluids; for example, mouth care, oropharyngeal suctioning, and vaginal care.

7. For medical regimens for HSV see Table 17-3. For medical regimens for VZV see Table 17-4 and Box 17-2.

BOX 17-2   PEDIATRIC CONSIDERATIONS
Herpes Zoster

Treatment
Acyclovir 15-30 mg/kg IV daily (in three divided doses)
Or
Acyclovir 1000 mg PO qd (in five divided doses)

Maintenance
Recommended if subsequent episodes are frequent or severe:
 Acyclovir 80 mg/kg IV qd (in three divided doses)

Oral Hairy Leukoplakia

■ DEFINITION AND ETIOLOGY

Oral hairy leukoplakia (OHL) is a white thickening of the oral mucosa, often with vertical folds or corrugations. It can appear on the buccal mucosa, soft palate, floor of the mouth, or tongue. The most common presentation, though, is on the lateral surface of the tongue. The lesions can be as small as a few millimeters, but if the tongue is involved, lesions can cover the entire dorsal surface.

Infection with the Epstein-Barr virus (EBV) or HPV can cause OHL. There is an increased incidence in smokers. OHL is a category B condition (category B conditions are described in Chapter 1), often appearing when the CD_4 cell count is between 200 and 500 cells/mm^3.

■ CLINICAL OVERVIEW

OHL rarely occurs in clients who are not immunosuppressed. Before the use of highly active antiretroviral therapy (HAART), its appearance suggested the progression of HIV disease. Clients are usually asymptomatic and not treated unless there is accompanying oral pain, altered voice, difficulty in chewing, or reduced or altered taste. Occasionally there may be spontaneous regression of the lesion.

■ DIAGNOSIS

The appearance of OHL may mimic pseudomembranous candidiasis, smoker's leukoplakia, epithelial dysplasia, oral cancer, white sponge nevus, or plaque from lichen planus. Diagnosis is made from clinical appearance and biopsy. A biopsy of suspected tissue will reveal epithelial hyperplasia with a thickened parakeratin layer showing surface irregularities. These irregularities are projections or hairs and vacuolated prickle cells (hence the origin of the term "hairy" in reference to this condition). There is no inflammation, and EBV can be iden-

Table 17-5	Medical Regimens

Oral Hairy Leukoplakia	Regimens
Prophylaxis	No known therapy.
Treatment	If lesions are symptomatic: Acyclovir 800 mg PO five times daily × 2-3 weeks. (Most times when acyclovir is discontinued, the lesions reappear; therefore, acyclovir maintenance therapy can be considered. Ganciclovir can also be used.) A one-time topical application of podophyllin resin may be used occasionally, though the FDA has not yet approved the use of podophyllin for this purpose.
Maintenance	No known therapy.

tified in the vacuolated prickle cells and in superficial epithelium. OHL is readily identifiable by a skilled clinician, making biopsy unnecessary.

■ MEDICAL MANAGEMENT

The lesions of OHL rarely cause any symptoms. In most cases treatment is not indicated. If symptoms accompany the lesions, then high doses of the drug acyclovir can reduce or eliminate the lesions. If acyclovir is subsequently discontinued, the lesions reappear.

■ NURSING IMPLICATIONS

1. If the mouth is painful, drinking from a straw may be helpful. The client can be instructed to use ice cream or popsicles to numb the lesion and provide some nutrition. The client may be instructed in the preparation of blenderized foods.
2. If the mouth is painful, the client should be taught to avoid hot and spicy foods that are poorly tolerated. Alcohol may exacerbate mouth pain, particularly if lesions are present.
3. For medical regimens see Table 17-5.

Progressive Multifocal Leukoencephalopathy

■ DEFINITION AND ETIOLOGY

Progressive multifocal leukoencephalopathy (PML) is an opportunistic infection caused by the Jamestown Canyon virus (JCV). JCV is a slow growing, neurotropic human papovavirus that has worldwide incidence. The majority of the population shows serologic evidence of exposure to this virus by teenage years.

Activated infection with JCV in clients with AIDS usually results in the selective destruction of white brain matter, resulting in the presence of multiple lesions. PML develops in approximately 2% to 4% of clients with AIDS. Frequently, active infection is the result of reactivation of the virus in severely immunosuppressed individuals. Typically, the onset of PML occurs when the CD_4 cell count is less than 200 cells/mm³. PML is recognized as an AIDS-indicator condition.

■ CLINICAL OVERVIEW

PML causes focal brain disorders involving the cerebral hemispheres. These focal symptoms have a subacute onset and evolve, in a steady but gradual progression, over a period of days, weeks, and months. Clients experience a progressive decline until death, which typically occurs 4 to 6 months after the onset of symptoms.

The focal signs, due to demyelination of cortical matter, can include homonymous visual field disturbances, hemiparesis, hemisensory disturbance, aphasia, apraxia, dysarthria, dystonia, diplopia, and other cortical dysfunctions depending on the location of the lesion. Basically, the client presents with weakness and progressively impaired speech, vision, and motor function. Level of alertness is preserved. There is no fever and no headaches. Changes in cognition, leading to dementia, can occur, but this would be a relatively late development. Spontaneous remission has been documented.

■ DIAGNOSIS

Three opportunistic infections in clients with AIDS commonly cause focal brain disease. These are cerebral toxoplasmosis (see Chapter 16), primary CNS lymphoma (see Chapter 15), and PML. When a client presents with symptoms suggestive of focal brain disease, it is necessary to consider the differential diagnoses.

Table 17-6 presents some factors to consider in making the diagnosis of various focal brain disorders. It is possible to detect JCV DNA in CSF using polymerase chain reaction (PCR) techniques, but the presence of viral DNA alone is not sufficient (although it may be necessary) for making the diagnosis of clinical PML. This is because the presence of JCV DNA in CSF does not prove that the virus is in brain tissue. A definitive diagnosis of PML is made from brain biopsy or autopsy. However, a careful health history, physical examination, and neuroimaging studies are usually sufficient to make the diagnosis. An indicative health history would reveal a gradual onset of focal symptoms, as opposed to an abrupt onset. An indicative physical examination would reveal the presence of focal symptoms, and neuroimaging studies (i.e., magnetic resonance imaging [MRI], computed tomography [CT]) would reveal single or multiple confluent, hypodense, nonenhancing lesions predominantly in the parietal-occipital white matter without a mass effect. In many cases, findings from the MRI are very characteristic and diagnostic.

Table 17-6	Differential Diagnosis of Focal Brain Disorders			
Disorder	**Relative Progression of Focal Symptoms from Onset**	**Level of Alertness**	**Fever**	**Lesions**
Cerebral toxoplasmosis	Most rapid	Reduced; related to generalized encephalopathy, which has a combination of both focal and generalized symptoms	Common	Multiple lesions in basal ganglia and cortex
Primary central nervous system (CNS) lymphoma	Intermediate	Variable	Absent	Few lesions, periventricular with subendymal spread
Progressive multifocal leukoencephalopathy (PML)	Slowest	Preserved	Absent	Multiple lesions located in subcortical, white matter

■ MEDICAL MANAGEMENT

There is no proven, effective therapy for the treatment of PML. The use of IV or intrathecal cytosine arabinoside (Ara-C) or alpha interferon might be helpful in some clients. At present, the best strategy is to maximize the use of antiretrovirals.

■ NURSING IMPLICATIONS

1. Routine screening for detection of JCV is not done because nearly everyone has been infected at some time.
2. If a client is receiving Ara-C for treatment of PML, the nurse should be aware of side effects. Ara-C causes bone marrow suppression and decreases lymphocyte, platelet, and red blood cell counts. Other bone marrow–suppressive drugs, such as AZT and ganciclovir, should be stopped during the course of Ara-C administration to avoid additive bone marrow toxicity. Nausea, vomiting, diarrhea, abdominal pain, oral sores, and abnormal liver function may all develop in response to Ara-C treatment. A few people experience a syndrome called *cytara-*

bine syndrome, which is characterized by fever, bone pain, chest pain, rash, inflammation around the eyes, and malaise, all occurring within 6 to 12 hours after injection. The administration of corticosteroids may be helpful in preventing this. Sometimes severe and fatal allergic reactions may occur to Ara-C.

3. It is important to support and counsel clients with PML, as well as their significant others, since the disease causes major losses of function, mobility, and self-care capacity. It also results in a decreased ability to communicate effectively. The disease is usually fatal and death can occur fairly quickly after onset of symptoms. It is important to discuss expected outcomes and to help in arranging for home care, hospice care, or nursing home placement. The nurse will be called on to provide anticipatory grief counseling and to support the family.

4. There is no effective medical regimen for PML. There are no specific, preventive drug therapies. Maintaining low viral loads through antiretroviral therapy seems to be the best strategy for preventing occurrence.

BIBLIOGRAPHY

Bartlett J: *Medical management of HIV infection,* Baltimore, 1997, Port City Press.
Centers for Disease Control and Prevention: 1997 USPHS/IDSA guidelines for the prevention of opportunistic infections in persons infected with human immunodeficiency virus, *MMWR* 46(RR-12):1, 1997.
Libman H, Witzberg R: *HIV infection: a primary care manual,* ed 3, Boston, 1996, Little, Brown & Co.
Sande M, Volberding P: *The medical management of AIDS,* ed 6, Philadelphia, 1999, Saunders.

Unit V   Frequently Asked Questions

Can I get sick from having contact with a household pet?

Yes, household pets can transmit a wide variety of zoonotic organisms. A zoonosis is a disease of animals that may be secondarily transmitted to humans. If you have HIV/AIDS and are severely immunosuppressed, the risk of acquiring an illness from a pet is greatly increased. The Centers for Disease Control and Prevention (CDC) estimates that a quarter of the AIDS-defining conditions involve pathogens that also infect animals. Moreover, many of the organisms that infect animals may be responsible for symptoms in immunosuppressed individuals. For example, diarrhea in clients with AIDS may be of zoonotic origin. Agents that occur in animals and cause diarrhea in humans include: salmonella, *Campylobacter* spp., cryptosporidia, and *Giardia* spp. Salmonella leads the list of zoonotic infections in clients with AIDS. Although salmonella is frequently acquired by eating contaminated animals and animal products, it can also be acquired from simply having contact with cats and dogs carrying the organism. If your cat or dog is having frequent diarrhea, this is an important warning sign that they may be infected with salmonella. Turtles, lizards, and snakes can also be sources of salmonella.

Dogs and cats, especially puppies and kittens, frequently excrete *Campylobacter* spp. in their stool. The occurrence of *Campylobacter* spp. in kitten and puppy feces can be as high as 35% to 42%. Many animals can be a reservoir for cryptosporidia, including fishes, reptiles, mice, rats, guinea pigs, birds, dogs, and cats. *Giardia* spp. can infect the gastrointestinal tract of dogs, cats, and horses.

I have had my pets for a long time and don't want to get rid of them. What precautions can I take to decrease the risk of getting sick from my pets?

We know that companion animals significantly improve the quality of life for people with HIV/AIDS. If you own a pet or would like to own one, you should take a variety of precautions to decrease its risk of acquiring zoonoses:

- Choose healthy animals as pets. Select an adult animal in preference to a puppy or kitten and have the pet examined by a veterinarian.
- Have the pet neutered. This prevents roaming behavior in both sexes, which increases the risk of acquiring infections, and in females, it prevents pregnancy (which can lower immunity and hence increase the potential for shedding zoonoses).
- Make sure all pets have routine health care, including a yearly physical examination, vaccinations, and fecal examination for parasites.
- Keep pets indoors as much as possible. Again, this is to decrease roaming behavior. It also prevents their ingestion of feces and carcasses of other animals, which can infect them. Walk dogs on a leash.
- Pets should not be fed raw or uncooked meat, fish, or eggs.

■ Clients should wash their hands after handling pets and avoid contact with animal excreta.

Before I started receiving combination therapy I used to get fungus in my mouth all the time. Does the fact that I am on a combination antiretroviral therapy have anything to do with the fact that I don't have any more fungal infections?

Untreated HIV-positive clients usually experience at least one episode of fungal infection. In fact, a fungal infection is often the first HIV-related opportunistic infection that is seen. Mucosal candidiases, either oropharyngeal in men or women or vaginal in women, are often the first indication of an impaired immune response. The severity of fungal infections increases as the immune system becomes more impaired and they can progress from a local to a life-threatening disease.

However, with the advent of combination antiretroviral therapy, especially with the use of protease inhibitors (PIs), there has been a dramatic decline in the incidence of fungal infection. Furthermore, in those who are already infected with a fungal infection and who then begin treatment with a PI, the condition clears rapidly. Some researchers believe that there may actually be a direct link between PIs and their effect on *Candida* spp.

I used Panretin gel for my Kaposi's Sarcoma but the lesions did not go away. Do you think I did anything wrong?

There are two possible reasons why your lesions did not respond to Panretin gel (a topical antitumor gel). The first reason you did not see a response may be a result of the length of time that you used the medication. The earliest response that was seen in clients who used this drug was within 2 weeks. Only 1% of the clients who participated in investigations of this drug had a response in 2 weeks. Some participants required over 14 weeks to respond; therefore you may not have used the medication long enough to see a response. Secondly, you may not have had a response because in investigations of this drug only one participant had complete clearance of the lesions under study.[1] In fact, a response (defined as 50% improvement in the appearance of the lesions) was only seen in about 36% of the participants.[2] This means that not everyone that uses this medication will see an improvement or decrease in the number of lesions; and furthermore, it is rare that anyone has complete disappearance of their lesions.

Will I ever be able to stop taking the medicine to prevent
Mycobacterium avium **complex (MAC)?**

The answer to this question depends on whether you are taking MAC for prophylaxis (for primary prevention) or to prevent recurrence of disseminated MAC disease. If you are taking medication for primary prophylaxis, you were probably started on the medicine when your CD_4 cell count dropped to 50 cells/mm^3 to prevent MAC infection. If you are taking antiretrovirals and your CD$_4$ cell count goes back up to 100 cells/mm^3 or more and stays there for at least 3 to 6 months, and your viral load remains suppressed, it would be reasonable for your provider to consider stopping the medicine.

If you are taking medication to prevent recurrence of disseminated MAC disease, it is currently believed that, because you have had MAC in the past, you should continue to receive the full doses of your medication for the rest of your life to prevent getting the disease again. As more people are studied and more information is learned, this recommendation may change at some time in the future.

A friend of mine said that he got herpes and had sores on his privates. He said the doctor gave him a medication and the sores went away. Does this mean he is cured and can't give it to someone else during sex?

No, right now there is no cure for herpes. There are medications that can make the sores go away more quickly and make the person feel better but the virus is still present in the body. It can still cause sores and other symptoms again in the future. In people whose immune system is not working well, herpes is more likely to cause symptoms again, and symptoms can be severe. Your friend could still give herpes to a sexual partner and he should always use a condom.

REFERENCES

1. Dman-Kein AF, Conant M: North American phase 3 study (protocol L1057T-31) of Panretin gel (LGD1057, ALRT1057) for cutaneous AIDS-related Kaposi Sarcoma, *International Conference on AIDS* 12:319 (abstract no. 619/22283), 1998.
2. Ligand Pharmaceuticals: Panretin product literature.

Unit VI

Special Topics
in HIV/AIDS

18

Dermatological Care of Clients with HIV/AIDS

Jill Handel

Certain conditions of the integument (i.e., skin, hair, mucous membranes, nails) are opportunistic illnesses and others are signs of immune system dysfunction in clients who are HIV-positive. These conditions may herald a new or previously unrecognized diagnosis or the progression of a disease that was detected earlier. The integument may be affected by a variety of factors in the setting of HIV/AIDS. These include: (1) immune dysfunction, (2) systemic infections, (3) pathogens, (4) neoplasms, and (5) therapies used to treat HIV disease. While most of the cutaneous manifestations observed in clients with AIDS are not specific to HIV infection, their clinical presentations are often modified by the associated immune dysfunction, altered inflammatory response, and confounding effects of complex therapy regimens.

The era of highly active antiretroviral therapy (HAART), which began in late 1995 with the first available protease inhibitor (PI), has greatly affected the spectrum of skin disorders in the HIV-positive client population. The frequency of certain conditions (e.g., Kaposi's sarcoma) has been dramatically reduced. Therefore, health care providers are challenged to recognize increasingly rare, but extremely important physical signs. HAART has also challenged clinicians because suddenly large numbers of clients are being treated with complex, multi-drug combinations that can be toxic to the integument. HIV/AIDS health care providers are frequently encountering novel adverse drug effects.

Some of the important disorders of the skin and adjacent structures are presented in this chapter with an emphasis on diagnosis, treatment strategies, and client education.

CUTANEOUS EFFECTS OF IMMUNE DYSFUNCTION

Psoriasis

■ DEFINITION AND ETIOLOGY

Psoriasis is a chronic inflammatory condition that undergoes periods of exacerbation and remission and tends to become more severe as immune function declines. Rapid cell turnover in the epidermal layer of the skin increases the number of epidermal cells, which creates scales and well-marginated, erythematous, psoriatic plaques. Although psoriasis may be diagnosed in anyone who is HIV-positive, 50% of those with psoriasis have a genetic predisposition.[1] In HIV-positive individuals, HIV-induced acceleration of previously diagnosed psoriasis is the most common presentation of this disorder.

■ CLINICAL OVERVIEW

Common skin findings are scaly papules (nummular), or plaques (classic), which may be thick and salmon- or silver-colored. The scalp, low back, knees, and nails are the most common sites involved. Nails may be crumb-like, thick, pitted, and discolored. Removal of scales reveals punctate bleeding points known as Auspitz's sign. Psoriatic lesions in HIV-positive clients tend to be more severe and less responsive to treatment than those in HIV-negative clients.[2]

■ DIAGNOSTIC TESTING

Diagnosis is made by the typical clinical appearance of thick, silvery-white plaques. When diagnosis is questionable, a skin biopsy may be useful. Differential diagnoses include seborrheic dermatitis or Reiter's disease.

■ MEDICAL MANAGEMENT

There is no cure for psoriasis and, therefore, the goal of therapy is suppression. Successful treatments reduce the rate of cell turnover and inhibit the inflammatory process, thereby decreasing symptoms. Treatments include the following:

- Topical corticosteroid preparations applied directly to the lesions. Potent preparations are generally used initially or during periods of exacerbation, and then are followed by a less potent steroid cream for maintenance. Occlusive nighttime dressings are sometimes helpful for recalcitrant cases.
- Glucocorticoid solutions and coal tar shampoos used for cases of scalp involvement.
- Ultraviolet light plus coal tar ointment or gel, which may be used when more than 10% of the skin surface is involved. Up to 6 weeks of treatment may be required.
- Systemic treatments, which are reserved for severe or resistant disease; they include methotrexate, cyclosporin, synthetic retinoids, and psoralen with psoralen ultraviolet A-range (PUVA) (i.e., ultraviolet A light therapy).

■ NURSING CONSIDERATIONS

1. The chronic, relapsing nature of the disease should be reviewed with the client so that expectations of therapy are realistic.
2. Treatment success depends on the client's compliance with prescribed treatment. The rationale for the treatment modality should be reviewed and treatment schedules should be provided in writing.

3. Clients with excessive scaling can enhance treatment results by warm (not hot) bathing and soft scrubbing before applying topical preparations.
4. Moderate amounts of sun exposure may reduce the need for topical treatment, although overexposure or sunburn may exacerbate psoriasis.
5. Keeping the skin well-hydrated should be emphasized. The client should be advised to drink a liter of water daily and to keep bathing to a minimum (e.g., once a day or less), as well as to avoid excessive use of soap, which can be very drying. Emollients should be applied to skin directly after showering or bathing; mineral oil applied thinly to wet skin is preferable.
6. The nurse should remind clients to avoid sunburn and other forms of skin trauma (e.g., vigorous scrubbing or scratching), which can stimulate the proliferative process.
7. Exacerbation may result from certain medications, local skin trauma, infection, alcohol consumption, physical and psychological stress, and sunlight deprivation.
8. Medications that may exacerbate psoriasis include systemic corticosteroids, lithium, chloroquine, beta blockers, and nonsteroidal antiinflammatory drugs (NSAIDs). Drug-induced exacerbation can be unpredictable and may occur months after use.[3]

Seborrheic Dermatitis

■ DEFINITION AND ETIOLOGY

While its pathogenesis appears to be primarily inflammatory, in some cases seborrheic dermatitis may be triggered by an allergic response to microorganisms colonizing the adnexal structures of the skin.

■ CLINICAL OVERVIEW

Seborrheic dermatitis is marked by pinkish-red patches and plaques with waxy scales or crusts. Seborrheic eruptions occur in areas where sebaceous glands are concentrated, namely the scalp, face, upper trunk, and body folds. Scalp involvement often presents as dandruff and progresses to erythematous, crusted plaques. It may also involve the ears and periauricular areas. Facial involvement typically affects the eyebrows, bridge of the nose, and nasolabial folds. On the trunk, special attention should be paid to the axillae and breast folds. In addition, perspiration often causes secondary infection in the perianal and vaginal regions. Lesions may be pruritic, leading to secondary lichenification caused by scratching trauma.

■ DIAGNOSTIC TESTING

Diagnosis is usually based on clinical presentation, but a biopsy or scraping for histologic studies will exclude other disease processes. Differential diagnoses include psoriasis, lichen simplex, pityriasis rosea, ringworm (particularly in body folds), candidiasis, erythrasma, and lupus erythematosus.

▓ MEDICAL MANAGEMENT

Suppression of symptoms is the goal of treatment, as seborrheic dermatitis has no cure. Treatments include the following:

- Scalp conditions are treated with medicated shampoos containing tar, selenium sulfide, or ketoconazole.
- Mild topical steroids such as 0.5% hydrocortisone ointment or 2% ketoconazole cream are used for acute episodes of the face and trunk.
- Ultraviolet B (UVB) therapy is implemented or a short course of systemic antifungal medications (e.g., ketoconazole or itraconazole) is administered orally for cases unresponsive to topical treatments.
- Unusually, severe and recalcitrant episodes may require systemic steroid treatment with a medication such as oral prednisone.

▓ NURSING CONSIDERATIONS

1. Seborrheic dermatitis is a chronic disease that undergoes periods of exacerbation and remission. Regular treatment may be required for months at a time.
2. Alcohol-based hair preparations or gels should be avoided, as they may be an irritant and precipitate exacerbation.
3. Washing regularly with soap and water decreases the presence of yeast, which can cause inflammation and secondary infection.
4. Exacerbation can be induced by excess sunlight, stress, and fatigue.

Aphthous Ulcers

▓ DEFINITION AND ETIOLOGY

Aphthous ulcers are painful ulcers in the mouth that occur in both immunocompetent and immunocompromised individuals. They appear singly or in groups and their exact cause is not clear, though an autoimmune etiology is suspected. In clients with HIV, diminished lymphocyte counts are strongly associated with recurrence and increased size.

▓ CLINICAL OVERVIEW

Aphthous stomatitis presents as painful ulcerations of the oral mucosa, commonly referred to as canker sores. Ulcerations vary in color from erythematous to white and may have a raised, rimlike periphery. There is little surrounding inflammation. On occasion, the ulcers may be "giant" (i.e., exceeding 1 cm in diameter) or may be destructive of adjacent tissue (e.g., the uvula or the gingiva). The condition may involve structures both in the anterior and posterior pharynx and ulcers can appear anywhere in the oral cavity as discrete single lesions or as multiple ulcers. Symptoms include painful swallowing, which can lead to poor nutritional intake and rapid weight loss. The severity of pain experienced by the client typically seems out of proportion to the visible signs of disease. Aphthous stomatitis can occur in all HIV-positive populations; ulcers may be larger and more frequent than in the HIV-negative population.[4]

■ CLINICAL OVERVIEW

EPF typically involves the anterior and posterior trunk and upper arms, as well as the neck. Eruptions are characterized by small pustules that are numerous and situated at the hair follicle; they may be pruritic. At first glance the condition is difficult to distinguish from acne vulgaris or bacterial folliculitis. The major differential diagnoses to be considered are acneiform eruption, atypical drug allergy, and bacterial folliculitis.

■ DIAGNOSTIC TESTING

The diagnosis of EPF is usually apparent from clinical inspection alone. Skin biopsy and special staining, which is rarely necessary, reveals an intense eosinophilic infiltrate that is characteristic of this condition.

■ MEDICAL MANAGEMENT

Treatment options include the following:
- Potent topical corticosteroids
- Systemic antihistamines
- Itraconazole
- PUVA light therapy

■ NURSING CONSIDERATIONS

1. The goals of therapy are to manage the client's symptoms (e.g., pruritis). There is no cure for this disorder.
2. The nurse should remind clients to avoid skin trauma (e.g., vigorous scrubbing, scratching). Application of topical corticosteroids or ingestion of systemic antihistamines can be useful.
3. Moderate sun exposure may help ameliorate the signs of the disease.

CUTANEOUS EFFECTS OF SYSTEMIC INFECTION
Herpes Simplex

■ DEFINITION AND ETIOLOGY

There are two distinct strains of herpes simplex virus (HSV): HSV-1 and HSV-2. HSV-1 generally involves the oral cavity and is transmitted via direct contact with oral mucous membranes and saliva. HSV-2 generally affects the anogenital area and is spread through sexual contact.[6] Shedding of the virus, particularly from anogenital sites, can occur without the presence of visible lesions. There is a 2- to 20-day incubation period for primary infection. Following primary infection at any site, the virus becomes latent and resides in the sensory nerve ganglia for the lifetime of the individual; thus recurrent outbreaks are common and are manifestations of systemic infection.

■ CLINICAL OVERVIEW

The clinical manifestation of HSV is the appearance of grouped vesicles on an erythematous plaque that can ulcerate. Vesiculoulcerative lesions can appear anywhere on the body, but facial (e.g., with HSV-1 infection), genital, and perianal sites (e.g., with HSV-2 infection) are most common.[6] Lesions of the mouth, often referred to as "cold sores," occur on the lips, tongue, or buccal mucosa and range from mildly painful to severely painful. When the oral mucosa is affected, the anterior portions of the oral cavity are most often involved. Genital HSV usually begins as a cluster of small papules that develop into painful vesicles. Recurrent lesions appear in the same area as the primary infection and may have a prodrome of burning, tingling, or itching before vesicular eruption. Recurrence of HSV ulceration is more likely as immunodeficiency progresses. Furthermore, clients with CD_4 cell counts of less than 200 cells/mm^3 are more likely to develop coalescence of ulcers that involve large areas of skin, and that do not heal without aggressive antimicrobial therapy.

■ DIAGNOSTIC TESTING

Diagnosis is usually made by visual inspection with confirmation by viral culture, Tzanck smear, or biopsy. Differential diagnoses include syphilitic chancre, fixed-drug eruption, chancroid, gonococcal erosion, folliculitis, pemphigus, aphthous stomatitis, erythema multiforme, and CMV.

■ MEDICAL MANAGEMENT

The goal of therapy is to shorten the time of active viral shedding and the duration of symptoms. (For an extensive discussion of HSV see Chapter 17). Treatments include the following:

- Oral antivirals (e.g., acyclovir, famciclovir, valacyclovir*) are particularly effective for the treatment of primary or recurrent clinical episodes.
- In recurrent episodes, there may be some benefit if therapy is begun at the onset of prodromal symptoms.
- Daily suppressive therapy with oral antivirals decreases the frequency of recurrent outbreaks.
- On rare occasions, parenteral therapy with intravenous acyclovir or foscarnet is required.

■ NURSING CONSIDERATIONS

1. Transmission occurs via skin-to-skin or skin-to-mucosa contact with an infected person actively shedding virus onto the broken skin or susceptible mucosal surfaces. HSV is inactivated at room temperature and transmission is unlikely to occur via fomites or aerosols.[6]
2. Meticulous handwashing should be emphasized to prevent secondary infection and autoinoculation. Health care providers or family members should wear gloves when treating, bathing, or inspecting lesions.

---

*Valacyclovir originally carried a black-box FDA warning against use for clients with AIDS. This reflected rare cases of Henoch-Schönlein purpura observed in premarketing clinical studies. Subsequently this warning was removed, but it is prudent to use this drug with caution.

3. Safer sexual practices should be reviewed to prevent spread and recurrence. Viral shedding can occur in infected individuals without the presence of a lesion.
4. Chronic antiviral therapy may be required to suppress recurrences of HSV, especially when they occur frequently.

Varicella Zoster Virus

■ DEFINITION AND ETIOLOGY

After primary infection, commonly called "chicken pox," varicella zoster virus (VZV) lies dormant in the dorsal root ganglia for years. Immunodeficiency or progression of immunodeficiency can incite reactivation at any stage of HIV disease, although reactivation more commonly occurs before profound immunosuppression. Recurrent or disseminated infection occurs more commonly in clients with CD_4 cell counts of less than 100 cells/mm^3.[6] Acute localized reactivations of VZV are also called "shingles."

■ CLINICAL OVERVIEW

Typically vesicles or pustules appear grouped on an erythematous base. These lesions are usually confined to an area of 1 to 2 dermatomes. The outbreak of lesions follows a prodromal phase of skin discomfort (i.e., pain, burning, tingling, tenderness). Malaise, lymphadenopathy, and rarely meningeal symptoms and low-grade fevers may accompany the eruptions, although clients with HIV may never develop an overt vesicular eruption. Vesicles crust and heal in 7 to 10 days. Many clients experience scars and painful postherpetic neuralgia that may persist for months.

■ DIAGNOSTIC TESTING

Presumptive diagnosis is reliable with the appearance of typical shingles. A culture of vesicle fluid, Tzanck preparation, or skin biopsy can be used to confirm the diagnosis. After acute stages of the disease have passed, a fourfold increase in VZV antibodies can confirm the diagnosis retrospectively.

■ MEDICAL MANAGEMENT

The goal of treatment is pain relief and prevention of dissemination and secondary infection (for an in-depth discussion see Chapter 17). Treatments include the following:

■ Oral antivirals (e.g., acyclovir, famciclovir, valacyclovir*), which shorten the period of viral shedding and promote healing of lesions.

---

*Valacyclovir originally carried a black-box FDA warning against use for clients with AIDS. This reflected rare cases of Henoch-Schönlein purpura observed in premarketing clinical studies. Subsequently this warning was removed, but it is prudent to use this drug with caution.

- Oral corticosteroids, which have been used in older adult clients to reduce the risk of postherpetic neuralgia. In the HIV/AIDS population, the risks of further immunosuppression must be weighed heavily.
- Mild analgesics (e.g., NSAIDS) or narcotics, which may be used for relief of pain and discomfort.
- Topical antibacterial ointment applied to lesions, which prevents secondary infection.
- Resistant strains of VZV may require treatment with IV foscarnet.

▓ NURSING CONSIDERATIONS

1. Herpes zoster is transmitted via direct contact with active lesions. Skin and wound precautions should be used until lesions have crusted. The use of gloves and strict handwashing should be emphasized for all care givers and family members.
2. Clients with AIDS who have not had chicken pox should be advised that primary varicella infection might result from exposure to either chicken pox or herpes zoster. Symptoms appear approximately 14 days after exposure.[6] In those few clients with HIV who have not had a primary infection with VZV as children, varicella zoster immune globulin can be effective in preventing primary disease should they become exposed to VZV. The globulin, however, has to be administered within 96 hours of exposure.
3. Symptomatic recurrence of VZV (in the same or other dermatomes) is more common in the HIV/AIDS population. Prodromal symptoms of pain or dysesthesia should be reviewed with clients; they should be taught to seek treatment if these occur.
4. Clients should be forewarned of postherpetic neuralgia and encouraged to seek early treatment if symptoms occur.
5. Shingles is a systemic viral illness; clients should be encouraged to rest during the acute phase.

Cytomegalovirus

▓ DEFINITION AND ETIOLOGY

CMV is a systemic infection that can reactivate in the setting of AIDS immunosuppression and cause a variety of illnesses, including retinitis, colitis, pneumonitis, and pancreatitis. (For a more extensive discussion of CMV see Chapter 17.) CMV may also cause skin disease as a sign of systemic infection.

▓ CLINICAL OVERVIEW

Skin disease caused by CMV usually presents as painful ulcerations of the anogenital region. The ulcers tend to be shallow, surrounded by an erythematous patch, and may be indistinguishable from HSV. Fever is commonly associated with CMV progenitalis. More rarely, CMV may cause ulceration of the oral mucosa. The ulcers are often solitary and chronic. They may be less painful than aphthous or HSV ulcers of the oral cavity.

■ DIAGNOSTIC TESTING

CMV should always be diagnosed appropriately, because treatment requires IV medications for extended periods. A skin biopsy should be done to detect typical cytomegalic intracellular inclusions, which are abnormal microscopic structures identified within a cell. Serologic tests are not helpful because of the very high prevalence of antibodies against CMV in the populations at-risk for HIV/AIDS.

■ MEDICAL MANAGEMENT

Treatment consists of systemic antimicrobial therapy because, when skin involvement occurs, there is a high prevalence of active CMV at other sites. Treatments include the following:

■ The three available therapies are ganciclovir, foscarnet IV, and cidofovir IV. Although ganciclovir is available as an oral preparation, it is poorly absorbed and is not reliable for primary therapy of CMV disease.

■ Topical antibacterial ointments may help reduce the risk of secondary infection.

■ Immune reconstitution with HAART can help control active disease and prevent recurrences.

■ NURSING CONSIDERATIONS

1. Clients should be educated as to the systemic nature of CMV infection.
2. The importance of adherence to CMV therapy, and reporting of any adverse drug events should be stressed.

PRIMARY INFECTIONS OF THE INTEGUMENT
Staphylococcus Aureus

■ DEFINITION AND ETIOLOGY

The most common bacterial skin pathogen found in clients with HIV is *S. aureus,* known to cause both primary cutaneous disease and secondary infection. The anterior nares frequently serve as a reservoir for the colonization of *S. aureus,* allowing continuous bacterial shedding.

■ CLINICAL OVERVIEW

The most common manifestation of *S. aureus* infection is furunculosis. Furuncles are commonly known as "boils" and present as large tender papules that involve the subcutaneous tissue. Folliculitis may also be caused by *S. aureus.* It may be widely distributed with an acnelike appearance, or it may present as small, inflamed papules or pustules surrounding a hair follicle, occurring on the chest, back, upper arms, head, or neck. These skin eruptions are not as intensely pruritic as those of EFP.

Folliculitis occurs more frequently when the CD_4 cell count is less than 200 cells/mm^3.[1] When folliculitis is caused by *S. aureus*, the finding of a bacterial reservoir in the anterior nares is quite common.

Impetigo is a contagious bacterial infection caused by *S. aureus*. It initially presents as painful, small, discrete, fluid-filled vesicles that rupture easily and form a honey-colored crust. The lesions typically erupt in locations of skin folds, such as the axillary and inguinal areas. In immunocompetent individuals, impetigo is found most often on the face.[7]

■ DIAGNOSTIC TESTING

Generally, clinical inspection will provide the diagnosis of these conditions. A biopsy may be necessary to differentiate bacterial and eosinophilic varieties. Culture of skin lesions or anterior nares is important not only for diagnosis, but also to exclude methicillin-resistant *S. aureus*. Differential diagnoses include allergic contact dermatitis, cutaneous drug reaction, scabies, atopic dermatitis, EPF, VZV, and HSV.

■ MEDICAL MANAGEMENT

Treatments include the following:

- Topical antibiotics such as clindamycin and antibacterial soaps, which are indicated for bacterial folliculitis and impetigo. If infection is widespread a systemic antibiotic may be used.
- Topical steroid preparations, such as hydrocortisone, which provide symptomatic relief of itching and resolution of lesions.
- Systemic antihistamines, such as Claritin or Benadryl, which also provide relief from itching but may induce somnolence.
- To eradicate the nasal carrier state, it may be necessary to use topical mupirocin or oral antibiotics. Combinations of betalactamase-resistant antibiotics with rifampin have the highest success rates. However, if rifampin is used, attention must be paid to drug interactions with antiretrovirals.

■ NURSING CONSIDERATIONS

1. Weeping impetiginous lesions are highly contagious; strict handwashing practices should be emphasized.
2. Impetigo usually does not scar but may be observed as a secondary infection in conditions that frequently scar, such as herpes zoster.
3. Recurrence is common with furunculosis, folliculitis, and impetigo; early recognition and treatment are keys to confining infection.

Oral Hairy Leukoplakia

■ DEFINITION AND ETIOLOGY

Oral hairy leukoplakia (OHL) is a benign condition. The lesions are caused by the HIV-facilitated replication of the Epstein-Barr virus (EBV) and become more common as the CD_4 cell count decreases below

200 cells/mm^3. OHL is an indicator of both HIV disease and immunodeficiency; it appears less frequently in children with HIV than in adults with HIV.[8] (For a more extensive discussion of OHL see Chapter 17.)

■ CLINICAL OVERVIEW

OHL presents with white plaques from which hairlike excrescences grow, which are aligned vertically on the lateral and inferior surface of the tongue, buccal mucosa, or soft palate. Hairy leukoplakia is not tender or painful, cannot be scraped off, and does not resolve with antifungal treatment.

■ DIAGNOSTIC TESTING

Diagnosis is usually made on the basis of clinical findings; a mucosal biopsy for histology may be performed if the diagnosis is uncertain. Differential diagnoses include hyperplastic oral candidiasis, condyloma, HIV-induced neoplasia (e.g., squamous intraepithelial lesions, SCC), geographic tongue, lichen planus, tobacco associated leukoplakia, mucous patch of secondary syphilis, and occlusal trauma.

■ MEDICAL MANAGEMENT

OHL is usually asymptomatic and no treatment is indicated. Resolution of lesions often occurs with HIV viral suppression using HAART. Treatments include the following:

■ Acyclovir, which may be used in high doses to treat symptomatic OHL.
■ Antifungal treatment, which may be needed to decrease superinfection with *Candida* spp. (see the next section and Chapter 14 for a discussion of candidiasis).

■ NURSING CONSIDERATIONS

1. The appearance of OHL may be anxiety provoking. Clients need to be reassured that it is benign and noncontagious and that resolution with effective treatment of HIV may take weeks to months.
2. Recurrence is common.

Oral and Esophageal Candidiasis

■ DEFINITION AND ETIOLOGY

Pseudomembranous candidiasis (also known as thrush) is caused by an overgrowth of *Candida* spp. (normal flora), which causes the symptoms. It is the most common fungal infection in clients with HIV. Symptoms increase in frequency as immunodeficiency progresses.

■ CLINICAL OVERVIEW

Pseudomembranous candidiasis presents as a white, curdlike coating on the tongue, buccal mucosa, gums, or hard palate. The coating can be partially scraped off with a tongue blade or dry gauze pad. Erythematous candidiasis appears as flat, red lesions. Clients may complain of altered taste sensation or sore throat. Painful swallowing, retrosternal pain, and nausea are signs of esophageal involvement.

◼ DIAGNOSTIC TESTING

A presumptive diagnosis is made by appearance and the ability to scrape off plaques. Pseudohyphae visualized on a potassium hydroxide (KOH) preparation of mucosal scrapings confirms the diagnosis. Esophageal involvement may require endoscopy with biopsy. Differential diagnoses include OHL, geographic tongue, occlusal trauma, and oral SCC.

◼ MEDICAL MANAGEMENT

Treatments include:
- Clotrimazole troches which are usually adequate for an acute flare-up of oral candidiasis.
- Chronic suppression with nystatin or clotrimazole, which is needed in clients with frequent recurrences. When infection is more recalcitrant, the use of ketoconazole, fluconazole, or itraconazole is indicated.

◼ NURSING CONSIDERATIONS

1. Thrush is a recurring disease; good oral hygiene can decrease candidal overgrowth.
2. Self-monitoring and early treatment can minimize the extent of involvement and discomfort.
3. Thrush may be precipitated by the use of inhaled corticosteroids or a prolonged course of antibiotic treatment.

Onychomycosis

◼ DEFINITION AND ETIOLOGY

Onychomycosis is a fungal infection of the nails and is a common finding among clients with HIV/AIDS. Although not specific to such clients, immunosuppression increases the number of nails involved and the extent of the involvement. Fungi that cause infection of skin and nails may be referred to as dermatophytes, and the causative organism is frequently *C. albicans*.

◼ CLINICAL OVERVIEW

Onychomycosis causes whitish-yellow discoloration of the fingernails and toenails. It may involve the entire nail plate and cause pain and secondary bacterial paronychias. Associated fungal intertrigo (i.e., "athlete's feet") is commonly observed.

◼ DIAGNOSTIC TESTING

The diagnosis is usually apparent from careful inspection. Occasionally, nail scrapings are sent for KOH preparation or culture to confirm the diagnosis. The differential diagnoses include toxicity of antiviral medications, psoriatic nail disease, or, rarely, nutritional deficiencies.

■ MEDICAL MANAGEMENT

Treatment must be matched to the extent of disease and the symptoms. Topical therapy is sufficient to keep the disease under control in many cases. When the condition affects the quality of life, long-term treatment (e.g., 6 to 12 weeks) with oral terbinafine, ketoconazole, or itraconazole may be considered. Attention must be paid to potential hepatotoxicity or drug-drug interactions with PIs if these medications are used. Generally, griseofulvin, which may cause bone marrow suppression, is not recommended for clients with AIDS.

■ NURSING CONSIDERATIONS

1. Clients should be instructed that dermatophytes are contagious and can be transmitted by contact with colonized surfaces (e.g., showers). They enter the skin through breaks in its integrity (e.g., hangnails, fissures); good foot hygiene is essential. Areas between toes must be dried after bathing and an antifungal foot powder may be useful.
2. Clients and partners should be informed that candidal infections are not spread via person-to-person contact.
3. The health care provider should help the client weigh the benefits and risks of different therapies so as to facilitate an informed decision about treatment.
4. Clients should be instructed on hygienic principles to avoid auto-inoculation of uninvolved nails.

Molluscum Contagiosum

■ DEFINITION AND ETIOLOGY

Molluscum contagiosum is caused by a poxvirus. Molluscum can occur in all populations regardless of HIV status but, in clients with HIV, the lesions tend to be larger, more numerous, and last months to years.[2]

■ CLINICAL OVERVIEW

Molluscum contagiosum are asymptomatic, dome-shaped, skin-colored, translucent papules with a central umbilication. Lesions may be pruritic if secondary infection with *S. aureus* is present. The most commonly affected areas are the face, neck, scalp, axillae, groin, and anogenital region; lesions are initially small in size and few in number but with autoinoculation and progression of immunodeficiency, they become larger and more numerous despite aggressive treatment. Molluscum can cause significant cosmetic disfigurement.

■ DIAGNOSTIC TESTING

The diagnosis is usually made clinically by appearance of the lesions; lesional biopsy confirms the diagnosis.

■ MEDICAL MANAGEMENT

Treatment usually requires destructive measures such as cryotherapy, curettage, or electrosurgery in multiple sessions until lesions are resolved. Recurrence is common.

■ NURSING CONSIDERATIONS

1. Molluscum can be sexually transmitted, particularly when pubic and anogenital lesions are present.
2. Clients should be warned against picking or shaving lesions to avoid spreading and secondary infection.
3. Clients should be advised that multiple treatments are required to completely remove molluscum and recurrence is common.
4. With successful viral suppression and increased CD_4 counts, molluscum may spontaneously regress.

Condyloma Acuminata

■ DEFINITION AND ETIOLOGY

Condyloma acuminata, or venereal warts, are sexually transmitted primary infections of the integument. They are caused by various strains of the human papilloma virus (HPV).

■ CLINICAL OVERVIEW

Condyloma acuminata commonly appear in the anogenital region but may be transmitted to the urogenital tract, the oral mucosa, and even the nares. Typically, multiple lesions are observed. They appear as cerebrated papules that are off-white and occasionally pedunculated. Recognition of these lesions is important for two reasons. First, they are contagious to uninvolved areas of the client's integument, and to sexual partners. Second, the chronic inflammation and cell transformations may predispose to cervical, anal, or oral SCC. (See Chapter 8 for a discussion of HPV infection in women.)

■ DIAGNOSTIC TESTING

The diagnosis is often made based on the clinical appearance of the lesions. Biopsy is necessary when the lesions must be distinguished from other forms of viral skin disease, skin tags, neurofibromata, or SCC.

■ MEDICAL MANAGEMENT

Treatment implications include the following:

- Excision, which is feasible when the number of lesions is small and the lesions are accessible.
- Topical ablation, which is possible with 5-fluorouracil, tincture of podophyllin, or trichloroacetic acid.
- Topical treatment with 5% Imiquimod, which is generally not effective when significant immunosuppression is present.

◼ NURSING CONSIDERATIONS

1. Clients should be informed of the contagious nature of this condition. Safe sexual practices designed to prevent HIV transmission may not adequately prevent transmission of HPV.
2. The cancer-promoting effect of HPV must be emphasized, as well as the need for frequent cervical and anal Pap smears.

NEOPLASMS

Kaposi's Sarcoma

◼ DEFINITION AND ETIOLOGY

AIDS-related Kaposi's Sarcoma (KS) is the most common neoplasm to develop in HIV-positive clients and can occur at any stage of the disease.[9] It is an AIDS-defining disease that is progressive but indolent. KS is not purely a cutaneous disease, as it may affect visceral organs including the lungs, gastrointestinal (GI) tract, spleen, and liver. While the etiology of KS remains unclear, the current theories include genetic and environmental factors and the human herpesvirus-8, or the KS herpes virus, as causal entities. (See Chapter 15 for further discussion of KS.)

◼ CLINICAL OVERVIEW

Cutaneous or subcutaneous lesions begin as nonpruritic, painless macular spots with smooth or jagged borders that may be pink, red, brown, or purple in color. The overall shape of the lesion is typically elliptical, with the long axis oriented along the skin bias or lines of Langer, which are the linear clefts in the skin that follow the fibers of the dermis. Over time the lesions may increase in size, darken, and become raised plaques, papules, or nodules. On occasion spontaneous remission of individual lesions may be observed.

The lesions appear most frequently in white and Hispanic men who have sex with men. Other groups at risk for HIV, including IV drug users, hemophiliacs and other blood product recipients, and women, rarely develop KS.[9] Still a hallmark of AIDS, the incidence of HIV-related KS (i.e., epidemic KS) has dramatically lessened in association with the use of PI-containing treatment regimens and continued safer sex practices.

◼ DIAGNOSTIC TESTING

Clinical diagnosis is confirmed via lesional punch biopsy. GI lesions are diagnosed by endoscopic visualization and biopsy. Pulmonary KS is diagnosed via bronchoscopy with transbronchial biopsy. Differential diagnoses include malignant melanoma, angiomas, cutaneous angiosarcomas, angiolipoma, dermatofibromas, pyogenic granulomas, and sarcoid nodules. Bacillary angiomatosis is caused by a dissemination of *Bartonella quintana* and can mimic KS (see Chapter 13 for discussion of bacillary angiomatosis). More aggressive KS may resemble lichen planus, sarcoidosis, urticaria pigmentosa, papular urticaria, eruptive xanthomas, disseminated secondary syphilis, and/or angiosarcomas.

■ MEDICAL MANAGEMENT

Treatments include the following:

- Complete suppression of HIV viral RNA with HAART, which may provide spontaneous resolution of early KS with few lesions.
- Topical cryotherapy (with liquid nitrogen) applied in repeated treatments to freeze off small individual lesions in new-onset KS.
- Intralesional injections of vinblastine or vincristine, which are used in treating individual lesions but may cause irritation, ulceration, and pain at the site of injection.
- Radiation therapy, which may be used particularly when limited numbers of lesions are causing localized symptoms.
- IV chemotherapy using liposomal doxorubicin (Doxil) or liposomal daunorubicin (DaunoXome), which are used to treat advancing KS.
- Subcutaneous interferon administered daily in increasing doses, which has been effective in early and advanced disease.

■ NURSING CONSIDERATIONS

1. Clients should be instructed to perform regular self-examination of skin and to point out suspicious lesions to health care providers.
2. In addition to being physically disfiguring, KS is an AIDS-defining illness and may be anxiety-provoking in an HIV-positive client.
3. All treated lesions and lesions of advanced KS should be monitored for wound infection.

Squamous Cell Carcinoma

■ DEFINITION AND ETIOLOGY

SCC affects the skin and mucous membranes with increased frequency in clients with HIV/AIDS. Skin on the face and sun-exposed areas of the trunk and the arms is most susceptible. HIV-positive clients also appear to be at increased risk for cervical SCC, anal SCC, and head and neck SCC. SCC is more prevalent in clients who are also infected with HPV (see p. 338). (See Chapter 8 for a discussion of SCC in women.)

■ CLINICAL OVERVIEW

Typically, skin cancers in HIV-positive clients are multiple, more aggressive than usual, and require more radical surgery to effect a cure. In the case of mucosal (anogenital and oral) disease, early local metastases to lymph nodes are common. On the skin, lesions appear as small, scaly plaques with little surrounding erythema. On mucosal surfaces, the disease may present either as a chronic ulceration or as a pale area of induration with overlying friability.

■ DIAGNOSTIC TESTING

Diagnosis requires a tissue biopsy. Differential diagnoses include premalignant lesions, carcinoma in situ, and nonneoplastic conditions such as eczema, scabies, contact dermatitis, and psoriasis.

■ NURSING CONSIDERATIONS

1. Clients should be instructed about self-examination of the skin. Instruction should include the warning signs of skin cancer—asymmetry of the lesion, irregular borders, color variations, and a diameter of greater than 6 mm.
2. Risk-reduction training is important to lessen the likelihood of subsequent episodes of the disease. Risk reduction education includes topics such as avoidance of excessive sunlight, and the use of sunscreens. The client should also understand the need for early detection measures, such as frequent Pap smears and ear, nose, and throat examinations.

INTEGUMENT TOXICITY CAUSED BY HIV THERAPIES

The widespread use of HAART has made dramatic inroads in converting AIDS from a fatal to a chronic, long-term condition. However, the use of polypharmacy has caused new and significant integumentary toxicity to appear in the clinical setting. Drug toxicity may occur either as a direct toxic effect or it may be mediated through the dysregulated immune response that is characteristic of HIV/AIDS.

DIRECT TOXIC EFFECTS

- Xerosis or pathologic dry skin may occur in clients treated with indinavir and other PIs, particularly during the dry winter months. Emollients are used to decrease itching and discomfort.
- Penile ulcers secondary to Foscavir treatment can result from high concentrations of Foscavir in the urine.
- Paronychia (i.e., "crix toe") initially appears unilaterally as tenderness and erythema around the cuticle of the great toe. Pressure applied to the area releases purulent drainage. PIs, as a class, inhibit retinoic acid metabolism, which directly affects skin and nails. Anecdotally, nails tend to grow faster in length as well as laterally. The mechanism for this is poorly understood. Treatment generally entails removal of nail overgrowth in the lateral margins.
- Hair growth may be affected by certain HIV medications. Lamivudine and hydroxyurea have been observed to cause hair loss. Generally, hair regrowth occurs when the offending drugs are discontinued. Hair loss resulting from the use of these drugs must be distinguished from telogen effluvium, which is hair loss following a long, febrile illness, in which case the amount of hair loss is proportional to the duration and severity of the precipitating illness.

IMMUNOLOGICALLY MEDIATED TOXICITIES

- Morbilliform or measleslike rashes are the most often encountered allergic skin eruptions. In most cases of hypersensitivity, a widespread maculopapular rash will occur within 8 to 12 days after initiating treatment; this may be accompanied by pruritus and fever. Rashes generally resolve within days of discontinuing the offending medication. The agents most commonly associated with allergic skin reactions in HIV-positive clients are trimethoprim-sulfamethoxazole, sulfadiazine, aminopenicillins, efavirenz, nevirapine, delavirdine, and abacavir.
- Stevens-Johnson syndrome is a severe allergic skin reaction characterized by fever and a blistering rash involving the skin and mucous membranes. This is a life-threatening condition that requires hospitalization.

Nursing Considerations

1. Clients should contact their health care provider in the event of rash or fever higher than 101° F.
2. At each health care examination, clients should present a written list of symptoms and concerns that occurred since their last visit. Symptoms such as dry skin may be easily forgotten and ingrown nails may be overlooked if shoes were not removed for the examination.
3. Potential side effects of all new medications should be reviewed and provided in writing to the client whenever possible.

REFERENCES

1. Berger TG: Dermatologic manifestations of HIV infection. In Cohen PT, Sande MA, Volberding PA, eds: *The AIDS knowledge base*, ed 2, Boston, 1994, Little, Brown & Co.
2. Aftergut K, Cockerell CJ: Update on the cutaneous manifestations of HIV infection, *Dermatologic Clinics* 17(3): Jul 1999.
3. Lowe NJ: Management of psoriasis. In Goroll AH, May LA, Mulley AG, eds: *Primary Care Medicine*, ed 3, Philadelphia, 1995, Lippincott.
4. Greenspan D, Greenspan JS: Oral cavity manifestations. In Mildvan D, ed: *Mandell's atlas of infectious diseases; vol. 1: AIDS*, ed 2, Philadelphia, 1997, Current Medicine.
5. Bickers DR, Pathak MA, Lim HW: The porphyrias. In Freedberg IM et al, eds: *Fitzpatrick's dermatology in general medicine; vol 2*, ed 5, New York, McGraw-Hill.
6. Erlich KS, Safrin S, Mills J: Herpes simplex virus. In Cohen PT, Sande MA, Volberding PA, eds: *The AIDS knowledge base*, ed 2, Boston, 1994, Little, Brown & Co.
7. Cockrell CJ, Friedman-Kien AE: Cutaneous manifestations of HIV infection. In Merigan TC, Bartlett JG, Bolognesi D, eds: *The textbook of AIDS medicine*, ed 2, Baltimore, 1999, Williams & Wilkins.

8. Greenspan D: The mouth: hairy leukoplakia and Epstein-Barr virus. In Cohen PT, Sande MA, Volberding PA, eds: *The AIDS knowledge base,* ed 2, Boston, 1994, Little, Brown & Co.
9. Miles SA: Kaposi's sarcoma and cloacogenic carcinoma: virus-initiated malignancies. In Merigan TC, Bartlett JG, Bolognesi D, eds: *The textbook of AIDS medicine,* ed 2, Baltimore, 1999, Williams & Wilkins.

19 HIV/AIDS Nutritional Management

Glenda Winson

AIDS WASTING

Wasting is caused by insufficient nutritional intake or a disturbance in metabolism that interferes with the effective use of nutrients, resulting in loss of lean body mass. Two types of malnutrition, *marasmus* and *kwashiorkor* can lead to wasting. The term *marasmus* refers to protein-calorie malnutrition and is associated with an insufficient intake of protein and total calories. It is characterized by depletion of body fat and skeletal muscle with preservation of visceral proteins. The term *kwashiorkor* refers to protein malnutrition that may occur with adequate total caloric intake. It is characterized by depletion of lean body mass, often with preservation of body fat; hypoalbuminemia and edema are additional features of this condition. In the client with AIDS, the loss of lean body mass is a primary cause of functional decline in wasting, resulting in increased risk of opportunistic infections, reduced quality of life, and reduced survival. The problem of wasting, and the ensuing debilitation, is one of the most devastating aspects of AIDS. It is well documented that when a client's weight is reduced to 60% of his or her ideal body weight, death may ensue, regardless of the underlying condition (e.g., AIDS).[1]

CONSEQUENCES

When clients are wasted, they grow weaker and are not able to perform their usual activities of daily living. As a result, the client may become depressed and may feel a loss of independence, social identity and self-esteem. Ultimately, the lack of vitality may persuade the individual that life is meaningless. These consequences, added to the original cause of the inadequate nutrition, precipitate a vicious downward spiral. When the progress of weight loss is arrested, the client gains a sense of control, which, in turn, improves quality of life.

DEFINITION AND ETIOLOGY

In 1993, the Centers for Disease Control and Prevention (CDC) revised its criteria for AIDS-defining illnesses to include involuntary weight loss of greater than 10% from baseline, with either chronic diarrhea or weakness

344

and fever for 30 days or longer.[2] These criteria represent the current clinical definition of HIV wasting.

There is no single etiology of wasting syndrome. A thorough client history, physical examination, and nutritional assessment may uncover one or several of the following etiologies:

Decreased Food Intake

Food intake may be inadequate because of conditions that cause mechanical difficulties, pain when eating (e.g., mucositis, dysphagia, odynophagia), or loss of appetite. The cause or causes of decreased food intake need to be identified. Common causes in clients with AIDS are fungal infections, such as *Candida albicans,* and esophageal ulcers of viral, bacterial, or neoplastic variety. Anorexia may be a side effect of various medicines or may result from a neurological disease, which could also impair swallowing. Psychological factors, such as depression and anxiety, can also contribute to anorexia. Delayed emptying of the stomach, which gives the feeling of fullness, is also common in AIDS.[3]

Intestinal Problems

Malabsorption.   Severe wasting is often associated with small intestine injury due to protozoal infections, producing a defective mucosal barrier. This defective mucosal barrier reduces the absorption of essential nutrients and is accompanied by an increase in stool volume; stool volume is related to food intake, especially of fats. Bowel movements occur four to eight times a day, so the client may stop eating in an effort to reduce the number of bowel movements. Cryptosporidia and microsporidia (see Chapter 16) are common parasites in clients with AIDS and are often implicated as the cause of malabsorption. When these organisms are present, they infiltrate the epithelial lining of the small intestines, causing increased epithelial cell loss, which leads to partial villus atrophy. As a result, there is a change in the morphology, shrinkage of the surface area for absorption, and a curtailing of the production of digestive enzymes (Figures 19-1 [normal villi] and 19-2 [abnormal villi]). Diarrhea and malabsorption of nutrients lead to precipitous weight loss, weakness, and severe malnutrition.

Large-Bowel Disease.   In HIV-positive clients, large-bowel disease usually takes the form of a generalized inflammatory disorder caused by viral, bacterial, or parasitic infections or by a neoplasm. The most common viruses that cause large-bowel disease are herpes virus and cytomegalovirus (CMV). Antibiotic-associated colitis may be observed as a complication of antibiotic therapy in clients with AIDS, as well as other clients. For example, *Clostridium difficile* is a common pathogen that results in antibiotic-associated colitis. The presence of *C. difficile* can be readily detected in a sample of stool that has been sent to a laboratory by identification of one of the two toxins produced by this organism. The colitis that results from *C. difficile* infection can be treated with oral

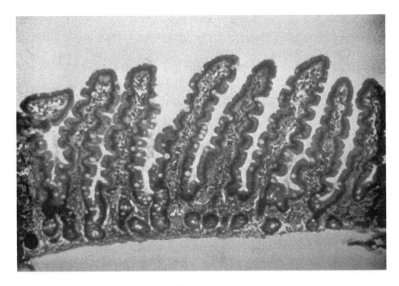

Figure 19-1. Normal villi.

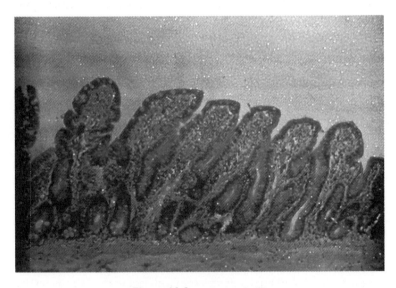

Figure 19-2. Abnormal villi.

BOX 19-1 CALCULATING NITROGEN BALANCE

Urinary urea nitrogen (UUN) is an indicator of nitrogen output and is used to estimate nitrogen balance. Nitrogen balance is calculated as follows:

$$\text{Nitrogen balance} = \text{protein intake (g)}/6.25 - (\text{UUN [g]} + 4)$$

The urine sample sent to the laboratory should be an aliquot drawn from an accurate 24-hour urine collection. The factor "4" is added as an empirical number to account for nonurinary nitrogen, such as that excreted in feces and sweat and lost through other normal causes.

Adapted from Shatsky F: *Nutritional support*. In Knoben JE, Anderson PO, eds: *Handbook of clinical drug data*, ed 7, Hamilton, Ill, 1993, Drug Intelligence.

vancomycin or metronidazole. All other antibiotics should be discontinued, if possible. It is essential to establish the cause of colitis and treat it appropriately. Eating often exacerbates the diarrhea; therefore clients often avoid food. In large-bowel disease, bowel movements are small, mucoid, and occur at regular intervals up to 30 times a day. To curb diarrhea, antimotility agents may help in the short term, but these agents can cause megacolon if used for prolonged periods. Salicylates, such as Asacol, may be effective in large-bowel disease, as they reduce inflammation in the colon.

Systemic Infections

Nitrogen is found in protein, and most adults in the United States normally eat more protein than is needed for body building and repair. Hence most adults are in positive nitrogen balance, meaning that they are anabolic, or capable of building up tissue. There is no storage for excess protein; the excess is excreted in urine and feces.

Clients with AIDS who have acute or chronic systemic infection have metabolic rates up to 40% above normal, which increase the body's need for nitrogen intake (protein) to as much as 2 g/kg/day (normal is 0.8 g/kg/day). If nitrogen intake (protein) does not meet daily requirements, a negative nitrogen balance results and they cannot build or maintain tissue (Box 19-1). When this happens, there is a loss of lean body mass, which is mobilized or broken down to meet the energy needs of the body. Metabolic alterations and increased body energy expenditure have also been noted in HIV-positive individuals without systemic infection.[4] Effective treatment of underlying infections has been shown to improve the client's nutritional status.[5]

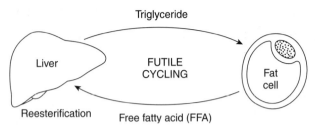

Figure 19-3. Lipolysis mobilizes fatty acid from peripheral fat cells. The fatty acid, rather than being oxidized to produce energy by the liver, is reesterified into triglyceride, resecreted into the blood, and returned to the fat cell.

Cytokines

Cytokines play multiple roles in the body's immune and inflammatory responses (see Chapter 1). Low levels are essential for host defense, but excessive amounts lead to metabolic disturbance. Normally, during lipolysis, fatty acids are mobilized from fat and oxidized to produce energy. Cytokines, especially tumor necrosis factor (TNF) alpha, stimulate increased hepatic synthesis of fatty acids. TNF rapidly mobilizes free fatty acids, which are reesterified into triglycerides in the liver and resecreted. Fatty acids thus move from fat tissue to the liver and back to fat tissue without being used for energy. This process, called *futile cycling* (Figure 19-3), might contribute to anorexia and weight loss.

Reduced Hormone Levels

Decreased levels of testosterone have been reported in 35% to 50% of HIV-positive men.[7] Testosterone has two distinct biological effects: (1) virilizing activity, or androgenic effect, and (2) protein-building activity, or anabolic effect. In HIV-positive men, lowered testosterone levels have been correlated with weight loss and possibly decreased survival time.[8] Because testosterone is an anabolic hormone, deficiency may cause a loss of body cell mass and contribute to HIV wasting. The role of gonadotrophic hormones in women with wasting is not well studied. Women who are wasted tend to lose a significant amount of body fat, but body cell mass is not significantly decreased. Men, on the other hand, tend to lose a significant amount of lean body mass, with preservation of fat (Table 19-1).[9]

The nursing assessment is important in identifying factors that place a client at risk for wasting. Box 19-2 lists factors that indicate high risk for wasting.

Diagnostic Tests for Wasting

Anthropometric Measurements

Assessment of protein compartments (muscle) can aid in the diagnosis of clients with wasting. The assessment begins by taking a diet history and performing a physical examination. This includes obtaining the client's

Table 19-1	Gender Differences in Body Composition in AIDS	

Men	Women
Body cell mass significantly decreased.	Body cell mass not significantly decreased.
Body fat not significantly decreased.	Body fat significantly decreased.

BOX 19-2   RISK FACTORS FOR WASTING

Wasting is likely when one or more of the following factors are present:

- Recent unintentional weight loss
- Altered sense of smell or taste affecting food intake
- Difficulty with chewing, swallowing, or poor dentition
- GI problems, such as diarrhea, nausea, vomiting, constipation, indigestion, flatulence, abdominal distention, and abdominal pain
- Living alone, poor food preparation abilities, or lack of cooking facilities and refrigeration in home
- Eating less than three well-balanced meals a day
- Financial difficulties affecting purchase and selection of foods
- Physical, mental, and emotional difficulties affecting shopping, cooking, or eating
- Consumption of alcohol or recreational drugs
- Prescribed dietary restrictions or restrictions that are self-imposed as a result of religious or ethnic beliefs
- Taking many prescribed medications, which may affect appetite
- Depression, grieving, or sadness, which may affect food intake
- History of eating disorders (e.g., anorexia, bulimia)

height and weight. Body weight should be measured at every visit. A significant change in body weight is considered to have occurred when the client loses 5% of body weight over a 3-month period or 10% or more over a 6-month period.

Assessment of the client's body mass index (BMI) uses the client's height and weight to determine if the weight is appropriate for the height; it is thus a measure of the degree of obesity. It is calculated by dividing the client's weight (kg) by the height squared (m^2) (Box 19-3).

The BMI, however, does not differentiate between the amount of weight from fat and the amount from fat-free mass and therefore is insensitive to the respective contribution of muscle and fat to the body

BOX 19-3 CALCULATING THE BODY MASS INDEX (BMI)

1. Measure the weight in kilograms.
2. Measure the height in meters.
3. Divide the weight by the height squared.

For example:
- Client's weight—68 kg
- Client's height—1.74 m

$$\text{BMI}—68/(1.74)^2 = 68/3.0 = 22.6$$

Table 19-2 Relationship of Degree of Obesity to Body Mass Index (BMI)

Degree of Obesity	BMI
Not obese	<25
Moderately obese	25-30
Obese	30-40
Morbidly obese	>40

---

weight. The BMI should therefore be cautiously interpreted. The values obtained suggest that the higher the BMI, the greater the fat (Table 19-2).

In studies on AIDS clients with wasting syndrome, the BMI was found to be significantly lower in clients with AIDS than in the control groups.[9] A BMI below 20 is indicative of wasting.

Triceps skinfold (TSF) thickness measurement or mid-upper arm circumference (MAC) can aid in assessing weight loss. TSF thickness is a measure of subcutaneous fat reserves. MAC provides an estimate of skeletal muscle mass and fat stores. Both TSF thickness and MAC are decreased in chronic and acute protein malnutrition. These measurements may also be influenced by shifts in hydration status.[10] They are also used to calculate mid-upper arm muscle circumference (MAMC), which estimates skeletal muscle reserves or the amount of lean body mass (Fig. 19-4).

A measurement of functional power, such as grip strength, is also useful as a means of identifying muscle weakness. Using a dynamometer (from Greek, meaning "power measure"), the nurse can measure a client's grip force in kilograms (Box 19-4). This measurement should be taken at a time when the client is clinically well and a comparison of scores should be recorded over time. Clients who are wasting have a decrease in grip

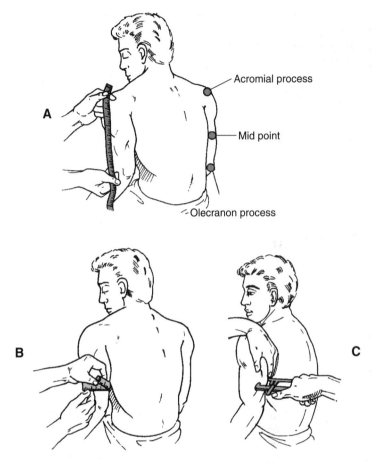

Figure 19-4. Measuring adipose and skeletal muscle tissue to estimate the client's reserves of protein and calories. **A,** Locate the midpoint of the client's relaxed, nondominant upper arm by palpating the acromial and olecranon processes and measuring the distance between the two points with a tape measure. Mark the posterior aspect of the arm at the midpoint with a pen. **B,** Measure mid-upper arm circumference (MAC) at the midpoint, keeping the tape measure level. **C,** Just above the midpoint at the posterior aspect of the arm, grasp the client's skin and subcutaneous tissue between thumb and index finger, freeing it from the underlying muscle mass. Place the calipers at the midpoint just below the fold of grasped tissue. Squeeze the calipers until they are equilibrated at the "measure" markings for approximately 3 seconds. Read the measurement to the nearest millimeter. Repeat the reading two more times, allowing a rest period of 3 seconds between readings. Calculate the average of the three readings for the TSF thickness.

Continued

Calculate the mid-arm muscle circumference (MAMC) using the following formula:
MAMC (in cm) = [MAC in cm] − [(0.314) × (TSF in mm)]

Measurement		Standard	90%	60%
Midarm circumference (MAC)	Men	29.3 cm	26.4 cm	17.6 cm
	Women	28.5 cm	25.7 cm	17.1 cm
Triceps skinfold (TSF)	Men	12.5 mm	11.3 mm	7.5 cm
	Women	16.5 mm	14.9 mm	9.9 mm
Midarm muscle circum-ference (MAMC)	Men	25.3 cm	22.8 cm	15.2 cm
	Women	23.2 cm	20.9 cm	13.9 cm

Figure 19-4, cont'd. D, Compare the client's values for MAC, TSF thickness, and MAMC to standard values to determine nutritional risk status. *Undernutrition* is indicated by a measurement below 90% of the standard. Protein calorie *malnutrition* is indicated by a measurement of less than 60% of the standard, especially for the MAMC. *Obesity* is indicated by a TSF thickness measurement 120% or more above the standard. (*From Black JM, Matassarin-Jacobs E:* Luckmann and Sorensen's medical-surgical nursing: a psychophysiologic approach, *Philadelphia, 1993, WB Saunders.*)

BOX 19-4 TIPS FOR SUCCESSFUL DYNAMOMETER MEASUREMENT

- The client should be in standing position.
- The grip size should be adjusted so that the subject has a good grasp on the apparatus.
- The client's wrist and forearm should be in a mid-prone position during the measurement.
- To obtain the measurement, the client should exert pressure maximally and quickly. Observe the client during measurement. The client should avoid jerking the dynamometer.

---

strength. As muscle strength improves (e.g., through the use of anabolic steroids) grip strength should improve.

Measurement of body composition should be performed, if possible, to establish lean body mass, percentage of body fat, percentage of body water, and bone density. However, not all facilities have the necessary equipment to carry out such specialized and detailed body composition measurement (Box 19-5). With increasing frequency, however, bioelectrical impedance analysis (BIA) is being used to measure body composition (Box 19-6). BIA measures resistance and reactance to salts, which are greater in lean tissue because it contains more water and electrolytes than

BOX 19-5   DETERMINATION OF DETAILED BODY COMPOSITION

Determination of detailed body composition involves determining the lean body mass, percentage of body fat, percentage of water, and bone density.

Lean Body Mass

Lean body mass is the part of the body that has no fat and is about 70% water and 30% solids. It can be assessed by measuring the total body potassium. The majority (97%) of potassium (K_{40}) is intracellular. K_{40} is a naturally occurring radioactive isotope and can be measured by using a whole-body liquid scintillation counter. From this measurement, the amount of intracellular K_{40} in the body can be calculated. Changes in the volume of intracellular K_{40} correlate with a change in lean body mass.

Body Fat

The percentage of body fat can be assessed by several techniques. Anthropometric measurements, such as TSF thickness measurement, are widely used but imprecise. Underwater weighing (hydrostatic weighing) and dual-energy x-ray absorptiometry (DXA) can also be used.

Bone Density

DXA, which was originally developed for early detection of osteoporosis, is often used to measure bone density. DXA has the added benefit of providing body composition data, specifically regarding body fat and lean mass.

Total Body Water

Water represents the largest single constituent of the body. Water makes up 55% to 65% of a person's body weight. Measurement of body water is important because the volume is altered with disease. Isotopes of water have an important role in the study of water; they can be used to define the amount of body water in different body compartments. Blood and saliva samples are obtained, and the amounts of isotopes in the samples are measured to provide information about the amount of body water.

BOX 19-6   CLIENT INSTRUCTIONS FOR BIOELECTRICAL IMPEDANCE ANALYSIS (BIA)

- Refrain from drinking alcohol for 12 hours before the procedure.
- Do not exercise or use a sauna within 8 hours of the procedure.
- Refrain from eating food for 4 hours before the procedure.
- Remove jewelry on hands and feet just prior to the procedure.
- Lie quietly and do not move during the procedure; the entire procedure time is less than 2 minutes.

| Table 19-3 | Laboratory Values in Protein Depletion | | | |

Parameter	Standard	Mild Protein Depletion	Moderate Protein Depletion	Severe Protein Depletion
Serum albumin	3.5-5.0 mg/dl	3.5-3.0 mg/dl	3.0-2.1 mg/dl	<2.1 mg/dl
Prealbumin	>20 mg/dl	20-15 mg/dl	15-10 mg/dl	<10 mg/dl
Total lymphocyte count	1800-3000	1800-1200	1200-800	<800
Transferrin	200-400 mg/dl	200-150 mg/dl	150-100 mg/dl	<100 mg/dl

Adapted from Shatsky F: *Nutritional support.* In Knoben JE, Anderson PO, eds: *Handbook of clinical drug data,* ed 7, Hamilton, Ill, 1993, Drug Intelligence.

adipose tissue. From these values, in addition to height, weight, age, and gender, body composition can be estimated. The technique is simple and requires minimal training.*

Laboratory Data

Measurement of complete blood count (CBC), serum electrolytes, and serum plasma proteins, such as albumin and transferrin, can support the diagnosis of wasting. Serum albumin, however, is not a sensitive indicator of acute change in a client's nutritional status due to its long half-life. Pre-albumin, which has a half-life of approximately 2 days, is a much more sensitive indicator of acute changes in nutrition. Transferrin, a protein synthesized by the liver, is also a more sensitive indicator of nutritional status. Serum proteins must be interpreted with caution; they can be low when a client has liver disease, nephrotic syndrome, or neoplastic disease. In many HIV-negative clients, the CBC result can aid in diagnosis because the total lymphocyte count contains a reduced number of lymphocytes in cases of malnutrition. However, in HIV-positive clients, the result may not be helpful because of the decreased lymphocyte count resulting from the disease. Electrolytes are important to monitor because a shift of fluid and solutes occurs between the intracellular and extracellular spaces in cases of malnutrition. (Important parameters are listed in Table 19-3.)

---

*For a complete review of BIA the nurse is referred to Swanson B, Keithley JK: Bioelectrical impedance analysis (BIA) in HIV infection: principles and clinical application, *J Assoc Nurs AIDS Care* 9(1), 1998.

Clients with diarrhea should have stool studies done to determine if the cause of wasting is an infectious source (see Chapter 16 and Figure 16-1 for discussion of diarrhea). To measure intestinal absorption, the D-xylose test can be performed. Xylose is a pentose sugar passively and completely absorbed from the small intestines. The client is given 25 grams of D-xylose orally. Blood samples for D-xylose are drawn, both 1 and 2 hours after ingestion. If the small intestines are absorbing well, almost all of the ingested xylose should be present in the serum. When serum sample results are below 20 mg/dl, they indicate that the intestines are not absorbing sufficiently and malabsorption is present.

MEDICAL MANAGEMENT

If infection has been determined to be a contributing factor to the client's wasting, the provider should focus on eradication of the offending organism. Effective treatment of infections has been shown to improve a client's nutritional status[5]. Gastrointestinal (GI) parasites such as cryptosporidia and microsporidia may cause unrelenting diarrhea in clients and contribute to the client's wasting. There is no cure for these parasites, but the medications albendazole, thalidomide, nitazoxanide (NTZ), and azithromycin are being used in trials and, in some cases, may reduce the number and volume of stools.

The use of appetite stimulants such as megestrol acetate (Megace) or dronabinol (Marinol) may help. Megace is a synthetic progestogen used to treat breast and endometrial cancer. It has been shown to increase body weight, but clients tend to gain fat rather than muscle mass, which is usually what is wasted, especially in men.[3] Dronabinol, the major psychoactive component of marijuana, has been noted to increase appetite and improve weight in a number of clients.[11]

Testosterone can be administered when testosterone levels are low. It has been shown to help increase lean body mass and weight.[7] Testosterone is given by intramuscular injection or transdermal patches. To combat wasting and increase lean body mass, anabolic agents are also being used. This approach was used in a limited number of clients with AIDS, and it was found that anabolic therapy reversed weight loss, improved strength, and increased an individual's sense of well-being.[12] Examples of anabolic steroids are oxandrolone (Oxandrin) and nandrolone decanoate (Deca-Durabolin). Human growth hormone (Serostim) is associated with an increase in protoplasm and thus an increase in protein, causing a positive nitrogen balance. This was demonstrated in a study that found that human growth hormone reverses protein wasting and results in an increase in lean body mass and improved nitrogen balance.[13] When using anabolic agents, an exercise program is beneficial, especially strength training, as it maintains muscle tone and improves appetite. Anticytokine therapy is being tried to reduce weight loss. The drugs most often used are thalidomide (Synovir) and pentoxifylline (Trental). (See Table 19-4 for additional information on medications used in HIV wasting.)

Table 19-4	Medications Used in HIV Wasting		
Generic Name (Trade Name)	**Maximum Dose**	**Route**	**Most Common Side Effects**
Marinol (Dronabinol)	15 mg/kg per day	PO	Irritability, insomnia, mood changes, hallucinations, anxiety, vision changes, hypotension
Megestrol acetate (Megace)	1200 mg per day	PO	Impotence, altered menstrual pattern, acne, loss of scalp hair
Testosterone (Depo-Testosterone)	200 mg per week	IM	Bladder irritability, frequent erections, altered mood, edema, pain at injection site
Testosterone (Testoderm Transdermal)	6 mg per day	Scrotal patch	As testosterone above; also scrotal skin irritation
Testosterone (Androderm Transdermal patch)	5 mg per day	Two skin patches	As testosterone above; also skin erythema
Oxandrolone (Oxandrin)	20 mg per day	PO	Increased liver function tests, testicular atrophy, oligospermia
Nandrolone decanoate (Deca-Durabolin)	100 mg per week	IM	As oxandrolone
Thalidomide (Synovir)	50-100 mg per day	PO	Sedation, neuropathy, severe congenital abnormalities in developing fetuses
Pentoxifylline (Trental)	1200 mg per day	PO	GI disturbances, dizziness, tachycardia, flushing
Recombinant human growth hormone (Serostim)	6 mg per day	SC	Salt and water retention, carpal tunnel syndrome, increased intracranial pressure

NUTRITIONAL SUPPORT

Nutritional counseling is vital to ensure that clients eat a well-balanced diet, with attention paid to micronutrients and macronutrients. It is helpful to ask clients to keep a detailed food diary of all food and drink consumed (including snacks) to assess their nutritional status. When taste sensation is altered, avoiding extremes in food temperature (e.g., extremely cold or hot drinks) may be helpful. Foods with a strong aroma, such as those containing curry, should be avoided. Clients with mouth sores or pain should avoid citrus fruits, spices, and abrasive foods. Short-term dietary modifications are necessary for clients with temporary oral problems. Individualized meal plans often stimulate intake and cater to personal tastes. Small, frequent meals are less overwhelming than larger

Table 19-5	**Teaching the Client about Food Safety**

Activity/Food	Recommendations
Grocery Shopping	Do not buy food past expiration date. Do not buy cracked eggs. Avoid soft cheeses. Always make sure fish and meat are fresh.
Food Preparation	Wash hands thoroughly with warm water and soap before food preparation and after handling raw meat or fish. Do not touch mouth and eyes while handling raw meat or fish unless hands are washed. Counters should be washed thoroughly. Wash all fruits and vegetables; peel when possible. Thaw frozen food in the refrigerator and not on the counter. Use wooden chopping boards instead of plastic boards when possible. Research has shown that plastic boards retain microorganisms.[14]
Food Cooking	Make sure all meat and fish are well cooked. Avoid foods containing raw or partially cooked eggs.
Leftovers	Refrigerate leftovers as soon as possible after eating.
Water, Soft Drinks, Juices	If CD_4 cell count is below 100 cells/mm^3, boil water for 1 minute or use a water filter that screens out particles down to 1 micron to filter out cryptosporidia. If bottled water is used, it must come from underground wells or springs to be safe. Poland Springs and Deer Park brands make that claim. Commercially bottled soft drinks and seltzers are safe. Bottled juices are safe if they have been pasteurized.

ones. The best way to establish food tolerance is by trial and error. Client education about food safety is of paramount concern, since enteric infections in AIDS often relapse or prove untreatable (Table 19-5).

Clients with small intestinal disease and malabsorption should be encouraged to eat small, frequent meals that are low in fat, lactose, and fiber and high in calories. They should avoid caffeine, as it stimulates motility and fluid secretion, which worsens diarrhea. Alcohol should also be avoided; it has a diuretic effect, causing the loss of additional water. Lactase is one of the many digestive enzymes produced by the small intestine. Clients who are malabsorbing are unable to digest lactose and therefore should eat yogurt and other active cultures that can help break down lactose. Many nutrients, such as fat-soluble vitamins, magnesium, calcium and potassium, may not be absorbed, so supplements may be needed. Whenever the distal part of the ileum is involved, vitamin B_{12} levels need to be monitored because signs of B_{12} deficiency, such as neuropathy, can occur (see Chapter 22). Clients with colonic disease should be encouraged to eat small, frequent meals that are low in fiber, fat, and residue to minimize the number of bowel movements.

Enteral Feeding

When the dietary needs of individuals cannot be met by a well-balanced diet, oral supplements should be introduced. A dietitian can assess the most appropriate type of supplement by considering GI function, length of time that supplementation will be required, cost of therapy, and client acceptance. The GI tract is the preferred route for nutrient delivery to maintain the structural and functional integrity of the GI mucosa. Intestinal mucosa can become significantly atrophied if the client takes nothing by mouth for extended periods of time. Enteral formulas are effective as supplements to oral intake, or they can be used as the sole source of nutrition. Enteral products fall into three categories—elemental formulas, polymeric formulas, and modular formulas:

1. *Elemental* formulas consist predominantly of monosaccharides, amino acids, and ditriglycerides. They are low in fat and residue and free of lactose, so they require little digestion, thus promoting maximal absorption. This is an important consideration for clients with malabsorption. Examples of elemental formulas are Alatra and Peptamen.

2. *Polymeric* formulas contain complex carbohydrates and are higher in fat than elemental formulas. Examples include Advera, Sustacal, Ensure, and Nubasics.

3. *Modular* or *single-nutrient* formulas are tailored for specific nutrient needs. Examples are Renalcal for renal clients and Replete for wound healing.

Enteral formulas are usually given orally. When oral feeding is not possible, these formulas can be given via nasogastric tube or percutaneous endoscopic gastrostomy (PEG) feeding tube. It has been clearly demonstrated that enteral feeding does result in weight gain in malnourished clients.[15] In a study comparing the effects of enteral feeding of elemental formula with the effects of total parenteral nutrition in clients with malabsorption, little difference was found.[16] Enteral feeding is obviously preferable because the risk of infection is high with parenteral nutrition, and intestinal mucosa quickly becomes atrophied if not used.

Parenteral Feeding

TPN involves supplying nutritional requirements via catheter directly into the vascular system. TPN may be used as the sole source of nutrition when enteral feeding is not feasible, such as when the GI tract is not functioning. However, in one study it was found that response to nutritional support can depend on clinical circumstances. The study's authors concluded that body mass repletion was possible in clients with AIDS in whom malabsorption was the major pathogenetic factor in producing malnutrition but was less successful in clients with serious ongoing systemic diseases.[17]

A peripheral vein can be used to deliver TPN. Peripheral parenteral nutrition (PPN) is appropriate when short-term nutritional support is needed to preserve lean body mass. Central parenteral nutrition (CPN) (i.e., delivered via central vein) is reserved for clients with prolonged dysfunction of the GI tract.

WASTING IN THE ERA OF PROTEASE INHIBITORS

With recent advances in antiretroviral therapies and the prophylaxis and treatment of disease complications, the long-term outlook of clients with HIV has markedly improved. Serious malnutrition is less prevalent. However, nutritional status does not return completely to normal, and a syndrome of truncal obesity and metabolic abnormalities has been described and is of concern. Characteristic alterations in body composition, notably the development of truncal (visceral) obesity and subcutaneous fat loss on the limbs and face (lipodystrophy), as well as hyperlipidemia and insulin resistance, have been reported in both men and women.[18] The cause of these changes is unknown. The presence of central obesity, buffalo hump, hyperlipidemia, and insulin resistance is a familiar constellation of findings in clinical medicine and occurs in several well-characterized syndromes (e.g., syndrome X).[19] Its development during the course of an infectious disease (e.g., HIV infection) is distinctly unusual. The presence of these changes is usually a predictor of accelerated atherogenesis. Indeed, an increasing number of reports are describing the development of cardiac disease with myocardial infarction in young HIV-positive clients with these changes.[20]

There are two general hypotheses to explain the changes. The first states that the changes are a side effect of therapy with protease inhibitors,[21,22] suggesting that the changes are indirectly related to therapy and somehow unmasked by protease inhibitors (e.g., by abolishing viral replication or promoting partial immune reconstitution). The second hypothesis is that the changes may represent an altered stress response with mild chronic hypercortisolism in some clients.[23] This is especially relevant in people who have developed the changes in the absence of protease inhibitor therapy. The whole topic is currently under active investigation.

Wasting has a disastrous effect upon a client's quality of life and may cause a feeling of loss of control. The provider needs to focus on the cause and individualize the nutritional program according to the client's specific needs. The myriad nutritional problems mandate sensitivity, resourcefulness, and creativity. Reversing the process can improve quality of life, revive body image, and increase the client's sense of well-being.

REFERENCES

1. Kotler DP et al: The magnitude of body cell mass depletion in the timing of death from wasting in AIDS, *Am J Clin Nutr* 50:444, 1989.
2. Centers for Disease Control and Prevention: 1993 revised classification for HIV infection and expanded surveillance case definition for AIDS among adolescents and adults, *MMWR* 41(RR17):1, 1992.
3. Kotler D: Malnutrition in HIV infections and AIDS, *AIDS* 3:175, 1989.

4. Melchair J et al: Resting energy expenditure in HIV patients: comparison with and without infection, *Am J Clin Nutr* 57:614, 1993.

5. Kotler D, Tierney A, Altilio D: Nutritional consequences of ganciclovir therapy on CMV infection in AIDS, *Clin Res* 25:368, 1987.

6. Grunfield C, Feingold KR: The metabolic effects of tumor necrosis factor and other cytokines, *Biotherapy* 3:143, 1991.

7. Coodley C, Loveless M, Nelson H: Endocrine dysfunction in HIV wasting, *J AIDS* 7:46, 1994.

8. Rabkin J, Rabkin R, Wagner C: Illness stage, concurrent medications and correlates with low testosterone levels in HIV infected men, *AIDS Hum Retrovirus* 8:204, 1995.

9. Kotler D et al: Studies of body composition in patients with HIV, *Am J Clin Nutr* 42:1255, 1985.

10. Lewis SM, Collier IC, Heitkemper MM: Medical-surgical nursing: assessment and management of clinical problems, ed 5, St Louis, 2000, Mosby.

11. Gorter R, Seefriend M: Dronabinal effects on weight in patients with HIV, *AIDS* 6:127, 1992.

12. Fox M, Minot A, Liddle G: Oxandrolone: a potent anabolic steroid of novel configuration. *J Clin Endocrinol* 22:921, 1962.

13. Salman F, Ross C: Effects of treatment with human growth hormone on body composition and metabolism in adults, *N Engl J Med* 321:1797, 1989.

14. Raloff J: Wood wins, plastic trashed for cutting meat, *Science News*, 143:84, 1993.

15. Kotler D et al: Effects of enteral feeding upon body cell mass in AIDS, *Am J Clin Nutr* 51:1449, 1991.

16. Kotler D, Tierney A, Folgeman L: Comparison of TPN and a semi-elemental diet in patients with malabsorption, abstract presented at Vancouver International AIDS Conference, 1994, *J Parenteral Nutr* 22:120, 1998.

17. Kotler D, Culpepper-Morgan J, Tierney A: Effects of home TPN upon body composition in AIDS, *J Parenteral Nutr* 14:454, 1990.

18. Carr A, Samaras K, Burton S: A syndrome of peripheral lipodystrophy, hyperlipidemia and insulin resistance in HIV patients receiving protease inhibitors, *AIDS* 12:F51, 1998.

19. Bjorntorp P: Abdominal obesity and the development of non-insulin dependent diabetes mellitus, *Diabet Metab Rev* 4:615, 1998.

20. Henry K, Melroe H, Huebsch J: Severe premature coronary artery disease with protease inhibitors, *Lancet* 351:1328, 1998.

21. Miller KD, Jones E, Yanovski JA: Visceral abdominal fat accumulation associated with the use of indinavir therapy, *Lancet* 351:871, 1998.

22. Carr A, Semaras K, Chisolm DJ: Pathogenesis of HIV-1 protease inhibitor–associated peripheral lypodystrophy, hyperlipdemia, and insulin resistance, *Lancet* 131:1881, 1998.

23. Miller KK, Daly PA, Sentochnick D: Pseudo-Cushing's syndrome in HIV-infected patients, *Clin Infect Dis* 27:68, 1998.

20 HIV/AIDS and Pregnancy

Deborah Sherman
Neal Sherman

During the past decade, HIV infection has become a leading cause of morbidity and mortality among women. Women accounted for 18% of the total number of AIDS cases reported to the Centers for Disease Control and Prevention as of the end of 1999.[1] Heterosexual transmission of HIV is the most common route of transmission to women worldwide, while intravenous drug use is the most common risk factor for acquiring HIV among HIV-positive pregnant women in the United States.[2] The incidence of HIV infection in women of childbearing age had resulted in increasing numbers of children infected through perinatal (mother-to-infant) transmission.[3] Perinatally-acquired AIDS, however, declined steeply in the United States during the 1990s because of the rapid implementation of the use of zidovudine (AZT) to prevent perinatal transmission.[1] Both in the United States and worldwide, there are many HIV-positive women who receive inadequate health care and substandard prenatal care, which jeopardizes the health of both mother and newborn.[4]

UNDERSTANDING THE HEALTH RISKS

Many HIV-positive women face difficult choices regarding pregnancy. The decision to become pregnant or to continue a pregnancy, given their health status, can be a source of considerable stress. Discussions among the pregnant woman, HIV specialists, and the obstetrician are important so that the woman understands the risk of perinatal HIV transmission (PHT) to the fetus or newborn, the potential effects of antiretroviral drugs on the fetus and newborn, and the recommended treatment to promote the mother's own health. Women should be informed that without treatment, there is a 20% to 30% chance of transmitting HIV infection to their fetus during pregnancy, labor, delivery, and breastfeeding, but that this risk can be reduced by two-thirds by taking the antiretroviral drug zidovudine (ZDV)[3] and by careful monitoring of maternal and fetal health through prenatal care. HIV-positive women should also avoid breastfeeding.

With the increasing incidence of HIV infection in women of childbearing age, health care providers are concerned about the effect of pregnancy on HIV progression, as well as the influence of disease on pregnancy outcomes. According to the American Medical Association, there is no evidence to date that suggests that HIV infection makes pregnancy more difficult to manage.[5] Furthermore, pregnancy does not appear to influence the rate of progression of HIV disease despite adjustments for age, exposure groups, CD_4 cell count or use of treatment.[6] Clearly the decision to use antiretroviral therapy to treat HIV-positive pregnant women must include consideration of the woman's health status, history of antiretroviral use, and personal choices regarding the risk to the fetus.[4]

HIV COUNSELING, TESTING, AND RELATED DECISIONS

In 1994, the results of a multicentered, randomized double-blind clinical trial (ACTG 076) demonstrated that ZVD chemoprophylaxis could reduce perinatal HIV-1 transmission by nearly 70%.[3] The U.S. Public Health Service therefore encourages all women to ascertain their HIV status through counseling and voluntary testing, ideally before becoming pregnant. Decisions related to infection and pregnancy include choices of continuation or termination, as well as choices regarding antiretroviral medications. Health providers should inform women that a child, at birth, will carry the mother's HIV-positive antibodies, and therefore may test falsely positive for infection if only antibody testing is done. Children usually lose their mother's antibodies by 18 months of age, and can be tested at that time to determine their own HIV-antibody status. HIV culture and polymerase chain reaction (PCR) tests can provide parents a definitive answer as to the HIV status of the infant within 48 hours of life. (See Chapter 21 for a discussion of HIV testing in newborns). Given the uncertainty of the fetus' HIV status, abortion should not be presumed to be the preferred option. Health care providers should provide a climate that allows open deliberation regarding the pregnancy, which includes discussion of personal, medical, economic, and religious issues; the risks of infection to the neonate; and the risks to the mother's own health. Women should also be informed of the factors related to disease progression in the neonate, including the timing of perinatal infection, the viral load, the newborn's immune response, and the virulence of the virus itself.[2] Early onset of symptoms and rapid progression of the disease in infants have been associated with high levels of plasma HIV RNA at birth and during the first 6 months of life, rapid and sustained loss of CD_4 cells, and in utero HIV infection.[2] Women should also be aware that HIV-positive children are at greater risk for health problems, developmental difficulties, and severe childhood illnesses. It should be reinforced that regardless of the demands of caring for her child, an HIV-positive mother must consider her own health and personal need for treatment. Maintaining the health of the mother is extremely important to the well-being of the newborn and family.

RISK FACTORS RELATED TO PHT

Viral, immunologic, and clinical factors in both mother and infant play a role in the process of vertical transmission from mother to baby. Evidence supports that the transmission of the HIV infection occurs in utero (before birth), intrapartum (during labor and delivery), and postpartum (after birth—breastfeeding).[2] *Early transmission* of the virus is defined as detection of HIV infection within the first 48 hours of life, followed by confirmation after the neonatal period (the first 28 days of life). *Late transmission* is defined as negative virologic evaluations during the first week of life, followed by HIV detection between 7 and 90 days of age.[7] Although the exact mechanisms associated with PHT are still unknown, it is believed that most PHT occurs during labor and delivery.[7] For those transmissions that occur in utero, the timing of the infection remains uncertain, though evidence suggests that infection most often occurs in late gestation.[3]

The risk of PHT is associated with a number of factors. Several studies have shown that women with advanced HIV disease, as evidenced by higher viral loads (greater than 50,000 copies/ml), are more likely to transmit HIV infection to their infants. Analysis of data from 551 participants in the NIH-sponsored Women's and Infants Transmission Study has recently confirmed that a lower viral load correlates with a lower risk of vertical transmission. In this study, among women receiving ZDV, the incidence of maternal HIV transmission ranged from 0% for the 22 women whose viral load was less than 1000 copies/ml to a high of 31.3% for those with 50,000 to 100,000 copies/ml. For women not receiving ZDV, none of the 35 women with a viral load of less than 1000 copies/ml transmitted the infection, while 31.6% of women with viral loads between 50,000 to 100,000 copies/ml and 68% of women with a viral load exceeding 100,000 copies/ml transmitted the infection. The findings suggest that aggressive treatment to lower the viral load in pregnant clients could reduce the risk of PHT.[8] This finding contrasts with former studies indicating that PHT occurs across a broad range of viral loads, including low levels of HIV RNA.[3] The immunologic status of the woman is also normally compromised during pregnancy. However, in the presence of HIV disease, a low CD_4 cell count (less than 200 cells/mm^3) is recognized as an additional risk factor for PHT. As with viral load, however, PHT has been shown to occur in low to high ranges of CD_4 counts. The current recommendation is therefore to regard high viral loads and low CD_4 cell counts, though not necessarily conclusive in terms of PHT risk, as indicators of the need for antiretroviral therapy to promote the mother's health.[9]

Additional risk factors in the progression of HIV disease and PHT are the presence of untreated sexually transmitted diseases (STDs) in women and their partners, as well as maternal intravenous drug use. Early detection and treatment of STDs, as well as counseling to reduce addiction behaviors in pregnancy, must be a priority of prenatal care.

Of further concern is the use of invasive obstetrical procedures during pregnancy and birth that may promote the transmission of HIV to the fetus. Specifically, fetal scalp blood sampling and the use of internal fetal monitoring during labor may increase the risk of PHT; lacerations of the neonate's skin may facilitate the transmission of HIV from infected maternal body fluids. Amniocentesis, external version, and forceps or vacuum extraction also place the fetus at increased risk of contact with maternal blood and therefore should be avoided in pregnancies complicated by HIV infection. Several studies also indicate that the rupture of a woman's membranes for more than 4 hours is associated with a significantly increased risk of PHT transmission. Therefore, it is recommended that labor not be artificially induced in HIV-positive women. Researchers have also examined the relationship between the route of delivery, specifically vaginal delivery versus cesarean section, and the associated risk of PHT. Data from the Twelfth World AIDS Conference (Geneva, 1998) indicates, based on two European studies, that elective cesarean section combined with ZDV treatment in pregnancy decreased the risk of vertical HIV transmission.[10-12] Furthermore, the results of a metaanalysis, which used data of individual clients from 15 prospective cohort studies to examine the mode of delivery and the risk of vertical transmission, indicate that elective cesarean section reduces the risk of transmission of HIV-1 from mother to child independently of the effects of treatment with ZDV. If clinicians were able to treat all HIV-positive pregnant women with ZDV and deliver the babies by elective cesarean section, the risk of PHT would be reduced to just 2%. Pregnant women infected with HIV-1 should be advised of the potential benefit of elective cesarean section and the risks associated with surgical delivery.[13]

During labor and delivery, health care providers must be reminded of the need for strict adherence to universal blood and body fluid precautions to prevent work-related HIV exposure. Water repellent gowns, goggles, gloves, and masks should be used for all deliveries and cesarean sections. Mouth-operated mucus traps to suction newborns of secretions must not be used and wall suction pressure should be kept under 140 mm Hg.[9]

MANAGEMENT OF HIV INFECTION IN PREGNANT WOMEN

Combination antiretroviral therapy is the recommended standard of care for nonpregnant HIV-positive women with a CD_4 cell count less than 500 cells/mm^3 and a viral load of HIV RNA greater than 10,000 copies/ml, or for women with clinical symptoms of HIV disease (see Chapter 4).[3] Guidelines suggest that optimal antiretroviral therapy and its initiation in pregnancy should be based on the woman's virologic and immunologic status, and that such therapy should not be withheld due to pregnancy, regardless of gestational age.[14]

The choice of antiretrovirals for the treatment of HIV-positive pregnant women does, however, require unique considerations, given the physiologic changes of pregnancy. Alterations in dosing requirements may be needed because of potential changes in drug absorption, distribution, biotransformation, and elimination. Furthermore, consideration must be given to the potential effects of agents on the fetus and newborn, although to date, safety studies regarding teratogenicity, mutagenicity, or carcinogenicity are unavailable for the majority of antiretroviral medications.[3] The potential harm to the fetus from the ingestion of antiviral drugs depends not only of the drug itself, but also on the dosage, gestational age at exposure, duration of exposure, interaction with other agents to which the fetus is exposed, and the genetic makeup of the mother and fetus.[3]

Contingent upon the assessment of the woman's health status and the potential risks of delaying therapy, a woman who is not on anti-retroviral therapy may be advised to delay the initiation of therapy in the first trimester of pregnancy. Antiretroviral therapy would then be administered after 14 weeks of pregnancy; that is, following the period of rapid organogenesis during which the embryo is most susceptible to the teratogenic effects of drugs. Additionally, nausea and vomiting, which are frequent symptoms of early pregnancy, may adversely affect the woman's ability to take and adequately absorb oral medications in the first trimester, and therefore are factors in determining the initiation of antiretroviral therapy.

Women who have begun antiretroviral therapy before pregnancy often express concern regarding the effects of medications on fetal growth and development, and thereby may elect to stop therapy in an attempt to protect their fetus. In a discussion of this concern, health providers should emphasize that there is insufficient data regarding teratogenic effects of the medications on the fetus and infant. It must also be explained that there is a significant possibility of rebound of the woman's viral load during the period of discontinuation of treatment, which presents an increased risk of PHT to the fetus, as well as the potential progression of HIV disease in the mother.[3] Women should be further informed that, if they discontinue antiretroviral medications for any reason, agents should be stopped simultaneously—and reinstituted simultaneously—to prevent the development of viral resistance.

ZDV—THE GOLD STANDARD IN PREVENTING PHT

To date the only drug shown in large studies to reduce the risk of PHT is ZDV, also referred to as AZT. In recent studies, nevirapine—given in a single dose, to both HIV-positive women and their newborn infants—also reduced PHT. ZDV prophylaxis given during the antenatal, intrapartum, and neonatal periods has been shown to consistently result in a 65% to 75% reduction in PHT rates, with no serious consequences to the mother. This risk reduction occurs regardless of the woman's viral load or CD_4 cell count. Therefore, researchers urge that health providers offer ZDV therapy to all pregnant HIV-positive women, regardless of the stage of disease.[3] Researchers believe that ZDV works by protecting the fetus against HIV infection. ZDV also has some ability to lower the maternal plasma viral load, though this is not considered the primary factor in the drug's efficacy. Researchers speculate that the effect of ZDV in reducing perinatal transmission may be due in part to the presence of the drug in utero at the time of delivery, providing the fetus with preexposure prophylaxis.[3] An expert panel convened by the National Institutes of Health in January 1997 concluded that the benefits of ZDV in reducing the risk of perinatal transmission outweighed the hypothetical risks of transplacental carcinogenesis.

Table 20-1	ACTG 076 Guidelines for ZDV Administration During Pregnancy

Pregnancy	Dosage and Timing of ZDV Administration
Antepartum	ZDV 100 mg PO five times daily (initiated at 13 to 34 weeks of gestation and continued throughout the pregnancy)
Labor and Delivery	ZDV, administered IV during labor in a 1-hour loading dose of 2 mg/kg of body weight **then** continuous infusion of 1 mg/kg of body weight per hour until delivery
Neonatal	ZDV, administered PO to the newborn in the first 6 weeks of life (ZDV syrup dose of 2 mg/kg of body weight q6h)

In accordance with the ACTOG 076 Guidelines, ZDV is administered as outlined in Table 20-1.[3] Given its effectiveness in reducing PHT, ZDV should be included as a component of all combination antenatal regimens. If a woman's personal choice or history of toxicity to ZDV precludes its antenatal use, intrapartum and/or newborn ZDV should still be recommended. Women who have a CD_4 cell count greater than 500 cells/mm^3 and a plasma HIV RNA count between 10,000 and 20,000 copies/ml can be offered ZDV as single-drug therapy during pregnancy; they are less likely to experience viral resistance because of limited viral replication and time-limited exposure to the drug.[3] However, for women with advanced disease or higher levels of HIV RNA, a combination antiretroviral regimen that includes ZDV is more effective in reducing the chance of resistance, reducing the risk of transmission to the fetus, and promoting the health of the mother, compared with the use of ZDV prophylaxis alone.[3] This is further supported by recent research, presented in Geneva at the Twelfth World AIDS Conference, that indicates that the use of triple drug antiretroviral combinations in pregnancy improves maternal health and reduces the rates of maternal-to-fetal transmission of HIV to a near-zero level.[15]

Given the minimal data available on the pharmacokinetics and safety of antiretroviral agents during pregnancy, choices should be individualized and based on available data from preclinical and clinical drug testing. 3TC, an antiretroviral, has been studied and appears to be well tolerated by pregnant women, demonstrating an ability to cross the placenta adequately. All nucleosides, except didanosine (ddI), have been tested in preclinical animal studies, which have indicated potential fetal risk and are classified as FDA pregnancy category C. In cases in which a woman has more advanced disease and for clients who are ZDV-experienced, many practitioners consider the combination therapy of ZDV and 3TC, given that this combination has the largest body of safety data. Preclinical and clinical data relevant to the use of antiretrovirals during pregnancy is presented on Table 20-2.

Table 20-2 Preclinical and Clinical Data Relevant to the Use of Antiretrovirals in Pregnancy

Antiretroviral Drug	FDA Pregnancy Category	Placental Passage (Newborn: Maternal Drug Ratio)	Long-term Animal Carcinogenicity Studies
Nucleoside Analogue Reverse Transcriptase Inhibitors (NRTIs)			
Zidovudine (ZDV)	C	Yes (human) [0.85]	Positive (in rodents, noninvasive vaginal epithelial tumors)
Zalcitabine (ddC)	C	Yes (rhesus) [0.30-0.50]	Positive (in rodents, thymic lymphomas)
Didanosine (ddI)	B	Yes (human) [0.5]	Negative (no tumors in lifetime rodent study)
Stavudine (d4T)	C	Yes (rhesus) [0.76]	Not completed
Lamivudine (3TC)	C	Yes (human) [~1.0]	Negative (no tumors in lifetime rodent study)
Nonnucleoside Reverse Transcriptase Inhibitors (NNRTIs)			
Nevirapine	C	Yes (human) [~1.0]	Not completed
Delavirdine	C	Unknown	Not completed
Protease Inhibitors (PIs)			
Indinavir	C	Yes (rats) Significant in rats, but low in rabbits	Not completed
Ritonavir	B	Yes (rats) [Mid-term fetus, 1.15; late term fetus, 0.15-0.64]	Not completed
Saquinavir	B	Unknown	Not completed
Nelfinavir	B	Unknown	Not completed

FDA pregnancy risk categories:

A Adequate and well-controlled studies of pregnant women fail to demonstrate a risk to the fetus during the first trimester of pregnancy (and there is no evidence of risk during later trimesters).

B Animal reproduction studies fail to demonstrate a risk to the fetus; adequate and well-controlled studies of pregnant women have not been conducted.

C Safety in human pregnancy has not been demonstrated and animal studies are either positive for fetal risk or have not been conducted; the drug should not be used unless the potential benefit outweighs the potential risk to the fetus.

D Positive evidence of human fetal risk based on adverse reaction data from investigational or marketing experiences; the potential benefits from the use of the drugs in pregnant women may be acceptable despite its potential risks.

X Studies in animals or reports of adverse reactions have indicated that the risk associated with the use of the drug for pregnant women clearly outweighs any possible benefit.

From Centers for Disease Control and Prevention: Public Health Service Task Force recommendations for the use of antiretroviral drugs in pregnant women infected with HIV-1 for maternal health and for reducing perinatal HIV-1 transmission in the United States, *MMWR CDC Morbid Mortal Wkly Rep* 47:1, 1998.

NNRTIS AND PIS IN PREGNANCY

Of the nonnucleoside reverse transcriptase inhibitors (NNRTIs), only nevirapine has been evaluated for use in pregnancy. Nevirapine is administered as a single 200 mg oral dose to the mother at the onset of labor and as a single dose to the infant of 2 mg per kg of weight at 2 or 3 days of age. Although data indicate that nevirapine is well tolerated as a single dose, crosses the placenta, and achieves neonatal blood concentrations equivalent to those in maternal blood, its mean half-life is longer than in nonpregnant women. The consequences for the mother and fetus are unknown.

Currently studies of combination therapy with protease inhibitors are being conducted in pregnant HIV-positive women to determine drug dosage, safety, and tolerance. In adults, indinavir is associated with hyperbilirubinemia and renal stones. This may also be problematic for the neonate if placental passage occurs or if the mother is given the drug close to the end of labor. Given the immaturity of the neonate's liver and the resultant increase in the half-life of indinavir, there is the potential for exacerbation of physiologic neonatal hyperbilirubinemia. Furthermore, given immature neonatal renal function and delayed elimination, theoretically the neonate may be predisposed to renal stones.[9] Although carcinogenicity and toxicity studies have been conducted on rats and mice using saquinavir and ritonavir, there are no well-controlled studies of these drugs in pregnant women.[3] It is further noted that ritonavir is associated with significant gastrointestinal upset, which may be particularly problematic given the occurrence of nausea in early pregnancy.

For a woman being treated with protease inhibitors before her pregnancy, the continuance of such agents in pregnancy is questionable given the lack of safety data. Nonetheless, the concern with discontinuance is the possibility of an increase in maternal viral load and the potential risk of developing viral resistance. The conservative approach may therefore be to delay initiation of protease inhibitors in early pregnancy, but this will depend on maternal health status.

An additional consideration in the use of protease inhibitors in pregnancy is the associated onset of diabetes mellitus or hyperglycemia or the exacerbation of existing diabetes mellitus in HIV-positive clients. This is particularly important given the adverse effects of gestational diabetes on the health of fetuses and neonates. Therefore, close monitoring of the glucose levels of HIV-positive women taking protease inhibitors is warranted, as is teaching the client the signs of hyperglycemia.[7]

The various clinical situations and recommendations for use of antiretrovirals to reduce PHT are presented in Table 20-3, including recommendations for (1) HIV-positive women without prior antiretroviral therapy, (2) HIV-positive women receiving antiretroviral therapy during a current pregnancy, (3) the use of antiretrovirals in HIV-positive women

Table 20-3	Clinical Situations and Recommendations for Use of Antiretroviral Drugs to Reduce PHT

Scenario	Recommendations for Use of Antiretroviral Therapy
HIV-positive pregnant women without prior antiretroviral therapy	HIV-positive pregnant women must receive standard clinical, immunologic, and virologic evaluation, and recommendations for the initiation and choice of antiretroviral therapy should be based on the same parameters used in nonpregnant individuals, with consideration and discussion of the known and unknown risks and benefits of such therapy during pregnancy.
	The 3-part regimen, which includes ZDV, should be recommended for all HIV-positive pregnant women to reduce the risk of perinatal HIV transmission (PHT). Women who are in the first trimester of pregnancy may wish to consider delaying initiation of therapy until at least after 10-12 weeks of gestation.
HIV-positive women receiving antiretroviral therapy during a current pregnancy	HIV-positive women receiving antiretroviral therapy in whom pregnancy is identified after the first trimester should continue therapy.
	Women receiving antiretroviral therapy in whom pregnancy is recognized during the first trimester should be counseled regarding the benefits and potential risks of antiretroviral administration during this period. Discontinuation of therapy should be considered.
	If therapy is discontinued during the first trimester, all drugs should be stopped simultaneously to avoid development of resistance.
	If the current therapeutic regimen does not contain ZDV, the addition of ZDV or substitution of ZDV for another nucleoside analogue antiretroviral is recommended after 14 weeks gestation. Intrapartum and newborn ZDV administration is recommended regardless of the antepartum antiretroviral regimen.
HIV-positive women in labor who have had no prior therapy	Administration of intrapartum intravenous ZDV should be recommended along with the 6-week newborn ZDV regimen.
	In the immediate postpartum period, the woman should undergo appropriate assessments (e.g., CD_4 cell count, HIV RNA copy count) to determine whether antiretroviral therapy is recommended for her own health.
Infants born to mothers who have received no antiretroviral therapy during pregnancy or intrapartum	The 6-week neonatal ZDV component of the ZDV chemoprophylaxis regimen should be discussed with mothers and offered for the newborn.
	ZDV should be initiated as soon as possible after birth, preferably within 12-24 hours after birth.
	Some clinicians may choose to use ZDV in combination with other antiretroviral drugs, particularly if the mother is known or suspected to be infected with ZDV-resistant virus. However, the efficacy of this approach is unknown for prevention of transmission and appropriate dosing regimen for neonates is incompletely defined.
	In the immediate postpartum period, the woman should undergo appropriate assessments (e.g., CD_4 cell count, HIV RNA copy count) to determine whether antiretroviral therapy is recommended for her own health.

From Centers for Disease Control and Prevention: Public Health Service Task Force recommendations for the use of antiretroviral drugs in pregnant women infected with HIV-1 for maternal health and for reducing perinatal HIV-1 transmission in the United States, *MMWR CDC Morbid Mortal Wkly Rep* 47:1, 1998.

in labor without a history of prior therapy, and (4) the use of antiretrovirals in infants born to mothers who have received no antiretroviral therapy during pregnancy or the intrapartum period.

CURRENT DRUG TRIALS

It is expected that combination antiretroviral regimens will become the standard of care in preventing PHT, as opposed to ZDV monotherapy. However, there are several considerations, specifically the increased risk of side effects, high cost of therapy, and complexity of the dosing schedule. There are several combinations of antiretroviral regimens that are now used in the standard care of women with HIV infection and that are being evaluated for their ability to prevent PHT. Such trials[4] include:

- ACTG 353: nelfinavir, ZDV, and 3TC
- ACTG 354: ritonavir, ZDV, and 3TC
- ACTG 357: abacavir, ZDV, and 3TC
- ACTG 358: indinavir, ZDV, and 3TC

MONITORING MATERNAL/FETAL HEALTH AND HIV PROGRESSION

PRENATAL CARE

1. A complete history should be taken during the initial evaluation of an HIV-positive pregnant woman, specifically:

   Menstrual history—including cycle length, duration and characteristics of menstrual flow, date of last menstrual period, and previous methods of contraception;

   Medical history—including history of STDs and symptoms of HIV/ AIDS, as well as family and genetic history;

   Obstetric history—including numbers of previous pregnancies, numbers of miscarriages or terminations, pregnancy and labor or delivery complications and outcomes, and neonatal outcomes;

   Social history—including occupational hazards, involvement of the father, expectations related to childbearing and childrearing, support system, and potential stressors, including financial status; and

   Habits—including alcohol and drug use, diet, and exercise.

2. Physical Examination—Height, weight, vital signs, examination of the thyroid, breast examination, and cardiovascular, respiratory, and abdominal assessments

3. Pelvic examination—Assessment of the external genitalia, vagina, and cervix for signs of STDs, performance of a bimanual examination to rule out adnexal abnormalities, and determination of uterine size and any deviations

4. Laboratory data—Tests for the initial visit and during pregnancy, as follows:

   - Initial visit—Pap test, complete blood count, urinalysis, screen for bacteriuria, ABO blood type, RH type, antibody screen, Venereal

Disease Research Laboratory (VDRL) test for syphilis, rubella antibody titer, and hepatitis B surface antigen (HBsAg); cervical cultures for gonorrhea and chlamydia, toxoplasmosis antibody testing, tuberculin skin testing, and cytomegalovirus titers should also be performed.[13] The American College of Obstetricians and Gynecologists' recommended intervals for routine and indicated tests during pregnancy[13] are:

Time (weeks)	Assessment
8-18	Ultrasonography
	Serum alpha fetoprotein (AFP)
	B human chorionic gonadotropin (B-HCG)
24-28	Blood glucose screen following 50 g of oral glucose
	Repeat antibody test of unsensitized D-negative clients
	Prophylactic administration of immune globulin D
32-36	Ultrasonography
	Repeat syphilis and gonorrhea screening
	Repeat hemoglobin or hematocrit measurement

5. Expected weight gain in pregnancy is 2 to 5 lbs in the first trimester and ¾ to 1 lb per week thereafter, with a total weight gain of an average of 25 to 35 lbs.[13]

INITIAL EVALUATION AND MONITORING OF HIV-POSITIVE PREGNANT WOMEN

In addition to the routine and recommended tests of pregnancy, initial evaluation and monitoring of an HIV-positive pregnant woman should include an assessment of HIV disease status by CD_4 cell count and of risk of disease progression by viral load—HIV RNA copy number, history of prior or current antiretroviral therapy, and determination of gestational age of the fetus.[3]

Normal physiologic changes experienced during pregnancy further confound the monitoring of HIV-positive pregnant clients. Normal variations in CD_4 cell counts during pregnancy may reflect physiologic changes, thereby making it difficult to determine the risk of opportunistic infections or the progression to AIDS. As such, CD_4 percentages appear to be more stable and accurate indicators of immune system functioning in pregnancy.[3]

The correlation of HIV RNA with disease progression in nonpregnant women suggests that HIV RNA should also be monitored closely. It is therefore recommended that CD_4 cell counts and HIV RNA levels be obtained every 3 to 4 months, or approximately once every trimester of pregnancy, to determine the need for initiation or alteration of antiretroviral therapy. As CD_4 counts become lower, prophylaxis against organisms, such as *Toxoplasma gondii* and *Mycobacterium avium*, should also be considered. It has been further documented that women, despite undetectable plasma HIV RNA, may have detectable HIV RNA levels in the genital tract. Therefore, plasma HIV RNA levels may not be an adequate indicator of risk to infants delivered vaginally.[3]

Women who are receiving ZDV in pregnancy should also be monitored monthly for associated hematologic and liver chemistry abnormalities. Hemoglobin of less than 8 g/dl, an absolute neutrophil count of less than 750 cells/μL, or aspartate aminotransferase (AST) or alanine aminotransferase (ALT) greater than five times the normal upper limit indicates ZDV toxicity, which may require interruption or cessation of ZDV use.[7] Antepartum fetal monitoring for women who receive only ZDV should be performed as clinically indicated; there is no evidence of increased risk of fetal complications. However, given the unknown effects of the drugs on pregnancy, women who are receiving combination antiretroviral therapy require more intensive monitoring with the use of level II ultrasound and continued assessment of fetal growth and well-being.[3]

CONCERNS RELATED TO POSTPARTUM—THE PHT RISK OF BREASTFEEDING

Comprehensive care and support services for HIV-positive women and their families should be made available in the postpartum period. Coordinated care between the client, the HIV specialist, and the obstetrician should continue with a focus on the continuity of antiretroviral treatment for those receiving combination therapy, or on the initiation of such treatment for women who only received ZDV chemoprophylaxis during pregnancy.

It should be noted that isolation of clients and their infants from other clients and staff is not recommended. However, universal precautions should be used for all interactions between women, newborns, and staff during the postpartum period to protect the health provider from infected blood and body fluids, including vaginal secretions and breast milk.[13]

Furthermore, worldwide studies indicate that breastfeeding is a significant cause of PHT with the risk estimated between 14% and 22% in some developing countries.[4] Studies conducted in South Africa indicate that breastfeeding until 18 months of age doubles the risk of PHT, as compared with formula feeding. Guidelines from the Centers for Disease Control and Prevention (CDC) strongly suggest the avoidance of breastfeeding in women who are HIV-positive.[3] Currently, there is interest in the timing of transmission through breastfeeding; that is, whether PHT is more likely to occur in the time immediately following birth, when the newborn may be breastfed, or during subsequent months in infants who are breastfed in the first year of life.

In light of concern about the role of breastfeeding in PHT, there are new initiatives to examine alternatives, specifically formula feeding and a reduction in breastfeeding duration to 6 months or less, particularly in underdeveloped countries. However, several factors make formula feeding an undesirable alternative, particularly in developing countries. These factors include the cost of maintaining a supply of infant formula and teaching mothers the techniques of bottle feeding to prevent infant colic, as well as maintaining a hygienically appropriate environment to prepare formula, including the ability to boil water and to mix the formula, and having clean water to wash the bottles. Unfortunately, to date there are no treatments to eradicate the HIV virus in breastmilk.

IDENTIFICATION AND TREATMENT OF STDS, CERVICAL DYSPLASIA, AND OPPORTUNISTIC INFECTIONS

The early identification and treatment of STDs is important for the health of the woman and her fetus or newborn. Pregnant women with primary genital herpes have a high rate of complications, particularly in the third trimester, including premature labor, intrauterine growth retardation, and congenital infection.[16] The treatment most often recommended for genital herpes is acyclovir. Data on human experience with acyclovir indicate no increased risk of birth defects to date in infants with in utero exposure.[13]

As the most commonly transmitted STD in the United States, chlamydia has been associated with preterm delivery and premature rupture of membranes. Pregnant women may be treated with 500 mg erythromycin base, or erythromycin ethylsuccinate, 800 mg orally four times daily for 7 days; or with amoxicillin, 500 mg orally three times daily for 7 days.

Given that gonorrhea and trichomoniasis are believed to be cofactors for increased sexual transmission and the progression of HIV, reassessment for these diseases is suggested during the last trimester of pregnancy. Gonorrhea is treated in pregnancy with ceftriaxone, 125 mg intramuscular (IM) injection in a single dose, or with cefixime 400 mg orally in a single dose. For clients who cannot tolerate a cephalosporin, spectinomycin 2 g IM can be given in a single dose. Vaginal trichomoniasis has also been associated with preterm delivery and premature rupture of membranes. The only approved treatment for trichomoniasis is oral metronidazole, but it is not recommended in the first trimester of pregnancy. After the first trimester, women may be treated with a single dose, 2 g orally.[16]

Bacterial vaginosis is not strictly classified as an STD. Pregnant women who are symptomatic can be treated in the first trimester with clindamycin cream (2%), one full applicator (5 g) intravaginally at bedtime for 7 days, or 300 mg orally twice daily for 7 days.[16] Clindamycin cream is recommended instead of the oral regimen because it limits fetal exposure to the medication. After the first trimester, metronidazole, 250 mg orally three times daily or 500 mg orally twice daily for 7 days, can be used for treatment. Alternatively, metronidazole 2 g orally in a single dose or clindamycin, 300 mg orally twice daily for 7 days, can be used.[16]

For women with advanced maternal HIV disease, studies indicate that higher viral loads (greater than 10,000 copies/ml) are more often associated with cancer-causing types of human papillomavirus (HPV). It is therefore recommended that women with higher viral loads should be more aggressively monitored for the development of precancerous cervical changes by Pap testing, followed by colposcopy if the results are abnormal.[3] See Chapter 8 for a discussion of HPV and precancerous cervical changes.

Protecting HIV-positive women from opportunistic infections during pregnancy is also of significant concern. The most frequent opportunistic infection seen in clients with AIDS is *Pneumocystis carinii* pneumonia. The risks of this infection to a pregnant woman far outweigh the risks to the fetus. Prophylaxis is therefore indicated in pregnant clients with CD_4 cell counts less than 200 cells/mm^3 and in those with symptoms of thrush or unexplained fever for greater than 2 weeks, regardless of CD_4 level. The U.S. Public Health Service Task Force recommends trimethoprim-sulfamethoxazole (TMP-SMX), administered daily as one double-strength tablet, as the first-line agent for prophylaxis against *P. carinii* pneumonia. Several alternative agents are available for TMP-SMX–intolerant clients with mild disease, such as atovaquone and clindamycin plus primaquine. These drugs have not been shown to be teratogenic to the fetus.[9]

Toxoplasmosis, an opportunistic infection caused by *T. gondii,* can be life threatening for both mother and fetus. However, tests for toxoplasmosis in pregnancy frequently indicate false positives, which may lead the practitioner to believe, erroneously, that a pregnant woman has been recently infected; antitoxoplasma antibody tests should be interpreted with caution. Before counseling a woman regarding risks to the fetus and the possibility of abortion, the FDA advisory board suggests repeated blood testing to differentiate recent from old infections. Toxoplasmosis should be treated with sulfadiazine and pyrimethamine isethionate.[9]

Another opportunistic infection commonly affecting HIV-positive women is vaginal candidiasis. (See Chapter 14 for a discussion of candidiasis). Pregnant women who are symptomatic of vaginal candidiasis should be treated with a topical antifungal medication.[14]

HIV-positive pregnant clients should also receive pneumococcal, influenza, and hepatitis B vaccinations.[9]

OTHER INTERVENTIONS FOR THE PREVENTION OF PHT

Testing is underway to identify antiviral agents for topical use.[4] For example, studies are examining the effect of vaginal and newborn cleaning after birth with an antiseptic solution of chlorhexidine. However, early results have produced conflicting findings. In one study, it was shown that 0.25% solution of chlorhexidine reduced the rate of PHT for women whose membranes ruptured for greater than 4 hours,[4] while another reported no effect in terms of PHT, based on a large sample of women in Africa.[2]

Immune-based therapies are also being investigated in an efficacy trial involving both HIV-positive women and their infants. In the ACTG

185 protocol, pregnant, HIV-positive women were rand
either ZDV with intravenous gamma immunoglobulin or Z
intravenous gamma immunoglobulin. Results indicate that there
tistically significant difference between groups with regard to PHT.

SUPPORTING THE IMMUNE SYSTEM
OF A HIV-POSITIVE PREGNANT WOMAN

Because of the concomitant negative effect of HIV disease and pregnancy on CD_4 functioning, support of the immune system is an extremely important consideration in women infected with the HIV virus who are pregnant. Perinatal education should include stress management, exercise, nutrition, and avoidance of alcohol, drugs, and smoking.

Stress management should be a focus of care to avoid the negative effect of stress on the immune system and the potential progression of the disease under conditions of duress. Assessment of the physical and emotional indicators and the identification of sources of stress are priorities. When women are anxious they tend to overbreathe or hyperventilate, which causes a carbon dioxide and oxygen imbalance that can be detrimental to the well-being of both mother and fetus. Symptoms of hyperventilation often include tingling sensations in the face and fingers and dizziness. Slow, deep breathing can assist the mother in regaining carbon dioxide balance. Use of relaxation techniques during pregnancy and labor are important in maintaining a sense of control and allaying the normal anxieties associated with pregnancy and delivery. Teaching clients problem-solving strategies, ways of reducing environmental causes of stress, and ways of managing stress through such techniques as imagery, relaxation exercises, biofeedback, music, yoga, massage, support groups, talking with family and friends, and therapy can also be very important in coping with the stresses of pregnancy.[17]

As with pregnant women, HIV-positive individuals have a number of physical and psychological stressors that contribute to a high rate of metabolism. In addition, physical inactivity and psychological factors contribute to muscle wasting, weakness, and fatigue.[18] Therefore, mild to moderate exercise during pregnancy is important for reducing stress, promoting muscle strength, improving circulation, and releasing the body's natural endorphins, which promote a sense of wellness both during pregnancy and as a part of the overall treatment program for individuals with HIV.[18] Furthermore, exercise has also been correlated with a transient increase in CD_4 cells and a reduction in opportunistic infections in clients with all stages of HIV infection.[18,19]

Although pregnant women can usually continue any exercise they performed before pregnancy, it is recommended that they not begin new sports during pregnancy. Exercise is recommended three times a week for approximately 20 to 30 minutes, with 5 minutes of gentle warm up and cool down. Women should be instructed to check their pulse rates during exercise to avoid rates greater than 140 beats per minute, which may

placenta and raise internal core tempera-
...ning are considered beneficial exercises in
...se of several muscle groups. As with other
...itive women should drink fluids to maintain
...avoid jumping and high impact motions, avoid
...tions that may divert maternal blood away from
...cises that may lead to abdominal injury (e.g., ski-
...oid exercise in hot weather, and observe for signs of
tiredne.... ...omen should stop exercising and notify their health
care provider ...ey experience any symptoms of vaginal bleeding or
fluid loss, pain, shortness of breath, palpitations, uterine contractions,
dizziness, or fainting.[17]

Literature indicates that nutritional status also plays a role in HIV
progression and immune system function.[20] Specifically, deficiencies in
nutrients such as iron, zinc, selenium, and vitamin A have been associated with HIV progression.[21] Decreased plasma levels of vitamins B_6, B_{12},
and A have also been correlated with alterations in immune response and
cognitive function.[22] Equally important is the vital role nutrition plays in
determining the health of the newborn child.[13] Nutrient facts related to
pregnancy, including the necessary nutrients, nutrient function, and best
sources (according to the March of Dimes Birth Defects Foundation) are
outlined in Table 20-4.

In general, the caloric intake of a pregnant woman should be approximately 30 to 35 kcal per kg per 24 hours, plus an additional 300 calories per day.[23] One of the most important nutrients for a pregnant woman
is protein, which provides the growth element for body tissues and contains iron and B vitamins. Pregnant women require an extra 30 g of protein per day, as well as 30 mg of elemental iron per day.[23] During pregnancy, a total of 2 to 3 servings of protein a day is recommended,
including lean meats, eggs, fish, poultry, and other protein-rich foods,
such as beans and tofu.

About 3 to 5 servings of vegetables, including green and yellow vegetables, and 2 to 4 servings of fruit are necessary to supply a pregnant
woman with adequate amounts of vitamins, particularly A and C. About
4 servings a day of milk and milk products are also suggested to ensure a
total calcium consumption of 1200 to 1500 mg per day, which is necessary
to strengthen bones and promote muscle and nerve response. Women
who are lactose intolerant may require calcium gluconate tablets (45 mg
Ca^+ per 500 mg tablet) or generic calcium carbonate (260 mg Ca_2^+ per
650 mg tablet).[23]

In addition, 6 to 11 servings of grain products are recommended to
ensure the adequate intake of fiber and B-complex vitamins. Any of the
following constitutes a serving: 1 slice of bread, ¾ cup of enriched cereal,
½ cup of oatmeal, ½ cup of rice, or ½ cup of spaghetti or noodles. Gastrointestinal side effects from antiretroviral medications, as well as the
common discomforts of pregnancy, such as nausea and heartburn, may

Table 20-4	Nutrition in Pregnancy	
Nutrient	**Function**	**Best Sources**
Calcium	Strengthens bone and teeth; helps blood clot; improves muscle and nerve response	Milk, cheese, green leafy vegetables, clams, oysters, almonds, legumes, tofu, softened bones of canned fish (sardines, mackerel, salmon)
Copper	Helps body use iron; aids energy metabolism	Liver, shellfish, nuts, legumes, water
Folic Acid	Essential for cell growth, hemoglobin formation, and DNA, RNA synthesis	Liver, eggs, leafy green vegetables, yeast, legumes, whole grains, nuts, fruits, vegetables, orange juice
Iron	Carries oxygen in blood	Liver, meat, dried fruit, enriched and whole grains, legumes, green leafy vegetables
Vitamin B_6	Essential for making DNA and for processing carbohydrates, lipids, and amino acids	Meats, liver, bananas, egg yolk, grains, legumes
Vitamin C	Helps make collagen in connective tissue; helps body use iron, calcium, and folic acid	Citrus fruits, broccoli, green pepper, strawberries, cabbage, tomato, cantaloupe, potatoes
Vitamin D	Regulates use of calcium in mother and baby	Fortified milk, green leafy vegetables, egg yolk, fish oils, butter, liver
Zinc	Aids synthesis of protein, DNA, and RNA	Oysters, seafood, meat, liver, eggs, whole grains, wheat germ

Modified from the March of Dimes Birth Defects Foundation: *Eating for two: nutrition during pregnancy, part 1*, 1992. http://www.noah.curry.edu/pregnancy/march_of_dimes/pre_preg.plan/eatingis.html

be overcome by having smaller, more frequent meals, eating crackers as snacks, and consuming liquids between rather than with meals. Prenatal vitamins, daily, are also recommended to ensure an adequate intake of vitamins and minerals, particularly of folic acid which may reduce the risk of neural tube defects in developing fetuses.[23]

Women should also be advised that alcohol, drugs, and smoking are not only harmful to their health, but also to the health of their developing baby. Excessive alcohol consumption can lead to fetal alcohol syndrome, while recreational drugs can cause a number of birth defects and/or childhood problems. Infants of women who smoke during pregnancy are smaller than infants of women who do not smoke during pregnancy, and also have a higher rate of stillborn and neonatal death.[17] Health care providers should therefore assess HIV-positive women for such substance use during pregnancy and provide counseling to reduce or eliminate consumption.

REFERENCES

1. Centers for Disease Control and Prevention: HIV/AIDS Surveillance Report, *HIV/AIDS Surveillance Report* 11(2):1, 1999.
2. Bryson YJ: *Advances in the prevention and treatment of perinatal HIV infection,* 1996, International AIDS Society, JAMA HIV/AIDS Information Center. http://www.ama-assn.com/bryson.htm
3. Centers for Disease Control and Prevention: Public Health Service Task Force recommendations for the use of antiretroviral drugs in pregnant women infected with HIV-1 for maternal health and for reducing perinatal HIV-1 transmission in the United States, *MMWR CDC Morbid Mortal Wkly Rep* 47:1, 1998.
4. Hanna L: Highlights from the conference on global strategies on the prevention of mother-to-child HIV transmission, BETA, 37, 1998.
5. American Medical Association: *Treatment center: perinatal transmission,* 1997, JAMA HIV/AIDS Information Center, The Association. http://www.ama-assn.org/aids
6. Alliegro M et al: Incidence and consequences of pregnancy in women with known duration of HIV infection, *Arch Intern Med* 157:2585, 1997.
7. Minkoff H: *HIV-infected women: transmission and management strategies,* Presentation at the Seventh Annual Clinical Care Options Symposium, 1997. http://www.healthcg.com/journa/june97/transmission.html
8. Bankhead C: HIV load predicts infant infection, *Obstetrician & Gynecologist Medical Tribune* 5(2):1, 1998.
9. American College of Obstetricians and Gynecologists: Human immunodeficiency virus infections in pregnancy, *ACOG Educational Bulletin* 232:1, 1997.
10. Mandelbrot L et al: *Decreased perinatal HIV-1 transmission following elective cesarean delivery with zidovudine treatment,* presentation at the Twelfth World AIDS Conference, Geneva, June 28-July 3, 1998.
11. Lutz-Friedrich R et al: *Decreased perinatal HIV-1 transmission following elective cesarean delivery with zidovudine treatment,* presented at the Twelfth World AIDS Conference, Geneva, June 28-July 3, 1998.
12. Zoler M: Strategies to reduce vertical HIV transmission, *OB-GYN News* 33(15):9, 1998.
13. The International Perinatal HIV Group: The mode of delivery and the risk of vertical transmission of human immunodeficiency virus type 1, *N Engl J Med* 340(13):977, 1999.
14. AIDS Institute New York Department of Health: *Criteria for the medical care of adults with HIV infection,* New York, 1993, New York Department of Health.
15. Beckerman K et al: *Control of maternal HIV-1 disease during pregnancy,* presentation at the Twelfth World AIDS Conference, Geneva, June 28-July 3, 1998.
16. American College of Obstetricians and Gynecologists: Antimicrobial therapy for obstetric patients, *ACOG Educational Bulletin* 245:1, 1998.
17. The March of Dimes Birth Defects Foundation: Fitness for two. In New York Online Access to Health, 1993. http://www.noah.cuny.edu/pregnancy/march_of_dimes/pre_preg.plan/fit42is.html
18. Cooper R: *Exercise and HIV,* 1994, AIDS Education Global Information System.
19. Laperrie A et al: Exercise and psychoneuroimmunology, *Med Sci Sports Exerc* 26(2):182, 1994.
20. Timbo B, Tollefson L: Nutrition: a cofactor in HIV disease, *J Am Diet Assoc* 94(9):1018, 1994.

21. Matulessy P, Forina M, Asmuni R: The role of nutrition on HIV infection and AIDS, *International Conference on AIDS* 10(2):226, 1994.
22. Baum M et al: Inadequate dietary intake and altered nutrition status in early HIV-1 infection. *Nutrition* 10(1):16, 1994.
23. Levy B, Brown P: Prenatal care. In Graber, ed: *University of Iowa family practice handbook,* ed 3, St Louis, 1999, Mosby.

21 Children with HIV/AIDS

Ann-Margaret Dunn

EPIDEMIOLOGY

INTERNATIONAL

An estimated 33.6 million persons worldwide were living with HIV/AIDS through 1999, as reported by the Pan-American Health Organization.[1] Women represent 14.8 million of these people, and children under the age of 15 years represent 1.2 million.[1] The Joint Nations Program on HIV/AIDS (UNAIDS) estimates that each year 350,000 children in developing countries are born with congenital HIV infection.[2] The Pan-American Health Organization estimates that there were 1.1 million AIDS deaths in women and 470,000 deaths in children under the age of 15 years in 1999.[1] Since the beginning of the epidemic, the total number of AIDS orphans (defined as children who lost their mothers or parents to AIDS when they were under the age of 15 years) is estimated to be 11.2 million.[1] This figure is probably grossly underreported, since accurate statistics on HIV infection depend on standardization of HIV-testing policies and reporting practices. Such standardization is essentially nonexistent in many developing countries.

UNITED STATES

In the United States, 733,374 persons (adults and children) with AIDS were reported to the Centers for Disease Control and Prevention (CDC) through December 31, 1999. Of this cumulative number, 8718 reported cases were in children less than 13 years of age.[3] The exposure category of 7943 of these reported pediatric cases was mothers with or at risk for HIV infection.[3] Hence, in the United States, perinatal transmission accounts for the majority of cases of HIV infection in children under 13 years.

In 1994, there was a significant reduction of perinatal transmission reported, which was secondary to zidovudine (ZDV) use by pregnant women and newborn infants. The effectiveness of ZDV in decreasing perinatal transmission was demonstrated in a study by the AIDS Clinical Trial Group (ACTG) 076, which was a "Phase III Randomized Placebo-Controlled Trial to Evaluate the Efficacy, Safety, and Tolerance of Zidovudine for the Prevention of Maternal-Fetal HIV Transmission." The ability to decrease the congenital transmission rate was the most significant clinical research breakthrough for pediatric HIV infection (for a detailed discussion see Chapter 20). This landmark study resulted in the Public Health Service (PHS) issuing guidelines for the use of ZDV to reduce perinatal transmission and for universal HIV counseling with voluntary testing of pregnant women in 1995.[4,5] Implementation of these guidelines resulted in a 39% decrease in the number of perinatally acquired AIDS cases (from 8.4 to 5.1 cases per 100,000 births) from the first half of the 1992 birth cohort to the first half of the 1995 birth cohort.[2]

In the United States during 1999, 88% of all pediatric AIDS cases occurred in children born to mothers with or at risk for HIV infection.[3] During the same period, 33% of AIDS cases in female adolescents (ages 13 to 19 years) were due to heterosexual transmission, and 33% of AIDS cases in male adolescents (ages 13 to 19 years) were transmitted by male-to-male sexual contact.[3] Injection drug use was the next most frequently cited exposure category for female adolescents. For male adolescents, the next most frequently cited categories were hemophilia/coagulation and heterosexual contact, which each accounted for 8% of the exposures. These statistics represent the ongoing transmission of a preventable fatal infectious disease and illustrate the need for intensified efforts aimed at prevention. It is true that HIV-infected children and adolescents are living longer with an improved quality of life due to earlier diagnosis and advances in treatment. Yet the most promising scientific advance would be an effective intervention to prevent transmission.

DIAGNOSING HIV INFECTION IN INFANTS AND CHILDREN

In adults, the enzyme-linked immunoabsorbent assay (ELISA) and Western blot assays are used to detect HIV antibodies in the serum; the presence of antibodies in adults indicates infection with HIV. HIV antibodies cross the placenta. Therefore, all infants born to HIV-positive mothers will test positive for maternal antibody at birth and for 9 to 18 months thereafter.[6] This complicates diagnosis of HIV infection in such infants when relying exclusively on standard antibody tests.[6] The HIV antibody tests are unreliable for diagnosis in children less than 18 months of age but do indicate maternal infection. By age 18 months, these maternal antibodies are not typically present in a child who is not infected with HIV.[7,8] In children younger than 18 months, HIV infection can be ruled out or confirmed by a qualitative test for HIV DNA, such as the polymerase chain reaction (PCR) test. Before availability of the PCR test, it could take 18 months or more for parents to learn whether their child was infected. The standard use of virological diagnostic assays, such as the HIV DNA PCR, has facilitated distinction between maternal and infant HIV infection.

The preferred virological test for diagnosing HIV in infancy is the HIV DNA PCR. In a metaanalysis of data from 271 HIV-infected children, 38% of the tested neonates had positive PCR tests by the age of 48 hours. There was no significant change in sensitivity noted during the first week of life, but sensitivity increased dramatically during the second week of life, with 93% of infants testing positive by the age of 14 days.[9]

HIV viral culture, another method used to diagnose HIV, has a sensitivity similar to that of DNA PCR in the diagnosis of HIV infection.[10] However, HIV viral culture is more complex and expensive to perform.[11]

p24 antigen tests are highly specific for HIV infection and have been used in the past to diagnose infection in children. However, the use of p24 antigen testing alone to diagnose HIV infection in infants under 1 month of age is not recommended because of the high frequency of false-positive assays during this period.[12]

HIV infection in children may be excluded in one of two ways. First, it may reasonably be excluded in children with two or more negative virological tests if two of these tests are performed at an age greater than 1 month and one is performed at an age greater than 4 months.[13] Second, HIV infection may reasonably be excluded in children with two or more negative ELISA tests (with an interval of at least 1 month between tests) performed at an age greater than 6 months, if the child is without any clinical signs of HIV infection. HIV infection can definitely be excluded in children with a negative HIV antibody test at an age greater than 18 months (in the absence of hypogammaglobulinemia), no clinical symptoms of HIV infection, and negative HIV virological assays.[6,11,14]

NURSING CONSIDERATIONS

1. HIV testing of the exposed infant using a virological test should be done before the infant is 48 hours old, at age 1 to 2 months, and at age 3 to 6 months. It may also be beneficial to perform HIV testing at 2 weeks of age to facilitate early diagnosis of infection.[11,14,15]

2. When collecting a specimen for HIV DNA PCR, cord blood should never be used for HIV testing of the newborn because of the potential for contamination with maternal blood.

3. To obtain an HIV DNA PCR, a minimum of 1 cc of blood (1.5 cc is preferred) must be collected via venipuncture into the ethylenediamine tetraacetic acid (EDTA) tube (with the lavender top) provided in the specimen collection kit. This volume permits for both HIV PCR and HIV antibody testing if required by state law.

4. The nurse must avoid overfilling the specimen tube and mix the specimen well to disperse the anticoagulant and prevent clotting. Specimens are often maintained at room temperature. For accurate specimen handling, the nurse should consult with laboratory personnel.

CDC CLASSIFICATION SYSTEM OF PEDIATRIC HIV INFECTION

The clinical, immunological, and virological manifestations of HIV disease in children with congenital HIV infection vary considerably from those in adults and adolescents. One of the primary reasons for these differences is thought to be the competence of the immune system at the time of infection. When congenital transmission occurs, the immature immune system of a fetus or neonate is affected at a critical time in its development. When an adult or adolescent is infected, the immune system is typically fully developed and competent.

In 1987, the differences in manifestations were recognized and subsequently translated into a classification system to help clinicians characterize the various clinical presentations of pediatric HIV disease. Two problems with this initial classification system were that: (1) it did not lend itself to prognostic assumptions and (2) it did not incorporate the immunological status of the child. Therefore, as additional knowledge of the progression of HIV disease in children was gained, a revision of this classification system was warranted. After ongoing collaboration with a working group of PHS representatives and other consultants convened by the CDC, a revised classification system was published in 1994.[6] This current system classifies children into mutually exclusive categories according to HIV infection status, clinical status, and immunological status.

The system was designed for children with congenital HIV infection who are less than 13 years of age. It uses a combination of a letter and a number to represent the clinical and immunological status of a child. The letter designates the clinical status; the number designates the immunological status. Once a child is classified into a more severe clinical or immunological category, he or she will always be classified into that category. Therefore, HIV-infected children may be classified into a more severe clinical or immunological category than their current status would suggest. They could even be without any signs of illness. In such cases, the classification would represent a past history of symptomatic disease or immunodeficiency. It is important to remember that the last published revision of this classification system was in 1994. This revision preceded many medical advances in the treatment of HIV disease, including highly active antiretroviral therapy (HAART). The current system of classification according to HIV-infection clinical and immunological status is discussed in detail in the following sections.

CLASSIFICATION OF HIV INFECTION STATUS

There are three possibilities for the HIV infection status of a child born to an HIV-positive mother: HIV-infected, HIV-exposed, and seroreverter (SR). *HIV-infected* designates an infant or child with confirmed HIV infection. *HIV-exposed* represents confirmed maternal infection, and indeterminate HIV-infection status of the infant or child. *Seroreverter* is a term used for a child who was exposed to maternal HIV infection but who is definitely not HIV-infected. (These possibilities for HIV infection status and the criteria for applying the diagnoses are outlined in Box 21-1.)

HIV-INFECTED INFANTS AND CHILDREN

Working definitions have been proposed for HIV infection acquired during the intrauterine and intrapartum periods. Infants with a positive

BOX 21-1 DIAGNOSTIC CRITERIA FOR THE DIAGNOSIS OF HIV INFECTION IN CHILDREN

HIV-Infected
Child <18 months of age
Known to be HIV seropositive or born to an HIV-positive mother
And
Having positive results on two separate determinations (excluding cord blood) from one or more of the following HIV detection tests:
- HIV culture
- HIV DNA PCR
- HIV antigen (p24)

Or
Meeting criteria for AIDS diagnosis based on the 1987 AIDS surveillance case definition
Child ≥18 months of age
Born to an HIV-positive mother or infected by blood, blood products, or other known modes of transmission (e.g., sexual contact)
And
HIV-antibody–positive by repeated reactive enzyme immunoassay (EIA) and confirmatory test (e.g., Western blot, immunofluorescence assay [IFA])
Or
Meeting any of the criteria for a child <18 months of age.

Perinatally Exposed (E)
Child who does not meet the aforementioned criteria
HIV seropositive by EIA and confirmatory tests (e.g., Western blot, IFA) performed at <18 months of age
Or
Having unknown antibody status but was born to a mother known to be infected with HIV

Diagnosis: Seroreverter (SR)
Child who is born to an HIV-positive mother
Having been documented as HIV-antibody–negative (i.e., two or more negative EIA tests performed at 6 to 18 months of age or one negative EIA test after 18 months of age)
And
Having had no other laboratory evidence of infection (i.e., has not had two positive viral detection tests, if performed)
And
Having not had an AIDS-defining condition

From Centers for Disease Control and Prevention: Revised classification system for human immunodeficiency virus infection in children less than 13 years of age, *MMWR* 43(RR-12):3, Sept 30, 1994.

virological test at or before 48 hours of age are considered to have early (intrauterine) infection. Infants with negative virological tests during the first week of life and subsequent positive tests are considered to have late (intrapartum) infection.[16] Some researchers have proposed that infants with early infection may experience a more rapid disease progression than those with late infection and should be treated more aggressively.[17,18] However, other data from prospective cohort studies indicate that, although there were early differences in HIV RNA levels between infants with positive HIV cultures within 48 hours of birth and those with positive cultures after 7 days, these differences are no longer statistically significant after 2 months of age.[19] The number of HIV RNA copies after the first month of life is more prognostic of rapid disease progression than is the time at which HIV culture tests initially become positive.[19]

Nursing Considerations

See p. 402 for selected nursing considerations for HIV-infected children.

PERINATALLY EXPOSED (E) INFANTS

Any infant born to an HIV-positive mother is classified as *perinatally exposed*. The infant remains classified as such until HIV diagnostic tests either confirm or rule out infection, as described previously. The time of indeterminate infection is often one of great anxiety for the family of the exposed infant or child. Families experience feelings of vulnerability because of not knowing whether or not the child has a chronic and ultimately terminal illness. This is a time when education, support, and preparation for the possibility of confirmed HIV infection in the child must be provided.

Exposed infants are given ZDV chemoprophylaxis, beginning 8 to 12 hours after birth at a dose of 2 mg/kg every 6 hours for 6 weeks to reduce the possibility of HIV infection; thus medical care of the HIV-exposed infant should be provided by a team of pediatric HIV clinicians.

Nursing Considerations

1. Parents must understand the importance of ZDV prophylaxis for their newborn. The nurse should review the dose, frequency, side effects, and duration of therapy (i.e., 6 weeks). The nurse should be certain that the parent has a sufficient supply of medicine to complete the regimen. It is essential for the nurse to assess and monitor adherence to the ZDV regimen during the first 6 weeks of the newborn's life.

2. HIV-exposed newborns receiving ZDV prophylaxis should undergo a complete blood count (CBC) at birth and at the completion of the 6-week course of therapy. Some clinicians recommend additional monitoring 3 to 4 weeks after starting therapy.[20] The frequency of monitoring ultimately depends on the hematological status of the infant. Anemic infants require closer follow-up.

3. CD_4 lymphocyte counts and percentages should be monitored at 1 and 3 months in all HIV-exposed infants. Infants whose diagnostic

status is unclear should continue to undergo monitoring of the CD_4 lymphocyte count and percentage at 3-month intervals (i.e., at 6, 9, and 12 months of age) or more frequently if the CD_4 lymphocyte count or percentage declines rapidly.

4. Quantitative immunoglobulins should also be measured by the time the infant is 4 to 6 months of age.[21]

5. Initiation of *Pneumocystis carinii* pneumonia (PCP) prophylaxis with Bactrim is indicated for HIV-exposed infants at 4 to 6 weeks of age.[13] Some clinicians may elect not to begin Bactrim in infants who have had 2 to 3 negative PCR test results. When Bactrim is administered, parents should be provided with education on the dose, administration, and importance of this medication. (See Chapter 16 and Box 16-3 for a discussion of PCP.)

6. HIV-exposed infants should receive standard pediatric immunizations (see Chapter 6).

7. It is important to note that protocols for long-term follow-up of HIV-negative infants with congenital HIV exposure vary according to the clinical practice site. However, the American Academy of Pediatrics (AAP) recommends continued follow-up with serological testing to document the disappearance of HIV antibodies for all HIV-exposed infants who are believed to be uninfected based on negative virological tests for HIV, such as DNA PCR or viral culture.[21]

SEROREVERTER (SR)

Seroreverter is a term applied to an infant or child born to a HIV-positive mother, but who is definitely not HIV-infected as evidenced by the absence of clinical or laboratory signs of HIV infection. (The specific criteria for seroreverter classification designated by the CDC are outlined in Box 21-1.)

Nursing Considerations

1. Some HIV centers recommend annual follow-up for HIV-negative seroreverters. This follow-up is to monitor the clinical effect of congenital exposure to an infectious disease and to any maternal antiretroviral therapy during the pregnancy. It also maintains the helping relationship formed during a difficult period in the family's life and offers the opportunity to discuss any lingering fears or questions regarding the child's HIV exposure.

2. There are many parents who experience some difficulty understanding the concept of seroreversion. They may need much reinforcement of the reality of this negative HIV diagnosis.

3. Continued follow-up with serological testing is indicated for all HIV-exposed children ages 12 months or older to document clearance of HIV antibodies.[21]

4. Seroreverters should receive standard pediatric immunizations when being immunized for diphtheria, pertussis, and tetanus; hepatitis B; *Haemophilus influenzae;* and inactivated poliovirus (IPV). An annual

influenza vaccination (each fall) should be administered if a serore-verter resides with HIV-positive household members. Annual testing for tuberculosis (TB) is also indicated for seroreverters residing with HIV-positive household members.[21] Varicella vaccine should be administered to varicella-susceptible seroreverters. If a varicella-vaccine rash develops, the HIV-positive household members need to avoid direct contact with the child for the duration of the rash.

CLINICAL CATEGORIES

Children with HIV infection or HIV exposure may be classified into one of four mutually exclusive clinical categories based on their signs, symptoms, or diagnoses related to HIV infection.[6] These clinical categories were defined to provide a staging classification and, therefore, they do have some prognostic significance. An infant or child classified into clinical category A, for example, would be less symptomatic than an infant or child classified into clinical category B (Box 21-2).

Category N: Not symptomatic. This category is applied to children who have no signs or symptoms considered the result of HIV infection or who have only one of the signs or symptoms listed under category A in Box 21-2.

Category A: Mildly symptomatic. This category is applied to children with two or more of the conditions listed under category A in Box 21-2. To be assigned to this category, the infant or child can have none of the conditions listed in the moderately symptomatic or severely symptomatic categories.

Category B: Moderately symptomatic. This category is applied to children who have one or more of the symptomatic conditions listed under category B in Box 21-2. All category B conditions must be directly related to HIV disease. Signs and symptoms related to causes other than HIV infection should not be used to classify the children. For example, a drug-related anemia would not cause a child to be classified into category B because the anemia should resolve with discontinuation of the drug.

Category C: Severely symptomatic. This category is applied to children who have any one of the conditions listed under category C in Box 21-2. This category is particularly important in that any HIV-positive child with a clinical category C condition meets the criteria for an AIDS diagnosis.

Although this clinical classification system is primarily used to categorize children with HIV infection, it may also be useful for infants and children exposed to HIV and with uncertain HIV-infection status. For example, application of the categories N and A to an HIV-exposed infant may help distinguish between those who are more or less likely to be infected with HIV. Therefore the prefix "E" for "exposed" is combined with N or A to describe the clinical signs and symptoms of the infant or child to offer some prognostic assistance. HIV-exposed infants in category A (EA) may be more likely to be infected with HIV than those infants in category N (EN).

BOX 21-2   1994 REVISED HIV PEDIATRIC CLASSIFICATION SYSTEM: CLINICAL CATEGORIES

Category N: Not Symptomatic

Children who have no signs or symptoms considered to be the result of HIV infection or who have only one of the conditions listed in category A.

Category A: Mildly Symptomatic

Children with two or more of the following conditions but none of the conditions listed in categories B and C:

- Lymphadenopathy (≥0.5 cm at more than two sites; bilateral findings count as one site)
- Hepatomegaly
- Splenomegaly
- Dermatitis
- Parotitis
- Recurrent or persistent upper respiratory infection, sinusitis, or otitis media

Category B: Moderately Symptomatic

Children who have symptomatic conditions other than those listed for category A or category C that are attributed to HIV infection. Examples of conditions in clinical category B include, but are not limited to, the following:

- Anemia (<8 gm/dL), neutropenia (<1000 cells/mm³), or thrombocytopenia (<100,000 cells/mm³) persisting for more than 30 days
- Bacterial meningitis, pneumonia, or sepsis (single episode)
- Candidiasis, oropharyngeal (e.g., thrush) persisting for 2 months in children aged 6 months
- Cardiomyopathy
- Cytomegalovirus (CMV) infection with onset before age 1 month
- Diarrhea (recurrent or chronic)
- Fever lasting 1 month
- Hepatitis
- Herpes simplex virus (HSV) stomatitis (recurrent [i.e., more than two episodes within 1 year])
- HSV bronchitis, pneumonitis, or esophagitis with onset before age 1 month
- Herpes zoster (i.e., shingles) involving at least two distinct episodes or more than one dermatome
- Leiomyosarcoma
- Lymphoid interstitial pneumonia (LIP)* or pulmonary lymphoid hyperplasia complex
- Nephropathy
- Nocardiosis
- Toxoplasmosis with onset before age 1 month
- Varicella (disseminated [i.e., complicated chickenpox])

Category C: Severely Symptomatic

Children who have any condition listed in the 1987 surveillance case definition for AIDS (with the exception of LIP, which is a category B condition*).†

---

* Although lymphoid interstitial pneumonia (LIP) is listed in category B, it is an AIDS-defining condition in children. It is not listed in category C because the prognosis for children with LIP is substantially better than children with category C conditions.
† For 1987 surveillance case definition see Centers for Disease Control and Prevention: Revision of the CDC surveillance case definition for AIDS, *MMWR* 36(Suppl):1, 1987.
Modified from Centers for Disease Control and Prevention: Revised classification system for human immunodeficiency virus infection in children less than 13 years of age, *MMWR* 43(RR-12):1, Sept 30, 1994.

Nursing Considerations

1. Parents of newly diagnosed children are often focused on whether their child has "AIDS." Only children with one or more of the clinical manifestations listed in category C (with the exception of lymphoid interstitial pneumonia [LIP]) have an AIDS-defining condition.

2. When the guidelines were revised in 1994, this new classification system aimed at providing clinicians with a framework to reflect the current or past history of disease severity. A child in category C is or has been more symptomatic than a child in category A or B.

3. Once a child is in a more severe clinical category, the child will always be in that clinical category. For example, a 6-month-old child who develops PCP will always be classified in clinical category C, even if the child then remains clinically and immunologically stable for years.

IMMUNOLOGICAL CATEGORIES

Three immunological categories have been established to categorize children by the severity of immunosuppression attributable to HIV infection. These age-specific categories are numbered as 1, 2, or 3 in order of worsening immunodeficiency (Table 21-1). The categories include both the absolute CD_4 count and CD_4 percentage of total lymphocytes. Although the CD_4 absolute number that identifies a specific level of immune suppression changes with age in each immunological category, the CD_4 percentage that defines each immunological category does not. Thus a change in CD_4 percentage, not the absolute number, may be a better marker to identify disease progression in children.[11,14,15] Knowledge of the immune status as evidenced by the CD_4 T lymphocyte count and percentage is essential when caring for HIV-infected infants and children. The CD_4 count or percentage value is used in conjunction with other measurements to guide antiretroviral treatment decisions and primary prophylaxis for PCP after 1 year of age.[11] It is important to remember that all HIV-infected infants remain on PCP prophylaxis for the first year of life, irrespective of CD_4 counts. The CD_4 count guides clinical decisions regarding prophylaxis for other opportunistic infections such as *Mycobacterium avium* complex (MAC). Therefore, CD_4 T lymphocyte values should be obtained as soon as possible after a child has a positive virological test for HIV, and every 3 months thereafter.[7,22]

There are some complexities in the interpretation of CD_4 T lymphocyte counts in children. CD_4 counts are normally higher in children than in adults, declining over the first few years of life.[23-27] Children may also develop opportunistic infections with higher CD_4 counts when compared to their adult counterparts.[28-30] In addition, CD_4 cell values can be associated with considerable intraclient variability. Even mild intercurrent illness or the receipt of vaccinations can produce a transient decrease in CD_4 cell number and percentage. Therefore CD_4 values are best measured when clients are clinically stable.[14,15] Immunological classification based on age-specific CD_4 counts appears to be clinically useful despite these complexities.[6]

Table 21-1 **Immunological Categories Based on Age-Specific CD$_4$ T Lymphocyte Counts and Percentage of Total Lymphocytes**

Immunological Category	Age of Child		
	<12 Months Lymphocytes (%)	1-5 Years Lymphocytes (%)	6-12 Years Lymphocytes (%)
(1) No evidence of suppression	≥1500 (>25)	≥1000 (≥25)	≥500 (≥25)
(2) Evidence of moderate suppression	750-1499 (15-24)	500-999 (15-24)	200-499 (15-24)
(3) Severe suppression	<750 (<15)	<500 (<15)	<200 (<15)

Modified from Centers for Disease Control and Prevention: Revised classification system for human immunodeficiency virus infection in children less than 13 years of age, *MMWR* 43(RR-12):1, Sept 30, 1994.

NURSING CONSIDERATIONS

1. If the absolute CD$_4$ T lymphocyte count and CD$_4$ percentage are not in the same immunological category, the child should be staged in the more severe immunological category.[6] CD$_4$ T lymphocyte percentages have less measurement variability than CD$_4$ absolute counts and therefore are the preferred value.[31] For example, if a 2-year-old child has an absolute CD$_4$ count of 525, but the CD$_4$ percentage is 13%, this child would be in immunological category 3.

2. Once a child is assigned to a more severe immunological category, the child will always be in this immunological category, even if there is a significant increase in his or her absolute CD$_4$ T lymphocyte count or percentage.

3. No modification in therapy should be made in response to a change in CD$_4$ values until the change has been substantiated by at least one additional determination, with a minimum of 1 week between measurements.[14,15]

4. Education of the parents and child using age-appropriate language on the function of the CD$_4$ T lymphocytes in the body is an important component of family-centered education.

NATURAL HISTORY OF HIV INFECTION IN CHILDREN

In children with congenital HIV infection, the HIV RNA copy number and its fluctuations differ from the pattern seen in infected adults. In adults, during the period of primary HIV infection, the HIV RNA copy number initially rises to peak levels. These levels decline 2 to 3 log$_{10}$ copies due to the body's humoral and cell-mediated immune response as the virological set point is established. This decline occurs 6 to 12 months following acute primary HIV infection and reflects the balance between ongoing viral production and elimination by the immune system.[32,33] In contrast, high HIV RNA copy numbers persist in HIV-infected children for prolonged periods.[34,35] In one prospective study,[19] HIV viral loads were low at birth (<10,000 copies/ml) and increased to high values by the age of 2 months. Most infants in this study had values that were >100,000 copies/ml with a range from undetectable to nearly 10 million copies/ml. Viral copies decreased slowly over the first year of life, with a mean HIV RNA level of 185,000 copies/ml. Also in contrast to the pattern observed in adults, after the first year of life, the HIV RNA copy number continues to slowly decline over the next few years.[19,36-38] This decline is most rapid in the first 12 to 24 months after birth, with an average decline of 0.6 $\log_{10}$ per year. This is followed by a slower decline until approximately 4 to 5 years of age, with an average decline of 0.3 $\log_{10}$ per year. These patterns are thought to illustrate the lower efficiency of an immature, developing immune system in containing viral replication; they may also represent a greater number of HIV-susceptible cells.[11]

High HIV RNA levels (i.e., >100,000 copies/ml) in infants have been associated with a high risk of disease progression and death, especially if the CD_4 percentage is less than 15%.[37,38] However, the predictive value of specific HIV RNA levels for disease progression and mortality for an individual child is moderate.[37] The interpretation of HIV RNA levels during the first year of life is especially complicated because of high viral RNA levels seen in many infants and because of the marked overlap in levels between children with and without rapid disease progression.[34] CD_4 T lymphocyte percentage and HIV RNA copy number (viral load) at baseline and serial measurements over time contribute to the prediction of mortality risk in infected children and, used together, may more accurately define the prognosis of the HIV-infected child.[37,38]

Due to these distinct virological patterns in children, the following recommendations have been made. Only changes in RNA copy number of greater than fivefold (0.7 $\log_{10}$) in infants less than 2 years of age and changes in RNA copy number greater than threefold (0.5 $\log_{10}$) in children 2 years old or older should be considered reflective of a biologically and clinically substantial change.[11,14,15] These values should be present on two or more measurements. Interpretation of HIV RNA levels for clinical decision-making in children needs to be done by or in consultation with an expert in pediatric HIV infection.

Viral burden in peripheral blood can be determined using quantitative HIV RNA assays.[15] Because of assay variation, it is important to use a consistent assay when performing viral RNA measurements. A single specimen tested by two different assays can differ by twofold (0.3 $\log_{10}$) or more.[11] To reduce the effect of assay variability in the clinical management of clients, two samples can be obtained at baseline, and the average of the two values can be used for comparison with future tests. No alteration in therapy should be made as a result of a change in HIV copy number unless the change is confirmed by a second measurement.[14] Choice of an HIV RNA assay for young children may be influenced by the amount of blood required for the assay[15]:

- The nucleic acid sequence–based amplification (NASBA) assay requires the least amount of blood (100 μL of plasma).
- The Amplicor HIV-1 monitor requires 200 μL of plasma.
- The Quantiplex assays require 1 ml of plasma.

TREATMENT OF PEDIATRIC HIV INFECTION

There are many complex, clinical challenges inherent in the treatment of the child with HIV infection. Perinatally infected children may have had prior exposure to various antiretroviral drugs used by the mother during the prenatal period or administered to the infant during the neonatal period.[4,39] In addition, drug pharmacokinetics change depending on the age of the recipient; this necessitates specific evaluation of drug dosing and toxicity in infants and children.[15] Adherence issues in the pediatric population present ongoing challenges to the health care team, as described on p. 397. Treatment of HIV disease is also rapidly evolving, particularly with regard to antiretroviral therapy. However, the availability of antiretroviral drugs for HIV-infected children has lagged behind the availability for infected adults.[15]

The rapidity and magnitude of HIV replication during all stages of infection are greater than was previously believed and account for the emergence of drug-resistant HIV variants when antiretroviral treatment does not maximally suppress replication.[40,41] Therefore, therapeutic strategies now focus on early initiation of antiretroviral regimens capable of maximally suppressing viral replication, preferably to undetectable levels. The goals of antiretroviral therapy are to preserve immune function, prevent disease progression, and reduce the development of drug-resistant strains of virus.[11,15] As with adults, combination therapy is recommended for all infants, children, and adolescents treated with antiretroviral agents. This is because, when compared with monotherapy, combination therapy slows disease progression, improves survival, results in greater and more sustained virological response, and delays the development of virus mutations.[14,15] Monotherapy with ZDV is only appropriate for prophylaxis of congenital HIV infection during the first 6 weeks of life. If the infant is diagnosed to be HIV-infected while receiving ZDV prophylaxis, the drug regimen should be changed to a combination antiretroviral drug regimen.[14,15]

Theoretically, the selection of the initial antiretroviral regimen for infected infants would seem to be influenced by the antiretroviral regimen(s) received by their mothers during pregnancy.[11,14,15] Yet data from Pediatric AIDS Clinical Trial Group (PACTG) protocol 076 indicate that ZDV resistance did not account for acquisition of the virus in most infants who became infected, despite maternal ZDV treatment.[42] In addition, data from PACTG protocol 185 indicate that duration of previous ZDV therapy in

BOX 21-3   INDICATIONS FOR INITIATION OF ANTIRETROVIRAL THERAPY IN CHILDREN WITH HIV INFECTION

- Clinical symptoms associated with HIV infection (i.e., clinical categories A, B, or C [see Box 21-2])
- Evidence of immune suppression, indicated by CD_4 T lymphocyte absolute number or percentage (i.e., immune category 2 or 3 [see Table 21-1])
- Age <12 months, regardless of clinical, immunological, or virological status. For asymptomatic children aged ≥1 year with normal immune status, two options are available:

Preferred Approach

Initiate therapy, regardless of age or symptom status.

Alternative Approach

Defer treatment in situations in which the risk for clinical disease progression is low and other factors (e.g., concern for the durability of response, safety, and adherence) favor postponing treatment. In such cases, the health care provider should regularly monitor virological, immunological, and clinical status. Factors to be considered in deciding to initiate therapy include:

High or increasing HIV RNA copy number

Rapidly declining CD_4 T lymphocyte number or percentage to values approaching those indicative of moderate immune suppression (i.e., immune category 2 [see Table 21-1])

Development of clinical symptoms

Indications for initiation of antiretroviral therapy in postpubertal HIV-positive adolescents should follow adult guidelines.*

---

* Office of Public Health and Science, Department of Health and Human Services: Availability of report of NIH panel to define principles of therapy of HIV infection and guidelines for the use of antiretroviral agents in HIV-positive adults, *Fed Register* 62:33417, 1997.

From Centers for Disease Control and Prevention: Guidelines for the use of antiretroviral agents in pediatric HIV infection, *MMWR* 47(RR-4):1, 1998.

Note: Consultation with an expert in pediatric HIV therapy is essential in the management of pediatric antiretroviral therapy.

---

women with advanced disease was not associated with diminished ZDV efficacy for the reduction of perinatal transmission.[43] Many women received prolonged ZDV therapy before pregnancy. These data do not suggest that the antiretroviral regimen for an infected infant should be chosen on the basis of maternal antiretroviral use.[14,15] However, it is crucial to monitor the frequency of perinatal transmission of antiretroviral-resistant isolates, because maternal treatment with combination antiretroviral therapy is becoming more common, and the prevalence of resistant viral strains in the HIV-positive population may increase over time.[14,15]

The pediatric doses and specifics of antiretroviral medications are listed in the color insert drug guide entitled "HIV/AIDS Medications." Boxes 21-3 through 21-5 review guidelines for the initiation of antiretroviral therapy and recommended antiretroviral regimens for initial ther-

BOX 21-4   RECOMMENDED ANTIRETROVIRAL REGIMENS FOR INITIAL THERAPY FOR HIV INFECTION IN CHILDREN

Preferred Regimen

There is evidence of clinical benefit and sustained suppression of HIV RNA in HIV-positive adults and children. Regimen considerations are as follows:
- The preferred regimen is one highly active protease inhibitor (PI) plus two nucleoside reverse transcriptase inhibitors (NRTIs).
- The preferred PI for infants and children who cannot swallow pills or capsules is nelfinavir or ritonavir. An alternative for children who can swallow pills or capsules is indinavir.
- Recommended dual NRTI combinations—The most data on use in children are available on the combinations of ZDV and didanosine (ddI) and ZDV and lamivudine (3TC). More limited data are available for the combinations of stavudine (d4T) and ddI, d4T and 3TC, and ZDV and zalcitabine (ddC).*
- If child can swallow capsules—Efavirenz (Sustiva) **plus** two NRTIs *or* Efavirenz **plus** nelfinavir and one NRTI

Alternative Regimen

The alternative regimens are as follows:
Nevirapine‡ and two NRTIs
Or
Abacavir in combination with ZDV and 3TC

Offer Only in Special Circumstances

The regimens are as follows:
Two NRTIs
Or
Amprenavir in combination with two NRTIs
Or
Amprenavir in combination with abacavir

Not Recommended

The following are not recommended because of evidence of overlapping toxicity and because use may be virologically undesirable:
Any monotherapy‡
d4T and ZDV
ddC and ddI
ddC and d4T
ddC and 3TC

---

* ddC is not available in a liquid preparation commercially, although a liquid formulation is available through a compassionate-use program of the manufacturer (Hoffman-LaRoche Inc., Nutley, New Jersey). The combination of ZDV and ddC is a less preferable choice for use in combination with a protease inhibitor.

† A liquid preparation of nevirapine is not available commercially, but it is available through a compassionate-use program of the manufacturer (Boehringer Ingelheim Pharmaceuticals, Inc., Ridgefield, Connecticut).

‡ Except for ZDV chemoprophylaxis administered to HIV-exposed infants during the first 6 weeks of life to prevent perinatal HIV transmission; if an infant is identified as HIV-positive while receiving ZDV prophylaxis, therapy should be changed to a combination antiretroviral drug regimen.

From Working Group on Antiretroviral Therapy and Medical Management of HIV-Infected Children: Guidelines for the use of antiretroviral agents in pediatric HIV infection, National Pediatric and Family HIV Resource Center (NPHRC), Health Resources and Services Administration (HRSA), and National Institutes of Health (NIH). http://hivatis.org/index.html
Note: Consultation with an expert in pediatric HIV therapy is essential in the selection and management of pediatric antiretroviral therapy.

BOX 21-5 CONSIDERATIONS FOR CHANGING ANTIRETROVIRAL THERAPY FOR HIV-POSITIVE CHILDREN

Virological Considerations*

- Less than a minimally acceptable virological response after 8 to 12 weeks of therapy. For children receiving antiretroviral therapy with two NRTIs and a protease inhibitor, such a response is defined as a less than tenfold ($1.0 \log_{10}$) decrease from baseline HIV RNA levels. For children receiving less potent antiretroviral therapy (e.g., dual NRTI combinations), an insufficient response is defined as a less than fivefold ($0.7 \log_{10}$) decrease in HIV RNA levels from baseline.
- HIV RNA not suppressed to undetectable levels after 4 to 6 months of antiretroviral therapy.†
- Repeated detection of HIV RNA in children who initially responded to antiretroviral therapy with undetectable levels of HIV RNA.‡
- A reproducible increase in HIV RNA copy number among children who have had a substantial HIV RNA response but still have low levels of detectable HIV RNA. Such an increase would warrant a change in therapy if, after initiation of the therapeutic regimen, a greater than threefold ($0.5 \log_{10}$) increase in copy number for children aged ≥ 2 years and a greater than fivefold ($0.7 \log_{10}$) increase for children aged <2 years is observed.

Immunological Considerations*

- Change in immunological classification (see Table 21-1)§
- For children with CD_4 T lymphocyte percentages of $<15\%$ (i.e., those in immune category 3), a persistent decline of 5% or more in CD_4 cell percentage.
- Rapid and substantial decrease in absolute CD_4 T lymphocyte count (e.g., a 30% decline in <6 months)

Clinical Considerations

- Progressive neurodevelopmental deterioration
- Growth failure defined as persistent decline in weight-growth velocity despite adequate nutritional support and without other explanation
- Disease progression defined as advancement from one pediatric clinical category to another (e.g., from clinical category A to B) (see Box 21-2)¶

---

* At least two measurements (taken 1 week apart) should be performed before considering a change in therapy.

† The initial HIV RNA level of the child at the start of therapy and the level achieved with therapy should be considered when contemplating potential drug changes. For example, an immediate change in therapy may not be warranted if there is a sustained 1.5 to 2.0 $\log_{10}$ decrease in HIV RNA copy number, even if RNA remains detectable at low levels.

‡ More frequent evaluation of HIV RNA levels should be considered if the HIV RNA increase is limited (e.g., when using an HIV RNA assay with a lower limit of detection of 1000 copies/ml, there is a $<0.7 \log_{10}$ increase from undetectable to approximately 5000 copies/ml in an infant aged <2 years).

§ Minimal changes in CD_4 T lymphocyte percentage that may result in a change in immunological category (e.g., from 26% to 24%, or 16% to 14%) may not be as great a concern as a rapid substantial change in CD_4 percentage within the same immunological category (e.g., a drop from 35% to 25%).

¶ In clients with stable immunological and virological parameters, progression from one clinical category to another may not represent an indication to change therapy. Thus, in clients whose disease progression is not associated with neurological deterioration or growth failure, virological and immunological considerations are important in deciding whether to change therapy.

From Centers for Disease Control and Prevention: Guidelines for the use of antiretroviral agents in pediatric HIV infection, *MMWR* 47(RR-4).1, 1998.

Note: Consultation with an expert in pediatric HIV therapy is essential in the management of pediatric antiretroviral therapy.

BOX 21-6   ESSENTIAL CONCEPTS IN TREATING CHILDREN WITH HIV INFECTION

- It is essential for an expert in the treatment of pediatric HIV to actively direct the child's care. If such a specialist is unavailable due to logistical or geographical difficulties, the general pediatric practitioner should regularly consult with an HIV expert.
- All antiretroviral drugs approved for the treatment of HIV infection may be used for children when indicated, irrespective of labeling notations.
- The complex and diverse needs of children and families infected with and affected by HIV disease require a multidisciplinary team approach. This team should ideally include physicians, nurse practitioners, nurses, pharmacists, home care agency staff, child life specialists, social workers, psychologists, psychiatrists, chaplains, nutritionists, and volunteers skilled in the treatment of HIV-positive families.
- Enrollment of pregnant HIV-positive women; their HIV-exposed newborns; and infected infants, children, and adolescents into clinical trials offers the best means of determining safe and effective therapies.
- Identification of HIV-positive women before or during pregnancy is critical in the provision of optimal therapy for infected women and their children. It is also essential in preventing perinatal transmission.
- Antiretroviral medication has to be administered for many years. The choice of an antiretroviral regimen should, therefore, include consideration of factors associated with the possible limitation of future treatment options, including the potential for antiretroviral resistance.
- When an antiretroviral regimen is selected by the pediatric HIV specialist, consideration of certain factors influencing adherence to therapy need to be considered. These include:
  - Availability and palatability of pediatric formulations.
  - Effects of the medication schedule on the quality of life.
  - Ability of the parent or adolescent to administer a complex regimen.
  - Potential for drug interactions with current medications.
  - Serial HIV RNA copy number and CD_4 T lymphocyte measurements are essential for monitoring and modifying antiretroviral regimens.

From Centers for Disease Control and Prevention: Guidelines for the use of antiretroviral agents in pediatric HIV infection, *MMWR* 47(RR-4):1, 1998; Working Group on Antiretroviral Therapy and Medical Management of HIV-Infected Children: *Guidelines for the use of antiretroviral agents in pediatric HIV infection,* National Pediatric and Family HIV Resource Center (NPHRC), Health Resources and Services Administration (HRSA), and National Institutes of Health (NIH). http://hivatis.org/index.html; Working Group on Antiretroviral Therapy and Medical Management of Infants, Children, and Adolescents with HIV Infection: Antiretroviral therapy and medical management of pediatric HIV infection, *Pediatrics* 102(4):1005, 1998.

apy, and also present considerations for changing an antiretroviral regimen. Box 21-6 contains the essential concepts that should be considered when treating HIV-infected children.

ADHERENCE TO ANTIRETROVIRAL THERAPY IN CHILDREN

Combination antiretroviral drug treatments are the current standard of care. It is not uncommon for clients with HIV infection who are clinically stable to require a total of five different antiretroviral/prophylactic medications with complicated dosing schedules every day. This often proves difficult for adults, and it becomes even more difficult for the HIV-infected child who is required to take antiretroviral medications that may be unavailable in pediatric formulations. Administering antiretroviral medications that are unavailable in liquid formulations or that have a poor palatability proves most difficult for parents. The issues of medication adherence for an HIV-infected child are diverse and challenging. However, addressing these issues is an indispensable component of the treatment plan, especially because of the potential for developing resistant strains of the HIV virus due to missed doses.[44] Box 21-7 contains information that serves as a guide for the nurse to support treatment adherence in the pediatric population.

COMMONLY ENCOUNTERED PROBLEMS

A parent reports that the child is not taking the medications. This is a very common but nonspecific complaint. If a parent communicates missed doses of medication, the nurse should ascertain the facts without making negative judgments. Families affected by HIV infection are quite sensitive to both the negative and positive opinions of their health care providers. Families who are penalized for honesty avoid speaking the truth.[45] A detailed history, as indicated by the following questions, is most important for discovering the etiology of the problem and the related solution[45]:

What—Which medication is not being taken as prescribed?

Who—Who usually gives the medications to the child? Are the missed doses occurring when a different person attempts to administer medications?

When—When are the missed doses occurring? How many doses are being missed? Is there a specific pattern to the missed doses? For example, does it happen on afternoons when the child is tired? Or does it occur during school hours due to inconsistent administration on the part of the child or school personnel?

Why—Why were doses missed? If there is a specific cause, intervention should be directed at this cause. For example, if a child or parent reports that morning doses are missed because the medication causes nausea, administration with food may ameliorate the problem, unless contraindicated.

BOX 21-7 ADHERENCE TO ANTIRETROVIRAL MEDICATIONS IN HIV-INFECTED CHILDREN: GUIDELINES FOR NURSING CARE

1. Possible side effects and adverse reactions related to the prescribed antiretroviral medications should be communicated to the child and family; unexpected side effects may result in the family's discontinuation of the medications.
2. The use of visual aides and educational materials (e.g., a written daily schedule that illustrates both doses and times) encourages adherence.
3. The nurse must not make assumptions about the family's understanding of the child's medications. The use of a syringe, pillbox, medicine cup, or any other tool given to the family must be demonstrated thoroughly. A return demonstration confirms the family's understanding of instructions; the family should restate the name, purpose, dose, and dosing time of each of their child's antiretroviral medications. This is a valuable measure for assessing comprehension. It is essential to tailor the treatment plan to meet the needs of both the child and family. If the plan is very labor intensive and difficult for the parent-child dyad, it is reasonable to expect that it will not be executed.
4. The nurse must be certain to explain to the child and family the immune system's function and the effect of HIV on the immune system. Any explanations of HIV disease presented to a child must be tailored to the child's age, development, and knowledge of his or her diagnosis. Concrete illustrations of actual increases in CD_4 counts and decreases in the viral load are a significant measure of success for the HIV-positive child and family. Whenever possible, the child and family should be provided with the actual reports.
5. The nurse should use the support of other professionals, such as pharmacists, visiting nurses, social workers, and child life specialists. The pharmacist is an integral part of the health care team, yet he or she is often overlooked due to logistical differences with the prescriber. Pharmacists are a key resource for medication information. They can review medication profiles, discuss potential drug interactions, provide medication consultation, and reinforce directions before dispensing the drug. The pharmacist may also have better access to bilingual teaching tools for the child and family. A visiting nurse is able to observe and monitor medication administration by the parent directly in the home environment. Home visits also offer the opportunity to identify any barriers to adherence and provide the necessary forum to offer appropriate education and support. Social workers help translate medical knowledge into a workable and understandable plan for the child and family. Child life specialists advocate for both the child and family by acting as intermediaries with the health care team.
6. Telephone support, encouragement, and positive feedback should be offered when indicated. A clinician should be available for ongoing support and education. A collaborative relationship with the family is unequivocally one of the best methods for fostering adherence.

From Dunn AM, Navarra JP, Cervia J: *Adherence to antiretroviral medications in HIV-infected children: a collaborative approach with guidelines for care,* The Twelfth World AIDS Conference, Geneva, Switzerland, June 28-July 3, 1998 (abstract, no. 32378).

Where—In what location are the medications usually given? Is it the same place that the missed doses are occurring? For example, if a family reports that the child is missing the 3 PM medications every day, it is important to learn where the child is at 3 PM. If the child is with a babysitter, for example, parents may be skipping afternoon medications for fear the babysitter will learn the diagnosis.

How—How are medications usually taken? Are medications given with milk, water, sucking candy, or on an empty stomach? Is a medication cup, pillbox, syringe, or spoon used? How are the missed medications supposed to be given?

A parent reports that the child hates the taste and refuses to take the medicine. The parent should be counseled to offer the child some real choices regarding how the medications are taken, considering that often choices are limited when coping with chronic illness.

A pharmacist may have some ideas about how to make the medication more palatable or fun to take. He or she may have specialized compounding skills and be able to flavor the medication, sweeten the medication, or entirely change the dosage form of the medication. These special formulations should only be administered in controlled environments with adequate parental supervision or to older children who are able to understand the difference between candy and medicine. The compounding of an antiretroviral or any other medication depends on the pharmacokinetics of the specific drug and therefore must be discussed with both the pharmacist and manufacturer of the medication.[45]

A parent reports that the child is being given his or her medications, but the nurse suspects that adherence is inadequate because of a deterioration of the child's clinical and immunological status. This may be a good time to call the pharmacist to determine if the parent is actually filling prescriptions on a regularly scheduled basis. The pharmacist has a complete record of the client's medication profile, including the time between refills. For example, if the parent is refilling a 30-day supply of medication every 60 days, there is an obvious problem with adherence. Additionally, the support of a home health care agency with visiting nurse services is invaluable in these situations.[45]

A parent with medical and or psychological/cognitive limitations is required to administer a complicated medical regimen at home. Children with congenital HIV infection may require between 5 and 25 different medications to treat their HIV and related conditions. If a parent cannot administer these medications, the use of home care nursing may be necessary. There are also many parents without any psychological/cognitive limitations who may require nursing assistance when the treatment plan is very complex.[45]

The parent reports that the child becomes very nauseated and sometimes vomits after taking medications. Administration of a medication with food, if not contraindicated, usually helps to prevent nausea. If food may not be given at the same time, a full 8-oz glass of water may help reduce gastric irritation and related nausea.[45]

A parent is fearful that the antiretroviral medications will harm the child in some way. This is one of the more difficult challenges that a clinician faces. The difficulties arise from two different and often opposing belief systems. The goal for this problem should be a win-win solution, in which (1) the family understands the recommendations and rationale for the treatment plan and (2) the clinician attains an understanding of the family's mistrust and anxiety. It is only through mutual empathy and collaboration that the belief systems of both clients and clinicians can be challenged to evolve and change. Patience, perseverance, and a non-judgmental attitude are essential attributes for the health care team caring for the family coping with chronic illness.[45]

Collaboration with the family is one of the most important components of the adherence plan. It is more important than ever for families to be active participants in medication and treatment decisions, especially families facing chronic, terminal illness. Collaboration supports adherence to medication schedules and improves self-esteem and, ultimately, the quality of life.[45]

NURSING CARE OF PARENTS AND HIV-POSITIVE INFANTS AND CHILDREN

PARENTAL CARE

This section presents nursing guidelines for the health education of parents of a newly diagnosed HIV-infected infant or child. The guidelines help facilitate optimal care of HIV-infected children and their families. It is not feasible to completely cover all aspects of these guidelines during a client's initial visit. The guidelines should instead be viewed as a framework for ongoing nursing care tailored to the emotional and intellectual capabilities of the parents. The nurse must also provide the parents with information in written form, especially information on administration of medications. When caring for the family unit the nurse should be mindful of the overwhelming guilt typically experienced by an HIV-positive mother. This guilt may be expressed as anger towards the health care team. The nurse should be aware that the initial clinic visits for many mothers of HIV-infected infants may be particularly stressful experiences. The mother may have recently learned of her own HIV diagnosis and now has to face the HIV diagnosis of her infant. When caring for the family unit the nurse should consider:

- Providing a mental health referral for the mother if indicated or requested.
- Screening for domestic violence during the psychosocial history and interview.
- Providing a referral for substance abuse treatment if indicated or requested.
- Providing a referral for home care (e.g., home health aide, homemaking services, visiting nurse services) if indicated or requested.

BOX 21-8 PLANNING FOR LONG-TERM CARE OF CHILDREN WITH ILL PARENTS

1. *Informal arrangements*—These arrangements are not legally binding.
2. *Power of attorney*—A person is designated to make decisions for the child on behalf of the parent. This arrangement is legally binding.
3. *Designation of a guardian in a will*—This establishes the parent's wishes for a guardian for the child. The named person is not required to accept guardianship. A judge decides who will become the legal guardian.
4. *Adoption*—The parent agrees to terminate parental rights permanently.
5. *Voluntary placement in foster care*—The parent requests out-of-home placement because of illness and because kinship care or nonrelative care are the only options. The parent retains the right to make permanency plans.
6. *Involuntary placement in foster care*—A child is removed based on documentation of abuse or neglect. Kinship care or nonrelative care are the available options. The parent still retains the right to make permanency plans.
7. *Emergency and respite care*—The parent retains parental rights, and the family receives support services.
8. *Standby guardianship*—The parent retains parental authority; the guardian assumes authority when the parent is incapacitated.

From Taylor-Brown S: Talking with parents about permanency planning. In Aronstein D, Thompson B, eds: *HIV and social work: a practitioner's guide,* New York, 1998, Harrington.

- Offering assistance with partner notification and counseling on the prevention of HIV transmission.
- Offering assistance and support in determining the HIV status of other children.
- Providing education on the risk for HIV transmission through breastfeeding and advising the mother not to breastfeed infants.[46]
- Offering anticipatory guidance on the frequency of clinic visits at the time of the initial visit.
- Discussing the potential for HIV discrimination and the need to be selective in discussing an HIV diagnosis.

The psychosocial difficulty encountered by families that include one or more HIV-positive members has enormous influence on the treatment plan. Children and infants with congenital HIV infection are typically cared for in the context of their mothers' ill health. Many HIV-positive mothers may also be simultaneously facing issues of poverty, substance abuse, mental illness, inadequate housing, and violence. There are many grandmothers caring for their HIV-infected grandchildren due to the illness, substance abuse, or death of the child's parent(s). The nurse must make sure that a social work referral is initiated to assess the family unit. Long-term permanency planning is an essential component of care, especially if the parent is critically ill. Although options vary by state, Box 21-8 identifies some of the options available to parents.[47]

BOX 21-9   CHILDREN AND VENIPUNCTURE: SUGGESTED NURSING INTERVENTIONS

Repeated and frequent venipuncture is extremely stressful. It often proves more difficult for the parent than the child; this may be related to the parent's unresolved guilt over congenital HIV transmission. A child who is agitated during a venipuncture poses a risk to the health care worker. To perform a safe and effective venipuncture in a child, the following nursing interventions should be utilized:

- Explain the purpose and significance of the various blood tests that are obtained.
- Eutectic Mixture of lidocaine and prilocaine (EMLA) cream (lidocaine 2.5% and prilocaine 2.5%) is a topical anesthetic demonstrated to be extremely effective in reducing the pain, trauma, and anxiety associated with invasive procedures such as venipuncture and immunizations in children.
- EMLA cream is applied to intact skin and covered with a Tegaderm dressing 1 hour before venipuncture for selected children with a medical order, as directed by the manufacturer.
- EMLA should not be used for those rare clients with congenital or idiopathic methemoglobinemia, in infants under the age of 12 months who are receiving treatment with methemoglobin-inducing agents, or in neonates with a gestational age less than 37 weeks.
- EMLA should also be used with caution in clients receiving Class I antiarrhythmic drugs because of potentially synergistic effects and in clients who may be more sensitive to the systemic effects of lidocaine and prilocaine.
- The child should be given as many choices as possible about care and treatment to promote a sense of control. For example, when giving an immunization or performing venipuncture, ask the child if he or she "wants the needle in the left or right arm." Another example of a question that helps promote a sense of control is: "Do you want to sit on mommy's lap or do you want to sit alone?"

From Cooper CM et al: EMLA reduces the pain of venipuncture in children, *Europ J Anasthesiol* 4:441, 1987; Hopkins CS, Buckley CJ, Bush GH: Pain free injection in infants, *Anesthesia* 43:198, 1988; and Taddio A et al: Use of lidocaine-prilocaine cream for vaccination pain in infants, *J Pediatr* 124:643, 1994.

THE HIV-INFECTED CHILD

The nursing care needs of children infected with HIV are vast and very dynamic. The following are selected nursing interventions specific to HIV-infected children:

1. CD_4 T lymphocyte values should be obtained as soon as possible after a child has a positive virological test for HIV and every 3 months thereafter.[7,22] More frequent CD_4 T lymphocyte measurements are indicated for infants and children with immunological, virological, or clinical signs and symptoms suggestive of HIV-disease progression. The nurse should anticipate that repeated venipuncture is an important and anxiety-provoking event for children and parents. (Box 21-9 describes the nursing approach for the child receiving a venipuncture.[49-51])

2. PCP prophylaxis (see Box 16-3) is indicated for all HIV-infected and HIV-exposed infants at age 4 to 6 weeks, irrespective of the CD_4 T lymphocyte count. This prophylaxis continues for the first year of life in HIV-infected infants. In HIV-exposed infants, it is continued until HIV infection has been excluded, as described earlier in this chapter. In children 1 year of age and older, PCP prophylaxis is indicated based on age-specific CD_4 T lymphocyte values, as outlined in Box 16-3. The nurse should provide parents with education on the purpose and importance of PCP prophylaxis. It is also essential to reinforce the information about PCP prophylaxis given by the HIV specialist.

3. Prophylaxis against MAC is initiated in HIV-positive infants and children per age-specific CD_4 T lymphocyte values (see Box 13-1). Education on MAC and MAC prophylaxis should be provided for parents.

4. The nurse should instruct parents on the need to contact the pediatric HIV specialist if any signs or symptoms of illness occur (e.g., fever, vomiting, diarrhea, changes in appetite or activity, rash). The parent should also contact the specialist if another family member develops a contagious illness or signs and symptoms of an illness that might prove to be contagious.

5. Both education and anticipatory guidance on the recommended immunization guidelines for HIV-infected infants and children should be provided (Box 21-10).

6. Monitoring growth and development is essential in the care of HIV-infected children. The neurodevelopmental status of infants and children with HIV infection needs to be monitored closely through the use of age-appropriate assessments and examinations. Growth delay affecting both height and weight is one of the earliest signs of HIV disease in both infants and children. Serial measurements of weight, height, and head circumference are essential to the diagnosis.[15] Growth failure and neurodevelopment deterioration may be specific manifestations of HIV infection. A significant number of children with HIV or AIDS develop clinical, neurological, and behavioral difficulties. See Box 21-11 for a review of neurodevelopmental criteria for central nervous system (CNS) disease progression in children.

7. Nutritional education should be integrated into the care plan, and interventions should be directed at the entire family unit.[15] Nutritional support is an intervention that affects immune function, quality of life, and bioactivity of antiretroviral drugs.[14,15]

8. If the child or another family member owns a pet, parents should have the child avoid contact with pet feces and wash his or her hands after handling the pet.[48] Regular veterinary care should also be provided to maintain the animal's health.

9. Available clinical trials and treatment options should be reviewed in collaboration with the health care team.

BOX 21-10 IMMUNIZATIONS IN HIV-INFECTED CHILDREN

Infants and children with HIV infection or exposure should receive standard pediatric immunizations per the AAP guidelines when being immunized with hepatitis B, diphtheria-pertussis-tetanus, and *H. influenzae* vaccines.[11] However, some important differences from the standard pediatric immunization guidelines are outlined here. (Immunizations with pediatric considerations are discussed in detail in Chapter 9.) Guidelines are as follows:

- IPV (as opposed to oral poliovirus vaccine) is generally recommended for all children. HIV-infected infants and children and other children residing in the home with an HIV-infected infant or child should receive IPV.
- Annual influenza vaccination is indicated for the HIV-infected infant beginning at 6 months of age. Annual influenza vaccination is also indicated for all household contacts of the HIV-infected infant or child.
- Pneumococcal vaccination is indicated for HIV-infected children (see Appendix D).
- Annual TB testing using the Mantoux test is indicated for the HIV-infected infant or child beginning between 9 months and 1 year of age.[15] Annual TB testing is also indicated for household contacts of the HIV-infected infant or child.
- Varicella vaccines can be considered for an asymptomatic, immunocompetent HIV-infected child. Varicella zoster immune globulin (VZIG) may be administered to varicella-susceptible HIV-infected infants and children after varicella zoster exposures in an attempt to prevent the disease (indications, administration, and dosages are discussed in Box 6-10).
- MMR vaccination is deferred in HIV-infected children with severe immunocompromise (immunological category 3; see Table 21-1).[52,53] Both symptomatic and measles-susceptible asymptomatic HIV-infected children should receive IG prophylaxis if exposed to measles (indications, administration, and dosages are discussed in Box 6-7 and Box 21-12).
- HBV vaccination should be administered to all infants born to HIV-infected women at birth. HBV immune globulin (HBIG) should also be administered if the mother tests infected for HBV surface antigen[21] (indications, administration, and dosages are discussed in Box 6-2).
- In the management of wounds classified as tetanus prone, children with HIV infection should receive intramuscular tetanus immune globulin (TIG) regardless of vaccination status. Because of the infrequency of TIG administration, the dosage range, and the lack of an established optimal therapeutic dose,[54] a pediatric infectious disease expert should be consulted.

PREVENTION AND TREATMENT OF DISEASE IN CHILDREN— INTRAVENOUS IMMUNE GLOBULIN

Many children with congenital HIV infection receive monthly infusions of intravenous immune globulin (IVIG). Its major therapeutic uses for HIV infection are prevention of serious bacterial infections and treatment of idiopathic thrombocytopenic purpura (ITP). Immune globulin is derived from the pooled plasma of adults by an alcohol-fractionation procedure. It primarily consists of IgG (95%), with trace amounts of immunoglobulins A (IgA) and M (IgM).[55] IVIG has antibodies against a

BOX 21-11 NEURODEVELOPMENTAL CRITERIA FOR CNS DISEASE PROGRESSION

In the absence of alternative explanations, HIV-associated neurological disease progression can be defined as: (1) a child who is neurologically normal at baseline but subsequently develops one of the major abnormalities (i.e., A, B, C); or (2) a child who possesses neurological or developmental abnormalities at baseline but subsequently develops two of the following major abnormalities (i.e., A, B, C):

A. Impairment of brain growth, in the absence of alternative etiologies, documented by 1, 2, 3, or 4 below; should be persistent or progressive as documented by two measures separated by at least 2 months:
   1. For infants <1 year of age, failure to attain above the 5th percentile head circumference growth curve (i.e., from the National Center for Health Statistics growth curves), with neither an alternative explanation nor a diagnosis of congenital microcephaly.
   2. For infants <3 years of age, crossing two major head circumference growth-curve percentiles from a baseline measurement without alternative explanation. Consider neuroimaging correlation that demonstrates atrophy and basal ganglia calcification.
   3. For any age, falling below the 5th percentile head circumference growth curve without an alternative explanation. Consider neuroimaging correlations.
   4. For any age, serial neuroimaging studies, performed under the same conditions and reviewed or compared simultaneously, documenting progressive and significant loss of cerebral parenchymal volume ("atrophy") without other cause.
B. Decline of cognitive function, documented by psychometric testing persistent on at least two individual valid assessments separated by at least 1 month.
   1. For infants from birth to 3 years, a fall of 2 standard deviation (SD) units on a standardized, nonscreening developmental assessment (e.g., Mental Developmental Index of the Bayley Scales of Infant Development).*†
   2. For children >3 years, a fall of ≥1 SD on a standardized test of intelligence.†
   3. At any age, loss of previously attained cognitive or language milestones, without alternative explanation, and confirmed by standardized testing.*†
C. Clinical motor dysfunction, without alternative explanation, documented to be progressive on two individual examinations separated by at least 1 month in:
   1. Loss or significant deterioration of motor skills attained previously or in any of the following subcriteria (2, 3, or 4).
   2. Diffuse and symmetrical loss or deterioration in power or strength that is not the result of a systemic, nutritional, or metabolic complication.
   3. Diffuse and symmetrical abnormalities of tone, including, but not limited to, hypotonia, hypertonia, or rigidity.
   4. Diffuse, symmetrical, and pathologically increased deep tendon reflexes.

---

* Scores corrected for prematurity may lead to factitious results. Thus, consider using uncorrected scores for premature infants.
† For children who start with developmental delay, or for those transitioning to a different standardized test, consult a psychologist to determine change over time.

From Working Group on Antiretroviral and Medical Management of Infants, Children, and Adolescents with HIV Infection: Antiretroviral therapy and management of pediatric HIV infection, *Pediatrics* 102(4, Part 2): 1005, 1998.

BOX 21-12 **ADMINISTRATION OF IMMUNE GLOBULIN**

- IG can be administered to prevent or modify measles in a susceptible person anytime during the first 6 days following exposure to measles.
- All HIV-infected, perinatally-exposed children who are exposed to measles should receive immune globulin (IG) prophylaxis 0.5 cc/kg (not to exceed 15 cc) IM or IVIG 400 mg/kg regardless of measles vaccination status.
- Children receiving monthly IVIG infusions whose last dose was received within 3 weeks of measles exposure may not need an additional dose of IVIG; however, some experts recommend that an additional dose be considered if 2 or more weeks have elapsed since the last dose of IVIG;
- IG preparations interfere with the serological response to measles vaccine for variable periods depending on the dose administered. The suggested interval between MMR or monovalent measles vaccination and IG preparations is as follows:
  - VZIG: 5 months
  - HBIG: 3 months
  - IVIG 400 mg/kg per dose: 8 months
  - IVIG 1000 mg/kg per dose: 10 months
  - IG for measles prophylaxis: 5 months for doses of 0.25 cc/kg; 6 months for doses of 0.5 cc/kg
- Blood products also interfere with the serological response to measles vaccine for variable periods depending on the blood product administered. Blood products and suggested intervals between their administration and the administration of MMR or monovalent measles vaccinations are specified below:
  - Red blood cells (RBCs) with adenine-saline added (10 cc/kg): 3 months
  - Plasma or platelet products (10 cc/kg): 7 months
  - Packed RBCs (10 cc/kg): 5 months
  - Whole blood (10 cc/kg): 6 months

From American Academy of Pediatrics: Measles. In Pickering LK, ed: *2000 red book: report of the Committee on Infectious Diseases*, ed 25, Elk Grove Village, Ill, 2000, American Academy of Pediatrics; and American Academy of Pediatrics: HIV infection. In Pickering LK, ed: *2000 red book: report of the Committee on Infectious Diseases*, ed 25, Elk Grove Village, Ill, 2000, American Academy of Pediatrics.

number of common pathogens and can protect against recurrent serious bacterial illness in children with HIV infection. This beneficial effect of IVIG was demonstrated in a randomized, placebo-controlled outpatient study conducted in 28 clinical sites. A reduction in serious and minor viral and bacterial infections was observed in children with entry CD_4 counts of at least $0.20 \times 10^9/L$.[56] Another randomized, double-blind, placebo-controlled trial conducted in 30 clinical sites also demonstrated the benefit of IVIG in children with advanced HIV disease who were receiving ZDV. There was a decreased incidence of serious bacterial infections in children who were not receiving prophylaxis with trimethoprim-sulfamethoxazole.[57] The usual IVIG dose for prophylaxis of bacterial infections is 400 mg/kg/dose, administered monthly.

Children with HIV-related thrombocytopenia might also be prescribed IVIG infusions, usually by a pediatric hematologist. Higher doses of IVIG are required for the treatment of ITP and are indicated for active bleeding or platelet counts less than $20 \times 10^9/L$. The usual dose for ITP is 1 to 2 g/kg/day over 1 to 3 days. Based on the client's platelet count, IVIG is then administered every 2 to 4 weeks as directed by a pediatric hematologist.[58]

One of the more challenging aspects of IVIG administration in pediatric clients is related to immunization administration; children should not be immunized with measles-mumps-rubella (MMR) or monovalent measles vaccine for 8 months after IVIG administration at the standard dose of 400 mg/kg/dose.[52] See Box 21-12 for waiting periods for the administration of other immune globulins and for additional information about IG administration.

The reported incidence of adverse reactions to IVIG ranges from 1% to 15% but is usually less than 5%.[55] Most of these reactions are mild and self-limited; severe reactions occur very infrequently. Adverse events include fever, chills, headache, myalgia, anxiety, lightheadedness, nausea, vomiting, flushing, tachycardia, change in blood pressure, aseptic meningitis, and hypersensitivity reactions.[55] Anaphylactic reactions induced by anti-IgA can occur in children with primary antibody deficiency and total absence of circulating IgA and antibodies to IgA. These reactions are rare, and screening for IgA deficiency is not routinely recommended.[55]

Nursing Considerations

1. Parents and children need to be educated on the frequency of IVIG treatment before initiation of therapy.
2. Parents may inquire about the safety of this product because it is pooled from plasma. An outbreak of HCV did occur in 1994 among recipients of products from a single domestic manufacturer in the United States. Procedures and requirements for the preparation of IVIG have been implemented to prevent transmission of HCV.[55]
3. The initial infusion is administered in the hospital setting so the child may be monitored for any adverse reactions. After the initial infusion, parents and children should be offered a choice as to where subsequent infusions will be administered. Some parents refuse home infusions for fear of neighbors learning the HIV diagnosis. If the parent and child agree, monthly IVIG may be provided in the child's home through the assistance of home care services. This will decrease the frequency of hospital or clinic visits.
4. Children must be screened for a past history of an adverse reaction to a previous IVIG infusion or any other medications before administration.
5. The protocol for administration of IVIG depends on the nursing policies and procedures of the given institution or facility. The nurse must adhere to the guidelines of his or her employer. However, there are

some basic considerations for administration of IVIG to be included in the nursing care plan, which include:

- Not shaking the vial (to avoid foaming).[59]
- Starting the infusion within 6 hours of opening the vial, and completing the infusion within 12 hours.[59]
- Before use, refrigerating the medication at 36° to 46° F.[59]
- Using filters according to institutional protocol (they are unnecessary, though some facilities may use them).[59]
- Administering IVIG infusions on a controller-type IV device to maintain a constant infusion rate.
- Administering IVIG infusions through a dedicated IV line.[59]
- Administering initial infusions slowly, with vigilant monitoring of vital signs before, during, and after IVIG infusion; frequency depends on the policy of the facility or institution.
- Maintaining the recommended rate of 0.01 to 0.02 ml/kg/min during the first 30 minutes of infusion.[59]
- Observing the client closely for signs (noted previously) of an adverse reaction to the IVIG infusion; epinephrine and other medications and equipment to treat an anaphylactic reaction must be available when infusing IVIG in the home or hospital.
- If no discomfort or signs of adverse reaction occur, the infusion rate may be increased to a maximum 0.06 ml/kg/min.[57] Other sources recommend a maximum rate of 0.08 ml/kg/min.[59] There should be gradual advancement to this rate, especially during the initial infusion.[57] Advancement to the maximum infusion rate may proceed more rapidly during subsequent infusions, once the child's tolerance has been determined.[57]

DISCLOSURE OF AN HIV DIAGNOSIS TO INFECTED CHILDREN

Disclosure of an HIV diagnosis to a child has proven to be one of the more challenging aspects of the treatment plan, especially as perinatally infected children and adolescents are living longer with HIV. During the early phases of the epidemic, pediatric HIV infection seemed universally fatal and, therefore, the question of how to inform a child of an HIV diagnosis seemed irrelevant.[60] However, recent medical advances resulting in improved quality of life have necessitated greater attention to disclosure. The difficulties surrounding disclosure of an HIV diagnosis to a child vary within the context of each family system. However, some common themes related to difficulties in disclosure have been identified[61]:

- It brings premature death into the consciousness.
- It involves the positive diagnosis of the mother of congenitally infected children.
- Parents fear that disclosure will harm the child in some way.
- There is maternal guilt regarding congenital transmission.
- There is a social stigma attached to a fatal infectious disease.

- Parents fear that the child will disclose the diagnosis to friends, classmates, or others.

In addition to these common themes, there are many other issues encountered by parents contemplating disclosure. Some parents fear their child will reject them if he or she learns about the behaviors of the parents that led to HIV infection.[62] There are other parents who choose not to disclose because of denial and difficulty in coping with their own illness.[63] Parents may not want to discuss their child's HIV illness because talking about it makes it real.[64] The secrecy surrounding HIV disease and disclosure within a family system has been described as both a protective function and an adaptive communication style.[60] Disclosure of HIV diagnosis to a child may be one of a number of family secrets not to be discussed. Understanding this should help limit the anger often experienced by health care professionals in response to a family's difficulties with disclosing a HIV diagnosis to a child.

Clinical research involving children with other life-threatening conditions such as cancer has revealed that children have an awareness of the serious nature of their illness. This is present even if adults have not informed the child of the seriousness.[65] A child's worst fears are often associated with abandonment, not death,[62] and this is an important premise to communicate to a parent who fears disclosing the name of a fatal illness. Health care professionals should educate parents on the benefits of disclosure for children. Children with a variety of chronic diseases, including cancer, exhibit better coping skills and fewer psychological problems when appropriately informed about their illness.[66,67] Preliminary studies indicate that children who know their HIV diagnosis have higher self-esteem than infected children who are unaware of their status.[63] Parents who had not revealed the HIV diagnosis to their child were found to be significantly more depressed than those who shared the diagnosis.[67] The risks of not disclosing, such as secrecy, deception, and inadvertent disclosure, should be addressed.[65] Children who overhear medical talk coupled with their parents being upset may suspect that they are more seriously ill than they are being told and develop inappropriate and hurtful fantasies about their illness.[62,63] If parental death were to occur before the disclosure of a HIV diagnosis, the opportunity for the child to discuss his or her diagnosis would be lost.[63] However, despite these reasons, contraindications to disclosure may appear at any point in the disclosure process,[60] and these vary according to the individual family. Full acceptance of the consequences of a child's HIV diagnosis involves a lengthy process for the entire family and warrants empathy, education, direction, and support from the health care team.

The AAP has published the following recommendations regarding disclosure of HIV/AIDS status to children and adolescents[63]:

- Parents and other guardians of HIV-infected children should be counseled by a knowledgeable health care professional about HIV disclosure to the child. This counseling may need to be repeated throughout the course of the child's illness.

■ Disclosure of the diagnosis to an HIV-infected child should be tailored to the child's cognitive ability, developmental stage, clinical status, and social circumstances.

■ Younger children with symptomatic disease do not need to be informed of their HIV diagnosis, but the illness should be discussed with them. If children are informed of their diagnosis, fears and misperceptions should be addressed.

■ The AAP strongly encourages disclosure of HIV infection status to school-age children. Older children have a better capacity to understand the nature and consequences of their illness. Symptomatic children requiring hospitalization should be informed of their HIV status because of the likelihood of inadvertent disclosure.

■ Adolescents should be informed of their HIV status. This knowledge permits appreciation of the consequences of the diagnosis for many aspects of their lives, including sexual behavior. It also enables them to make appropriate decisions about treatment and participation in clinical trials.

Nursing Considerations

1. The health care team should anticipate and plan for eventual disclosure of HIV diagnosis to the child; this disclosure plan should be part of the overall treatment plan.

2. Disclosure requires a multidisciplinary approach, including collaboration with the child and family. It is not an exclusive dialogue between the medical practitioner and family. Other professionals crucial for this process include, but are not limited to, social workers, child life specialists, chaplains, and psychiatrists.

3. Disclosure is an evolving process rather than an isolated event in time. Disclosure of an HIV diagnosis does not begin or end with naming the disease. Naming the illness is only one moment along the continuum of communication.[64]

4. It is important to ask the child what he or she knows "about why they come to the clinic every 2 months" and proceed from there. Often, the focus is on providing the child with information, with little attention directed at understanding what the child already understands of the illness. Some children are either surprisingly informed or misinformed about their HIV diagnosis.

5. The timing of disclosure should vary among children, and disclosure to an individual child at a particular time may not be ideal for any number of reasons. However, communication should not come to a halt. Other aspects of HIV disease may be discussed without naming the illness. For example, discussion of the child's medications and "how they are helping to keep the soldiers [CD_4 T lymphocytes] in the blood strong" is an example of ongoing communication related to disclosure. Simultaneously, the mental health team can help manage the issues precluding full disclosure.

6. Disclosure-related decisions made by the multidisciplinary team and the child's family always must be guided by the best interest of the child.
7. Disclosure-related interventions for the child must be done within the context of the family and not apart from it. The child and family must both be prepared for the disclosure of an HIV diagnosis for optimal outcomes to occur. If the disclosure process does not include the parents, the child will experience isolation upon leaving the clinic or hospital setting.
8. Support, counseling, and education on the benefits of disclosure should be provided to families struggling with disclosure. The health care provider should avoid engaging in an oppositional relationship.
9. Parents should be encouraged to discuss any anxiety or guilty feelings attached to disclosure. Referrals to available HIV-infected parent groups may offer considerable peer support.

ADOLESCENTS WITH PERINATAL HIV INFECTION

The provision of optimal care to an HIV-infected adolescent depends upon both an understanding and an appreciation of the key developmental aspects of adolescence. Management of a teenager's HIV disease cannot be provided in isolation of his or her adolescence. This section provides a general overview of the essential psychosocial components inherent in effective nursing management of the perinatally-infected adolescent.

Adolescence is a time of growth and transition between childhood and adulthood.[68] Although changes can vary widely from individual to individual, three phases of adolescence have been described—early, middle, and late (Box 21-13). It is important to remember that these phases offer guidelines when caring for the adolescent. Categories may overlap or occur at different ages than those listed. Progress through these stages differs by gender, race, and culture and may frequently be delayed by physical and psychosocial stresses such as chronic illness, family dysfunction, abuse, learning disorders, substance abuse, poverty, and sexual identity struggles.[68] There are some children with advanced HIV disease who present with delays in growth, development, and onset of puberty. Other children progress normally into adolescence, and still others present with delays in their cognitive or emotional development.[68]

The developmental tasks of adolescence are in direct opposition to effective HIV treatment. Adolescents characteristically need increased independence from their parents and are increasingly dependent on peer and opposite-sex relationships. They also may demonstrate risk-taking behaviors, rebellion toward authority figures, and, possibly, experimentation with sex, drugs, and alcohol. A developmentally oriented approach is fundamental when conducting psychosocial assessments in the HIV-infected adolescent. The HEADDS assessment in Box 21-14 is one example of such an approach. An advantage of the HEADDS assessment is that it moves from less to more personal questions. Since trust is extremely important to an adolescent, the clinician should review the policy on con-

BOX 21-13   ADOLESCENT DEVELOPMENT

Early: 10-13 Years of Age

- Pubertal changes and resulting concerns (e.g., "Am I normal?")
- Wide mood swings
- Intense feelings
- Low impulse control
- Role exploration
- Concrete thinking
- Little ability to anticipate long-term consequences of actions
- Literal
- Estrangement
- Need for privacy
- Increased importance and intensity of same sex relationships

Middle: 14-16 Years of Age

- End of pubertal changes
- Sense of invulnerability
- Risk-taking behavior peaks
- Ability to conceptualize the idea of abstract images such as love, justice, truth, and spirituality
- Peak of parental conflicts
- Rejection of parental values
- Peak of peer conformity
- Increased importance of opposite sex relationships

Late: 17 Years of Age and Older

- Sense of responsibility for one's health
- Increasing sense of vulnerability
- Ability to consider others and suppress own needs
- Less risk taking
- Formal operational thought
- Ability to compromise and limit set
- Understand others' thought and feelings
- Improved communication
- Acceptance of parental values
- Peers decrease in importance
- Mutually supportive, mature, intimate relationships increase in importance

From Samples C, Goodman E, Woods E: Epidemiology and medical management of adolescents. In Pizzo PA, Wilfert CM, eds: *Pediatric AIDS: the challenge of HIV infection in infants, children, and adolescents*, ed 3, Baltimore, 1998, Williams & Wilkins.

fidentiality of information communicated by the adolescent before beginning the HEADDS assessment. Most clinicians inform the adolescent that any information communicated will be kept confidential unless it involves intent to harm the self or others, situations of abuse or violence, or other information that the provider must report. In addition, before beginning the HEADDS assessment or any psychosocial assessment, it is

BOX 21-14   MODIFIED **HEADDS** ASSESSMENT FOR THE **HIV**-INFECTED TEENAGER*

Home (H)—Where are you living? How long have you been living there? Tell me about the neighborhood you are living in. Do you feel safe in your neighborhood? With whom do you live? (Do not assume the teen is living with two parents.) Do you all get along with each other? Have there been any problems in your home that you are worried about? (Screening for domestic violence and substance abuse should be included.)

Education (E)—Are you attending school at this time? If yes, what school do you attend? How do you like the school? If no, when did you stop attending school? Tell me about what stopped you from attending school? Are there any problems in the school (e.g., violent crime, substance abuse)? What grade are you in? What are your favorite subjects? What are the classes you do not like? What are your grades like? Are you thinking about college? If yes, what would you like to study in college? (Be sure to offer positive feedback for the teen's successes; problem-solve with the teen in areas needing improvement.)

Activities (A)—Tell me about your friends. Do you have a best friend? If yes, what do you like to do with him/her? What kind of music/dance do you like? Do you or any of your friends drive? (If yes, review car safety such as seat belts) Do you play any sports? (Review bike safety, including the use of a bike helmet.) Are you able to discuss your HIV diagnosis with your best friend or any of your friends? Who else can you talk to about your HIV (e.g., guidance counselor, family member)?

Drugs (D)—Some of the teenagers I care for smoke cigarettes. Do any of your friends smoke cigarettes? Have you ever smoked a cigarette? If yes, do you smoke every day? How many cigarettes do you typically smoke in a day? Sometimes, teens drink beer at parties or when they are hanging out with their friends. What do your friends drink at parties? What do you like to drink at a party? Have you ever been drunk? How much did you drink to make you drunk? A lot of drugs are sold in schools today. What drugs are sold in your school? What drugs do your friends use? How do you handle it when your friends are using drugs in front of you? Have you ever tried any drugs? What kinds of drugs have you tried? Have you ever been high from drugs? If yes, how many times, and what drugs made you high? How many times a week do you get high? (Health teaching and referral to smoking cessation or substance abuse counseling should be done as appropriate.)

---

* Note: Additional questions relevant to HIV infection have been added.

Continued

BOX 21-14   MODIFIED HEADDS ASSESSMENT FOR THE HIV-INFECTED TEENAGER—CONT'D

Depression (D)—Dealing with HIV is tough for many of the teens I care for. How do you handle being HIV-positive? Do you ever feel sad or afraid because of your HIV? Have you lost anyone close to you as a result of HIV? If yes, can you tell me about it? Do you worry about becoming very sick from HIV? Have you ever thought of hurting yourself when you were feeling down? If yes:
- How did you plan on hurting yourself or have you ever tried to hurt yourself in the past?
- Has anyone in your family ever tried to kill him or herself?
- Have any of your friends ever tried to kill or hurt themselves?
- Are you thinking about hurting yourself now? (If yes, seek immediate consultation with a mental health professional.)

To whom can the teen talk when feeling down? Does he or she need you to find someone he or she can talk to on a regular basis?

Sexuality (S)—Are you dating anyone at this time? (Do not assume a heterosexual identity for the teen). If yes, where did you meet, and how long have you been dating? Where do the two of you like to go when you are together, and what do you enjoy doing? Does he or she know your HIV diagnosis? Many teens are having sexual intercourse today, and there are also may teens who have chosen not to have sex. How have you chosen to handle this? (If the teen is sexually active, inquire about age of onset of sexual activity, number of partners, history of pregnancy, birth control, abortions, sexually transmitted diseases, and menstrual history.†) Have you ever felt pushed or forced into sexual intercourse or any other type of sexual activity?‡

---

† Sexually active females should be referred for gynecological care, and the date of the last Pap smear should be determined. Assessment for a history of abnormal Pap smears should also be obtained. This is an excellent point to rereview HIV prevention and the importance of consistent condom use. Screening for sexual abuse should also be done. Education on masturbation, nocturnal emissions, and spontaneous erections may also be provided. These topics need to be reviewed as a normal part of adolescent development, and teenagers should be encouraged to ask any relevant questions

‡ Be sure to counsel the teen on what to do should he or she feel forced or coerced into any type of sexual activity. Nurses should be aware of institutional, state, and federal laws for reporting sexual abuse of minors in case a minor reports an event to the nurse.

From Neinstein LS: The office visit and interview techniques. In Neinstein LS, ed: *Adolescent health care: a practical guide*, ed 2, Baltimore, 1991, Urban & Schwarzenberg.

crucial to inform the adolescent that, although some of the questions may be personal, they are being asked so that the information obtained can be used to provide the most appropriate care.

A pediatric HIV specialist and a multidisciplinary health care team are vital to the successful treatment of an adolescent with congenital HIV infection. Typically, general recommendations regarding antiretroviral treatment for adolescents with congenital HIV infection are not made. Treatment decisions are made by the pediatric HIV specialist and tailored to the individual medical and social needs of the adolescent. This is because of the likelihood of exposure to numerous antiretroviral medications beginning early in life and also because of the complex psychosocial issues that invariably affect treatment. Doses of antiretroviral and other medications should be prescribed according to Tanner's stages of puberty[69] and not on the basis of age.[7] To determine drug dosages for adolescents in early puberty (Tanner stages I and II), the prescriber should use pediatric schedules; for adolescents in late puberty (Tanner stage V), the prescriber should follow adult dosing schedules. Adolescents in their growth spurt (Tanner III in females and Tanner IV in males) should be closely monitored for medication efficacy and toxicity when either adult or pediatric dosing guidelines are used.[14]

Adherence to antiretroviral medications for HIV-infected adolescents presents unique challenges for the clinician. Selection of a potent antiretroviral regimen needs to include a realistic assessment of the existing and potential support systems to facilitate adherence. Asymptomatic HIV-infected teenagers may find it difficult to adhere to a complicated antiretroviral regimen, especially if the medications have side effects; this is reflective of the concrete thought process characteristic of adolescence.[14]

There are obvious stresses inherent in living with chronic HIV disease. Generally speaking, chronic illness is vastly different from acute illness; it drains the victim and the entire family over an indefinite period.[70] HIV has been described as a multigenerational family disease that intersects with psychosocial and societal issues, life events, and lifestyle choices in ways that other chronic illnesses do not.[71] Youths with perinatal HIV infection are often orphans or living with one sick parent by the time they reach adolescence.[68] There are also many grandmothers caring for their HIV-infected teenaged grandchildren. These grandmothers can be overwhelmed by the demands of a grandchild's care. Problem-solving for these challenges is ongoing, because most HIV-infected children are now surviving into adolescence. As the new millennium begins, college preparation, career counseling, and support for dating and socialization are just a few of the new challenges to be addressed in the care of HIV-infected adolescents.

Nursing Considerations

1. An essential component of the treatment plan for adolescents is to develop creative adherence strategies that do not interfere with peer activities. Adherence to complex regimens is particularly challenging for the HIV-infected adolescent who does not want to appear different from his or her peers.[15] For example, if peer activities interfere with a three times daily medication regimen, it may be possible to substitute a twice daily regimen.

2. It is important to avoid documentation during the psychosocial interview, especially if the teen is discussing sensitive issues such as sexuality or loss.

3. The psychosocial development of an adolescent with perinatal infection may be affected by multiple losses.[68] HIV-infected adolescents may be in foster care, orphans, or living with a sick parent. Consistent medical providers are an important source of stability for the adolescent. Changes in the health care professionals caring for the adolescent should not be made without consulting him or her first. Adolescents should also be informed when a health care professional is leaving the facility; opportunities for closure of the relationship should be provided.

4. All sexually active adolescents should be counseled about the correct and consistent use of condoms.[53] It is also helpful to actually show the teen a condom and illustrate its correct use. (For correct condom use, see p. 144.)

5. Assistance with partner notification should be offered to the sexually active adolescent.

6. Body image is of utmost importance to HIV-infected adolescents. However, many of them face alterations in body image because of short stature, wasting, dermatological conditions, central adiposity because of protease inhibitors, and indwelling devices such as gastrostomy tubes and central lines. Every effort should be made to preserve the adolescent's body image and integrity.

7. Nurses should be aware that adolescents may experience delayed onset of puberty because of chronic illness and should be prepared to support the adolescent and discuss concerns.

8. Ongoing education and anticipatory guidance should be directed at risk reduction because of the experimentation and risk-taking behaviors observed in adolescents.

REFERENCES

1. Pan American Health Organization–Working Group on Global HIV/AIDS and STD Surveillance: *AIDS surveillance in the Americas,* biannual report, June 1999.

2. Centers for Disease Control and Prevention. Update: perinatally acquired HIV/AIDS: United States, 1997, *MMWR* 46(46):1086, 1997.

3. Centers for Disease Control and Prevention.: U.S. HIV and AIDS cases reported through December 1999, *HIV/AIDS Surveillance Report* 11(2):1, 1999.

4. Centers for Disease Control and Prevention: Recommendations of the U.S. Public Health Service Task Force on the use of zidovudine to reduce perinatal transmission of human immunodeficiency virus, *MMWR* 43(RR-11):1, 1994.

5. Centers for Disease Control and Prevention: U.S. Public Health Service recommendations for human immunodeficiency virus counseling and voluntary testing for pregnant women, *MMWR* 44(RR-7):1, 1995.

6. Centers for Disease Control and Prevention: Revised classification system for human immunodeficiency virus infection in children less than 13 years of age, *MMWR* 43(RR-12):1, Sept 30, 1994.

7. U.S. Department of Health and Human Services: *Clinical practice guideline no. 7: evaluation and management of early HIV infection,* AHCPR Publication No. 94-0572, Rockville, Md, 1994, The Association.

8. Johnson JP et al: Natural history and serological diagnosis of infants born to human immunodeficiency virus–infected women, *Am J Dis Child* 143:1147, 1989.

9. Dunn DT et al: The sensitivity of the HIV-1 DNA polymerase chain reaction in the neonatal period and the relative contributions of intra-uterine and intra-partum transmission, *AIDS* 9:F7, 1995.

10. McIntosh K et al: Blood culture in the first six months of life for the diagnosis of vertically transmitted human immunodeficiency virus infection, *J Infect Dis* 170:996, 1994.

11. Centers for Disease Control and Prevention: Guidelines for the use of antiretroviral agents in pediatric HIV-infection, *MMWR* 47(RR-4):1, 1998.

12. Nesheim S et al: Diagnosis of perinatal human immunodeficiency virus infection by polymerase chain reaction and p24 antigen detection after immune complex dissociation in an urban community hospital, *J Infect Dis* 175:1333, 1997.

13. Centers for Disease Control and Prevention: 1995 Revised guidelines for prophylaxis against *Pneumocystis carinii* pneumonia for children infected with or perinatally exposed to human immunodeficiency virus, *MMWR* 44 (RR-4):1, 1995.

14. Working Group on Antiretroviral Therapy and Medical Management of HIV-Infected Children: *Guidelines for the use of antiretroviral agents in pediatric HIV infection,* National Pediatric and Family HIV Resource Center (NPHRC), Health Resources and Services Administration (HRSA), and National Institutes of Health (NIH). http://hivatis.org/index.html

15. Working Group on Antiretroviral Therapy and Medical Management of Infants, Children, and Adolescents with HIV Infection: Antiretroviral therapy and medical management of pediatric HIV infection, *Pediatrics* 102(4):1005, 1998.

16. Bryson YJ et al: Proposed definitions for in utero versus intrapartum transmission of HIV-1, *N Engl J Med* 327:1246, 1993.

17. Mayaux MJ et al: Neonatal characteristics in rapidly progressive perinatally acquired HIV-1 disease, *JAMA* 275:606, 1996.

18. Dickover RE et al: Rapid increases in load of human immunodeficiency virus correlate with early disease progression and loss of CD_4 cells in vertically infected infants, *J Infect Dis* 170:1279, 1994.

19. Shearer WT et al: Viral load and disease progression in infants infected with human immunodeficiency virus type 1, *N Engl J Med* 336:1337, 1997.

20. AIDS Institute: *Prevention of perinatal transmission,* 1998, New York State Department of Health.

21. American Academy of Pediatrics, Committee on Pediatric AIDS: Evaluation and medical treatment of the HIV-exposed infant, *Pediatrics* 99(6):909, 1997.

22. Wilfert CM et al: Quality standard for enumeration of CD_4^+ T lymphocytes in infants and children exposed to or infected with human immunodeficiency virus, *Clin Infect Dis* 21(suppl 1):S134, 1995.

23. Erkeller-Yuksel FM et al: Age related changes in human blood lymphocyte sub-populations, *J Pediatr* 120:216, 1992.

24. Denny T et al: Lymphocyte subsets in healthy children during the first 5 years of life, *JAMA* 267:1484, 1992.

25. McKinney RE, Wilfert CM: Lymphocyte subsets in children younger than 2 years old: normal values in a population at risk for human immunodeficiency virus infection and diagnostic and prognostic application to infected children, *Pediatr Infect Dis J* 11:639, 1992.

26. The European Collaborative Study: Age-related standards for T lymphocyte subsets based on uninfected children born to human immunodeficiency virus-1–infected women, *Pediatr Infect Dis J* 11:1018, 1992.

27. Waecker NJ et al: Age-adjusted CD$_4$ lymphocyte parameters in healthy children at risk for infection with the human immunodeficiency virus—the military pediatric HIC consortium, *Clin Infect Dis* 17:123, 1993.

28. Leibovitz E et al: *Pneumocystis carinii* pneumonia in infants infected with the human immunodeficiency virus with more than 450 CD$_4$ T lymphocytes per cubic millimeter, *N Engl J Med* 323:531, 1990.

29. Connor E et al: Clinical and laboratory correlates of *Pneumocystis carinii* pneumonia in children infected with HIV, *JAMA* 265:1693, 1991.

30. Kovacs A et al: CD$_4$ T lymphocyte counts and *Pneumocystis carinii* pneumonia in pediatric HIV infection, *JAMA* 265:1698, 1991

31. Raszka WV et al: Variability of serial absolute and percent CD$_4$ lymphocyte counts in healthy children born to HIV-infected parents, *Lancet* 13:70, 1994.

32. Katzenstein TL et al. Longitudinal serum HIV RNA quantification: correlation to viral phenotype at seroconversion and clinical outcome, *AIDS* 10:167, 1996.

33. Henrard DR et al: Natural History of HIV-1–cell-free viremia, *JAMA* 274:554-558, 1995.

34. Palumbo PE et al: Viral measurement by polymerase chain reaction-based assays in human immunodeficiency virus infected infants, *J Pediatr* 126:592, 1995.

35. Abrams EJ et al: *HIV viral load early in life as a predictor of disease progression in HIV-infected infants*, XI International Conference on AIDS, Vancouver, B.C., Canada, July 7-12, 1996 (abstract We.B.311).

36. McIntosh K et al: Age- and time-related changes in extracellular viral load in children vertically infected by human immunodeficiency virus, *Pediatr Infect Dis J* 15:1087, 1996.

37. Mofenson LM et al: The relationship between serum human immunodeficiency virus type 1 (HIV-1) RNA level, CD$_4$ lymphocyte percent, and long term mortality risk in HIV-1–infected children, *J Infect Dis* 175:1029, 1997.

38. Palumbo PE et al: Disease progression in HIV-infected infants and children: predictive value of quantitative plasma HIV RNA and CD$_4$ lymphocyte count, *JAMA* 279:756, 1998.

39. Centers for Disease Control and Prevention: Public Health Service Task Force recommendations for the use of antiretroviral drugs in pregnant women infected with HIV-1 for maternal health and for reducing perinatal HIV-1 transmission in the United States, *MMWR* 47(RR-2):1, 1998.

40. Perelson AS et al: HIV-1 dynamics in vivo: virion clearance rate, infected cell life span, and viral generation time, *Science* 271:1582, 1996.

41. Havlir DV, Richman DD: Viral dynamics of HIV: implications for drug development and therapeutic strategies, *Ann Intern Med* 124:984, 1996

42. Eastman PS et al. Maternal viral genotypic zidovudine resistance and infrequent failure of zidovudine therapy to prevent perinatal transmission of human immunodeficiency virus type 1 in pediatric AIDS Clinical Trials 076, *J Infect Dis* 177:557, 1998.

43. Mofenson L et al: Efficacy of zidovudine (ZDV) in reducing perinatal transmission in HIV-1 infected women with advanced disease. In *Abstracts of the 37th Interscience Conference on Antimicrobial Agents and Chemotherapy,* Toronto, Ontario, Sept 28-Oct 1, 1997 (abstract 1-117).

44. Dunn AM, Navarra JP, Cervia J: *Adherence to antiretroviral medications in HIV-infected children: a collaborative approach with guidelines for care,* 12th World AIDS Conference, Geneva, Switzerland, June 28-July 3, 1998 (abstract #32378).

45. Cervia J, Peters V: Supportive care issues for children with HIV infection. In Cunningham SC, George C, Gorospe M, eds: *Criteria for the medical care of children and adolescents with HIV infection,* ed 3, New York, 2000, AIDS Institute, New York State Department of Health.

46. American Academy of Pediatrics, Committee on Pediatric AIDS: Human milk, breastfeeding, and transmission of human immunodeficiency virus in the United States, *Pediatrics* 96:977, 1995.

47. Taylor-Brown S: Talking with parents about permanency planning. In Aronstein D, Thompson B, ed: *HIV and social work: a practitioner's guide,* New York, 1998, The Harrington.

48. Centers for Disease Control and Prevention: 1997 USPHS/IDSA guidelines for the prevention of opportunistic infections in persons with infected with human immunodeficiency virus, *MMWR* 46(RR-12):1, 1997.

49. Cooper CM et al: EMLA reduces the pain of venipuncture in children, *Europ J Anasthesiol* 4:441, 1987.

50. Hopkins CS, Buckley CJ, Bush GH: Pain free injection in infants, *Anesthesia* 43:198, 1988.

51. Taddio A et al: Use of lidocaine-prilocaine cream for vaccination pain in infants, *J Pediatr* 124:643, 1994.

52. American Academy of Pediatrics: Measles. In Peter G, ed: *1997 red book: report of the Committee on Infectious Diseases,* ed 24, Elk Grove Village, Ill, 1997, American Academy of Pediatrics.

53. American Academy of Pediatrics: HIV infection. In Peter G, ed: *1997 red book: report of the Committee on Infectious Diseases,* ed 24, Elk Grove Village, Ill, 1997, American Academy of Pediatrics.

54. American Academy of Pediatrics: Tetanus. In Peter G, ed: *1997 red book: report of the Committee on Infectious Diseases,* ed 24, Elk Grove Village, Ill, 1997, American Academy of Pediatrics.

55. American Academy of Pediatrics: Passive immunization. In Peter G, ed: *1997 red book: report of the Committee on Infectious Diseases,* ed 24, Elk Grove Village, Ill, 1997, American Academy of Pediatrics.

56. Mofenson L et al: Prophylactic intravenous immunoglobulin in HIV-infected children with CD_4 counts of 0.20×10^9 L or more, *JAMA* 268(4):483, 1992.

57. Spector S, Gelbert R, McGrath MS et al: A controlled trial of intravenous immune globulin for the prevention of serious bacterial infection in children receiving zidovudine for advanced HIV infection, *N Engl J Med* 331(18):1181, 1994.

58. Wood L: Immunomodulation and immune reconstitution. In Pizzo PA, Wilfert CM, eds: *Pediatric AIDS: The challenge of HIV infection in infants, children, and adolescents,* ed 3, Baltimore, 1998, Williams & Wilkins.

59. *Nurse Practitioner's drug handbook,* ed 2, Springhouse, Penn, 1998, Springhouse.

60. Lipson M: Disclosure of diagnosis to children with human immunodeficiency virus or acquired immunodeficiency syndrome, *J Dev Behav Pediatr* 15(3):S61, 1994.

61. Lipson M: What do you say to a child with AIDS?, *Hasting Center Rep* 23(2):6, 1993.

62. Wiener LS, Septimus A, Grady C: Psychosocial support and ethical issues for the child and family. In Pizzo PA, Wilfert CM, eds: *Pediatric AIDS: the challenge of HIV infection in infants, children, and adolescents,* ed 3, Baltimore, 1998, Williams & Wilkins.

63. American Academy of Pediatrics, Committee on Pediatric AIDS: Disclosure of illness stature to children and adolescents with HIV infection, *Pediatrics* 103(1):164, 1999.

64. Lipson M: Disclosing HIV status to HIV-infected children, *The AIDS Reader,* 5(6):204, Nov-Dec 1995.

65. Schonfeld DJ: Informing children of their human immunodeficiency virus infection, *Arch Pediatr Adolesc Med* 151:976, 1997.

66. Slavin LA et al: Communication of the cancer diagnosis to pediatric patients: impact in long term adjustment, *Am J Psychiatr* 139:179, 1982.

67. Wiener L et al: The HIV-infected child: parental responses and psychosocial implications, *Am J Orthopsychiatr* 64(3):485, 1994.

68. Samples C, Goodman E, Woods E: Epidemiology and medical management of adolescents. In Pizzo, Wilfert, eds: *Pediatric AIDS: the challenge of HIV infection in infants, children, & adolescents,* ed 3, Baltimore, 1998, Williams & Wilkins.

69. Schneider MB: Physical examination. In Friedman SB et al, eds: *Comprehensive adolescent health care,* ed 2, St Louis, 1998, Mosby.

70. Battle CU: Chronic physical disease, *Pediatr Clin North Am* 22(3):525, 1975.

71. Lewis SY, Haiken HJ, Hoyt LG: Living beyond the odds: a psychosocial perspective on long-term survivors of pediatric human immunodeficiency virus infection, *J Dev Behav Pediatr* 15(3):S12, 1994.

72. Neinstein LS: The office visit and interview techniques. In Neinstein LS, ed: *Adolescent health care: a practical guide,* ed 2, Baltimore, 1990, Urban & Schwarzenberg.

22

Neurological Disorders in HIV/AIDS

- *AIDS dementia*
- *Peripheral neuropathy*

Kenneth Zwolski

AIDS Dementia

■ DEFINITION AND ETIOLOGY

AIDS dementia is also referred to as HIV-associated cognitive motor complex. This latter designation is the term preferred by the World Health Organization (WHO) and the American Academy of Neurology (AAN). AIDS dementia is the most common central nervous system (CNS) complication of infection with HIV-1. Its frequency is estimated to be from 20% to 33% in all adults with AIDS and up to 50% in all children with AIDS. However, the early use of zidovudine (ZDV) and other antiretrovirals is reducing the prevalence of AIDS dementia. When AIDS dementia does occur, it typically presents late in the course of infection (i.e., a CD_4 cell count less than 200 cells/mm^3) and often occurs in association with other opportunistic infections. It is uncommon in clients who are systemically well.

AIDS dementia is a complex constellation of signs and symptoms. It includes aspects of dementia, as well as aspects of impaired motor function and, at times, characteristic behavioral changes. The disease does not generally cause alterations in the level of consciousness, neuropathies, or functional psychiatric disturbances.

From a pathophysiological perspective, it is thought that HIV-1 binds to macrophages in the brain. These macrophages then overrespond by releasing a variety of neurotoxic substances such as glutamate, free radicals, and arachidonic acid, which subsequently damage brain tissue. Some of these toxins overstimulate N-methyl-D-aspartate (NMDA) receptors, resulting in increased levels of neuronal calcium ion. This can produce injury similar to that seen in stroke or trauma.

■ CLINICAL OVERVIEW

AIDS dementia is characterized by a triad of cognitive, motor, and behavioral dysfunction that slowly progresses over a period of weeks to months. The cognitive changes are mostly a mental slowing and inattention. In the early stages, using normal assessment techniques, it is often difficult to document these cognitive impairments. Clients, or those close to the client, will begin describing difficulties with concentration and memory. Clients will, typically, lose track of their train of thought. They may complain of "slowness in thinking." Complex tasks become difficult and take more time to complete. They may miss appointments and find that they have to resort to keeping lists of daily chores and other duties. As the condition progresses, the clinician can begin to document poor performance on various assessments of cognitive function, such as the "serial sevens" test. In the later stages of AIDS dementia, the accentuated combination of inattention, reduced concentration, and forgetfulness may result in what can be described as global dementia.

The symptoms of motor dysfunction ordinarily develop after those of cognitive impairment. They include: poor balance or coordination (e.g., more frequent tripping and falling, dropping things more frequently), slower hand activities (e.g., writing, eating), hyperreflexia, and development of release signs such as snout, glabellar, and grasp reflexes. As the disease progresses, the client may develop spastic ataxia and leg weakness that can limit walking. In the latest stages, bladder and bowel incontinence can develop and paraplegia is a possibility. Motor symptoms can usually be detected on physical examination, even in the earlier stages. A test of alternating rapid movements is appropriate for the assessment of motor performance.

Behavioral changes include an apathetic affect with poor insight and an indifference to illness. The level of arousal is usually preserved. Even in the very terminal stages, when the client may be vegetative, he or she will still appear awake. Mutism may characterize the later stages. Psychological depression is infrequent. Even though clients appear uninterested and lack initiative, they do not have dysphoria. Some clients may become irritable and hyperactive; occasionally they may become overtly manic, but there is always an element of confusion present.

WHO and AAN have introduced a classification system for HIV-associated cognitive motor complex (Box 22-1). In this classification system, two major categories are established: HIV-1–associated minor cognitive disorder and HIV-associated dementia/HIV-associated myelopathy. This latter category is further divided into subcategories. In addition, this latter category introduces two new terms, either one of which can be used depending on whether the clinical presentation is more related to cognitive (HIV-associated dementia) or motor (HIV-associated myelopathy) abilities.

■ DIAGNOSIS

Diagnosis of AIDS dementia is made on the basis of nonfocal neurological findings, certain identifying clinical characteristics, and the exclusion of other conditions. Neuroimaging may be necessary to exclude other

BOX 22-1   WHO/AAN CLASSIFICATION OF HIV-ASSOCIATED COGNITIVE-MOTOR COMPLEX

HIV-1–Associated Minor Cognitive Disorder Is Defined by:

Symptoms—Two of five types of client symptoms in the cognitive, motor, behavioral sphere

Examination—Neurologic or neurophysiologic examination abnormalities

Mild impairment of work or activities of daily living (ADLs)

HIV-Associated Dementia and HIV-Associated Myelopathy

Mild

Impaired work and ADLs

Capable of basic self care

Ambulatory, but may need a single assistive device

Moderate

Unable to work or function unassisted or cannot walk unassisted

Severe

Unable to perform ADLs unassisted

Confined to bed or wheelchair

From Price R: Management of the neurological complications of HIV-1 infection and AIDS. In Sande M, Volberding P, eds: Medical management of AIDS, ed 5, Philadelphia, 1997, Saunders.

---

neurological conditions that may share certain signs and symptoms with AIDS dementia. These include cerebral toxoplasmosis, primary CNS lymphoma, progressive multifocal leukoencephalopathy (PML), cytomegalovirus (CMV) encephalitis, and cryptococcal meningitis. Imaging with computed tomography (CT) scans or magnetic resonance imaging (MRI) almost always shows cerebral atrophy with widened cortical sulci and enlarged ventricles. The basal ganglia are often reduced in volume.

An examination of the cerebrospinal fluid (CSF) will show abnormalities 50% to 70% of the time. But these are nonspecific changes often seen in other CNS opportunistic infections and CNS lymphoma. Abnormalities include indications of immune activation such as elevations in beta 2 microglobulin and neopterin levels (see Chapter 2 for discussion of these immune markers), the presence and concentration of which may serve as measures of the severity of dementia. An increase in white blood cells and an increase in protein are often seen as well.

■ MEDICAL MANAGEMENT

Treatment decisions can be made more appropriately if the disease has been staged. Price and Brew (1988) developed a classification system for AIDS dementia (Box 22-2).

In treating AIDS dementia, there is a good response to ZDV, but optimum dosing has not been established. There are not any current guide-

BOX 22-2 SYSTEM OF CLASSIFICATION FOR AIDS DEMENTIA SYMPTOMS

Stage 0: Normal

Stage 0.5: Subclinical or equivocal

Minimal or equivocal symptoms
Mild (soft) neurological signs
No impairment of work or activities of daily living

Stage 1: Mild

Unequivocal intellectual or motor impairment
Able to do all but the more demanding work of activities of daily living (ADLs)

Stage 2: Moderate

Cannot work or perform demanding ADLs
Capable of self-care
Ambulatory but may need a single assistive device

Stage 3: Severe

Major intellectual disability
Cannot walk unassisted

Stage 4: End stage

Nearly vegetative
Rudimentary cognition
Paraplegic or quadriplegic

From Price R, Brew B: The AIDS dementia complex, *J Infect Dis* 158:1079, 1988.

lines regarding the efficacy or use of other antiretrovirals. However, reducing viral load by use of antiretrovirals and protease inhibitors (PIs) seems promising. Nimodipine, a calcium channel–blocker, and memantine, an NMDA receptor inhibitor, have been the focus of early-phase clinical trials because they appear to block the neurotoxicity of HIV-1 gp 120 in cell culture.

If a client is suspected of having AIDS dementia, a typical work-up would include obtaining serum measurements of CD_4 cell counts and viral load, cryptococcal antigen, serum toxoplasmosis IgG titer, thyroid function studies, serum B_{12}, folate and albumin, complete blood count (CBC) with differential, a chemistry panel, and the rapid pPlasma reagin (RPR) test or the venereal disease research laboratories (VDRL) test. Also, obtaining either a CT scan or MRI with contrast and doing a lumbar puncture is indicated.

Psychotropic drugs may be initiated in small doses (which can then be titrated upward) for treatment of agitation, anxiety, mania, hypomania, and psychomotor slowing. Certain drugs are used with caution.

These include the benzodiazepines (for the treatment of anxiety or insomnia), because they have sedative properties and can impair memory; drugs with strong anticholinergic side effects, because they can precipitate delirium; and amitriptyline, because it can precipitate mania in predisposed clients.

■ NURSING CONSIDERATIONS

1. It is important to keep in mind that an accurate diagnosis is often difficult. Clients with AIDS dementia may have other coexisting organic brain diseases, so they may not fit the clinical picture of AIDS dementia only. Depression and even psychosis may be present either by themselves or coexistent with AIDS dementia.
2. The need for supervision must be carefully assessed. A home safety assessment should be conducted. The nurse should check for the presence of reality orientation cues such as calendars and clocks, and ensure that hallways and living areas are brightly lit, walkways are clear and free of electrical wiring or unstable furniture, and potentially dangerous objects, such as sharp objects, chemicals, poisons, and power tools, are safely stored away. Knobs should be removed from stoves to prevent confused clients from inadvertently burning themselves or setting fire to the house.
3. The nurse should attend to the well-being of the client's family and other caregivers. As the disease progresses, clients may become less communicative. Of all the complications faced by a caregiver, communication difficulties are often the most frustrating. The nurse should encourage the caregivers to take breaks from care and monitor them for signs of depression and burnout.
4. The use of drugs with CNS toxicity should be minimized.
5. Caring for clients with dementia is a collaborative effort between the client, family, and health care providers. The nurse seeks assistance from social workers, nutritionists, psychologists, and others in helping the client and family live with this disease and make appropriate choices as the disease progresses.

Peripheral Neuropathy

■ DEFINITION AND ETIOLOGY

Peripheral neuropathies are diseases that affect the peripheral nervous system. They can affect sensory, motor, or autonomic nerves. Peripheral neuropathy can involve the spinal root (radiculopathy), a single peripheral nerve (mononeuropathy), or widely distributed individual nerves (polyneuropathy). The symptoms of peripheral neuropathy can range from mild sensory disturbances to life-threatening paralytic disorders, as in cases of Guillain-Barré syndrome.

The symptoms associated with peripheral neuropathies occur as a result of either damage to the myelin sheath (demyelination) or axonal degeneration. Sometimes, combinations of both types of damage exist. Generally speaking, demyelination occurs secondary to inflammatory and/or autoimmune processes, whereas axonal degeneration occurs secondary to toxic or metabolic processes. Infection with HIV-1 can result in both demyelination and axonal degeneration. Many of the antiretroviral drugs used to treat HIV-1 infection are toxic to neurons, leading to a type of toxic peripheral neuropathy. Prominent among these antiretrovirals are didanosine (ddI), zalcitabine (ddC) and stavudine (d4T).

The different types of peripheral neuropathy most likely to occur in clients with HIV-1 infection are stratified according to the stage of HIV-1 infection. During the time of seroconversion or later (i.e., during the asymptomatic, clinically latent period with CD_4 cell counts greater than 500 cells/mm^3), an acute demyelinating polyneuropathy (i.e., Guillain-Barré syndrome) can occur. On occasion, a chronic inflammatory demyelinating polyneuropathy may develop during the asymptomatic phase.

When the CD_4 cell count ranges between 200 and 500 cells/mm^3, a herpes zoster neuropathy and/or a mononeuropathy designated as "mononeuritis multiplex, benign type" may arise. These tend to have a benign outcome and often remit spontaneously. In late-phase HIV-1 infection (i.e., CD_4 cell counts less than 200 cells/mm^3), several types of peripheral neuropathies occur. These include: CMV mononeuritis, CMV polyradiculopathy, autonomic polyneuropathy, distal sensory polyneuropathy (DSPN), and toxic peripheral neuropathy. DSPN is the most common of all peripheral neuropathies in clients with HIV-1. Its pathogenesis is uncertain, but it may be caused by infection of either the dorsal root ganglion of the involved nerve or the nerve itself. It involves cytokine dysregulation and axonal toxicity.

■ CLINICAL OVERVIEW

When sensory nerves are involved in peripheral neuropathy, symptoms can include numbness, localized tingling, hypesthesia or anesthesia, loss of vibration and position sense, and decreases in pain and temperature appreciation. Motor nerve dysfunction primarily manifests as weakness. It may also result in foot drop, muscle cramps, fasciculations, muscle atrophy, diminished muscle tone, and loss of reflexes. With autonomic dysfunction, the most common complaints are lightheadedness and syncope. In addition, clients may experience constipation, urinary incontinence, and impotence.

CMV polyradiculopathy presents as a severe ascending polyradiculopathy. It begins with painful lumbosacral root involvement (i.e., pain in back and legs) and progresses rostrally to involve sensory, motor, and autonomic components. Autonomic neuropathy presents with symptoms ranging from mild positional hypotension to cardiovascular collapse during invasive procedures. It may also contribute to chronic diarrhea. DSPN or sensory polyneuropathy is difficult to distinguish from toxic peripheral neuropathy. In both cases clients present with complaints of numb or burning feet and the inability to walk (not because of weakness or sensory ataxia but because of discomfort). The physical examination in these cases shows hyperesthesia, decreased pain and vibratory sensation, and decreased or absent Achilles reflexes (i.e., "ankle jerks").

■ DIAGNOSIS

On the basis of clinical features alone it is difficult to distinguish peripheral neuropathies that have mostly a demyelinating pattern of injury (i.e., Guillain-Barré syndrome; acute inflammatory, chronic inflammatory, or CMV polyradiculopathy) from those that have an axonal pattern of injury. This is important because demyelinating patterns of injury are treated somewhat differently than axonal patterns of injury. Two types of electrodiagnostic tests are available that can help in differentiation: electromyography (EMG) and nerve conduction velocity (NCV) tests.

In the case of CMV polyradiculopathy, the finding of polymorphonuclear pleocytosis in CSF and increased spinal fluid protein makes the diagnosis. A cytologic examination can sometimes demonstrate CMV inclusions in the CSF. In the case of Guillain-Barré syndrome and chronic inflammatory peripheral neuropathy, pleocytosis is also present in the CSF.

It is also difficult to differentiate DSPN from toxic polyneuropathy. In these cases electrodiagnostic tests are of little use. The best approach is to stop antiretroviral drugs or switch therapy. If the symptoms disappear, then the diagnosis of toxic peripheral neuropathy is confirmed.

■ MEDICAL MANAGEMENT

In clients presenting with signs and symptoms of peripheral neuropathy, other causes besides infection with HIV-1 need to be ruled out. Clients should be evaluated for alcoholism, diabetes, B_{12} deficiency, and thyroid dysfunction. If any of these conditions are present, they should be treated accordingly. Besides antiretrovirals, other neurotoxic drugs may cause peripheral neuropathy. These include metronidazole, isoniazid (INH), vitamin B_6, vincristine, and dapsone.

DSPN does not respond to treatment with ZDV or other antiretroviral drugs. Treatment in these cases depends on symptom management with tricyclics and various analgesics, including narcotics in severe cases. Toxic peripheral neuropathies often present dose-related symptoms. Antiretroviral drugs thought to be responsible should be discontinued and a new regimen instituted. Symptoms are usually reversible if recognized and treated early. In some cases, after withdrawal of the drug, symptoms may worsen for a few weeks. This phenomenon is referred to as "coasting." If the neuropathy is secondary to infection with CMV, then treatment is initiated with anti-CMV medications, such as ganciclovir and foscarnet (see Chapter 17). If the peripheral neuropathy is of a demyelinating

Table 22-1	Medical Regimens

Peripheral Neuropathy	Regimens
Mild	Ibuprofen 600 mg PO tid
Moderate	Nortriptyline 10-25 mg PO hs, increase prn, not to exceed to 75 mg (it may take 2-3 weeks before a response is seen) *Or* If no response: Phenytoin 200-400 mg PO qd *Or* If no response: Carbamazepine 200-400 mg PO bid *Or* Amitriptyline, mexiletine, baclofen, or clonazepam
Severe	Methadone, titrate up to 20 mg PO qid *Or* Fentanyl patch 25-100 µg qod *Or* Morphine sulfate

pattern, treatment options include plasmapheresis, corticosteroids, or IV immunoglobulins.

■ NURSING CONSIDERATIONS

1. Early recognition of toxic peripheral neuropathy is very important because discontinuation of responsible drugs in the early stages can bring about reversal of symptoms. Hence the nurse needs to be aware of the symptoms of sensory peripheral neuropathy and assess for them at each interaction, especially in clients receiving ddI, ddC, or d4T.

2. Weakness, a major problem associated with many of the peripheral neuropathies, can cause the client to have difficulty with routine chores such as carrying groceries or brushing teeth and hair. Proximal leg weakness can make it difficult to get out of a chair. The nurse needs to assess for difficulties in this area and proper interventions should be planned. Foot drop can cause clients to trip on their shoelaces, possibly resulting in falls and other injuries. The home situation should be evaluated for safety. The client should be encouraged to avoid trips that require extensive walking.

3. Clients experiencing sensory discomfort can be advised to avoid tight footwear and to soak their feet in ice. Capsaicin-containing ointments (Zostrix) have been found to be helpful in some cases, though in many instances they are not tolerated well.

4. For medical regimens see Table 22-1.

BIBLIOGRAPHY

Bartlett J: *Medical management of HIV infection,* Baltimore, 1997, Port City Press.

Libman H, Witzberg R: *HIV infection: a primary care manual,* ed 3, Boston, 1996, Little, Brown & Co.

Sande M, Volberding P: *The medical management of AIDS,* ed 6, Philadelphia, 1999, Saunders.

23

Health Care Worker Risk Reduction in HIV/AIDS Care

Dorothy Talotta

HEALTH CARE WORKERS AND BLOODBORNE PATHOGENS

The most life-threatening risk faced by health care workers is exposure to bloodborne pathogens.[1] In the United States, an estimated 8.8 million persons work in health care professions, and approximately 6 million persons work in hospitals.[2] The exact number of percutaneous injuries and other exposures occurring annually in the United States is unknown, but current estimates range between 590,000 and 800,000 annually.[3] These incidents include exposures that occur via needlesticks, sharps injuries, and lacerations, among others.[4,5] Eighty percent of contacts with blood occur via needlesticks, making these the most common cause of exposure to bloodborne pathogens among health care workers. Needlestick injuries are believed to be widely underreported. More than 20 pathogens, including HIV, hepatitis B virus (HBV), hepatitis C virus (HCV), syphilis, and malaria, can be transmitted by small amounts of blood.[5] This chapter primarily focuses on health care worker exposure to HIV. However, since nurses who care for clients with HIV may also be exposed to HBV, HCV, and tuberculosis (TB), exposure to these pathogens is also covered.

ROLE OF FEDERAL AGENCIES

In the United States, there are federal agencies that play roles in the prevention and management of infectious diseases. Two very important ones are the Centers for Disease Control and Prevention (CDC) and the Occupational Safety and Health Administration (OSHA).

The CDC is an agency of the Public Health Service and is responsible for providing leadership and direction in preventing and controlling diseases and other preventable conditions. It offers guidelines and recommendations related to controlling the spread of various diseases and conditions and is concerned with protecting both health care workers and clients. The CDC does not play a role in enforcement, but its guidelines and recommendations are used as standards for government regulation.[6]

OSHA is a branch of the United States Department of Labor that develops safety standards, inspects workplaces, and monitors job-related illnesses. Its standards are legally enforceable, and it protects not only health care workers but also other workers from job-related illnesses and accidents.[6] OSHA focuses on preventing the exposure of workers to hazards. It expects employers to use engineering controls wherever possible to reduce or eliminate a hazard at its source.[7] In health care facilities, engineering controls include conveniently placed, puncture-resistant, disposal containers for sharps, as well as safer needle devices that attempt to eliminate or minimize needlestick injuries.[4]

When it is impossible to prevent the exposure of employees to the hazard through the use of engineering controls, measures such as administrative and/or work practice controls must be used.[7] Examples of work practice controls are handwashing, disinfection, sterilization, and prohibition of manual handling of needles. The employer is responsible for providing and enforcing work practice controls, but the health care worker is responsible for using them.[6]

After these controls, if the hazard still exists, personal protective equipment (PPE) must be used for employee protection. PPE includes gloves, face shields, and reinforced gowns to protect employees from contact with blood and body fluids. Employers must provide appropriate PPE to employees at no cost and require employees to use it. Employers must also clean, repair, and replace such equipment when necessary.[8]

Employers are also required to provide information and training to all employees who could reasonably be anticipated to come into contact with blood or other potentially infectious material as a result of performing job duties. Such employees should receive information and training at the time of initial assignment and annually thereafter from persons knowledgeable about the subject. The information provided must include the epidemiology, modes of transmission, and symptoms of bloodborne diseases; an explanation of the facility's exposure control plan and how to obtain a copy; protective measures to minimize the risk of occupational exposure; how to report an exposure incident; who to contact in the event of an emergency; and other required information. Retraining must take place when new tasks or changes in tasks affect occupational exposure.[8]

STANDARD PRECAUTIONS

In 1987, the CDC issued a recommendation emphasizing the need for all clients to be considered potentially infected with HIV or other bloodborne pathogens. Therefore the CDC emphasized rigorous adherence to blood and body fluid precautions for all clients.[9] The use of blood and body fluid precautions for all clients was later labeled *universal precautions*.[10] Universal precautions are used by health care workers to prevent exposure to bloodborne pathogens. Since the publication of these guidelines, periodic modifications have been made. See Box 23-1 for selected precautions for all clients.

The most recent guideline was developed by the CDC and the Hospital Infection Control Practices Advisory Committee (HICPAC) in 1996.[11]

BOX 23-1 SELECTED INFECTION CONTROL PRECAUTIONS FOR ALL CLIENTS

Hands must be washed promptly and thoroughly:
- Between client contacts.
- After contact with blood, body fluids, secretions, or excretions.
- After contact with equipment or articles contaminated by blood, body fluids, secretions, or excretion.
- After removing gloves.

Gloves must be worn:
- When touching blood, body fluids, secretions, excretions, mucous membranes, or nonintact skin. Gloves must not be washed or disinfected.

The following must be worn when splashes or sprays of blood, body fluids, secretions, or excretions or large quantities of infective material are likely:
- A mask that covers nose and mouth
- Goggles or face shield
- Impermeable gown
- Leg coverings
- Boots or shoe covers

The nurse must use great care in handling needles and other sharp instruments, as follows:
- Do not bend, break, or recap used needles by hand.
- Do not remove used needles from syringes by hand.
- Do not manipulate used needles in any way by hand.

See the text for additional information on standard precautions. Further precautions are as follows:
- Dispose of used needles, syringes, scalpel blades, and other sharps in puncture-resistant containers.
- Place puncture-resistant containers as close as possible to the area of use.
- Do not exceed the recommended fill line of sharps containers.
- Have sharps containers replaced as soon as filled.
- Do not force sharp instruments into sharps containers.
- Do not use sharps containers for anything other than sharps.
- Check carefully for protruding sharps before handling sharps containers.

Garner JS, Hospital Infection Control Practices Advisory Committee: Guideline for isolation precautions in hospitals, *Infect Control Hosp Epidemiol* 17(1):54, 1996; United States Department of Health and Human Services, Public Health Service, Centers for Disease Control: *Guidelines for prevention of transmission of human immunodeficiency virus and hepatitis B virus to health-care and public-safety workers,* DHHS (NIOSH) Publication No. 89-107, Feb 1989; Morrison A: Sharps containers: take these steps to avoid getting stuck, *Nurs 98* 28(10):73, 1998.

The guideline recommends the use of a two-tier system of isolation precautions. The first tier includes precautions to be used in the care of all clients in hospitals. These are called *standard precautions* (SPs) and are seen as the primary strategy in the successful control of nosocomial infections. In the second tier are *transmission-based precautions,* which are designed only for the care of particular clients with known or suspected infections that can be transmitted by airborne, droplet, or contact modes. Airborne transmission occurs by dissemination of droplet nuclei or dust particles that contain the infectious organism. Droplet transmission differs from airborne transmission; it occurs when droplets generated from the infected person (e.g., during coughing, sneezing, or suctioning) are propelled a short distance through the air and deposited on the host's nasal mucosa, mouth, or conjunctiva. Contact transmission can occur via direct or indirect contact. Direct contact transmission involves a physical transfer of microorganisms through body surface–to–body surface contact. Indirect contact transmission involves a susceptible host contacting a contaminated object, such as contaminated instruments, dressings, or gloves.[11]

SPs incorporate the major components of universal precautions and a system of precautions called *body substance isolation.* (Body substance isolation is a system of infection precautions focused on the isolation of all potentially infectious fluid and solid body substances of all clients.[12]) SPs are also used for all clients and apply to: (1) blood; (2) all body fluids, excretions, and secretions *whether or not they contain visible blood,* with the exception of sweat; (3) nonintact skin; and (4) mucous membranes. According to the authors, the recommendations in the guideline are primarily intended for use in acute-care hospitals, but may also be applicable in extended-care or subacute-care facilities.[11]

SPs include prompt and thorough handwashing before and after contact with clients; after contact with blood, body fluids, excretions, or secretions; and after contact with contaminated articles or equipment. Gloves are worn to provide a protective barrier between hands and blood, body fluids, excretions, secretions, mucous membranes, and nonintact skin. They are also worn to prevent gross contamination of the hands of personnel and to decrease the likelihood of transmission of organisms present on the hands of personnel to clients. In addition, gloves are worn to prevent transmission of microorganisms from one client to another. Therefore, gloves must be changed between contacts with clients. Wearing gloves does not negate the need for washing hands. Hands should be washed after removing gloves.[11] The CDC emphasizes that neither surgical nor examination gloves should be washed or disinfected. Washing may enhance penetration of liquids through undetected holes in gloves. The use of disinfecting agents may cause deterioration of gloves.[10]

Gloves made of natural rubber latex have been considered the gold standard[13] and, according to studies, provide the best available protection from biohazardous substances.[14] However, there is no perfect glove, and gloves do not offer absolute protection against blood contact, even though their quality has been considerably enhanced.[14] For example, a recent study of the barrier integrity of gloves found latex glove failure rates of 0% to 4% after manipulation intended to simulate in-use conditions.[13] The Food and Drug Administration (FDA) mandates acceptable quality levels for gloves and has recently proposed that surgeon's gloves and gloves for client examination be reclassified to make them subject to additional controls. If the proposed rule is adopted, these gloves would be categorized as Class II, instead of Class I, medical devices. Devices in Class II are subject to special controls in addition to the general controls of Class I. According to the FDA, reasons for the proposed reclassification of such gloves include concerns about barrier integrity, contamination, and degradation of glove quality during storage. The proposed rule, if adopted, would also require expiration dating of gloves.[15]

Some studies have shown that, in surgical suites, rates of blood contamination of surgeons' hands were significantly lower in double-gloved surgeons when compared with those who were single-gloved.[16,17] In studies of surgeons and surgical personnel, double- and triple-gloving has also been shown to significantly decrease the risk of perforation of the inner glove.[18,19] However, in one study of the barrier integrity of gloves that used a protocol designed to mimic client care activities, there was essentially no difference in leakage rates for single or double latex gloves. These authors concluded that there is little advantage to double-gloving during routine procedures when there is minimal stress on latex gloves.[20]

The increased use of latex gloves as part of universal precautions has been implicated in the growing numbers of nurses and other health care workers with latex allergy.[2,21] A complete discussion of latex allergy is beyond the scope of this chapter; however, a few points should be noted. Avoiding latex products is the cornerstone of preventing both sensitization and reactions to latex. However, because latex proteins can be aerosolized when donning and removing powdered gloves, symptoms may not be alleviated by avoiding the latex products, particularly if coworkers continue to use powdered latex gloves.[2] An important additional purpose of the proposed FDA rule mentioned previously is to reduce adverse health effects from allergic reactions to latex gloves and glove powder.[15]

It is critical to note that vinyl gloves should not be used if there is risk of contact with infectious material, because barrier protection could be compromised.[22,23] Several studies have shown that vinyl gloves do not provide as effective of a protective barrier as latex gloves.[13,24] Latex gloves have a molecular structure that allows for rigorous manipulation activities while maintaining integrity and rebound (return to the original shape). Vinyl gloves, on the other hand, lack the ability to stretch when snagged or stressed, and they readily fracture, tear, or separate at the molecular level, resulting in barrier loss.[13]

As a result of the increased reports of latex allergies, there is interest in developing synthetic alternatives to latex that would provide comparable barrier protection. Nitrile is a recent synthetic that exhibits the rubberlike characteristics of tensile strength and elasticity. In a recent study comparing the barrier effectiveness of latex, vinyl, and nitrile gloves,[13] the researchers stated that no previous studies had evaluated the effectiveness of nitrile as a barrier to bloodborne pathogens. In this study, nitrile gloves were found comparable to latex gloves in terms of barrier performance characteristics, with failure rates of 1% to 3%.

SPs also include wearing face shields, goggles, and various types of masks to provide protection during activities that are likely to produce splashes or sprays of blood, body fluids, excretions, or secretions. In such situations, hospital personnel should wear masks that cover both mouth and nose, and goggles or a face shield to protect mucous membranes of the eyes, nose, and mouth. In certain situations (e.g., when there are or may be splashes or large quantities of infective material), impermeable gowns, leg coverings, boots, or shoe covers provide greater skin protection.[11] OSHA mandates wearing gloves, masks, face shields, and eye protection, as well as gowns and other protective apparel, in certain circumstances to decrease the risk of exposure to bloodborne pathogens.[25] For example, the use of eye protection and a mask or face shield to prevent contamination of the mucous membranes of the eyes, nose, and mouth is necessary when it can reasonably be anticipated that there will be spattering or generation of droplets.

The CDC emphasizes the importance of decreasing the risk of injury to health care workers from needles or other sharp instruments. Workers should take precautions when cleaning instruments and handling sharps after procedures. Precautions must also be taken during the disposal of used needles to prevent needlestick injuries. Used needles should not be recapped or manipulated by hand. Disposable sharps should be placed in puncture-resistant containers located as closely as possible to the area of use.[26]

In 1992, OSHA stated that, if a needle absolutely must be recapped and no alternative is feasible, a device that protects the hand from accidental puncture or the one-handed "scoop" method must be used. *The two-handed method of recapping must never be used.* Needles must not be removed from syringes or other devices by hand.[27] In 1996, OSHA stated: "Recapping, removing, or bending needles is prohibited unless the employer can demonstrate that no alternative is feasible or that such action is required by a specific medical procedure. When recapping, bending, or removing contaminated needles is required by a medical procedure, this must be done by mechanical means, such as the use of forceps, or by a one-handed technique. Shearing or breaking contaminated needles is not permitted."[8] In 1992, OSHA stated that it was most preferable to use devices that offer an alternative to needles, such as stopcocks, needleless systems, self-sheathing needles, and needle-protected systems.[27] Recently, a new OSHA directive addressed the mandatory use of such devices[3] (see p. 439).

In addition, nurses should be attentive to containers for sharps, which, if used properly, can prevent needlestick injuries. However, used improperly, they can create a serious hazard. The recommended fill line should not be exceeded. Overfilled containers present a hazard, and containers should be replaced as soon as filled. Sharp instruments should not be forced into containers, and containers should be used only for sharps. Nurses should check carefully for protruding sharps before handling containers and should read and attend to cautionary statements on such containers.[28] Box 23-1 provides a list of precautions to be used with all clients.

TYPES OF INJURIES

The CDC collects data from hospitals that participate in the CDC National Surveillance System for Hospital Health Care Workers (NaSH). According to this data, of nearly 5000 percutaneous injuries reported between June 1995 and July 1999, 62% were associated with hollow-bore needles, primarily hypodermic needles attached to disposable syringes (29%), and winged-steel ("butterfly") needles (13%). Intravenous (IV) stylets accounted for 6% of these injuries, phlebotomy needles for 4%, and other hollow-bore needles for 10%. Of percutaneous injuries with hollow-bore needles, 27% occurred while manipulating the needle in a client. Devices other than hollow-bore needles involved in percutaneous injuries were glass, suture needles, and other sharps, which accounted for 17%, 15%, and 6%, respectively. Approximately 38% of percutaneous injuries occurred during use of a needle or other sharp device, while 42% occurred after use and before disposal. Although two-handed recapping of needles has been prohibited for some time, recapping still accounts for 5% of needlestick injuries.[29]

Needlestick injuries occur in a variety of ways. For example, needles attached to a length of tubing, such as butterfly needles or needles attached to IV tubing, can be difficult to place in sharps containers and, therefore, can present a hazard. Injuries that involve needles attached to IV tubing can occur when a nurse inserts a needle into or withdraws a needle from an IV port. Injuries can also occur if the nurse tries to decrease the needlestick hazard by inserting the needle into an IV port or bag, a drip chamber, or bedding. When a nurse transfers blood or other body fluids from a syringe to a specimen container, he or she may miss the target and sustain an injury.[30] Nurses and all health care workers must exercise care when handling trash and dirty linens, because these activities are also associated with percutaneous injuries.[3]

Sharps containers, if used improperly, can create serious hazards. Overfilling containers, forcing lids onto overfilled containers, and forcing sharp instruments into containers can lead to injuries. Materials other than sharps placed into sharps containers can prevent needles from falling to the bottom. Needles protruding from sharps containers present a hazard.[28]

HEALTH CARE WORKER SAFETY LEGISLATION

While OSHA has indicated, in the past, that devices that offer alternatives to needles are preferred,[27] there have been efforts, including those of the American Nurses Association (ANA), to mandate the use of such devices through legislation.[31] In 1998, California became the first state to pass legislation requiring the use of safety-needle devices by all California health care workers. In 1999, New Jersey, Hawaii, Maryland, Tennessee, and Texas enacted some type of needle safety legislation. According to the ANA, 40 needle safety bills were introduced in 22 states in 1999.[32]

On the federal level, the Health Care Worker Needlestick Prevention Act of 1999 (HR 1899) was introduced by Representatives Pete Stark and

Marge Roukema on May 20, 1999. A few days later, Senators Barbara Boxer and Harry Reid introduced an identical bill, S. 1140. The act, if passed, would amend OSHA's bloodborne pathogens standard so as to require that all health care facilities use sharps and needle systems with engineered protections (e.g., retractable needles). Among other provisions, the act would establish a new clearinghouse within the National Institute for Occupational Safety and Health (NIOSH) to collect data on engineered safety technology.[33] As of this writing, ANA is continuing to lobby for the passage of this bill.

In the meantime, on November 5, 1999, OSHA issued a directive that stated that "where engineering controls will reduce employee exposure either by removing, eliminating, or isolating the hazards, they must be used."[3] The ANA believes that the directive will have a life-saving effect for nurses and indicates that it will work with State Nurses Associations to ensure that health care institutions implement the safer devices as required.[31] However, OSHA has not allocated additional funds for the enforcement of the directive. Passage of the Health Care Worker Needlestick Prevention Act of 1999, which is more comprehensive and far-reaching, is still needed.

HEALTH CARE WORKERS AND HIV

Despite the use of precautions, exposures to blood and/or body substances do occur. By December 1999, there were 56 reported cases of health care workers in the United States with documented occupational transmission of HIV and 136 cases that are considered possible occupational transmissions. Of the 56 documented cases, 49 occurred in workers exposed to HIV-positive blood. Of the 56, 23 were nurses, 16 were clinical laboratory technicians, and 6 were nonsurgical physicians. The remainder of the cases occurred in 3 nonclinical laboratory technicians, 2 surgical technicians, 2 housekeeper/maintenance workers, a dialysis technician, a respiratory therapist, a health aide/attendant, and an embalmer/morgue technician.[34]

An *exposure,* which may put a health care worker at risk for HIV infection, is defined by the CDC as[35]:

1. A percutaneous injury (e.g., needlestick, cut with a sharp).
2. Contact of mucous membrane or nonintact skin (e.g., dermatitis, chapping, abrasion), with blood, tissue, or other body fluids.
3. Contact of intact skin with blood, tissue, or other body fluids when there is either:
   - Prolonged duration of contact (defined as several minutes or more), or
   - Involvement of an extensive area.
4. Direct contact with concentrated HIV (e.g., in a research laboratory).

These situations require consideration of treatment with HIV antiretroviral therapy, also known as *postexposure prophylaxis* (PEP).[35] Examples of activities that may place a nurse at risk for percutaneous exposure include giving an injection and inserting an IV line. Mucous membrane exposure or exposure of nonintact skin can occur (for example) from a splash of peritoneal dialysis fluid when the nurse is changing the drainage bag. Blood could contact extensive areas of a nurse's intact skin during bloody procedures (e.g., resuscitation of a trauma victim).

The average risk of HIV transmission following percutaneous exposure to infected blood is estimated at 0.3%.[36] Following a mucous membrane exposure, it is estimated to be 0.09%.[37] The risk of transmission after skin exposure is not precisely known but has been estimated to be less than that following mucous membrane exposure.[38] The risk of transmission following exposure to fluids or tissues other than blood is also not precisely known.[35]

One case control study identified factors associated with increased risk of HIV transmission to a health care worker following percutaneous exposure to infected blood.[39] These factors included deep injury (a deep puncture or wound with or without bleeding), injury with a device that was visibly contaminated with blood, and a procedure involving a needle placed in a vein or artery. The researchers state that these three factors may be indicators of the quantity of blood transmitted. When needlesticks with hollow-bore needles were analyzed, there was a weak association between large-diameter needles (gauge of less than 18) and an increased risk of seroconversion. Another factor that affected the risk of transmission was exposure to blood from a client in the terminal phase of the disease. This factor may be related to a higher viral burden in the client's blood, but it may also be related to characteristics of the virus in the terminal phase of illness. The researchers estimated that the risk of transmission is probably higher than 0.3% when the exposure involves relatively large amounts of blood, especially if the client's viral burden is high. Elsewhere, it has been suggested that the risk of transmission of HIV may be affected by the host's defenses (i.e., the host's immune response may sometimes be able to prevent the establishment of HIV infection following a percutaneous exposure).[35]

POSTEXPOSURE TREATMENT AND REPORTING

In an effort to guide health care agencies in providing care to exposed health care workers, the CDC issued guidelines for the management of health care workers with occupationally related exposures to HIV.[35] OSHA requires that the employer provide postexposure evaluation and follow-up to employees according to current CDC recommendations.[3] According to the CDC guidelines, each health care organization should have written protocols to be followed in the event of occupational exposures to bloodborne pathogens.[35] (While this discussion focuses on HIV infection, other bloodborne pathogens such as hepatotropic viruses must also be considered. See the discussion later in this chapter.) It is critical that nurses be familiar with the protocols in their own institutions, clarify any questions, and know where to find the protocols so that appropriate first aid and reporting can begin immediately after an exposure occurs. While protocols for HIV exposure may vary from institution to institution, all should include mechanisms for prompt reporting, worker evaluation and counseling, postexposure treatment, and guidelines for follow-up.[35]

Prior to the new CDC guidelines, there were earlier recommendations by other authors to vigorously scrub parenteral injury sites with 10% povidone iodine solution for 10 minutes and promote bleeding by milking the wound site. The same authors also recommended that contaminated mucous membranes be irrigated with normal saline for 15 minutes. The authors admitted to an absence of data indicating that first aid measures influence transmission risk, but they made recommendations on the premise that these vigorous measures might help remove infected cells.[40]

The most recent CDC guidelines, however, recommend that a nurse or any health care worker who has a possible exposure to potentially infectious fluids wash the contact site with soap and water. If the site is a mucous membrane, it should be flushed with water. According to the CDC, antiseptics are not contraindicated, although there is no evidence that their use reduces the risk of transmission of HIV. Neither is there evidence that squeezing the wound to express fluid reduces the risk. The CDC does not recommend the use of caustic agents such as bleach, nor does it recommend injecting antiseptics or disinfectants into the wound.[35]

The nurse should report the exposure immediately to the appropriate individual(s). These usually include the responsible nurse manager and occupational medicine department, employee health service, or emergency department. PEP, if indicated, should begin within a few hours.[35] It is therefore critical that reporting be done immediately. OSHA requires that postexposure evaluation and follow-up be provided as soon as possible. An exact time is not stated because time limits on the effectiveness of PEP can vary depending on the infection to which the employee is exposed. However, the standard uses the term "immediately" to emphasize the importance of prompt medical evaluation and prophylaxis.[3] Regardless of how minimal the injury or exposure may seem, the nurse should follow the agency's exposure plan and report the incident to the appropriate department. (As noted earlier, needlestick injuries are believed to be widely underreported.[5] NIOSH, citing several studies, indicates that about half of needlestick and other percutaneous injuries go unreported.[30])

The nurse manager usually must be made aware of the exposure to ensure care for the injured nurse's assigned clients while the nurse reports to the occupational medicine or other appropriate department. In addition, the nurse manager may need to provide immediate counseling and reassurance to the client involved as well as other staff aware of the exposure. Other departments, such as those responsible for safety and for quality assurance, may also be notified depending on the protocols of the institution. Many exposed workers are inclined to tell colleagues about the occurrence. However, it has been recommended by some that the exposure not be discussed broadly since, if HIV infection does result, the worker may prefer that as few people as possible are aware of it.[40]

In most institutions, the occupational medicine department, employee health service, or emergency department has the responsibility for evaluating and managing an occupational exposure. The institution's policies or protocols should be followed regarding who should approach the source person (i.e., the person whose blood or body fluids are the source of the exposure) to obtain information that may be useful in evaluating the exposure. In most cases, the exposed nurse should not approach the source person following the incident.

POSTEXPOSURE EVALUATION

Critical services in postinjury management include evaluation of the injury, review and/or repeat of first aid, and initiation of psychological and medical therapy.[40] As part of postexposure evaluation, the following details surrounding the exposure incident are needed:

- When (date and time), where, and how the exposure occurred
- Type of device involved, as well as when and how the exposure occurred during the handling of the device
- Type and amount of fluid or material involved
- Severity of the exposure—for example, if the exposure was percutaneous; the depth of the injury and whether or not fluid was injected; if the exposure was via skin or mucous membrane; the estimated volume of material, duration of contact, and condition of skin[35]

Other helpful information includes the amount of time that elapsed between the time the needle or sharp was removed from the client and the occurrence of the exposure. The nurse should also report the type of first aid (e.g., duration of wound cleansing) and its timing following the injury.[40] In the event of a needlestick injury, the length and gauge of the needle, the route by which an injection was given, and whether or not visible blood was apparent on the needle may be considered in the evaluation.

There has to be an evaluation of the source person for HIV infection. Information to be used in the evaluation may come from the medical record or the person. The person's history, admitting diagnosis, and laboratory results are useful in determining the likelihood of HIV infection. Possible HIV exposures may be noted in a person's sexual and substance-use history or his or her history regarding receipt of blood or blood products prior to 1985. If the source person is known to be HIV-positive, additional information such as the stage of the disease, CD_4 count, viral load, and current and previous antiretroviral therapy should be obtained for use in choosing an appropriate postexposure prophylactic medication regimen. In the event that such information is not readily available, the initiation of the prophylactic regimen, if indicated, should not be delayed; changes can be made later, if appropriate. If it is not known whether the source is HIV-positive, the person should be told of the occurrence by the appropriate agency personnel and have consent obtained for HIV testing.[35]

OSHA requires that the employer test the source individual's blood after consent is obtained. The employer is required to ask for the source person's consent or that of anyone legally authorized to consent on the person's behalf. In jurisdictions where the individual's consent is not required, available blood may be used for testing.[3] State and local laws should be followed in regard to testing a source person if consent cannot be obtained.[35] The result of the source person's testing must be made available to the employee in accordance with applicable state and federal laws and regulations regarding medical privacy and confidentiality.[3]

Follow-up counseling, medical evaluation, and postexposure testing should be performed for health care workers who have had an occupational exposure to HIV. The worker should be offered HIV testing to establish a baseline.[35] However, OSHA requires that the consent of the employee be obtained prior to collecting and testing his or her blood. In addition, employees are not required to make an immediate decision regarding HIV testing; OSHA also requires that employees have the opportunity for future testing of blood drawn after the exposure. If involved in an exposure incident, employees have at least 90 days following baseline blood collection to decide if they want to have the blood tested for HIV. This requirement is intended to encourage employees to allow blood collection at the time of exposure. Employers are required to preserve blood that the employee consents to have drawn for at least 90 days if it was not tested for HIV initially.[3]

If the source of the exposure is HIV-negative, it is normally not necessary to perform baseline testing or further follow-up of the health care worker. However, if the source recently engaged in high-risk behaviors, baseline testing of the worker and follow-up testing should be considered. All workers who are concerned about a possible exposure to HIV should have access to serological testing. Testing for HIV antibodies should be performed for a minimum of 6 months following the exposure. Testing may be done, for example, at 6 weeks, 12 weeks, and 6 months postexposure. In certain circumstances, the follow-up period may be extended to 1 year or more.[35] The 1-year test has been recommended for three reasons: (1) the possibility that antiretroviral drugs may delay manifestations of seroconversion, (2) occasional reports of delayed seroconversions occurring more than 6 months following sexual exposure, and (3) the additional reassurance that this final test offers to the worker. It may help provide closure to the episode.[40]

POSTEXPOSURE HIV PROPHYLAXIS

Following an occupational exposure, there should be an evaluation of the need for PEP for HIV. (The employer is required to follow current guidelines at the time of the exposure to determine if PEP is medically indicated.[3]) If PEP is being considered, pertinent information about the health of the worker should be evaluated, including medications being taken, medical conditions, and pregnancy. Recommendations regarding the use of PEP should be implemented in consultation with an expert in anti-

Table 23-1	Postexposure Prophylaxis Regimens for Occupational Exposures to HIV	

Regimen Category	Application	Regimen
Basic	Exposures for which there is recognized transmission risk	ZDV 600 mg daily in divided doses (e.g., 300 mg bid, 200 mg tid, or 100 mg q4h) *And* Lamivudine 150 mg bid × 28 days
Expanded	Exposures that pose increased risk for transmission (e.g., larger volume of blood, higher virus titer in blood)	Basic regimen plus one of the following: Indinavir 800 mg q8h *Or* Nelfinavir 750 mg tid

Adapted from Centers for Disease Control and Prevention: Public Health Service guidelines for the management of health-care worker exposures to HIV and recommendations for postexposure prophylaxis, *MMWR* 47(RR-7):21, May 15, 1998.

retroviral therapy and HIV transmission when possible. Information about recommendations should be explained to the exposed worker. This explanation should include the information that the worker can decline any or all PEP drugs. The choice of a PEP regimen should consider the risk presented by the exposure and information about the source person, such as past response to antiretroviral drugs, CD_4 count, viral burden, and the stage of the disease.[35]

The drug regimens presented in Table 23-1 are those recommended by the CDC at the time of this writing. However, it is important to note that as new drugs and more information become available, recommended regimens may change. The nurse may also find recommendations for PEP other than those of the CDC being used, for example, those of a state health department. At the present time, the CDC states that a regimen of two drugs is appropriate in most cases of exposure, while the use of a third drug (usually a protease inhibitor) should be considered when the exposure poses an increased transmission risk or there is suspicion or knowledge of drug resistance. The two-drug regimen usually consists of zidovudine (ZDV) and lamivudine; for the three-drug regimen, usually indinavir or nelfinavir is added.[35]

In selecting a PEP regimen, the risk of infection must be balanced against the possible toxicity of the drugs used. According to the CDC, the use of PEP is not justified for exposures that present only a negligible risk because of its potential toxicity. According to the CDC, exposure to the saliva (in the absence of visible blood in the saliva) of an HIV-positive individual is not considered a transmission risk, nor is exposure to sweat, tears, or nonbloody urine or feces , and these exposures do not require postexposure follow-up for HIV.[35]

The PEP regimen should begin as soon as possible (i.e., within a few hours) after the exposure. In order to ensure this, an occupational exposure should be considered an urgent medical situation. However, if appropriate for the exposure, PEP should be started even if the time since exposure exceeds 36 hours since, according to the CDC, the time interval after which there is no benefit from PEP is not defined for humans. The CDC also states that the initiation of PEP even after 1 to 2 weeks may be considered if the exposure represents increased transmission risk, because even if HIV infection is not prevented, early treatment may be beneficial. The optimal duration of therapy is not known; the CDC states that PEP, if tolerated, should probably be administered for a 4-week period.[35]

In certain situations, the initiation of PEP requires consideration on a case-by-case basis. These situations include when the HIV status of the source is unknown, when the source is HIV-negative but may have recently been exposed to HIV, and when the exposure source is unknown.[35]

The worker should receive advice about the prevention of secondary transmission during follow-up, especially during the first 6 to 12 weeks following exposure because this is the time during which most people would be expected to seroconvert. The worker should abstain from sex or use condoms and should avoid pregnancy. In addition, the worker should not donate blood, plasma, tissue, semen, or organs during the follow-up period. The worker who is breastfeeding should consider discontinuing it, especially if the exposure was a high-risk one. Discontinuation of breastfeeding should also be considered while a health care worker is taking PEP. If any acute illness occurs during follow-up, the HCW should seek medical evaluation; such an illness may indicate acute HIV infection, but it may also indicate a drug reaction or medical condition.[35] (See Chapter 1 regarding signs and symptoms of acute HIV infection).

The health care worker should be advised of the importance of adhering to the PEP regimen, possible drug interactions and side effects, and drugs that should be avoided while receiving PEP. Workers who receive PEP should be monitored for drug toxicity. Efforts should be made to promote adherence to the regimen by managing side effects. The HCW should be informed of measures to decrease side effects and ways of monitoring for toxicity, as well as the need to seek immediate care for certain symptoms, such as pain in the back, in the abdomen, or upon urination; hematuria; and symptoms of hyperglycemia, such as polydipsia and polyuria.[35] (See the drug guide [color insert] for common side effects of the currently approved antiretrovirals.)

Special consideration regarding PEP is needed in certain situations. When there is drug resistance, special care is required in selecting the PEP regimen. When a health care worker is pregnant, she must receive full information about potential benefits and risks to herself and her fetus so that she can make an informed decision about using PEP.[35]

An important element of postexposure management for the employee is access to persons knowledgeable about occupational HIV transmission who can deal with the many concerns HIV exposure raises.[35]

PSYCHOSOCIAL CONSIDERATIONS

When an exposure occurs, a health care worker can experience extraordinary emotional and psychological stress. An occupational exposure to HIV creates profound anxiety. The exposed worker's immediate emotional response may be "extreme, gut-wrenching anxiety."[40] Therefore, during the initial postexposure evaluation, the worker's anxiety level should be evaluated, and he or she should receive counseling within the context of the relative risk of infection. The anxiety level of the worker at the time of the initial counseling session may be such that the worker is unable to comprehend or retain information received. Therefore, written information may be given and another appointment scheduled. The counseling process may be ongoing, and the worker may need help regarding counseling of a spouse, family member, or significant other.[40]

Many of the recommendations discussed previously (e.g., avoiding pregnancy, avoiding sexual practices that could infect a partner) can have profound implications. For example, a female nurse who has been trying very hard to become pregnant may find a wait of 6 months to a year unacceptable. Discussing abstinence or the use of barrier precautions with a sexual partner may be fraught with problems. The chance development of symptoms of an upper respiratory infection during the follow-up period could lead the exposed worker to believe that HIV infection has occurred. Because of these and many other possible problems and concerns, the exposed worker should have access at all times to personnel qualified in occupational medicine who can provide emotional and psychological support.[40]

RESOURCES AND REGISTRIES

The following resources and registries are available for health care providers:

1. Clinicians seeking consultation on PEP in managing an occupational exposure should utilize local experts whenever possible. In addition, the "PEP line" or National Clinician's Post-Exposure Prophylaxis Hotline is available to assist.
   Telephone: (888) 448-4911
2. The CDC encourages health care providers to enroll health care workers who receive PEP in the HIV Postexposure Prophylaxis Registry. The purpose is to assess toxicity.
   HIV PEP Registry
   1410 Commonwealth Drive, Suite 215
   Wilmington, NC 28405
   (888) PEP-4HIV

3. Any unusual, unexpected, or serious toxicity should be reported to the drug manufacturer and/or to the FDA.
   Telephone: (800) 332-1088
4. Instances of prenatal exposure to antiretroviral agents should be reported by the health care provider to the Antiretroviral Pregnancy Registry. The purpose is to assess potential teratogenicity.
   Antiretroviral Pregnancy Registry
   1410 Commonwealth Drive, Suite 215
   Wilmington, NC 28405
   Telephone: (800) 258-4263 or (800) 722-9292 ext. 39437
   Fax: (800) 800-1052
5. HIV seroconversion in a health care worker who received PEP can be reported to the CDC.
   Telephone: (404) 639-6425

HEALTH CARE WORKERS AND HEPATITIS

Hepatitis is a communicable disease that also presents a health hazard for health care workers. HBV and HCV are the two most common hepatotropic viruses that pose the greatest infection risk. In the United States, it is estimated that in 1995, 800 health care workers became infected with HBV, a 95% decline from the 17,000 new infections estimated in 1983.[41] The widespread immunization of health care workers with HBV vaccine and the use of universal precautions and other measures mandated by OSHA is largely responsible for the decline.[30]

In the United States, HCV infection is the most common chronic bloodborne infection; approximately 4 million people are infected with HCV.[42,43] The prevalence of HCV infection among health care workers is similar to that in the general population (1% to 2%),[42] and the number of workers with occupationally acquired HCV is unknown.[30] Of the total acute cases of HCV infection that occur annually, approximately 2% to 4% occur among health care workers exposed to blood in the workplace.[30] Only 5% to 10% of individuals who contract HBV will develop chronic HBV infection, compared with the 85% of individuals who contract HCV who will go on to develop chronic HCV infection.[44] However, individuals chronically infected with HBV also have a risk of developing chronic liver disease (e.g., chronic active hepatitis, cirrhosis), and their risk of developing primary hepatocellular carcinoma is substantially higher than that of those chronically infected with HCV.

Clearly, protection of health care workers from infection with HBV and HCV is essential. Exposure by percutaneous injury accounts for the majority of hepatotropic infections among health care workers. As with HIV, protection from infection is enhanced through the use of engineering controls, administrative and work practice controls, and personal protective devices, as described earlier in this chapter.

To further protect health care workers from HBV infection, HBV vaccination is now a standard of care. OSHA mandates that HBV vaccinations be made available, at the employer's expense, to all health care personnel who are at risk for exposure to blood or other potentially infectious materials. The first dose of vaccine must be made available to employees after required training and within 10 working days of their initial assignment. Part-time and temporary employees are also included.[3] The second dose of vaccine is administered 30 days after the first, the third dose 6 months after the initial dose. Employees may decline the vaccine by signing a declination form. However, the employer must provide the vaccine to the employee at a later date if the employee wishes.[3]

OSHA requires that employers follow current CDC guidelines regarding HBV vaccination.[44] The guidelines recommend that employees who have an ongoing risk for contact with bloodborne pathogens have postvaccination testing for antibodies to HBV surface antigen (HBsAg), such testing to be performed 1 to 2 months after completing the vaccine series. Workers who do not respond to the series must be revaccinated with a second series of three doses and retested. An employee who does not respond to the vaccine must be medically evaluated.[3]

Hepatitis B antibodies wane over time, and 60% of people who initially respond to the vaccine will lose detectable antibodies over the next 12 years.[45] However, according to the CDC, studies with adults indicate that vaccine-induced immunity continues to prevent clinical disease or detectable HBV viremia despite decreasing serum levels of the antibody.[44] At this time, employers are not required to provide routine boosters of the vaccine because these are still being assessed.[3]

Regarding HCV, OSHA requires that employers provide postexposure evaluation and follow-up to exposed employees, as recommended by the CDC. The CDC guidelines for postexposure follow-up of such employees include baseline testing of the source person for HCV antibodies. For the exposed health care worker, testing includes both baseline and follow-up testing for HCV antibodies and alanine aminotransferase (ALT). All positive HCV antibody results should be confirmed by supplemental testing.[42]

Treatment for HCV infection requires a liver biopsy to determine the extent of infection and genotype of the virus so as to predict response to treatment. Limited organ damage and genotypes 2 and 3 respond more favorably to treatment. Other factors, such as comorbidities and HCV viral load, may also affect response to treatment.

Currently, HCV is treated with a combination of interferon alfa-2b and ribavirin. The former is given as an injection three times weekly, the latter as a pill administered twice daily. Treatment is generally offered for a period of 6 months, at which time response to treatment is reevaluated. An unfavorable response generally results in lengthier treatment times. There are many side effects associated with treatment: headache, fatigue, psychiatric events, insomnia, irritability, and depression are the most common. Nausea, alopecia, anorexia, and flulike syndrome have also been reported.[46] Paradoxical worsening of liver disease has also occurred with interferon therapy. This exacerbation is thought to be an autoimmune reaction and it can be severe and even fatal.[43]

HEALTH CARE WORKERS AND TUBERCULOSIS

TB is a recognized hazard in health care facilities. The CDC has issued guidelines and recommendations to prevent the spread of TB in health care facilities, and OSHA enforces workplace requirements to protect health care workers from TB transmission.

According to OSHA, all health care facilities should have a TB protection program that incorporates the following:

1. A protocol for the early identification of clients with active TB.
2. A medical surveillance program of employees.
3. Evaluation and management of employees with a positive purified protein derivative (PPD) test or active TB.
4. Effective isolation of persons with suspected or confirmed TB.
5. Appropriate employee training.[7]

Health care facilities must have a protocol for early identification of persons with active TB. In facilities where clients with TB are encountered frequently, those who greet clients can ask simple screening questions regarding symptoms of TB such as cough, hemoptysis, weight loss and night sweats.[7] The index of suspicion for TB varies depending on its prevalence in a particular geographical area and population. When active TB is suspected, TB precautions should be implemented.[47] (See Chapters 7, 10, and 13 for additional information on TB and TB infection control.)

Employees of the health care facility, as well as attending staff, students, and volunteers (including those who have a history of bacille Calmette-Guérin [BCG] vaccination) should receive baseline and periodic PPD screening.[7] (Those with a documented history of a positive PPD, adequate prophylactic therapy, or adequate treatment for disease should be exempt from routine PPD testing.) If a health care worker has not had a documented negative PPD during the last 12 months, the two-step "booster" method may be used, depending on the frequency of boosting in the institution.[47] (See Chapter 7 for more on two-step testing.) Subsequent testing should be performed annually for all employees in health care facilities and every 6 months for those at higher risk of exposure, including those potentially exposed to the exhaled air of persons with suspected or confirmed TB and those exposed to high-hazard procedures, such as sputum induction and aerosolized medication treatments performed on clients with confirmed or suspected TB.[48] In addition, health care workers should be tested if they have been exposed to a client with TB without the use of appropriate precautions. PPD test results are to be recorded in a worker's health record and kept confidential.[47] The health care institution must evaluate and manage workers with a positive PPD, those who convert from negative to positive, and those exhibiting symptoms of active TB. TB testing, evaluation, and management must be provided by the institution at no cost to the employee.[48]

Health care workers who have pulmonary or laryngeal TB pose a risk to clients and other workers while infectious. They must be excluded from the facility until they are noninfectious. Before returning to the workplace the worker must have documentation of adequate therapy, resolution of cough, and three negative sputum smears collected on 3 consecutive days. It is not necessary to restrict the work activities of workers receiving prophylactic treatment for latent TB.[47]

When clients with suspected or confirmed TB are identified, they must be isolated in a TB isolation room, and health care workers coming in contact with the client must wear personal protective equipment (see Chapter 10).

OSHA requires that employees receive training and information about TB that is appropriate for their occupational group.[48] This training should include the pathogenesis of TB, situations that increase the risk of exposure, and infection control practices to reduce transmission, as well as other appropriate information. Health care workers should be taught to seek care if they experience a PPD test conversion or symptoms that could be related to TB.[47]

Health care workers should know if they have a medical condition or are receiving a treatment that may impair their cell-mediated immunity. Those who are at risk for HIV should voluntarily seek testing and know their HIV status. This knowledge allows the worker to take appropriate preventive measures and voluntarily seek work reassignment if appropriate. The measure that provides the most protection against TB for the severely immunocompromised worker is limiting exposure to TB clients. Workers who are severely immunocompromised have the option to transfer voluntarily to areas where there is a low risk for TB exposure. PPD testing at least every 6 months should be considered for those with potential exposure to TB because of the risk of rapid progression if TB infection occurs. If workers provide information regarding their immune status or request voluntary work reassignment, the facility must maintain confidentiality.[47]

REFERENCES

1. Jagger J, Perry J: Shield staff from occupational exposure, *Nurs Manage* 30(6):53, 1999.
2. Bolyard EA et al: Guideline for infection control in health care personnel, *Am J Infect Control* 26(3):289, 1998.
3. U.S. Department of Labor, Occupational Safety, and Health Administration: *Enforcement procedures for the occupational exposure to bloodborne pathogens*, OSHA instruction, directives number CPL 2-2.44D, Nov 5, 1999. http://www.osha-slc.gov/OshDoc/Directive_data/CPL_2-2_44D.html

4. Porta C, Handelman E, McGovern P: Needlestick injuries among health care workers: a literature review, *AAOHN J* 47(6):237, 1999.
5. Needle stick injuries: are nurses safe?, *Michigan Nurse* 72(4):20, 1999.
6. Schaffer SD et al: *Pocket guide to infection prevention and safe practice,* St Louis, 1996, Mosby.
7. Decker MD: Special report: OSHA enforcement policy for occupational exposure to tuberculosis, *Infect Control Hosp Epidemiol* 14(12):689, 1993.
8. U.S. Department of Labor, Occupational Safety, and Health Administration: *Occupational exposure to bloodborne pathogens,* OSHA 3127, 1996 (revised). http://www.osha-slc.gov/Publications/Osha3127.pdf
9. Centers for Disease Control and Prevention: Recommendations for prevention of HIV transmission in health-care settings, *MMWR* 36(2S):1, 1987.
10. Centers for Disease Control and Prevention: Update: Universal precautions for prevention of transmission of human immunodeficiency virus, hepatitis B virus, and other bloodborne pathogens in health-care settings, *MMWR* 37(24):377, June 24, 1988.
11. Garner JS, Hospital Infection Control Practices Advisory Committee: Guideline for isolation precautions in hospitals, *Infect Control Hosp Epidemiol* 17(1):54, 1996.
12. Lynch P et al: Implementing and evaluating a system of generic infection precautions: body substance isolation, *Am J Infect Control* 18(1):1, 1990.
13. Rego A, Roley L: In-use barrier integrity of gloves: latex and nitrile superior to vinyl, *Am J Infect Control* 27(5):405, 1999.
14. Heller ET, Greer CR: Glove safety: summary of recent findings and recommendations from health care regulators, *South Med J* 88(11):1093, 1995.
15. United States Department of Health and Human Services, Food and Drug Administration: Surgeon's and patient examination gloves: reclassification and medical glove guidance manual availability; proposed rule and notice, *Fed Register* 64(146):41709, July 30, 1999.
16. Cohn GM, Seifer DB: Blood exposure in single versus double gloving during pelvic surgery, *Am J Obstet Gynecol* 162(3):715, 1990.
17. Quebbeman EJ et al: Double gloving: protecting surgeons from blood contamination in the operating room, *Arch Surg* 127(2):213, 1992.
18. Bennett B, Duff P. The effect of double gloving on frequency of glove perforations. *Obstet Gynecol* 78(6):1019, 1991.
19. Rose DA et al: Usage patterns and perforation rates for 6396 gloves from intraoperative procedures at San Francisco General Hospital (abstract), *Infect Control Hosp Epidemiol* 15(5):349, 1994.
20. Korniewicz DM et al: Barrier protection with examination gloves: double versus single, *Am J Infect Control* 22(1):12, 1994.
21. Health and safety on the job: nurse, protect thyself, *Am Nurs* 29(5):1, Sept/Oct 1997.
22. Burt S: What you need to know about latex allergy, *Nurs 98* 28(10):33, 1998.
23. Gliniecki CM: Management of latex reactions in the occupational setting, *AAOHN J* 46(2):82, 1998.
24. Neal JG et al: Latex glove penetration by pathogens: a review of the literature, *J Long Term Effect Med Implant* 8(3-4):233, 1998.
25. United States Department of Labor, Occupational Safety, and Health Administration: Occupational exposure to bloodborne pathogens: final rule, *Fed Register* 56(235):64175, Dec 6, 1991.

26. United States Department of Health and Human Services, Public Health Service, Centers for Disease Control: *Guidelines for prevention of transmission of human immunodeficiency virus and hepatitis B virus to health-care and public-safety workers,* DHHS (NIOSH) Publication No. 89-107, Feb 1989.

27. United States Department of Labor, Occupational Safety and Health Administration: *Enforcement procedures for the occupational exposure to bloodborne pathogens standard,* OSHA directive CPL 2-2, 44C 29 CFR 1910.1030, Mar 6, 1992.

28. Morrison A: Sharps containers: take these steps to avoid getting stuck, *Nurs* 98 28(10):73, 1998.

29. Centers for Disease Control and Prevention, cited in United States Department of Health and Human Services, Public Health Service, Centers for Disease Control, National Institute for Occupational Safety and Health: *NIOSH alert: preventing needlestick injuries in health care settings,* Publication #2000-108, Nov 1999.

30. United States Department of Health and Human Services, Public Health Service, Centers for Disease Control, National Institute for Occupational Safety and Health: *NIOSH alert: preventing needlestick injuries in health care settings,* Pub. # 2000-108, Nov 1999.

31. ANA's "Safe Needles Save Lives" campaign scores important victory with release of new OSHA directive, American Nurses Association press release, Nov 5, 1999. http://www.nursingworld.org

32. American Nurses Association Legislative Branch: *2000 state legislative trends: needlestick injury prevention,* Jan 2000. http://www.nursingworld.org

33. American Nurses Association Legislative Branch, 106th Congress: *Health care worker needlestick prevention act of 1999,* H.R. 1899/S.1140. http://www.nursingworld.org

34. Centers for Disease Control and Prevention: HIV/AIDS surveillance report: year-end edition, *HIV/AIDS Surveillance Report* 11(2):26, 1999.

35. Centers for Disease Control and Prevention: Public Health Service guidelines for the management of health-care worker exposures to HIV and recommendations for postexposure prophylaxis, *MMWR* 47(RR-7):1, May 15, 1998.

36. Bell DM: Occupational risk of human immunodeficiency virus infection in healthcare workers: an overview, *Am J Med* 102(suppl 5B):9, 1997.

37. Ippolito G et al: The risk of occupational human immunodeficiency virus infection in health care workers, *Arch Intern Med* 153(12):1451, 1993.

38. Fahey BJ et al: Frequency of nonparenteral occupational exposures to blood and body fluids before and after universal precautions training, *Am J Med* 90(2):145, 1991.

39. Cardo DM et al: A case-control study of HIV seroconversion in health care workers after percutaneous exposure, *N Engl J Med* 337(21):1485, Nov 20, 1997.

40. Fahey BJ et al: Managing occupational exposures to HIV-1 in the healthcare workplace, *Infect Control Hosp Epidemiol* 14(7):405, 1993.

41. Centers for Disease Control and Prevention, cited in Department of Health and Human Services, Public Health Service, Centers for Disease Control, National Institute for Occupational Safety and Health: *NIOSH alert: preventing needlestick injuries in health care settings,* Pub. #2000-108, November 1999.

42. Centers for Disease Control and Prevention: Recommendations for prevention and control of hepatitis C virus (HCV) infection and HCV-related chronic disease, *MMWR* 47(RR-19):1, 1998.

43. National Institutes of Health: *National Institutes of Health consensus development statement online: management of hepatitis C,* 15 (3):1, Mar 24-26, 1997. http://odp.od.nih.gov/consensus/cons/105/105_statement.htm

44. Centers for Disease Control and Prevention: Immunization of health-care workers: recommendations of ACIP and HICPAC, *MMWR* 46(RR-18):1, Dec 26, 1997.

45. Centers for Disease Control and Prevention, cited in: Immunization of health-care workers: recommendations of ACIP and HICPAC, *MMWR* 46(RR-18):1, Dec 26, 1997.

46. Adapted from Rebetron: *Interferon alfa-2b and ribavirin,* product information, Schering Corporation, Kenilworth, NJ.

47. Centers for Disease Control and Prevention: Guidelines for preventing the transmission of mycobacterium tuberculosis in health-care facilities, *MMWR* 43 (RR-13):1, Oct 28, 1994.

48. Clark RA: OSHA enforcement policy and procedures for occupational exposure to tuberculosis, *Infect Control Hosp Epidemiol* 14(12):694, 1993.

24 Sexually Transmitted Diseases

Carl A. Kirton

Despite public health and individual provider efforts to teach healthy sexual behaviors, the spread of sexually transmitted diseases (STDs), including HIV, continues to affect all segments of the population. Overall, though the national rates of STDs are declining, certain groups continue to be affected disproportionately, namely African Americans, women, and adolescents.

HIV-positive individuals are still considered at high risk for acquiring and transmitting STDs.[1,2] health departments continue to report new cases of gonorrhea and syphilis among HIV-positive individuals.[3,4] This suggests that HIV-positive individuals continue to engage in activities that further the spread of HIV. As a part of routine health care, health care providers must take a sexual history and be prepared to discuss and teach clients about safer sexual activities, regardless of a client's presumed risk factors for STDs and HIV. Also, clients must be taught about barrier methods for preventing the spread of STDs and HIV. Male and female condoms are effective barriers in the transmission of most STDs when used consistently and correctly. However, both men and women should understand that condoms are not without their limitations; they do not cover all areas of the genitalia, and some STDs may be spread by skin-to-skin contact of unexposed areas (e.g., condylomata acuminatum).

Two reasons why it is important to identify STDs early are as follows: (1) STDs are more readily treatable in the early stages; and (2) it has been identified that STDs can facilitate the transmission of HIV infection by increasing the client's infectiousness or susceptibility.[5] During client examination, the genital and perineal areas should be checked regularly for any signs of STDs, such as ulcers or warts.

REPORTING STDS

Nurses and other health care providers should be aware that, in every state, clients with syphilis, gonorrhea, and AIDS must be reported to local health authorities. The reporting of clients with chlamydia or HIV may or may not be required, depending on locality. Therefore, health care providers must be aware of which diseases require reporting and which do not. Reporting responsibility resides primarily with diagnosticians, laboratories, and health care facilities. The role of the nurse is to make sure that clients whom they treat are aware that their infections may be reported to state agencies. The nurse should inform the client that, in an effort to curtail the spread of STDs, local and state health departments work with health care providers to ensure that clients and their sexual partners are treated for STDs appropriately. States have partner notification programs for cases in which a client has difficulty notifying his or her sexual partners.

Chlamydia

■ CLINICAL OVERVIEW

Infection with chlamydia occurs as a result of sexual transmission of *Chlamydia trachomatis*. This is the most common STD in the United States today. *C. trachomatis* is also implicated in other STDs such as lymphogranuloma venereum (LVG), nongonococcal urethritis, mucopurulent cervicitis, pelvic inflammatory disease, and epididymitis. The incubation period of the organism is typically 1 to 2 weeks but can be longer.

■ CLINICAL MANIFESTATIONS

All sexually active adults who do not use barrier protection for intercourse should be screened annually for infection with chlamydia. This is especially important for women because asymptomatic infections often occur in this group. Superficial inflammation of the mucosa in the affected area may be the only sign present. Symptoms that are likely to occur in men are dysuria, urethral discharge, epididymitis (causing unilateral scrotal pain, swelling, tenderness, fever) or proctitis (causing painful defecation). In women, there may be a mucopurulent endocervical discharge. The cervix may be edematous and may bleed easily. When the urethra is involved in women, it may cause symptoms similar to a male urethral infection.

■ DIAGNOSIS

The diagnosis of chlamydia is made by obtaining a urethral culture of the male penis or of a woman's endocervix. Sediments of the first-catch urine specimen can also aid in the diagnosis. The organism can also be detected by antigen detection techniques, such as direct fluorescent antibody (DFA) and enzyme-linked immunoassay (EIA), which are less expensive than culture techniques. Clients with chlamydia should also be tested for gonorrhea.

■ MEDICAL MANAGEMENT

Treatment should not be delayed while awaiting test results. History and physical examination findings should guide treatment decisions. Early diagnosis and treatment is important because complications such as infer-

Table 24-1	Medical Regimens	
Chlamydia	**Regimens**	
Treatment	Azithromycin 1 g PO × 1 dose *Or* Doxycycline 100 mg PO bid × 7 days *Or* Erythromycin 500 mg PO qid × 7 days	

tility and pelvic inflammatory disease can result from infection. Evidence of cure is not necessary if symptoms are not present.

■ NURSING CONSIDERATIONS

1. Ensure that the client understands the treatment prescribed for infection.
2. Inform the client that all sexual partners within the last 60 days should be told about the infection and advised to seek treatment from their health care providers even if they are not having symptoms.
3. Instruct client to refrain from sexual intercourse until 1 full week after they have completed the prescribed therapy.
4. Be prepared to discuss and assess the client's knowledge about safer sex practices and the use of condoms and other barriers to limit future exposure and transmission of STDs, as well as HIV.
5. Chlamydia infection may be a state-reportable infection. Hence, providers must check with their local or state health department about this requirement.
6. Encourage clients of unknown HIV status to consider HIV testing.
7. For medical regimens see Table 24-1.

Gonorrhea

■ CLINICAL OVERVIEW

Infection with gonorrhea occurs as a result of the sexual transmission of *Neisseria gonorrhea*. This organism is spread by direct contact with a person infected with the organism during sexual activity (vaginal, oral, or anal). The incubation period of the organism is typically 2 to 7 days.

■ CLINICAL MANIFESTATIONS

The manifestations of gonorrhea depend on the site of infection. In the majority of cases in men, manifestations are found in the urethra.

Gonorrhea presents as a profuse, purulent discharge, accompanied by dysuria. Women often have asymptomatic infection but may have changes in menstruation that prompt medical evaluation. Infrequently, women will present with vaginal discharge. Typically, upon examination the examiner will find redness and swelling of the cervix, the site of infection. Clients with anorectal gonorrhea often have no symptoms, so any client who practices anal intercourse should be assessed. Oral erythema or pharyngitis may be the only symptoms of pharyngeal infections.

■ DIAGNOSIS

Urethral culture of the male penis or culture of the female endocervix is used for the diagnosis of gonorrhea. Special media (Thayer-Martin plates) are used to grow gonococcus. These are chocolate-appearing plates that resemble a small piece of candy. Gonorrhea cultures can also be obtained simultaneously with *C. trachomatis* when DNA detection methods are used.

■ MEDICAL MANAGEMENT

Treatment should not be delayed while awaiting test results. History and physical examination findings should guide treatment decisions. Clients treated for gonorrhea should also simultaneously be treated for *C. trachomatis,* as these two infections often coexist. Complications, such as infertility from tubal scarring and pelvic inflammatory disease, can result from infection. Infection localized to a specific site such as the pharynx, rectum, or urethra is considered an uncomplicated gonorrheal infection (UGI). Disseminated gonorrheal infection (DGI) results in a bacteremia and often requires hospitalization, as intravenous antibiotics are generally indicated.

■ NURSING CONSIDERATIONS

1. Ensure that the client understands the treatment prescribed for infection.
2. Instruct the client that all sexual partners within the last 60 days should be told about the infection and advised to seek treatment from their health care providers even if they are not having symptoms.
3. Instruct the client to refrain from sexual intercourse until 2 to 4 weeks after they have completed the prescribed therapy.
4. Be prepared to discuss and assess the client's knowledge about safer sex practices and use of condoms and other barriers to limit future exposures and transmission of STDs, as well as HIV.
5. Inform clients that gonorrhea infection must be reported to local or state health departments.
6. Encourage clients of unknown HIV status to consider HIV testing.
7. For medical regimens see Table 24-2.

Table 24-2	Medical Regimens

Gonorrhea	Regimens
Treatment	**Uncomplicated Gonococcal Infections** Cefixime 400 mg PO × 1 dose (except for pharyngeal infections) *Or* Ceftriaxone 125 mg IM × 1 dose *Or* Ciprofloxacin 500 mg PO × 1 dose *Or* Ofloxacin 400 mg PO × 1 dose **plus** Azithromycin 1 g PO × 1 dose *Or* Doxycycline 100 mg PO bid × 7 days **Disseminated Gonococcal Infection** Ceftriaxone 125 mg IM or IV q24h *Or* Cefotaxime 1g IV q8h *Or* Ceftizoxime 1g IV q8h IM or IV therapy continues 24 to 48 hours after clinical improvement. Therapy can then be switched to 1 week of oral therapy: Cefixime 400 mg PO bid *Or* Ciprofloxacin 500 mg PO bid *Or* Ofloxacin 400 mg PO bid

Anogenital Herpes

■ CLINICAL OVERVIEW

Herpes is a viral disease caused by the herpes simplex virus (HSV). Anogenital herpes can be caused by Type 1, which primarily infects the oral cavity, or Type 2 HSV; most cases of anogenital herpes are caused by HSV-2. Infection occurs through contact with an infected person via mucous membranes or nonintact skin. Infection may go unrecognized. Often the virus establishes itself in the sensory nerve ganglion, innervating the site of initial infection.[6] The virus can remain dormant in the nerve ganglion and may never recur. However, often it does recur, especially during periods of stress, such as during anxiety, fatigue, or other illnesses. Because HSV is never eradicated from the body, an infected person is considered infected for life.

■ CLINICAL MANIFESTATIONS

Classic signs of an impending herpes eruption are burning, numbness, or tingling at the site. Eruptions typically present as vesicles. These vesicles contain viral particles. Shortly after their appearance, the vesicles rupture, releasing viral particles and leaving the area ulcerated. Associated symptoms are pain and inflammation at the site of involvement. Lymphadenopathy surrounding the area is often present. If the cervix is involved, the woman may have vaginal discharge.

■ DIAGNOSIS

The diagnosis of herpes is often made by clinical inspection of the characteristic lesion. Tzanck preparation, viral cultures, or antigen detection techniques are helpful to confirm a suspected diagnosis, but are rarely necessary. Previous infection with HSV can be detected by HSV serum antibodies, but this has no value in determining active infection or prediction of future outbreaks.

■ MEDICAL MANAGEMENT

Drug therapy for herpes does not eradicate the virus and is only beneficial in shortening the duration of the illness. Suppressive therapy may prevent reoccurrence of future outbreaks of the disease.

■ NURSING CONSIDERATIONS

1. Ensure that the client understands the treatment prescribed for infection. Treatment is either for active infection or for suppression of the virus to prevent reactivation. The two treatment strategies differ significantly; the client should understand the differences.
2. The client should understand that the treatment does not eliminate the virus, it merely speeds the process of healing. The client should also understand that since herpes infection is considered a chronic disease, future outbreaks might occur.
3. The client should be instructed to refrain from sexual intercourse when lesions are present or when numbness or tingling, which generally precedes vesicular eruption, is present.
4. The client should understand that viral spread is possible even when there are no visible lesions present.
5. The client should be educated about living with a chronic disease. Efforts should be made to diffuse any negative feelings associated with having a chronic STD. The client should be instructed in the use of condoms or other barrier methods as mechanisms to reduce transmission to a sexual partner. The client should be instructed to inform any sexual partners about their infection, as transmissibility is possible even without any evidence of lesions. Transmission can occur even when barrier methods are used.
6. Recurrent episodes can occur. Hence, clients should be instructed to take their medication when numbness or tingling is first noticed or within 1 day of vesicular eruption. Many health care providers supply clients with a prescription for medication for recurrent episodes.

Table 24-3	Medical Regimens

Anogenital Herpes	Regimens
Prophylaxis	See daily suppressive therapy below.
Treatment	**First Episode** Acyclovir 200 mg PO 5 per day × 7-10 days (may be given for longer periods) *Or* Acyclovir 400 mg PO tid × 7-10 days *Or* Famciclovir 250 mg PO tid × 7-10 days *Or* Valacyclovir 1000 mg PO bid × 7-10 days **Recurrent HSV Episodes** Acyclovir 400 mg PO bid × 5 days *Or* Acyclovir 200 mg PO 5 per day × 5 days *Or* Acyclovir 800 mg PO bid × 5 days *Or* Famciclovir 125 mg PO bid × 5 days *Or* Valacyclovir 500 mg PO bid × 5 days **Daily Suppressive Therapy** Acyclovir 400 mg PO bid *Or* Famciclovir 250 mg PO bid *Or* Valacyclovir 250 mg bid *Or* Valacyclovir 500 mg qd *Or* Valacyclovir 1000 mg qd

7. Suppressive therapy is necessary if the client has more than six outbreaks in a year. Therapy can continue for as long as 6 years, but is generally given for 1 year, at which time it is stopped and the client then observes for outbreaks. If outbreaks occur after this, therapy is continued.
8. Encourage clients of unknown HIV status to consider HIV testing.
9. For medical regimens see Table 24-3.

Syphilis

■ CLINICAL OVERVIEW

Syphilis is a disease caused by the organism *Treponema pallidum*, which is transmitted by direct contact with an infectious lesion. The organism is easily transmitted through mucous membranes or nonintact skin. The incubation period of syphilis is between 1 and 3 weeks. Clinically, unrecognized disease can have devastating cardiovascular and neurological sequelae.

■ CLINICAL MANIFESTATIONS

The course of syphilis is divided into three stages: primary, secondary, and tertiary (latent) syphilis. Each stage is recognizable by distinct clinical manifestations.

Primary Syphilis

Approximately 3 weeks after exposure to the infecting organism, the client develops a chancre at the site where the organism entered the body. It initially presents as a papule that, subsequently, exhibits necrosis and then ulcerates with serous exudate. Most ulcers go unnoticed, as they are usually painless and cause few symptoms. The ulcer generally resolves within 2 to 6 weeks.

Secondary Syphilis

The organism disseminates and, approximately 2 months after initial infection, the client may experience a generalized maculopapular skin eruption. Papules may also be noticed on the oral mucosa. The client may have symptoms suggestive of a viral influenza. These symptoms will often resolve within 2 to 8 weeks. Clients left untreated at this stage may develop tertiary syphilis.

Tertiary Syphilis

If untreated, after the rash has subsided the client may enter the third phase, called tertiary or latent syphilis. Clients with latent syphilis can remain completely asymptomatic and noninfectious to others. Sometimes, clients with latent syphilis can have complications 3 to 20 years after infection. These complications are due to the presence of gummas (areas of internal tissue granulation) that are not directly a result of the organism but of the inflammatory response triggered by the organism's presence. Gummas can result in severe, irreparable damage to bone, the liver, and the skin. They can cause cardiovascular complications that lead to the destruction of cardiac valves and the development of vascular aneurysms. The most severe complications, though, result in sensory-motor problems, loss of vision, paresis, and degenerations of brain tissue. These latter problems comprise what is termed neurosyphilis.

■ DIAGNOSIS

Clinical examination for the chancre typical of primary syphilis and the cutaneous eruption of secondary syphilis aid in the diagnosis of syphilis. Serologic studies are the most widely used methods for the diagnosis of syphilis and are classified as either nontreponemal or treponemal tests. The Venereal Disease Research Laboratory (VDRL) and the rapid plasma reagin (RPR) tests are two nontreponemal antibody tests commonly used to screen clients for syphilis. Two weeks after the appearance of a chancre these tests will be positive. All positive nontreponemal tests, though, should be confirmed with a treponemal test such as the flourescent treponemal antibody, absorbed (FTA-ABS), or the microhemagglutination–*Treponema pallidum* (MHA-TP) assay. Confirmation is necessary because false positives can occur with nontreponemal tests if a client is elderly; is pregnant; or has hepatitis, infectious mononucleosis, a recent smallpox vaccination, collagen disease, or narcotic addition.[6] The direct visualization of *T. pallidum* obtained from a chancre can be used to confirm the diagnosis of syphilis but is rarely performed.

Results of the nontreponemal test are reported quantitatively as a ratio that correlates to the amount of replicating spirochete. Adequate treatment may result in a negative titer, but some clients may have a low viral titer despite adequate treatment. Quadrupling of the titer is considered indicative of reactivated disease.

◼ MEDICAL MANAGEMENT

Adequate drug therapy results in eradication of syphilis. The organism is highly responsive to penicillin and other drugs. Primary syphilis may go undetected resulting in a systemic disease. Untreated clients may have infection of the central nervous system and develop symptomatic disease at any time. All clients with latent syphilis (seropositive and asymptomatic) should be evaluated for neurosyphilis. This includes a comprehensive neurological examination and a lumbar puncture for examination of the cerebrospinal fluid (CSF) for VDRL-CSF and other CSF–immune system parameters. Clients with evidence of CSF involvement should be evaluated by lumbar puncture every 6 months until CSF normalizes. Clients with persistent CSF abnormalities after 2 years should be retreated.

◼ NURSING CONSIDERATIONS

1. Ensure that the client understands the treatment prescribed for infection.
2. The client should be instructed to refrain from sexual intercourse when lesions are present.
3. Recurrent episodes can occur. Hence, clients treated for syphilis should be evaluated, at minimum at 3, 6, and 12 months. Syphilis serologies should be monitored. A fourfold increase indicates reactivated syphilis.
4. Clients with a fourfold increase should be retreated with three weekly injections of penicillin.
5. Clients who are penicillin allergic should be treated as follows:
   Doxycycline 100 mg PO bid × 2 weeks
   Or
   Tetracycline 500 mg PO qid × 2 weeks

Table 24-4	Medical Regimens	

Syphilis	Regimens
Prophylaxis	None indicated.
Treatment	**Primary Infection and Early Syphilis** Benzathine penicillin 2.4 million units IM × 1 dose *Or* Doxycycline 100 mg PO bid × 14 days **Late Latent Syphilis, Latent Syphilis of Unknown Duration, or Tertiary Syphilis** Benzathine penicillin 2.4 million units IM once weekly × 3 weeks **Neurosyphilis** Aqueous crystalline penicillin G, 3-4 million units IV q4h × 2 weeks

6. Inform clients that syphilis infection must be reported to local or state health departments.
7. Encourage clients of unknown HIV status to consider HIV testing.
8. For medical regimens see Table 24-4.

Trichomoniasis

▨ CLINICAL OVERVIEW

Infection with trichomoniasis often occurs as a result of sexual transmission of *Trichomoniasis vaginalis.* Although this organism mostly resides in the female reproductive tract it can also reside in the male prostate.

▨ CLINICAL MANIFESTATIONS

Infection in men rarely causes symptomatic infection. Sometimes, it may cause a mild urethritis. In contrast, woman may have malodorous vaginal discharge, pruritus, dysuria, dyspareunia, urinary frequency, and abdominal pain. Examination of the cervix often reveals petechial hemorrhages, called "strawberry cervix."

▨ DIAGNOSIS

The diagnosis of trichomoniasis is made using microscopic examination of the protozoan prepared on a wet-mount slide. However, clinical suspicion and physical examination findings are sufficient for a presumptive diagnosis.

▨ MEDICAL MANAGEMENT

Treatment should not be delayed while awaiting test results. History and physical examination findings should guide treatment decisions.

Table 24-5	Medical Regimens	
Trichomoniasis	**Regimens**	
Treatment	Metronidazole 2 g PO × 1 dose *Or* Metronidazole 500 mg PO bid × 7 days	

■ NURSING CONSIDERATIONS

1. Ensure that the client understands the treatment prescribed for infection.
2. Teach the client that alcohol must be avoided during treatment.
3. Inform the client that all sexual partners within the last 60 days should be told about the infection and should be advised to seek treatment from their health care providers, even if they are not having symptoms.
4. Instruct the client to refrain from sexual intercourse until therapy is completed.
5. Be prepared to discuss and assess client's knowledge about safer sex practices and use of condoms and other barriers to limit future exposures and transmission of STDs, as well as HIV.
6. Encourage clients of unknown HIV status to consider HIV testing.
7. For medical regimens see Table 24-5.

Condylomata Acuminata

■ CLINICAL OVERVIEW

Infection with the human papilloma virus (HPV) can result in infection of the genitalia and the anorectal area, causing genital warts. HPV enters the body through skin that has been abraded and subsequently infects the epithelial cell and causes a warty growth with a cauliflower appearance. Infection with HPV in the anorectal area is often caused by HPV type 6 or type 11. Once infection occurs, the incubation period can vary from several weeks to as long as 2 years.

The lesions associated with HPV vary, from small and microscopic to large and visibly apparent. Infection may be short-lived and require only conservative treatment.[7] Treatment of the lesions does not confer cure and the lesions may recur.

Cervical infections with HPV types 16 and 18, among others, are associated with cervical dysplasia and cervical neoplasia.

■ CLINICAL MANIFESTATIONS

Generally HPV infections are asymptomatic, but they may be cosmetically displeasing to clients and their sexual partners. The lesions are rarely painful and pruritic.

■ DIAGNOSIS

The diagnosis of condylomata acuminata is often made by direct visualization of typical lesions. Methods of amplification or detection of the HPV DNA in a biopsied tissue are available when it is necessary to differentiate the lesions of condyloma from those of other growths.

Acetowhitening can by used to aid in the diagnosis of subclinical infection, but this technique is not specific to lesions of HPV. This technique is comprised of soaking the suspected area with 5% acetic acid (white vinegar) for at least 5 minutes, and then inspecting the suspected areas, with intensive lighting and magnification, for whitening of the suspected lesions. The usefulness of this test is uncertain and is not currently recommended as a screening test for HPV infection.[8]

■ MEDICAL MANAGEMENT

Treatment focuses on removal of the visible warts. The type of treatment used is highly dependent on the location and number of warts and the provider's experience with wart removal intervention. For clients with a large number of warts, removal of all warts is rarely done in one session. No one treatment methodology is superior to another. Client response to treatment should guide the provider in determining the success and failure of a treatment. It may be necessary to use a variety of modalities.

■ NURSING CONSIDERATIONS

1. Ensure that the client understands the treatment prescribed for infection. Treatment employs acids, electrodissection, freezing, or excision.
2. Some treatment modalities result in local tissue inflammation. Therefore, instruct the client to keep irritated areas uncovered, dirt-free, and dry. Application of acids to the area can result in intense pain. The acid can be neutralized by the application of baking soda or talcum powder to the affected area.
3. Instruct the client in posttreatment wound care. Advise the client to keep the area clean and dry, and that applying a small amount of antimicrobial ointment may be helpful.
4. Instruct the client to refrain from sexual intercourse until all of the lesions are well healed.
5. Be prepared to discuss and assess the client's knowledge about transmission of HPV during sexual activities. Clients should be counseled about the use of condoms and other barriers to limit future exposures to this and other sexually transmitted diseases.

Table 24-6	Medical Regimens

Condylomata Acuminata	Regimens
Treatment	**Podofilox 0.5% Solution or Gel** Applied to wart for 3 days, followed by no therapy for 4 days. Clients should treat areas in this manner for no more than 1 month. **Imiquimod 5% Cream** Applied to wart three times a week. The client should wash the area with soap and water 6 to 10 hours after application of the cream. Clients should treat areas in this manner for no more than 4 months. It may weaken condoms; avoid sexual contact while cream is on. **Cryotherapy** Performed by an experienced provider using liquid nitrogen. Areas can be treated every 1 to 2 weeks until resolution. **Podophyllin Resin 10% to 25%** Applied to an area by an experienced provider. The client should wash treatment area with a mild soap and water 1 to 4 hours after application. **Trichloroacetic Acid (TCA) 80% to 90%** Applied by an experienced provider. Treatments may be repeated weekly. **Surgical Removal** Should be done only by a provider trained in such therapy.

6. Inform the client that condoms do not necessarily protect from exposure to HPV, as the virus is transmitted by skin-to-skin contact.
7. Clients in stable, monogamous sexual relationships should discuss with their partners the risk of infection. Clients and their partners should be instructed to use a barrier method when warts are visible.
8. Encourage clients of unknown HIV status to consider HIV testing.
9. For medical regimens see Table 24-6.

REFERENCES

1. Kissinger P et al: Incidence of three sexually transmitted diseases during a safer sex promotion program for HIV-infected women, *J Gen Intern Med* 11(12):750, 1996.
2. Afferty WE, Hughes JP, Handsfield HH: Sexually transmitted diseases in men who have sex with men: acquisition of gonorrhea and nongonococcal urethritis by fellatio and implications for STD/HIV prevention, *Sex Transm Dis* 24(5):272, 1997.

3. Belongia EA et al: A population based study of sexually transmitted disease incidence and risk factors in human immunodeficiency virus–infected people, *Sex Transm Dis* 24(5):251, 1997.

4. Torian LV et al: Trends in HIV seroprevalence in men who have sex with men: New York City Department of Health sexually transmitted disease clinics, 1988-1993, *AIDS* 10(2):187, 1996.

5. Centers for Disease Control and Prevention: HIV prevention through early detection and treatment of other sexually transmitted diseases—United States, *MMWR* 47(No. RR-12):2, 1998.

6. Luft J, Carnago LC: Nursing role in management of sexually transmitted disease. In Lewis, Collier, Heitkemper, eds: *Medical-surgical nursing: assessment and management of clinical problems,* St Louis, 1996, Mosby.

7. Ho GYF et al: Natural history of cervicovaginal papillomavirus infection in young women, *N Engl J Med* 338(7):423, 1998.

8. Centers for Disease Control and Prevention: 1998 guidelines for treatment of sexually transmitted diseases, *MMWR* 47(No. RR-1):94, 1998.

25

Complementary Therapies in HIV/AIDS Care

Kenneth Zwolski

Alternative medicine is often defined as "unorthodox therapeutic systems." However, what is alternative in one culture may be central or primary in another culture or context. Also, many people who use so-called unorthodox treatments or therapies use them to complement the more orthodox therapies of mainstream culture. Hence the term complementary alternative medicine (CAM) has evolved to describe those practices that do not form a part of the dominant system for managing health and disease.

Most CAM differs from traditional Western approaches in that it tends to focus on the host rather than the pathogenic organism. This is particularly true of theoretical systems such as traditional Chinese medicine (TCM), Ayurvedic medicine, and homeopathy. The aim of many CAM practices is an attempt to support the immune system. This is done through the use of nutrition, exercise, vitamins, stress-reduction and management techniques, spiritual practices and meditation, bodywork and massage, detoxification practices, use of herbs, and also the use of a variety of miscellaneous substances thought to have antiviral properties. TCM uses a combination of acupuncture, herbs, and movement and meditation practices such as Qi Gong to achieve its therapeutic ends.

Psychosocial interventions are very important. Four psychosocial strategies that have been found to increase the survival of HIV/AIDS clients are (1) healthy self-care, (2) maintaining connectedness, (3) having meaning or purpose, and (4) maintaining perspective.[1] Also, any intervention, belief, or practice that can reduce stress is very important. The scientific evidence for the efficacy of these psychosocial interventions and for the physiological value of reducing stress comes largely from the field of psychoneuroimmunology (PNI). Research from PNI has shown that the mind and body are connected. In fact, they cannot be separated and thus references to "body-mind" are common by practitioners of several modalities. This holistic perspective dominates most CAM approaches.

A study done by Eisenberg and his colleagues[2] has shown that CAM is used extensively in this country. The study also found that 83% of those using alternative therapies for serious medical conditions also sought treatment from a physician; 75% of those using CAM did not inform their traditional western provider and those with poorer health used more unconventional medicine than those with better health. A study done by Singh and others[3] showed that approximately 30% to 50% of clients with HIV have tried some form of alternative therapy.

There are many reasons why clients with HIV/AIDS use complementary alternative therapies. These include:

■ The paucity of consistently effective therapies for managing symptoms of HIV/AIDS and various related illnesses.

■ The search for meaning and human solace (inherent in this is the belief that CAM has a spiritual, psychological dimension for many people that they do not find in many traditional methods. This may derive from cultural contexts, religious contexts, or a theoretical-philosophical striving for wholeness).

■ An attempt to strengthen the body's resistance and delay the progression of the disease (often clients feel that alternative regimens are safe but not likely curative).

■ An effort to counter the side effects of medications.

■ A means of reducing stress.

USE OF VITAMINS

Those with HIV/AIDS frequently use vitamins, often in unconventional ways (e.g., in doses that exceed the recommended daily allowance [RDA]). Vitamin supplements are taken to replace decreased levels of vitamins due to the disease process itself, to increase the amount in the body above normal levels, and to counter certain symptoms. Table 25-1 provides information about various vitamins, including recommended daily allowances, natural sources, and usefulness, as well as general comments.

The disease process may decrease the number of vitamins available to the body, increase the need for vitamins, or both. Therefore it is difficult to assess exactly what the right amount of vitamin is for a client with HIV/AIDS. There is probably little danger of toxicity from large doses of water-soluble vitamins, but the fat-soluble vitamins (A, D, E, and K) can be retained in the body, and hence it is important to monitor for potential toxicities in any client who is taking megadoses.

Clients with HIV/AIDS may take megadoses of vitamins particularly to address problems of fatigue, weight loss, nerve pain, and muscle cramps. The B vitamins are numerous and, if the client wishes to supplement B vitamin intake, it is probably best if he or she takes a single multivitamin B complex tablet rather than trying to dose each B vitamin individually. Vitamins A, C, E, and D are antioxidants (i.e., substances that neutralize free radicals). Free radicals can damage the immune system. It is thought, therefore, that any antioxidant ingested can offer protection to the immune system. Studies have shown that deficiency of vitamin A in HIV-positive people may increase disease progression and mortality[4] and increase the probability of vertical transmission.[5] Another study looked at vitamin E levels in men with HIV and found that those men with the

Text continued on p. 472

Table 25-1 Overview of Vitamins

Vitamin	RDA or EMDR	Natural Sources	Use	Comments
Biotin (vitamin B₇ or vitamin H)	**EMDR** 30-100 μg	Cheese, kidneys, salmon, soybeans, sunflower seeds, nuts, broccoli, sweet potatoes	Needed for healthy skin, hair and nails	One can become biotin deficient through long-term use of antibiotics or by eating large quantities of raw egg whites. Signs of biotin deficiency include a scaly, oily skin rash, hair loss, nausea, vomiting, muscle pain, loss of appetite, red inflamed tongue, and fatigue
Niacin (vitamin B₃)	**RDA** Men: 19 mg Women: 15 mg Pregnant women: 17 mg	Liver, poultry, lean meats, fish, nuts, peanut butter, enriched flour	Useful for maintaining skin, nerves, and blood vessels, supporting the GI tract, stabilizing mental health, and detoxifying certain drugs and chemicals; helps insulin regulate glucose levels and can lower blood cholesterol and triglycerides, dilate blood vessels, and alleviate depression, insomnia, and hyperactivity	Signs of niacin deficiency are indigestion, diarrhea, muscle weakness, loss of appetite, dermatitis that is worsened by exposure to the sun, mouth sores, red, inflamed tongue, headaches, irritability, anxiety, depression, and diarrhea
Thiamine (vitamin B₁)	**RDA** Men: 1.5 mg Women: 1.1 mg	Lean pork, milk, whole grains, peas, peanuts, soybeans	Helps maintain proper nerve functioning, normal appetite, muscle tone, and mental health	Deficiency may result in fatigue, loss of appetite, nausea, moodiness, confusion, anemia and possibly heart arrhythmias; alcohol suppresses thiamine; large doses (up to 100 mg) may relieve itching from insect bites

	RDA		
Riboflavin (vitamin B₂)	**RDA** Men: 1.7 mg Women: 1.3 mg Pregnant women: 1.6 mg	Helps maintain healthy skin, hair, nails, and mucous membranes; aids in the manufacture of red blood cells, corticosteroids, and thyroid hormones; necessary for proper functioning of nerves, eyes, and adrenal glands	Alcoholics and older adults are prone to deficiency; signs of deficiency include oily, scaly skin rash, sores, especially on the lips and corners of the mouth, swollen, red, painful tongue, sensitivity to light, and burning or red itchy eyes; can be helpful in treating depression
Pyridoxine (vitamin B₆)	**RDA** Men: 2 mg Women: 1.6 mg Pregnant women: 2.2 mg	Supports immune functioning; nerve impulse transmission, especially in the brain; energy metabolism; and red blood cell production	Deficiencies can occur secondary to lactose intolerance, celiac disease, diabetes, and oral contraceptive use; deficiencies can cause acne, inflamed skin, insomnia, muscle weakness, nausea, irritability, depression, and fatigue
Cobalamin (vitamin B₁₂)	**RDA** Adults: 2 μg Pregnant women: 2.2 μg	Important for synthesis of red blood cells, converting fats, protein, and carbohydrates into energy, and for the synthesis of myelin	Deficiency is very common among those with HIV disease and often occurs early; deficiency can lead to sore tongue, weakness, weight loss, body odor, back pains, tingling arms and legs, anemia, fatigue, lesser forms of memory loss, tinnitus, and dementia
Folic acid (vitamin B₉)	**RDA** Men: 200 μg Women: 180 μg Women of childbearing age: 400 μg	Supports immune functioning and may help slow down atherosclerosis, as well as some cancers of the mucous membranes	Long-term use of aspirin and oral contraceptives may increase need; high doses are not toxic but may mask the symptoms of vitamin B₁₂ deficiency; deficiency can lead to megaloblastic anemia; insomnia; diarrhea; and red, inflamed tongue; alcoholics are highly susceptible to deficiencies

Continued

Table 25-1	Overview of Vitamins—cont'd			
Vitamin	RDA or EMDR	Natural Sources	Use	Comments
Vitamin A (retinol); beta carotene is a precursor to vitamin A	**RDA** Men: 5000 IU (or 3 mg beta carotene) Women: 4000 IU (or 2.4 mg beta carotene)	Orange and yellow vegetables and fruits, dark green leafy vegetables, whole milk, cream and butter, liver	Beta carotene acts as an antioxidant and supports immune function, increases resistance to infection; may help lower cholesterol; vitamin A is essential for good vision (especially night vision); healthy skin, hair, and mucous membranes; proper growth and development of bones and teeth; and stimulating wound healing	Too much vitamin A can cause headaches, vision problems, nausea and vomiting, dry and flaking skin, diarrhea, and an enlarged liver or spleen
Ascorbic acid (vitamin C)	**RDA** Adults: 60 mg Pregnant women: 70 mg	Citrus fruits, rose hips, bell peppers, strawberries, broccoli, cantaloupes, tomatoes, leafy greens	An antioxidant considered to be the first line of defense against free-radical damage; may inhibit viral replication; can raise the levels of intracellular glutathione; helps in the synthesis of collagen (a connective tissue); may protect against atherosclerotic heart disease, and common colds	More than the RDA is needed in times of physical and emotional stress; deficiency causes weight loss, fatigue, bleeding gums, easy bruising, reduced resistance to colds and other infections, and reduced wound healing; large doses may cause diarrhea, nausea, reduced selenium and copper absorption, excessive iron absorption, increased kidney stone formation, and false-positive reaction to diabetes tests

	RDA	Sources	Functions	Deficiency/Toxicity
Vitamin E	**RDA** Women 12 IU (8 mg) Men or pregnant or nursing women: 15 IU (10 μg)	Vegetable oils, nuts, dark green leafy vegetables, organ meats, seafood, eggs, avocados	A powerful antioxidant, required for proper functioning of the immune system, endocrine system, and sex glands; slows down atherosclerosis, accelerates wound healing, protects lung tissue from inhaled pollutants, prevents premature aging of skin	Deficiency can lead to anemia, fluid retention
Vitamin D (cholecalciferol, ergocalciferol)	**RDA** Adults: 200 IU (5 μg) Children, adolescents, and pregnant women: 400 IU (10 μg)	Fatty fish, such as herring, salmon, and tuna; dairy products; exposure to sunshine	Regulates the absorption and balance of calcium and phosphorous, which promotes healthy bones and teeth and fosters normal muscle contraction and nerve function	Deficiency can cause nervousness, diarrhea, insomnia, and muscle twitches and worsen osteoporosis; too much can raise calcium level, which can lead to headache, nausea, loss of appetite, excessive thirst, muscle weakness, and heart, liver, or kidney damage
Vitamin K (menadione, phytonadione)	**RDA** Men: 80 μg Women: 65 μg	Spinach, cabbage, broccoli, turnip greens, other leafy vegetables, beef, liver, green tea, cheese, oats; also produced by bacteria living in the GI tract	Necessary to form proteins needed for blood clotting; also aids kidney functioning and bone metabolism	Deficiencies rarely occur; megadoses higher than 500 μg can be toxic or cause allergic reactions; large doses of vitamin E may interfere with vitamin K's blood-clotting ability

Table 25-2	**Miscellaneous Substances Used in the Treatment of HIV/AIDS**		

Substance	Description	Action/Use	Comments
Boxwood (SPV-30)	Evergreen extract	Antiviral action	May increase CD_8 cell counts
DNCB (dinitro-chloroben-zene)	Physical agent used as a sensitizing chemical in photography	Once used to treat Kaposi's sarcoma, it is now used mostly for purported immune enhancing effect	Painted on the skin at regular intervals in 2- to 4-inch patches on the forearm; it creates a poison ivy like reaction; as the body's sensitivity increases, weaker solutions are used
Compound Q (tricosantin) (GLQ223)	Herbal extract from the root tuber of a Chinese cucumber	Shown to kill HIV-infected macrophages and block replication of viruses in CD_4 cells in vitro	Used in China as a cancer treatment and to induce abortions; usually given by intravenous infusion; common side effects include muscle aches and fatigue, which may be minimized by pretreating with antiinflammatory drugs such as ibuprofen; more serious side effects include disorientation, hallucinations, and coma; anyone with a CD_4 cell count less than 100 cells/mm³ should use extreme caution

highest blood levels of the vitamin had a 34% reduction in the risk of having disease progression as compared with men with the lowest levels of vitamin E.[6] The researchers of this latter study point out that it is still not clear whether the higher vitamin E level was responsible for the slowed disease progression or vice versa. Also, higher blood levels of vitamin E may be associated with other health factors that are responsible for the slowed disease progression rather than the vitamin itself.

MISCELLANEOUS SUBSTANCES THOUGHT TO HAVE ANTIVIRAL PROPERTIES

Many substances not classified as either herbs or approved medications are used by clients with HIV/AIDS because of their purported action as

Table 25-2	Miscellaneous Substances Used in the Treatment of HIV/AIDS—cont'd		
Substance	**Description**	**Action/Use**	**Comments**
Bitter melon	Extract of bitter melon (*Momordica charantia*)	Described as a kinder, more gentle Compound Q	It is a medicinal folk remedy used by Asians, especially Filipinos, often administered as an enema due to its bitter taste; a common side effect is diarrhea
Curcumin (curry)	Major active component of the spice tumeric	Purported to slow progression of HIV and block HIV LTR activity	Used mostly by people of Indian descent in Trinidad; it is not water soluble and very little has been detected in the blood stream of animals after feeding (hence, raises question of bioavailability); high doses have produced gastric ulceration in rats
N-acetyl-cysteine (NAC)	Antioxidant	Can increase levels of glutathione in blood cells (lower levels of glutathione in CD_4 cells can increase death of these cells); can inhibit HIV replication by blocking the effects of tumor necrosis factor (TNF) in HIV-infected cells	Clients with HIV often have decreased glutathione levels; NAC is available in an aerosolized form as a mucolytic treatment for bronchitis in Europe; in the United States it is administered for management of acetaminophen overdosage as Mucomyst
Ketotifen	Antihistamine	Purported to have anti-TNF activity	Used to treat wasting; sedation is a side effect

Continued

antiviral agents. These agents are often readily available through buyers' clubs. Many of these agents are currently being tested or have been tested for scientific efficacy with mixed results. Unlike many herbal preparations or vitamins, some of these substances may be truly harmful if taken in excessive amounts. Table 25-2 lists the most commonly used substances and provides a description of each.

| Table 25-2 | Miscellaneous Substances Used in the Treatment of HIV/AIDS—cont'd | | | |

Substance	Description	Action/Use	Comments
Shark Cartilage	Animal product	Soft bones of sharks contain natural antibiotics and other substances that may slow the growth of new blood vessels in tumors (i.e., may be an angiogenesis inhibitor)	Smells foul, difficult to take orally, causes nausea and vomiting, and is poorly absorbed by stomach; usually taken as an enema
Kobucha	Manchurian mushroom	Purported to have immune-enhancing and antibiotic properties	It is a growing colony of fungal and bacterial elements brewed and taken as a tea. Caution clients that other disease-producing organisms such as *Aspergillus* spp. may also be growing in the brew and, therefore, this could be dangerous to those with a suppressed immune system.
Dehydro-3-epiandrosterone (DHEA)	Adrenal steroid	Found to be present in decreased amounts in persons with HIV; has been shown to have anti-retroviral and immunomodulatory effects in vitro	Used to treat wasting; no consistent side effects noted

TRADITIONAL CHINESE MEDICINE

TCM is used by more than 20% of the world's population. It is a system of medicine that focuses on the whole person. It combines acupuncture, herbal treatment, and movement and meditation art, such as Qi Gong. Although just certain aspects of TCM can be used to provide relief of specific symptoms, it is best seen as an integrated system. The best results are achieved when the entire system is embraced. For westerners this frequently means making some major lifestyle changes.

At the core of TCM is the concept of energy, or Qi. Qi is the universal energy that is channeled from nature and runs through each individual. The Qi flows through well-defined meridians or channels within the body. Within the individual the terms yin and yang are used to describe the location, movement, function, and quality of the Qi. Yin and yang are polarities. Yin is described as passive, internal, cold, and feminine in nature; yang is active, external, hot, and masculine in nature. Disease is seen as a disharmony, an imbalance between yin and yang. The imbalance can cause Qi to be excessive or deficient. The disharmony can result from Qi being stagnant. Therapies are aimed at restoring harmony, promoting balance, and mobilizing stagnant Qi. Hence herbs, which are characterized as either yin or yang in their inherent properties, can be prescribed to remedy a yin or yang excess or deficit. Acupuncture, through manipulation of the meridians, can unblock stagnant Qi. Qi Gong combines aerobic, isometric, and isotonic exercise with the relaxation response, meditation, and guided imagery to keep Qi balanced and flowing.

Chinese herbs can be used individually or they can be compounded by an herbalist into an herbal formulation (i.e., a blend containing several different herbs). Some of the herbs that are thought to be effective in treating HIV/AIDS, because they either strengthen the person in general or more specifically enhance the immune system, include:

- Astragalus *(Astragalus membranaceus)*—strengthens the system
- Ganoderma *(Ganoderma lucidum)*—strengthens the system
- Asian ginseng *(Panax ginseng)*—strengthens the system
- Licorice *(Glycrrhiza glabra)*—enhances the immune system and inhibits the herpes virus; used in china as a tonic for low blood pressure and as an antiinflammatory

Three popular herbal formulas frequently used by clients with HIV/AIDS are "Resist," "Clear Heat," and "Enhance." These can be obtained by clients directly from an herbalist or through mail order.

In a study, conducted by San Francisco General Hospital, 30 HIV-positive clients without a prior diagnosis of AIDS were enrolled in a double-blind, placebo-controlled pilot study to obtain information on the efficacy of Chinese herbal therapies. The herbal concoction they were given was based on "Enhance" and "Clear Heat." The subjects took 28 pills per day for 12 weeks. Adherence was good—only one subject had to discontinue the regimen because of the development of diarrhea. At the end of the trial no significant changes were seen in any of the major outcome variables studied (i.e., mean changes in CD_4 cell counts, mean increase in weight). But those in the active group had the number of symptoms reduced and reported a higher median life satisfaction score change compared with the placebo group.[7] Practitioners of TCM have expressed concern about the trial's short duration, the lack of a Chinese diagnosis, which typically includes assessment of a client's pulse and tongue along with a comprehensive history, the lack of the use of acupuncture, and the fact that the herbs used were taken as extracts rather than whole preparations.

HERBS AND OTHER TREATMENTS

Some herbs used frequently by clients with HIV/AIDS include the following:

- Echinacea (*Echinacea* spp.)— thought to increase immune system functioning by stimulating T cells (it should be noted that it may not be effective in treating AIDS, since stimulation of T cells can lead to increased replication of HIV)
- Garlic *(Allium sativum)*—has antibacterial and antiviral properties
- Hyssop *(Hyssops officinalis)*—may be useful in treating Kaposi's sarcoma; can be applied externally as an ointment for skin irritations
- St. John's wort *(Hypericum perforatum)*—contains hypericin, a chemical that has been shown to inhibit the growth of the virus that causes one form of leukemia; it is also said to have broad-spectrum antiviral activity against HIV, herpes, CMV, and EBV; not effective if drunk as a tea, since a more powerful extract is needed for antiviral activity

Acupressure and aromatherapy may be useful in helping to reduce stress. Acupressure involves applying pressure with the fingers to the same points used in acupuncture to relieve a variety of symptoms. For example, massage of gall bladder 21, from the highest point on and then the shoulder muscle midway between the outer tip of the shoulder and the spine, can reduce stress. Aromatherapy involves the skilled and controlled use of essential oils to promote physical and emotional health. Each oil has both a physical and psychoemotional benefit, which can be experienced through direct application or inhalation. For example, lavender *(Lavendulin officinalis)* is useful for skin inflammation and muscle pain yet also balances the emotions and relieves nervous tension and stress. Other therapies, such as homeopathy and body work, are also frequently used by clients with HIV/AIDS.

Heat therapy is sometimes used by clients with HIV/AIDS. In heat therapy, clients combine hot baths with hot drinks and wrap themselves in blankets based on the theory that benefits can be derived from raising body temperature, which generally boosts immunity. Caution is indicated for any client attempting this therapy, however. It should only be done under supervision. Additionally, raising body temperature may actually be counterproductive because it may stimulate HIV replication.

Clients with HIV/AIDS may choose to avail themselves of any of the herbs, miscellaneous medications, or other practices that are considered to be part of the unorthodox approach to treating HIV/AIDS in an effort to alleviate a specific symptom or in the hope of slowing down the progression of the disease. Some clients, however, embrace complementary therapies as a means of bringing about meaningful lifestyle changes, an attempt to better integrate mind, body, and spirit. One study attempted to evaluate whether a standardized program that incorporated many complementary therapies combined with an appropriate course of standard medical therapy would have a measurable effect on the course of HIV disease.[8] Although the study can be justifiably criticized because of the small sample size (i.e., 10), its findings nonetheless are both interesting and encouraging. The experimental group for this study were followed for 30 months. They all agreed to adhere to the following protocol during this time: to follow a diet of adequate protein and calories, consisting primarily of whole grains, fruits, vegetables, fish, poultry, eggs, seeds, nuts, herbs, and spices; take on a daily basis high-potency multivitamin and mineral capsules (i.e., 2000 mg of vitamin C, 800 units of vitamin E, 25,000 units of beta carotene, two capsules of acidophilus, and large amounts [four capsules 3 times daily] of "Resist"); exercise no less than 3 times per week; refrain from cigarettes, marijuana, alcohol, and other recreational drugs; listen to a 15-minute stress reduction tape twice daily; meet in a professionally facilitated emotional support group monthly; and continue all standard medications.

All clients at the beginning of the trial were HIV-positive and asymptomatic. At 30 months they were compared to a control group (the comparison group included asymptomatic clients with HIV who were being followed at the same laboratory during an identical period of time and who had the same medical tests performed as the experimental group). The experimental group had only a 4% drop in CD_4 count as compared to the control group who experienced a 49% drop. Also the mean CD_8 count rose by 28% in the experimental group. No mortality in the experimental group occurred. The authors of this research study concluded that clients who are presented good counseling on nutrition, vitamin supplementation, stress reduction, and exercise and who involve themselves in the community can potentially continue to live asymptomatic lives that in quality and length exceed the lives of those not presented such counseling.

REFERENCES

1. Ironson G et al: Psychosocial factors related to long term survival with HIV/AIDS, *Clin Psychol Psychother* 2:249, 1995.
2. Eisenberg DM et al: Unconventional medicine in the United States: prevalence, costs and patterns of use, *N Engl J Med* 328(4):246, 1993.
3. Singh N et al: Determinants of nontraditional therapy use in patients with HIV infection, *Arch Intern Med* 156(2):197, 1996.
4. Semba R et al: Increased mortality associated with vitamin A deficiency during human immunodeficiency virus type 1 infection, *Arch Intern Med* 153(18): 2149, 1993.
5. Semba R et al: Maternal vitamin A deficiency and mother-to-child transmission of HIV-1, *Lancet* 343(8913):1593, 1994.
6. Tang A: Vitamin E slows aids progression, *AIDS* 11:613, 1997.
7. Burack JH et al: Pilot randomized controlled trial of Chinese herbal treatment for HIV-associated symptoms, *J Acquir Immune Defic Syndr* 12(4):386, 1996.
8. Kaier J, Donnegan E: Complementary therapies in HIV disease, *Altern Ther Health Med* 2(4):42, 1996.

Unit VI   Frequently Asked Questions

My health care provider started me on a regimen of trimethoprim-
sulfamethoxazole (Bactrim). Shortly after starting the medication,
I developed a rash, and it seems to be worse when I am in the sun.
How come my health care provider didn't change the medication like
when I developed a rash while taking a protease inhibitor?

One of the most common reactions from this medication is a change in the
skin. About half of the people treated with this medication report some
type of changes. For some people, this rash will disappear with continued
treatment and for others it will get worse. The skin often becomes red-
dened, dry, scaly, and sometimes there may be small eruptions. There is no
way to predict how your skin will eventually respond to this medication.
Bactrim is one of several medications that are known as photosensitizers;
that is, skin gets worse in sun-exposed areas. Sometimes these changes will
resemble a simple sunburn or may become scaly patches that itch. Unlike
the rash associated with some antiretrovirals, which can be severe, the rash
associated with Bactrim is rarely life-threatening. Because of the superiority
of this medication over all other medications in preventing *Pneumocystis
carinii* pneumonia (PCP) your provider did not stop it when you developed
the rash. Most clients obtain relief by applying an emollient to skin one or
two times a day. You can also protect the skin by minimizing its exposure to
the effects of the sun. You and your provider should monitor the skin because a life-threatening skin condition, although rare, is possible.

Now that I have this weight gain around my belly (i.e., central obesity) and at the back of my neck (i.e., buffalo hump), can I exercise and diet to get rid of it?

The symptoms you describe are characteristic of HIV-associated adipose
redistribution syndrome, or lipodystrophy. It does not appear that diet
and exercise are helpful in ameliorating this problem. However, diet and
exercise are important to your overall health. Because the exact reason as
to why this condition develops in persons with HIV taking antiretrovirals is unknown, there are no known approved therapies. Some researchers have found that subcutaneous injections of human growth hormone have a significant positive effect on this condition.[1] Other
researchers have found that discontinuing a client's protease inhibitor regimen and switching to a nonnucleoside-based regimen has been associated with improvement in this type of obesity.[2] You may be given other
medications to treat this syndrome because other abnormalities such as
increases in cholesterol often occur.

Will I be asked to participate in a drug study given that I am HIV-positive and pregnant?

Health care providers who are treating HIV-positive pregnant women are
encouraged to report cases of prenatal exposure to antiretroviral drugs,

either administered alone or in combination, to the Antiretroviral Pregnancy Registry. This registry is a collaborative project whose members include practitioners from obstetrics and pediatrics, governmental staff from the National Institute of Health and the Centers for Disease Control and Prevention, and staff from pharmaceutical companies. The research aim is to collect observational, nonexperimental data on antiretroviral exposure during pregnancy to assess the safety of antiretroviral medications in pregnancy and in pregnancy outcomes. You are referred to the Antiretroviral Pregnancy Registry, Post Office Box 13398, Research Triangle Park, NC 27709-3398; 1-800-258-4263.

I have been using many different medications to help control my neuropathy with minimal relief. Would you recommend nondrug therapies for this condition?

Treatment of peripheral neuropathy is very challenging and can often require the use of many different classes and strengths of medications—sometimes without improvement. Your primary care provider will continue to modify your drugs or drug dosages to manage the symptoms you are experiencing. There are few studies that compare the effects of nondrug therapies to drug therapies. In studies that evaluate nondrug therapies, it appears that individuals tend to feel much better and have some improvement in their physical strength. However, the long-term benefit of these therapies is unknown.[3] Certainly nondrug therapies such as thermal therapies, acupuncture, and reflexology are effective means of relief for a variety of conditions. Their direct effect on neuropathic pain is unknown. It is reasonable for you to consider using these therapies as adjuncts to your drug therapy.

Can a nurse refuse to take care of me because I have AIDS?

Absolutely not. Nurses have the obligation to provide care to all clients regardless of their age, color, creed, disability, gender, health status, lifestyle, nationality, race, religion, or sexual orientation. The American Nurses Association (ANA), a professional organization representing the nation's entire registered nurse population, supports the provision of skilled, knowledgeable, and compassionate nursing care, which respects client conscience and integrity, cultural values, beliefs, relationships, and the right to make choices.[4] When caring for clients with HIV, however, there is the risk of transmission of HIV and other pathogens to the nurse when performing direct care duties. Hospitals and other health-related facilities provide ongoing training about infectious diseases and the appropriate care of clients with infectious disease. They also provide nurses and other health care personnel with personal protective equipment (PPE) to prevent the accidental exposure of the nurse to potentially infectious material. Should you feel that you are not cared for appropriately or if a nurse refuses to care for you, you should ask to speak with the nurse manager about your concerns.

My partner and I are HIV-positive, and he does not like to use condoms. Can I use the female condom to protect myself from being reinfected with HIV?

Yes. The female condom (i.e., Reality) is a soft, loose-fitting polyurethane sheath that lines the vagina. Polyurethane is a strong, thin material that is an effective barrier to sexually transmitted diseases (STDs), including HIV. It is estimated to reduce the risk of HIV infection for each sex act by 97.1% when used consistently (every time) and correctly. This condom has a soft ring at each end. The ring at the closed end is used to put the device inside the vagina and to hold it in place during sex. The other ring stays outside the vagina and partly covers the labia. If you choose to use this barrier method, it is important to use the device correctly. First, inspect the condom and make sure it is completely lubricated on the outside and the inside. While holding the sheath at the closed end, grasp the soft, flexible inner ring and squeeze it with your thumb and middle finger (the fingers that you snap with) so it becomes long and narrow. With the other hand, separate the outer lips of your vagina. Gently insert the inner ring into your vaginal canal. You should feel the inner ring go up and move into place. Next, place your index finger on the inside of the condom, and push the inner ring up as far as it will go. Be sure the sheath is not twisted. The outer ring remains on the outside of your vagina. It is now in place and ready for use with a partner. You should gently guide the penis into the sheath's opening with your hand, to ensure that it enters properly. Be sure that the penis is not entering to the side of the sheath. It is important to use enough lubricant so that the condom stays in place during sex. If the condom is pulled out or pushed in, there is not enough lubricant; add more to either the inside of the condom or the outside of the penis. To remove the condom, twist the outer ring and gently pull the condom out. Do this before standing up to avoid any spillage. Throw the condom out in the garbage.[5]

Are there any herbal treatments that can interfere with the pharmacological treatment of HIV/AIDS?

In a recent study[6] carried out at the U.S. National Institutes of Health it was found that St. John's wort (hypericum perforatum), an herb frequently used to treat depression, can reduce the overall blood levels of indinavir (Crixivan), a PI, by an average of 57%. Based on these findings, the FDA has recommended that St. John's wort not be used concomitantly with PIs. The concern is that the reduction in the level of PIs may cause them to be ineffective, and it could also result in the development of HIV resistance (just as if too little of the drug had been taken). Although the study only examined the effect of St. John's wort on indinavir, the FDA advises caution in the concurrent use of St. John's wort with other anti-retroviral drugs, particularly other PIs and nonnucleoside reverse transcriptase inhibitors (NNRTIs) because these drugs are metabolized in a fashion similar to indinavir. Since there is little research in this area, not much is known about whether or not other herbal treatments may interact with antiretroviral medications.

I am HIV-positive. Should I avoid Tylenol?

Large doses of Tylenol or Tylenol taken over a long period of time may be harmful to clients with HIV because of the effect that acetaminophen has in depleting the body of glutathione. Glutathione plays an important role in the body's physiology; its main value is that of an antioxidant, which helps the body clean up intracellular toxins. In one study[7] it was actually shown that people with HIV who have lower glutathione levels have a much lower probability of surviving over the course of 3 years than do people with HIV with normal glutathione levels. N acetyl cysteine (NAC) is already taken by many clients with HIV. NAC is effective because it can increase glutathione levels. NAC in non-HIV contexts is used as an antidote to treat acetaminophen overdose. In other words, avoiding Tylenol might be a good idea. Other glutathione-depleting factors include exposure to ultraviolet radiation (usually from the sun) and drinking alcohol.

Can stress affect HIV progression?

A commonly held belief is that emotional stress does often translate into physical problems. Many people who are HIV-positive turn to more holistic therapies and lifestyles in an attempt to find meaning and reduce stress in their everyday lives. They see this as a positive step in keeping healthy. Because stress is so hard to quantify, and because so many other variables are always present that are hard to control, scientific evidence for these beliefs is difficult to obtain. One recent study, however, provides evidence that levels of stress may serve as predictors of early progression of HIV to AIDS.[8] In this study, 93 HIV-positive men who have sex with men were observed for a period of 42 months. The researchers found that stressful life events associated with depression can worsen HIV infection. The more severe the stress, the greater the likelihood of early progression to AIDS. For each severe stress per 6-month period (e.g., the death of a loved one) the risk of early disease progression doubled. However, stress levels common to everyday living did not appear to affect HIV progression.

REFERENCES

1. Wanke C et al: Recombinant human growth hormone improves the fat redistribution syndrome (lipodystrophy) in patients with HIV. *AIDS* 13(15):2099, Oct 1999.
2. Martinez E et al: Reversion of metabolic abnormalities after switching from HIV-1 protease inhibitors to nevirapine, *AIDS* 13(7):805, May 1999.
3. Galantino ML et al: Use of noninvasive electroacupuncture for the treatment of HIV-related peripheral neuropathy: a pilot study, *J Altern Complement Med* 5(2):135, 1999.

4. American Nurses Association: *AIDS/HIV disease and socioculturally diverse populations*, 1993 (position paper).
5. Reality package insert, instructions.
6. Piscitelli SC et al: Indinavir concentrations and St. John's wort, *Lancet* 335:547, 2000.
7. Herzenberg LA et al: Glutathione deficiency is associated with impaired survival in HIV disease, *Proceedings of the National Academy of Sciences of the United States of America* 94(5):1967, Mar 1997.
8. Evans DL et al: Severe life stress as a predictor of early disease progression in HIV infection, *Am J Psych* 154(5):630, 1997.

Appendix A

*Resistance Testing: A Primer For Clinicians**

The remarkable ability of HIV to evolve resistance to specific antiretroviral agents is among the major factors leading to failure of therapy. While the choice of antibiotics in treatment of a serious bacterial infection is often guided by antimicrobial susceptibility testing, management of HIV-positive clients with virologic failure has meant switching to as many new drugs as possible based upon the treatment history and known patterns of cross-resistance. The availability of resistance testing in clinical practice brings with it the possibility that therapeutic choices can be guided and refined to ultimately improve virologic and clinical outcomes. This article will discuss how resistance is detected in the clinical laboratory, situations in which resistance testing makes sense, situations where it may fall short, and how it can currently be used in clinical management.

HOW RESISTANCE EVOLVES

Variations in HIV RNA are generated, on average, at a rate of 1 nucleotide per replication cycle, meaning that if 10 billion viral particles are made daily, every possible drug mutation is generated daily. Thus, viral polymorphism (i.e., the presence of variants composed of different genetic material but which presumably have the same overall "fitness") is common in persons with established HIV infection. In the presence of selection pressure exerted by antiretroviral drugs, any preexisting virus with mutations conferring greater fitness emerges as the predominant strain. For some antiretroviral agents (e.g., 3TC, nonnucleoside reverse transcriptase inhibitors [NNRTIs]), a single-point mutation leads to high-level resistance. For other drugs (e.g., AZT, protease inhibitors [PIs]) high-level resistance requires the accumulation of multiple resistance mutations.

Evidence implicating a point mutation as the cause of drug resistance arises from two lines of data. First, in vitro passage of HIV-1 in culture in the presence of drug leads to the development of mutations. Second, viral geno-

---

*Article reproduced with permission from Erbelding EJ: Resistance testing: a primer for clinicians, *Hopkins HIV Report* 11(3), 1999; Courtesy of the Johns Hopkins University on behalf of its Division of Infectious Diseases and AIDS Service, Baltimore, Maryland.

types from many clients receiving a specific drug who experience virologic rebound have characteristic mutations. For most reverse transcriptase (RT) and protease (Pr) mutations outlined in Table A-1, the clinical and in vitro data correlate well. In standard resistance nomenclature, the first letter denotes the wild-type amino acid for that codon, the number represents the codon of interest, and the ending letter represents the amino acid coded for by the mutated codon. Thus K103N detected in the RT gene means that asparagine has been substituted for lysine at the 103 codon. Table A-2 lists the single-letter codes relating to amino acids in this system.

LABORATORY TESTING METHODS

GENOTYPE ANALYSIS

Genotypic assays depend upon amplification by RT-coupled PCR of either the Pr or RT genes isolated from viral RNA in plasma. The amplicons generated are then sequenced using automated DNA sequencing techniques. The amino acid sequence of the RT or Pr can then be inferred. Multiple-point mutations that code for amino acid substitutions do not necessarily coincide within the same viral particle, but each mutation identified must be present in at least 20% of circulating viral particles in order to be detected with this process. Thus genotypic analysis can only detect mutations that predominate at the time of sampling and is insensitive to mutations caused by drug pressure that have developed in the past but that are not currently predominant. Genotype analysis is also often insensitive to the T69SSS insertion, a mutation associated with resistance to all nucleoside analogues. Genotypic assays are technically difficult to perform when the viral copy count is less than 1000 copies/ml. The cost associated with genotypic testing varies from $360 to $480 per gene. The test is not currently licensed by the Food and Drug Administration (FDA) for clinical use, which means that commercial insurers, including Medicaid, might not reimburse the cost of the test.

PHENOTYPE ANALYSIS

The growth properties of an isolated virus in the presence of varying drug concentrations are assessed through phenotypic analysis in a fashion analogous to traditional susceptibility testing in clinical microbiology. Rather than assessing growth characteristics of primary viral isolates, however, currently available techniques insert the RT and Pr genes into a molecular HIV clone with standardized envelope and accessory genes. The phenotypic characteristics of the Pr and RT from the clinical isolate are then assessed in the presence of varying drug concentrations. The amount of drug required to inhibit viral growth by 50%, 90%, or 95% is determined. A four-fold or higher shift in IC50* (compared to wild type Pr and RT genes) cor-

---

*The inhibitory concentration (IC) serves as a quantitative measure of a drug's activity against infectious organisms. On the basis of the IC an organism may be designated as "susceptible," "moderately susceptible," "conditionally susceptible," or "resistant" to the agent tested.

Table A-1 Guide to Antiretroviral Resistance Mutations

These tables give an overview of mutations associated with resistance to antiretrovirals. While the interaction between mutations is complex and cannot be fully represented in a concise table format, these tables may still aid in the interpretation of genotypic analysis results. The tables list mutations that are seen frequently or are considered significant. Results of genotypic testing always indicate mutations in the majority virus population only (i.e., >20%). Mutations caused by previous antiretrovirals may only be present in minority virus populations and thus may not be detected; such mutations may reemerge if the drugs in question are resumed. Any mutations reported on previous genotypic testing of a given client should be taken into account when deciding on future treatment.

How To Read These Tables

Bold underlined—Major mutation frequently associated with high-level resistance
Bold—Common mutation that can be associated with resistance
Italicized—Not always associated with resistance; possible polymorphism

Nucleosides

	41	67	**69***	70		75	**151**	178	**184**	210	**215**	219	**333**	
AZT	**41**	67	**69***	70			**151**				**215**	219	**333**	184 restores AZT sensitivity in the presence of 41 and 215.
3TC			**69***				**151**		**184**				**333**	333 is likely resistant to AZT and 3TC
ddI		65	**69***		74		**151**		*184*					
ddC		65	**69***		74		**151**		**184**					Incomplete data
d4T	*50*		**69***			*75*	**151**	178						Multiple AZT mutations Questionable d4T resistance
ABC		65	**69***		74		**151**		**115**	**184**				Multiple mutations required

AZT = Zidovudine; 3TC = Epivir; ddI = Didanosine; ddC = Zalcitabine; d4T = Stavudine; ABC = Abacavir; 69* refers to 69SS insertion, which, along with other mutations in reverse transcriptase (RT), leads to cross-resistance for the class and is difficult to identify in genotypic testing; 151 mutation leads to cross-resistance to the NRTI class when present with ≥3 mutations.

Continued

Table A-I Guide to Antiretroviral Resistance Mutations—cont'd

Nonnucleoside Reverse Transcriptase Inhibitors

DLV		103				181				**236**	NNRTI resistance occurs quickly if viral suppression is incomplete. K103N and Y181C are the most common mutations and lead to cross-resistance. Y181C alone may not lead to EFV resistance.
EFV	**100**	103		**108**	**179**	**181**	**188**	**190**	**225**		
NVP	**100**	103	**106**	**108**		181	**188**	**190**			

DLV = Delavirdine; *EFV* = Efavirenz; *NVP* = Nevirapine.

Protease Inhibitors

APV	*10*						*36*	*46*	**47**	**48**	50	**54**	*63*	*71*			**82**	**84**			1° mutation: 150V; 88 increases APV sensitivity
IDV	*10*	**20**	**24**		**32**		*36*	46		*48*		**54**	*63*	*71*	**73**	*77*	82	**84**		**90**	≥3 mutations needed for high level resistance
NFV	*10*			30			*36*	*46*		*48*				*71*		*77*	**82**	**84**	88	**90**	1° mutation: D30N
RTV	*10*	**20**			**32**	**33**	*36*	*46*				**54**	*63*	*71*		*77*	82	**84**		**90**	Multiple mutations required
SQV	*10*	**20**	**24**	**30**			*36*	*46*		48		54	*63*	*71*	**73**	*77*	82	**84**		90	1° mutations: G48V and L90M

APV = Amprenavir; *IDV* = Indinavir; *NFV* = Nelfinavir; *RTV* = Ritonavir; *SQV* = Saquinavir. Primary mutations are 30, 48, 54, 82, 84, and 90. Resistance to all protease inhibitors is likely if 2 or more of these mutations are present.

Table A-2	Amino Acids and Corresponding Single-Letter Codes Used in Describing Genotypes

Letter Code	Amino Acid
A	Alanine
C	Cytosine
D	Aspartic acid
E	Glutamic acid
F	Phenylalanine
G	Glycine
H	Histidine
I	Isoleucine
K	Lysine
L	Leucine
M	Methionine
N	Asparagine
P	Proline
Q	Glutamine
R	Arginine
S	Serine
T	Threonine
V	Valine
W	Tryptophan
Y	Tyrosine

relates reliably with drug resistance. As with genotype analysis, the assays are difficult to perform if the viral copy count is less than 1000 copies/ml. As is also true with genotypic testing, the phenotypic assay is insensitive to resistant strains that do not represent at least 20% of the quasispecies. Thus clinical isolates from clients who are not receiving any therapy may not reflect resistance or cross-resistance acquired during time exposed to drugs in the past. Rather, as with genotypic analysis, the quasispecies that occurs without therapy is likely to be wild-type HIV. Phenotypic testing is also unlicensed for clinical use at this time. Phenotypic testing is more expensive (at about $900 per test) and time consuming than genotypic testing, and commercial availability in the United States is limited to one supplier.

The Effect of Genotypic Testing in Clinical Management

Though genotypic analyses are now relatively easy to obtain in clinical practice, many questions remain regarding their appropriate use and the amount of useful information they add to what can be inferred from the treatment history. To date, management of virologic rebound has meant switching all components of the "failing" regimen if possible. However, data generated in the past year from ACTG 343, the Trilege study, and from Merck clinical trials strongly suggest that genotypic analysis at the time of rebound may implicate only a single drug as failing rather than the whole regimen.[1] In rebound occurring with AZT/3TC/IDV (or with IDV alone following AZT/3TC/IDV), the M184V RT mutation conferring 3TC resistance was the most common mutation seen, while none had mutations associated with IDV resistance. Similarly, in clients with virologic rebound on IDV/EFV, the K103N RT mutation associated with NNRTIs was the single mutation identified most often. Thus genotypic testing at the time of initial virologic rebound may suggest that part of the combination is still working and that it may be more appropriate to modify or intensify the regimen than to change it completely. These strategies need to be evaluated prospectively in clinical trials to further assess whether resistance is present in the quasispecies but in a low prevalence (i.e., less than 20% of circulating viral clones).

This question of added utility was prospectively evaluated in CPCRA 046 (Baxter, et al: *6th Retrovirus Conf*, LB8). In this randomized controlled clinical trial, 153 clients with virologic rebound receiving a combination of 2 nucleoside reverse transcriptase inhibitors (NRTIs)/PIs were randomized to either of two management strategies for the selection of a salvage regimen. In Group I, the clinician received genotypic reports along with expert recommendations for antiretroviral management; in Group II, the regimen selection was guided by treatment history. The genotypic testing revealed a major RT and Pr mutation in 75% of clients, and a major RT mutation with no Pr mutation in 20% of clients. No major mutations were identified in 5% of cases. Less than half of clients in Group II (management guided by history) received 3 active new drugs, compared with 86% in Group I (management with genotype available, along with expert opinion). Initial viral load declines were more pronounced in Group I (i.e., -1.17 log) compared with Group II (i.e., -0.62 log; $p = 0.0001$). Though these early results support the use of genotypic testing in designing salvage regimens, it is important to use some caution in applying these findings broadly in clinical practice. The design of the trial makes the relative contribution of the genotype analysis unclear. It is possible that expert recommendations without the genotype data would have given the same results; viral load declines were significantly greater at sites that adhered to expert recommendations.

As with any clinical laboratory test, resistance assays will likely be most useful when ordered to answer a very specific question. Based upon current data, specific indications for the use of resistance testing included the following:

- Determining drug resistance in newly-infected persons, especially those who are experiencing acute retroviral syndrome. With many mutations, in the absence of selection pressure exerted by the presence of drug, there is a reversion to wild-type virus. Thus as HIV infection becomes established, resistance testing may become less useful.

- Defining the NRTI resistance pattern in those failing their first NRTI-containing combination. The detection of multi-drug–resistant virus may be an important consideration in subsequent therapy.
- Defining efavirenz resistance in clients failing therapy with other NNRTIs. The presence of the K103N mutation in this situation indicates that resistance to efavirenz (Sustiva) is also present.
- Defining the extent of PI resistance in those taking a PI-based combination. As described above, some clients failing PI combinations will have no Pr mutations.

SUMMARY

Resistance assays are now commercially available and use is expanding. Resistance testing has proven to be useful in predicting therapeutic failure. However, because such testing is insensitive to resistant strains present at low quantities, the documentation of wild-type virus by resistance testing is less useful in predicting drug success. As with any clinical laboratory test, the result is likely to be more useful in therapy decisions if the test was ordered with a clear question in mind linked to a specific management strategy. Management strategies incorporating the use of resistance testing need to thoroughly be tested prospectively in clinical trials.

RESISTANCE TESTING: CASE STUDIES

CASE 1

A 30-year-old woman was diagnosed to be HIV-seropositive in 1997. At that time, her CD_4 cell count was 270 cells/mm^3 and her HIV RNA was 152,000 copies/ml. She initiated treatment with AZT/3TC/IDV. Her CD_4 cell count increased to 602 cells/mm^3 within 10 months and her viral load was maintained at less than 400 copies/ml, until 6 weeks ago when it was measured at 1500 copies/ml despite her reports of no missed doses of therapy. The viral load was repeated after 4 weeks and found to be 2340 copies/ml. A genotype analysis revealed the following:

RT—M184V

Pr—Wild-type sequence

Commentary

This case illustrates what has been recently documented in clinical trials from clients taking similar regimens, that high-level 3TC resistance (M184V) seems to appear first in a person receiving a 3TC-containing regimen along with another nucleoside and a PI. This genotype provides useful clinical management information because it suggests that no Pr- or AZT-associated mutations had evolved on therapy. The regimen was intensified with abacavir and the client had a viral load at less than 40 copies/ml, documented at 6 weeks follow-up.

CASE 2

A 45-year-old man with HIV infection diagnosed in 1989 was started on a regimen of AZT in 1991 when his CD_4 cell count was measured at 310 cells/mm³. He continued until 1995 when 3TC was added. His CD_4 cell count at that time was 190 cells/mm³, but then began to slowly decline. In mid-1996, HIV RNA was measured at 92,000 copies/ml and CD_4 cell count was 120 cells/mm³. Therapy was switched to RTV/ddI/d4T. He developed neuropathy after 12 weeks. He was switched to RTV/SQV/NVP, but developed an exfoliating rash that was attributed to NVP; nevertheless, neuropathic symptoms improved. He continued on RTV/SAQ/d4T (reduced dose d4T), with one initial HIV RNA measured at 6 weeks follow-up, which showed less than 400 copies/ml, but subsequent measurements increased over the next 6 months to 9600 copies/ml. CD_4 counts were maintained in the range of 250 cells/mm³. He tolerated his medications relatively well. A genotypic analysis revealed the following:

RT—Wild-type sequence
Pr—M46L, G48V, G73S, V82T, L90M

Commentary

The fact that he had no RT mutations identified should come as no surprise, given that he is not currently taking any NRTIs with associated mutations identified by sequence analysis. With the exception of the insertion mutation denoted as T69SSS, genotypic correlates of d4T resistance are poorly defined, and not all genotypic analyses detect insertion mutations. Therefore, it could have been predicted that an RT genotype would add nothing to the history at this point in time. The protease sequence identified primary mutations associated with both ritonavir (at codons 46 and 82) and with saquinavir (at codons 48, 73, and 90). Though his remaining options for therapy included efavirenz (NVP was discontinued due to toxicity rather than virologic failure, implying that NNRTI-resistance may not have had a chance to evolve), there were few additional potent drugs to add. After discussion, the client and his physician elected to continue the current regimen as long as tolerated, waiting for new options to become available to combine with efavirenz to enhance the chances of a successful salvage.

CASE 3

A 29-year-old man presents for care because he intends to initiate antiretroviral therapy. He reports a positive HIV result through a home test kit 1 year ago. He believes that he became seropositive at the time of a mononucleosis-like illness 2 years ago after ending a sexual relationship with a man known to be HIV-infected. A confirmatory HIV serologic test is reactive, and his CD_4 count is 490 cells/mm³ with an HIV RNA count of 75,000 copies/ml. Because he inquires about the possibility of having acquired a resistant strain of HIV, genotypic testing is ordered and shows the following:

RT—Wild-type sequence

Pr—Wild-type sequence

Comment

Because this client has an established infection, the HIV genotype is not likely to give results that would aid in management and may not have been a prudent use of health resources. In the absence of selection pressure exerted by antiretroviral agents, the genotype shows no drug-associated mutations, even though it is possible that the client acquired drug-resistant virus. Had the blood test been done at the time of seroconversion (when the circulating quasispecies is more likely to reflect the transmitted strain), the results may have been more likely to show any resistance characteristic of the transmitted strain.

REFERENCES

1. Gallant J: Antiretroviral therapy in experienced patients, *Hopkins HIV Report* 11(2):1, 1999.

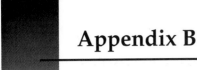

Appendix B

Internet Resources in HIV/AIDS

Carl A. Kirton
David Williams

PROFESSIONAL ORGANIZATIONS FOR HIV/AIDS PROVIDERS

- Association of Nurses in AIDS Care (ANAC)
  http://www.anacnet.org/
- Canadian Association of Nurses in AIDS care (CANAC)
  http://www.canac.org/
- European Association of Nurses in AIDS care (EANAC)
  http://www.uwcm.ac.uk/uwcm/ns/EANAC/
- International Association of Physicians in AIDS Care (IAPAC)
  http://www.iapac.org/

COMPREHENSIVE EXPERT HIV/AIDS INFORMATION

- AIDS Education Global Information System (AEGIS)
  http://www.aegis.com
  AEGIS is the largest online HIV/AIDS knowledge base in the world, with more than 341,000 files on its server—including, but not limited to, the National Library of Medicine's AIDSDRUGS, AIDSLINE, and AIDSTRIALS.
- AIDS Research Information Center
  http://www.critpath.org/aric/index.html
  The AIDS Research Information Center provides a public outreach program, the AIDS Medical Information Service (AMIS). This service operates an AIDS Medical Information Hotline via mail, email, and telephone that answers specific HIV/AIDS treatment questions from people with HIV/AIDS and/or their care and service providers. The Center also offers *pro bono* and reduced-rate publishing and design services to other AIDS organizations. A gallery of examples of some of their published graphic work is available for online viewing. Finally, it provides *free* webpage publishing to local AIDS organizations through their Web Access Program, allowing organizations that otherwise might not be able to use the remarkable networking potential of the internet to do so quickly, easily, and for *free*.

- CDC National Prevention Information Network
  http://www.cdcnpin.org/
  The CDC National Prevention Information Network (NPIN) is the U.S. national reference, referral, and distribution service for information on HIV/AIDS, STDs, and TB, sponsored by the Centers for Disease Control and Prevention. All of NPIN's services are designed to facilitate the sharing of information and resources among people working in HIV, STD, and TB prevention, treatment, and support services. NPIN staff serve a diverse network of constituents who work in international, national, state, and local settings.

- Center for AIDS Prevention Studies
  http://chanane.ucsf.edu/capsweb/
  The Center for AIDS Prevention Studies (CAPS) at the University of California at San Francisco is committed to maintaining a focus on prevention of HIV disease, using the expertise of multiple disciplines and an applied and community-based perspective within a university setting.

- Centers for Disease Control and Prevention Division of HIV/AIDS Prevention
  http://www.cdc.gov/hiv/dhap.htm
  This excellent site sponsored by the Centers for Disease Control and Prevention (CDC) should be visited frequently by anyone who desires high-quality, timely HIV/AIDS information. Information regarding basic science, surveillance, prevention, research, vaccines, and funding are among its many offerings. Downloadable slide sets from the CDC are also available.

- HIV/AIDS Information Network Online
  http://www.hivline.com
  This site is for HIV/AIDS providers and allied healthcare professionals who treat or counsel persons living with HIV/AIDS or who need constant updates on the latest advances in basic research and clinical management strategies. The goal of the HIV Information Network is to help meet this need by providing timely, relevant information. It includes a management tip of the day. There are links to newsletters written by leaders in HIV/AIDS research, and it is possible to ask questions of leaders in HIV/AIDS.

- HIV/AIDS Treatment Information Service
  http://www.hivatis.org
  The HIV/AIDS Treatment Information Service (ATIS) provides information about federally approved treatment guidelines for HIV and AIDS. ATIS is staffed by bilingual (English and Spanish) health information specialists who answer questions on HIV treatment options using a broad network of federal, national, and community-based information resources.

- HIV InSite
  http://hivinsite.ucsf.edu
  HIV InSite is an innovative website that has been developed by the

UCSF Center for AIDS Prevention Studies and the AIDS Program at San Francisco General Hospital. This site offers comprehensive information about HIV disease and AIDS, from prevention to clinical management and from reports on recent research data to discussion of social and ethical issues.

■ Immunet
http://www.immunet.org/immunet/home.nsf/page/homepage
This site provides easy access to a wide variety of information from several excellent HIV/AIDS resources.

■ The Johns Hopkins University Division of Infectious Diseases
http://www.hopkins-aids.edu/
This site, maintained by the Johns Hopkins University Division of Infectious Diseases, is a comprehensive site providing information about all aspects of HIV/AIDS care. The complete *1998 Medical Management of HIV Infection* by John G. Barlett, MD, is available online.

■ The Journal of the American Medical Association's HIV/AIDS Information Center
http://www.ama-assn.org/special/hiv/
Comprehensive information including HIV/AIDS news, and a complete library of full text articles on HIV/AIDS. Treatment standards and policy information make this a site to visit frequently.

■ Justice Resource Institute
http://www.infoweb.org/
This site is an online library containing HIV- and AIDS-related information. It provides information for clients with HIV, caregivers, and medical providers; includes legal and advocacy issues; and has comprehensive links to newsletters and magazine subscriptions.

■ Medscape's AIDS Page
http://hiv.medscape.com/Home/Topics/AIDS/AIDS.html
An excellent clinical site edited by Dr. Jeffrey Laurence and Dr. Jay Dobkin that includes case studies of clients with AIDS (CME credit available).

■ National Institute of Allergy and Infectious Diseases
http://www.niaid.nih.gov/
The National Institute of Allergy and Infectious Diseases (NIAID) provides the majority of support for scientists conducting research aimed at developing better ways to diagnose, treat, and prevent the many infectious, immunologic, and allergic diseases. The NIAID is responsible for conducting and supporting basic research on the pathogenesis of the human immunodeficiency virus (HIV), which causes acquired immunodeficiency syndrome (AIDS); developing new drug therapies; conducting clinical trials of promising experimental drugs for HIV infection and related opportunistic infections and cancers; carrying out epidemiologic studies to assess the effects of HIV on the populations most severely affected by the epidemic; and developing and testing HIV vaccines.

- United States Food and Drug Administration—HIV/AIDS
  http://www.fda.gov/oashi/aids/hiv.html
  This a comprehensive site for information from the Food and Drug Administration (FDA) on HIV/AIDS. It includes a timeline of milestones in the HIV/AIDS epidemic. This is the site to check to know if and when a drug was approved by the FDA.

TUBERCULOSIS

- Centers for Disease Control and Prevention, National Center for HIV, STD and TB, Division of Tuberculosis Elimination
  http://www.cdc.gov/nchstp/tb
  This site provides comprehensive information about TB and links to other sites.
- The Francis J. Curry National Tuberculosis Center
  http://www.nationaltbcenter.edu/
  This is one of three Model Tuberculosis Centers funded by the Division of Tuberculosis Elimination of the Centers for Disease Control and Prevention. It is based in San Francisco and its goal is to decrease tuberculosis morbidity.

PEDIATRIC AIDS

- Comprehensive Pediatric Resources
  http://mail.med.upenn.edu/~jstoller/pedaids.html
  Maintained by University of Pennyslvania medical student Jason Stoller with great links to pediatric organizations, facts, articles, and essays.
- The Elizabeth Glaser Pediatric AIDS Foundation
  http://www.pedaids.org/
  The Elizabeth Glaser Pediatric AIDS Foundation is the leading U.S. national nonprofit organizations dedicated to identifying, funding, and conducting basic pediatric HIV/AIDS research. The Foundation's goals include reducing HIV transmission from HIV-positive mothers to their newborns, prolonging and improving the lives of children living with HIV, eliminating HIV in infected children and promoting awareness and compassion about HIV/AIDS worldwide.
- The National Pediatric & Family HIV Resource Center
  http://www.pedhivaids.org/
  The National Pediatric & Family HIV Resource Center at University of Medicine and Dentistry of New Jersey is a nonprofit organization that serves professionals who care for children, adolescents, and families with HIV infection and AIDS. Founded in 1990, the Center offers education, consultation, technical assistance, and training for health and social service professionals.

CLINICAL TRIALS INFORMATION

- The Adult AIDS Clinical Trials Group (AACTG)
  http://aactg.s-3.com/

Funded by the Division of AIDS, National Institute of Allergy and Infectious Diseases, National Institutes of Health. The Adult AIDS Clinical Trials Group, the largest HIV clinical trials organization in the world, plays a major role in setting standards of care for HIV infection and opportunistic diseases related to HIV/AIDS in the United States and the developed world. The AACTG has been pivotal in providing the data necessary for the approval of therapeutic agents, as well as the treatment and prevention strategies for many opportunistic infections and malignancies. The AACTG is composed of and directed by leading clinical scientists in HIV/AIDS therapeutic research.

- AIDS Clinical Trials Information from the CDC
  http://www.actis.org/
  This site is a database of all open AIDS clinical trials for adults and children in the United States. It includes client inclusion and exclusion criteria, laboratory values at entry, drug information, and names and contact phone numbers for all participating clinics.

- Canadian HIV Trials Network (in English and French)
  http://www.hivnet.ubc.ca/ctn.html
  The Canadian HIV Trials Network (CTN) is a federally funded, non-profit, national organization created to facilitate HIV/AIDS clinical trial activity in Canada. A cornerstone of the federal government's *National AIDS Strategy*, the Network was established in response to the needs and concerns of Canadian clinical investigators, persons living with HIV/AIDS, the pharmaceutical industry, community physicians, specialists, and laboratories. The CTN is funded by Health Canada, and jointly sponsored by The University of British Columbia and St. Paul's Hospital, Vancouver.

- CenterWatch Clinical Trials List
  http://www.centerwatch.com/
  This site lists treatment trials available across the country by state, with very brief descriptions, contact names and phone numbers. There are profiles of the centers conducting the trials. The information is not just for HIV/AIDS.

- Terry Beirn Community Programs for Clinical Research on AIDS
  http://www.cpcra.org/
  The Terry Beirn Community Programs for Clinical Research on AIDS (CPCRA) was established in 1989 to broaden the scope of the AIDS research effort of the National Institute of Allergy and Infectious Diseases (NIAID) to include clinical trials conducted in community-based settings. The main goal of the CPCRA is to obtain evidence to properly inform healthcare providers and people living with HIV about the most appropriate use of available HIV therapies in diverse populations across the spectrum of HIV disease.

NEWLETTERS

- AIDS Treatment News (ATN)
  http://www.thebody.com/

ATN is published twice monthly by John James and provides excellent, up-to-the-minute information on experimental and standard treatments.

■ AIDS Treatment News Online
http://www.immunet.org/atn
This internationally recognized newsletter is an excellent resource for persons living with HIV/AIDS who are looking for information on new therapies. All articles are fully searchable and indexed.

■ GMHC Treatment Issues
http://www.gmhc.org/living/treatmnt.html
This is an excellent newsletter read by many providers and clients alike, now available online.

INFORMATION FOR CLIENTS

Many of these sites contain basic information. Issues covered include how to choose a provider, legal rights, insurance considerations, and information to consider when deciding whether to join a clinical trial. Community resources can be found at selected sites.

■ AIDS Action Committee of Massachusetts
http://www.aac.org
AIDS Action is New England's oldest and largest provider of AIDS services, education, and advocacy. Organized in 1983 by a small group of volunteers, the community-based organization provides support services to people living with AIDS and HIV, as well as the people who love and care for them; educates the general public, health care professionals, and individuals whose behavior puts them at high risk for HIV infection; and advocates at the local, state, and federal levels for fair and effective AIDS public policy and funding.

■ AIDS Glossary of Medical and Statistical Terms
http://www.smartlink.net/~martinjh/ch_glos.htm
The site's name is self-explanatory. It is very comprehensive.

■ Ask NOAH About: AIDS
http://www.noah.cuny.edu/aids/aids.html
NOAH seeks to provide high-quality full-text health information for consumers that is accurate, timely, relevant, and unbiased. NOAH currently supports English and Spanish.

■ AVERT Home Page
http://www.avert.org/
AVERT's website focuses on information about education to prevent infection with HIV, information for HIV-positive people, and the latest news and statistics. Details on AVERT's publications are also included.

■ The Body
http://www.thebody.com/learning.html
Written for a broad-based audience, much of The Body's treatment information is geared toward people with AIDS. It provides excellent articles on understanding HIV, working with a doctor, first steps to treatment, telling others, and women-specific treatment issues.

- Children's Animated Television HIV/AIDS Info
  http://www.qcfurball.com/cat/aids.html
  Children's Animated Television (CAT) provides educational information using all available technology including a computer bulletin board, website, and other electronic media. CAT supplies knowledge for children, parents, and educators to enable our society to develop ideas and solutions for a better tomorrow.

- Critical Path AIDS Project
  http://www.critpath.org/
  The Critical Path AIDS Project was founded by persons with AIDS (PWAs) to provide treatment, resource, and prevention information in wide-ranging levels of detail—for researchers, service providers, treatment activists, but, first and foremost, for other PWAs who often find themselves in urgent need of information quickly and painlessly. Critical Path provides easy access to the full range of potentially life-extending or life-saving AIDS prevention, treatment, and referral information. Critical Path makes it easier for individuals and their health care providers to make informed treatment decisions, based on the very latest, most complete and accurate treatment information and clinical trials findings available.

- Gay Men's Health Crisis (GMHC)
  http://www.gmhc.org/
  This site contains information on medical care and treatment, nutrition, mental health and counseling services, support groups, financial matters, legal concerns, alcohol and drug use, insurance, and emergency services from New York's premier AIDS service organization.

- New York Academy of Medicine HIV/AIDS Information Outreach Project
  http://www.aidsnyc.org/
  The HIV/AIDS Information Outreach Project is founded on the premise that information will support and strengthen those people affected by HIV/AIDS and those who work to provide for their needs. This site provides a wealth of community information for those in the New York City area.

- Positive Living from AIDS Project Los Angeles
  http://www.apla.org/
  This site includes treatment updates, information for clients, legal issues, resources, a calendar of events in the Los Angeles area, and an exhaustive list of resources from the West Coast's leading AIDS service organization.

- We the People
  http://www.critpath.org/wtp
  The only Philadelphia area organization created and run by and for people living with HIV disease and AIDS. The site includes their monthly newspaper, *Alive & Kicking!* and information about their weekly TV broadcast on health care in the age of AIDS: Positive Health.

- Women Alive
  http://www.thebody.com/wa/wapage.html
  This is a coalition of, by, and for women living with HIV/AIDS. It aims to help women connect with each other, exchange information, decrease isolation, and take charge of their lives.
- WORLD
  http://www.womenhiv.org/
  WORLD provides information and support for women with HIV. This site is currently under construction but lists a phone number contact.

ADVOCACY/POLICY

- AIDS Action Council
  http://www.aidsaction.org/
  AIDS Action, named by the New York Times as "among the country's most powerful advocacy groups," is a network of 3200 national community-based organizations and the one million HIV-positive Americans they help serve. Founded in 1984, AIDS Action is the only organization singularly dedicated to responsible federal policy for improved care and services, medical research, and effective prevention.
- AIDS Project Los Angeles
  http://www.apla.org/
  AIDS Project Los Angeles, the largest AIDS service organization in California and the second-largest in the United States, provides direct support services to men, women, and children living with HIV/AIDS in Los Angeles County. In addition, the agency provides HIV prevention and risk-reduction education to reduce the incidence of HIV infection and advocates for fair and effective HIV/AIDS-related legislation on the local, state, and federal levels.
- National AIDS Treatment Advocacy Project
  http://www.natap.org/
  This site includes information on drug development, position papers, and conference reports.
- Political Action Alerts from The Body
  http://www.thebody.com/govt.html
  This site is a compendium of treatment policies, health insurance policies, and funding and appropriation issues, and includes several links to activist organizations. It is valuable to clinicians and laypersons as well.
- Project Inform
  http://www.projinf.org
  Project Inform is a national, nonprofit, community-based organization working to end the AIDS epidemic. Its mission is to provide vital information on the diagnosis and treatment of HIV disease to HIV-positive individuals, their caregivers, and their healthcare and service providers; to advocate for enlightened regulatory, research, and funding policies; to effect the development of, access to, and delivery of effective treatments; to fund innovative research opportunities; and to

inspire people to make informed choices amidst uncertainty and choose hope over despair.

■ Social Security Administration: A Guide To Social Security and SSI
http://www.ssa.gov/pubs/10020.html
Disability Benefits for People with HIV Infection

CAREGIVER AND FAMILY RESOURCES

■ AIDS Resource List (by Celine)
http://www.teleport.com/~celinec/aids.shtml
This is a compendium of interesting HIV/AIDS sites, mainly for the lay person.

■ The Caregivers Guide
http://www.teleport.com/~celinec/caregivers/
Written by a mother who cared for her HIV-positive son, Bruce, Elizabeth's self-published, nonprofit book on being a caregiver of someone who is terminally ill (especially those with HIV/AIDS) is, as the book's subtitle suggests, a "labor of love." *The Caregivers Guide* is not a medical book, but rather is written for those who have to deal with the day-to-day practical needs and emotions.

■ CDC Guide to Caring for Someone with AIDS at Home
http://www.hivatis.org/caring
This site provides basic information about HIV—how to give care, protect against infections, recognize symptoms, make decisions, and provide emotional support.

■ Children with AIDS Project [of America]
http://www.aidskids.org/
Children with AIDS (CWA) offers a variety of services for children infected with or affected by AIDS or drug-exposed infants who will require foster or adoptive families. CWA works to create adoptive, foster, or family-centered care programs that are both effective and compassionate.

■ The Park Community, Inc.
http://www.the-park.com/shelter/
The park is based in San Francisco. This site offers information and links to other sites regarding many health-related issues, including HIV/AIDS.

DRUG INFORMATION

■ Antivirals from The Body
http://www.thebody.com/treat/antivir.html
This page contains general guidelines for the use of protease inhibitors and reverse transcriptase inhibitors, as well as information on viral load testing.

■ Medical Sciences Bulletin
http://pharminfo.com/pubs/msb/msbmnu.html
This is a database searchable by generic and trade names. It includes not just AIDS-related drugs.

ALTERNATIVE THERAPIES

- Bastyr University AIDS Research Center
  http://www.bastyr.edu/research/buarc/
  Based in Seattle, Bastyr is studying the use of alternative medicines to treat AIDS, with a multilevel survey of HIV-positive individuals using alternative health practices.
- Keep Hope Alive
  http://www.keephope.net/
  This site contains information on nutritional, bio-oxidative, and alternative therapies for the immunocompromised.

THE SCIENCE OF HIV

- The Garry Laboratory (all the Virology on the WWW)
  http://www.tulane.edu/~dmsander/garryfavweb.html
  All the Virology on the WWW is a resource for virology information on the internet. Collected here are all the virology-related websites that might be of interest to virologists and others interested in learning more about viruses.
- HIV Sequence Database from the Los Alamos National Laboratory
  http://hiv-web.lanl.gov/
  This site includes retroviral genetic sequence data for human retroviruses and AIDS. There is a searchable database of HIV sequences.
- The Internet Pathology Laboratory for Medical Education
  http://www-medlib.med.utah.edu/WebPath/webpath.html
  This site contains pictures of HIV, *Pneumocystis carinii*, cytomegalovirus (CMV), and other infectious agents.

JOURNALS

Because they rely on subscriptions and advertising to cover operating expenses, scientific and medical journals typically do not provide full-text articles on the Internet. However, many journals are beginning to provide abstracts or news releases of articles, and some include selected full text articles as well. However, journals published by the U.S. government are in the public domain and are widely available on the Internet.

- *American Family Physician*
  http://www.aafp.org/afp/index.html
  American Family Physician is the official journal of the American Academy of Family Physicians. The website contains full text and pictures of the current articles. Full text articles of back issues are available. While not specific to HIV, many articles relate to care of HIV-positive clients.
- *British Medical Journal (BMJ)*
  http://www.bmj.com/index.shtml
  This site contains abstracts or press releases for most of the journal's articles; some full text articles are available. Online registration is free of charge.

- Exeter University
  http://www.ex.ac.uk/~SJMacwil/lib/hivbib/bib2.html
  This site provides bibliographical details of articles, letters, and editorials on HIV/AIDS that have appeared in *BMJ* or *Lancet* since September/October of 1992.
- *JAMA* HIV/AIDS Library
  http://www.ama-assn.org/special/hiv/library/library.htm
  This site contains full text of selected HIV-related articles from the *Journal of the American Medical Association (JAMA)* and other specialty journals.
- *Morbidity and Mortality Weekly Report (MMWR)*
  http://www2.cdc.gov/mmwr/
  This site contains full text of all issues from 1993 on, which are now available in text-only versions. Adobe Acrobat Reader software (including graphics) is required to view issues.
- *Nature*
  http://www.nature.com/
  Online registration allows access to summaries of all articles and selected full-text articles.
- *Science*
  http://science-mag.aaas.org/
  This site includes full text and abstracts of all articles, as well as a database of back issues searchable by author, title, subject, or word.

CONFERENCE CALENDARS

- Immunet
  http://www.immunet.org/confcalendar
  This page contains an exhaustive list of conferences in the United States and abroad. It is searchable by date, location, or title.

OTHER HIV/AIDS—RELATED INTERNET SITES

- HealthWeb's AIDS Page
  http://www.uic.edu/depts/lib/health/hw/aids/
  HealthWeb is an electronic resource guide. It provides the convenience of daily 24-hour access and short reviews that accompany given resources. The majority of resources presented are hypertexted links to information on AIDS and HIV. Additional text-only resources have been added to round out the information provided. This site offers individuals experienced in HIV issues a new information avenue and also provides basic tools to broaden the knowledge base of those new to HIV/AIDS topics.
- HIVDENT
  http://www.hivdent.org/
  HIVDENT is a not-for-profit coalition of concerned health care professionals committed to ensuring access to high quality oral health care

services for adults, adolescents, and children living with HIV disease. HIVDENT disseminates state-of-the-art treatment information and shares expertise in advocacy, development, training, integration, and evaluation of oral health services for the HIV-positive population.

■ HIV Medication Guide
http://www.jag.on.ca/asp_bin/main.asp
This site, maintained by J. Antony Gagnon, contains drug-drug interactions, scheduling, and other medication information.

■ Marty Howard's HIV/AIDS home page
http://www.smartlink.net/~martinjh/
This site has just about everything related to HIV/AIDS.

■ Native American HIV/AIDS Homepage
http://www.sfo.com/~denglish/naap/naap.htm
This is the only website of its kind, dedicated to the topic of HIV/AIDS in Native Americans.

■ Project Open Hand
http://www.openhand.org/
Project Open Hand provides nutrition services to thousands of men, women, and children living with symptomatic HIV and AIDS in San Francisco and Alameda counties, as well as seniors living in San Francisco.

■ Rural Prevention Center
http://www.indiana.edu/[aids/backgr.html
The major focus of the Rural Center for AIDS/STD Prevention (RCAP) is the promotion of HIV/STD prevention in rural America, with the goal of reducing HIV/STD incidence. The RCAP develops and evaluates educational materials and approaches, examines the behavioral and social barriers to HIV/STD prevention that can be addressed by prevention programming, and provides prevention resources to professionals and the public. The center, which began operations in March, 1994, and is headquartered at Indiana University, is a joint project of Indiana University and Purdue University.

■ TB/HIV Research Laboratory
http://www.brown.edu/Research/TB-HIV_Lab
The TB/HIV Research Laboratory is dedicated to research into the prevention and treatment of two infectious diseases of global importance—human immunodeficiency virus (HIV) and tuberculosis (TB).

■ Twelfth International Conference on AIDS Welcome Page
http://www.aids98.ch/
This is the online news service for the Twelfth International Conference on AIDS held in Geneva, Switzerland.

■ Thirteenth International Conference on AIDS Welcome Page
http://www.aids2000.com/
This is the online news service for the Thirteenth International Conference on AIDS held in Durban, South Africa.

- The Yoga Group
  http://www.yogagroup.org/
  Since 1988, the Yoga Group, a Colorado nonprofit organization, has provided free Yoga classes and information to persons living with HIV/AIDS and has helped other Yoga teachers start similar programs.

SPIRITUALITY AND HIV

- The Ark of Refuge
  http://www.sfrefuge.org/ark.html
  The staff of The Ark of Refuge, Inc., has been working together since 1988 when they collectively designed a program that became a Northern California model for promoting AIDS education in the African-American community, targeting high-risk groups. A component defining the program's uniqueness was and continues to be a "train-the-trainer" peer outreach approach to the religious and lay communities.
- Computerized AIDS Ministries
  http://gbgm-umc.org/cam/
  Health and Welfare Ministries works on a community-wide basis to assist in the establishment of comprehensive community-based primary health care programs. Its extensive work in HIV/AIDS Ministries includes the Computerized AIDS Ministries.

Appendix C

Guide to Common Symptoms and Possible Etiologies

Kenneth Zwolski

Table C-1	Guide to Common Symptoms and Possible Etiologies

Symptoms Requiring Attention	Possible Causes
Dyspnea	1. Pulmonary infections (e.g., pneumonia—bacterial or fungal) 2. Invasive pulmonary disease (e.g., pulmonary Kaposi's sarcoma) 3. Obstructive airway disease 4. Emphysema 5. Severe anemia
New Fever or Change in Fever Pattern	1. Central nervous system (CNS) mass lesion—Often accompanied by headache 2. Meningitis—Also characterized by neurologic changes 3. Sinusitis—Also characterized by tenderness on percussion 4. Esophagitis—Often accompanied by dysphagia and odynophagia 5. Lymphoma—Often accompanied by adenopathy 6. Fungal infections—Often characterized by hepatomegaly; if respiratory, characterized by cough 7. *Mycobacterium avium* complex (MAC)—Often accompanied by chronic diarrhea and abdominal pain 8. Bacterial parasites—*Clostridium difficile*, cytomegalovirus (CMV), often accompanied by diarrhea 9. Pneumonia—Often accompanied by dyspnea 10. Tuberculosis—Often accompanied by dyspnea 11. Pneumocystis—Often accompanied by cough 12. Drug reactions 13. Advanced HIV disease

Continued

| Table C-1 | Guide to Common Symptoms and Possible Etiologies—cont'd |

Symptoms Requiring Attention	Possible Causes
New or Persistent Headache	1. Medications 2. CNS lymphoma 3. Cryptococcus 4. Meningitis 5. Toxoplasmosis
Altered Mental State	1. AIDS dementia 2. Complex CNS infection 3. Tumors
Seizures or Loss of Consciousness	1. CNS lymphoma 2. Medications 3. AIDS dementia 4. Toxoplasmosis
Peripheral Neuropathy	1. Medications 2. HIV infection 3. CMV 4. Herpes Zoster
Visual Changes	1. CMV retinitis (most common) 2. VZV 3. HSV 4. Toxoplasmosis 5. Syphilis
New or Persistent Diarrhea	1. Medications 2. Diet 3. Bacterial infections—Salmonella, shigella, campylobacter, *C. difficile* 4. Parasites—Cryptosporidia, Isospora, Giardia, Amoeba 5. Invasive diseases affecting the bowel—*M. avium-intracellulare*, lymphoma, CMV 6. Wasting syndrome
Gastrointestinal Bleeding	1. Herpes simplex 2. CMV 3. Candida 4. Kaposi's sarcoma 5. Lymphoma 6. Cryptosporidium 7. Salmonella 8. *C. difficile*
Dysphagia and Odynophagia	1. Candidiases 2. Herpes simplex 3. CMV 4. Neurologic impairment
Edema	1. Obstruction of venous or lymphatic vessels (e.g., from Kaposi's sarcoma, venous thrombosis, lymphoma) 2. Hypoalbuminemia 3. Renal failure 4. Congestive heart failure 5. Liver disease

Table C-1	Guide to Common Symptoms and Possible Etiologies—cont'd

Symptoms Requiring Attention	Possible Causes
Nausea and Vomiting	1. Medications 2. Infections 3. Massive disease of GI tract 4. CNS disease 5. Adrenal insufficiency
Inadequate Oral Intake	1. Anorexia 2. Nausea and vomiting 3. Dysphagia 4. Odynophagia 5. Inadequate access to food 6. Altered nutrition
Skin, Mucous Membrane Lesions	1. Drug reactions 2. Dry skin 3. Viral infections—Molluscum, herpes simplex or zoster 4. Bacterial infections—Bacillary angiomatosis, folliculitis, impetigo, ecthyma, abscesses 5. Fungal infections—Tinea, candida 6. Malignancy—Kaposi's sarcoma 7. Pressure ulcers

Appendix D

HIV Drug Interactions

Table D-1 Drugs That Should Not Be Used with Antiretrovirals

Drug Category	Indinavir	Ritonavir*	Saquinavir
Ca++ Channel Blocker	(None)	Bepridil	(None)
Cardiac	(None)	Amiodarone Flecainide Propafenone Quinidine	(None)
Lipid-lowering Agents	Simvastatin Lovastatin	Simvastatin Lovastatin	Simvastatin Lovastatin
Antimyco-bacterial	Rifampin	(None)	Rifampin/ Rifabutin‡
Antihistamine	Astemizole Terfenadine	Astemizole Terfenadine	Astemizole Terfenadine
Gastrointes-tinal	Cisapride	Cisapride	Cisapride
Neuroleptic	(None)	Clozapine/ Pimozide	(None)
Psychotropic	Midazolam Triazolam	Midazolam Triazolam	Midazolam Triazolam
Ergot Alka-loids (vaso-constrictor)	Dihydroer-gotamine (D.H.E. 45) Ergotamine (various forms)†	Dihydroer-gotamine (D.H.E. 45) Ergotamine (various forms)†	Dihydroer-gotamine (D.H.E. 45) Ergotamine (various forms)†

Suggested Alternatives

Simvastatin, lovastatin: atorvastatin, pravastatin, fluvastatin, cerivastatin (alternatives should be used with caution)
Rifabutin: Clarithromycin, azithromycin (MAI prophylaxis); Clarithromycin, ethambutol (MAI treatment)
Astemizole, terfenadine: loratidine, fexofenadine, cetirizine
Midazolam, triazolam: temazepam, lorazepam

*Some of the contraindicated drugs listed are based on theoretical considerations. Thus, drugs with low therapeutic indices yet with suspected major metabolic contribution from cytochrome P450 3A, CYP2D6, or unknown pathways are included in this table. Actual interactions may or may not occur in clients.
†This is likely a class effect.
‡May be used in certain situations.

Nelfinavir	Amprenavir	Nevirapine	Delavirdine	Efavirenz
(None)	Bepridil	(None)	(None)	(None)
(None)	(None)	(None)	(None)	(None)
Simvastatin	Simvastatin	(None)	Simvastatin	(None)
Lovastatin	Lovastatin		Lovastatin	
Rifampin	Rifampin	(None)	Rifampin	(None)
			Rifabutin	
Astemizole	Astemizole	(None)	Astemizole	Astemizole
Terfenadine	Terfenadine		Terfenadine	Terfenadine
Cisapride	Cisapride	(None)	Cisapride	Cisapride
			H$_2$ Blockers	
			Proton pump inhibitors	
(None)	(None)	(None)	(None)	(None)
Midazolam	Midazolam	(None)	Midazolam	Midazolam
Triazolam	Triazolam		Triazolam	Triazolam
Dihydroer-gotamine (D.H.E. 45)	Dihydroergot-amine (D.H.E. 45)	(None)	Dihydroergota-mine (D.H.E. 45)	Dihydroergota-mine (D.H.E. 45)
Ergotamine (various forms)†	Ergotamine (various forms)†		Ergotamine (various forms)†	Ergotamine (various forms)†

Drug Interactions Between Antiretrovirals and Other Drugs—Protease Inhibitors (PIs)

Drug Interactions Requiring Dose Modifications or Cautious Use

Drugs Affected	Indinavir	Ritonavir
Antifungals **Ketoconazole**	Levels—Indinavir ↑ 68% Dosage—Indinavir 600 mg tid	Levels—Ketoconazole ↑ 200% Dosage—Use with caution; do not exceed 200 mg ketoconazole qd.
Antimycobacterials **Rifampin**	Levels—Indinavir ↓ 89% Contraindicated.	Levels—Ritonavir ↓ 35% Dosage—No data. Increased liver toxicity possible.
Rifabutin	Levels—Indinavir ↓ 32% Rifabutin ↑ 100% Dosage—Rifabutin ↓ to 150 mg qd Indinavir 1000 mg tid	Levels—Rifabutin ↑ 300% Dosage—Rifabutin ↓ to 150 mq qod *or* dose three times per week
Clarithromycin	Levels—Clarithromycin ↑ 53% No dose adjustment.	Levels—Clarithromycin ↑ 77% Dosage adjust for renal insufficiency.
Oral **Contraceptives**	Levels—Norethindrone ↑ 26% Ethinylestradiol ↑ 24% No dosage adjustment.	Levels—Ethinylestradiol ↓ 40% Use alternative or additional method.
Lipid-lowering **Agents** **Simvastatin** **Lovastatin**	Levels—Potential for large increase in statin levels. Avoid concomitant use.	Levels—Potential for large increase in statin levels. Avoid concomitant use.
Anticonvulsants **Phenobarbitol** **Phenytoin** **Carbamazepine**	Unknown, but may decrease indinavir levels substantially. Monitor anticonvulsant levels.	Unknown; use with caution. Monitor anticonvulsant levels.
Methadone	No data.	Methadone ↓ 37%, may require dosage increase.
Miscellaneous	Grapefruit juice—Indinavir ↓ by 26% Sildenafil ↑ 200%-1100% Do not exceed 25 mg in a 48-hr period.	Desipramine ↑ 145%, reduce dosage. Theophylline ↓ 47%, monitor theophylline levels. Many possible interactions. Sildenafil ↑ 200%-1100%. Do not exceed 25 mg in a 48-hr period.

*Some drug interaction studies were conducted with invirase; the results of which may not necessarily apply to use with fortovase.

Drugs in which plasma concentrations may be decreased by coadministration with Norvir: anticoagulants (warfarin), anticonvulsants (phenytoin, divalproex, lamotrigine), antiparasitics (atovaquone).

Drug Interactions Requiring Dose Modifications or Cautious Use

Saquinavir*	Nelfinavir	Amprenavir
Levels—Saquinavir ↑ 200% Dosage—Standard.	No dose adjustment necessary.	Levels—Amprenavir ↑ 31% Ketoconazole ↑ 44%. Combination under investigation.
Levels—Saquinavir ↓ 84% Contraindicated.	Levels—Nelfinavir ↓ 82% Contraindicated.	Levels—Amprenavir ↓ 82% No change in rifampin level. Avoid concomitant use.
Levels—Saquinavir ↓ 40% Not recommended.	Levels—Nelfinavir ↓ 32% Rifabutin ↑ 100% Dosage—Rifabutin ↓ to 150 mg qd Nelfinavir ↑ dosage to 1000 mg tid	Levels—Amprenavir ↓ 15% Rifabutin ↑ 193% Dosage—No change in amprenavir dosage; rifabutin ↓ to 150 mg qd dosage
Levels—Clarithromycin ↑ 45% Saquinavir ↑ 177% No dosage adjustment. No data.	No data.	Levels—Amprenavir ↑ 18% No change in clarithromycin level. No dosage adjustment.
	Levels—Norethindrone ↓ 18% Ethinylestradiol ↓ 47% Use alternative or additional method.	Levels—Potential for metabolic interactions; use alternative or additional method.
Levels—Potential for large increase in statin levels. Avoid concomitant use.	Levels—Potential for large increase in statin levels. Avoid concomitant use.	Levels—Potential for large increase in statin levels. Avoid concomitant use.
Unknown, but may decrease saquinavir levels. Monitor anticonvulsant levels.	Unknown, but may decrease nelfinavir levels substantially. Monitor anticonvulsant levels.	Unknown, but may decrease amprenavir levels substantially. Monitor anticonvulsant levels.
No data.	No data.	No data.
Grapefruit juice increases saquinavir levels. Dexamethasone decreases saquinavir levels. Sildenafil ↑ 200%-1100%. Use a 25 mg starting dose of sildenafil.	Sildenafil ↑ 200%-1100%. Do not exceed 25 mg in a 48-hr period.	Sildenafil ↑ 200%-1100%. Do not exceed 25 mg in a 48-hr period.

Table D-3 — Drug Interactions: Protease Inhibitors and Nonnucleoside Reverse Transcriptase Inhibitors—Effects of Drug on Levels/Dosage

Drug Affected	Ritonavir	Saquinavir*	Nelfinavir
Indinavir	Levels—Indinavir ↑ 100%-400% Dosage—Limited data for indinavir 400 mg bid + ritonavir 400 mg bid *or* indinavir 600 mg bid + ritonavir 200 mg bid *or* indinavir 800 mg bid + ritonavir 100 or 200 mg bid	Levels—Indinavir: no effect Saquinavir ↑ 300%-600% Dosage— Insufficient data.	Levels—Indinavir ↑ 50% Nelfinavir ↑ 80% Dosage—Limited data for indinavir 1200 mg bid + nelfinavir 1250 mg bid
Ritonavir	N/A	Levels—Ritonavir: no effect Saquinavir ↑ 1900%†‡ Dosage—Invirase or fortovase 400 mg bid + ritonavir 400 mg bid	Levels—Ritonavir: no effect Nelfinavir ↑ 50% Dosage—Limited data for ritonavir 400 mg bid + nelfinavir 500-750 mg bid
Saquinavir	No data.	N/A	Levels—Saquinavir ↑ 200%-400% Nelfinavir ↑ 20%‡ Dosage—Standard nelfinavir dosage. Fortovase 800 mg tid
Nelfinavir	No data.	No data.	N/A
Amprenavir	No data.	No data.	No data.
Nevirapine	No data.	No data.	No data.
Delavirdine	No data.	No data.	No data.

*Several drug interaction studies have been completed with saquinavir given as invirase or fortovase. Results from studies conducted with invirase may not be applicable to fortovase.
†Conducted with invirase.
‡Conducted with fortovase.

Amprenavir	Nevirapine	Delavirdine	Efavirenz
Levels— Amprenavir ↑ 33% Dosage—No change.	Levels—Indinavir ↓ 28% Nevirapine: no effect Dosage—Indinavir 1000 mg q8h	Levels—Indinavir ↑ >40% Delavirdine: no effect Dosage—Indinavir 600 mg q8h Delavirdine— standard.	Levels—Indinavir ↓ 31% Dosage—Indinavir 1000 mg q8h
Levels— Amprenavir ↑ 250% Dosage— Insufficient data.	Levels—Ritonavir ↓ 11% Nevirapine: no effect Dosage—Standard.	Levels—Ritonavir ↑ 70% Delavirdine: no effect Dosage— Delavirdine: standard. Ritonavir: no data.	Levels—Ritonavir ↑ 18% Efavirenz ↑ 21% Dosage—Ritonavir 600 mg bid (500 mg bid for intolerance)
Levels— Amprenavir ↓ 32% Dosage— Insufficient data.	Levels—Saquinavir ↓ 25% Nevirapine: no effect Dosage—No data.	Levels—Saquinavir ↑ 400%† Delavirdine: no effect Dosage—Fortovase 800 mg tid Delavirdine: standard (monitor transaminase levels).	Levels—Saquinavir ↓ 62%† Efavirenz ↓ 12% Coadministration not recommended.
Levels— Amprenavir ↑ 150% Dosage— Insufficient data.	Levels— Nelfinavir ↑ 10% Nevirapine: no effect Dosage—Standard.	Levels—Nelfinavir ↑ 100% Delavirdine ↓ 50% Dosage—No data (monitor for neutropenic complications).	Levels—Nelfinavir ↑ 20% Dosage—Standard.
N/A	No data.	No data.	Levels— Amprenavir ↓ 36% Dosage— Amprenavir 1200 mg tid as single PI *or* 1200 mg bid + ritonavir 200 mg bid
No data. No data.	N/A No data.	No data. N/A	No data. No data.

Table D-4

Drug Interactions Between Antiretrovirals and Other Drugs—Nonnucleoside Reverse Transcriptase Inhibitors (NNRTIs)

Drug Interactions Requiring Dose Modifications or Cautious Use

Drugs Affected	Nevirapine
Antifungals	
Ketoconazole	Levels—Ketoconazole ↓ 63% Nevirapine ↑ 15%-30% Not recommended.
Antimycobacterials	
Rifampin	Levels—Nevirapine ↓ 37% Not recommended.
Rifabutin	Levels—Nevirapine ↓ 16% No data for Rifabutin dosage.
Clarithromycin	Levels—Nevirapine ↑ 26% Clarithromycin ↓ 30% No dosage adjustment.
Oral Contraceptives	No data.
Lipid-Lowering Agents	
Simvastatin	No data.
Anticonvulsants Phenobarbitol Phenytoin Carbamazepine	Unknown; use with caution. Monitor anticonvulsant levels.
Methadone	Levels—Nevirapine unchanged Methadone ↓ significantly Titrate methadone dosage to effect.
Miscellaneous	No data.

Drug Interactions Requiring Dose Modifications or Cautious Use

Delavirdine	Efavirenz
No data.	No data.
Levels—Delavirdine ↓ 96% Contraindicated. Levels—Delavirdine ↓ 80% Rifabutin ↑ 100% Not recommended.	Levels—Efavirenz ↓ 25% No dosage adjustment. Levels—Efavirenz unchanged Rifabutin ↓ 35% Dosage—Rifabutin ↑ to 450 mg **or** 600 mg qd
Levels—Clarithromycin ↑ 100% Delavirdine ↑ 44% Adjust dosage for renal failure. No data.	Levels—Clarithromycin ↓ 39% Alternative recommended. Levels—Ethinylestradiol ↑ 37% No data on other component. Use alternative or additional methods.
Levels—Potential for large increase in statin levels. Avoid concomitant use. Unknown, but may decrease delavirdine levels substantially. Monitor anticonvulsant levels.	No data. Unknown; use with caution. Monitor anticonvulsant levels.
No data.	No data.
May increase levels of dapsone, warfarin and quinidine. Sildenafil—Potential for increased concentrations and adverse effects. Do not exceed 25 mg in a 48-hr period.	Monitor warfarin when used concomitantly.

Table D-5	Drug Interactions Between Antiretrovirals and Other Drugs—Nucleoside Reverse Transcriptase Inhibitors (NRTIs)

Drug Interactions Requiring Dose Modifications or Cautious Use

Drugs Affected	Zidovudine	Stavudine	Didanosine
Methadone	No data.	Levels—Stavudine ↓ 27% Methadone unchanged. No dosage adjustment.	Levels— Didanosine ↓ 41% Methadone un- changed. Consider didano- sine dosage increase.
Miscellaneous	Ribavirin inhibits phosphorylation of zidovudine; this combina- tion should be avoided if possible.	No data.	No data.

Appendix E
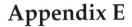

Recommendations for the Prevention of Pneumococcal Infections in HIV-Positive Children

Carl A. Kirton

Heptavalent pneumococcal conjugate vaccine (PCV7 or Prevnar) was approved by the Food and Drug Administration (FDA) in February 2000 and is recommended for universal use in children 23 months of age and younger. Recommendations have also been made for use of 23-valent pneumococcal polysaccharide (23PS) vaccine in children at high risk to expand serotype coverage.

NURSING CONSIDERATIONS

1. Each 0.5 ml dose of a pneumococcal conjugate vaccine is administered IM.
2. The initial 2-month dose should not be administered before 6 weeks of age.
3. It is safe to administer the pneumococcal vaccine with all other childhood vaccines using a separate syringe for the injection of each vaccine and administering each vaccine at a different site.

Table E-1 Recommended Schedule of Doses for Pneumococcal Conjugate Vaccine (PCV7) or 23-Valent Pneumococcal Polysaccharide (23PS) Vaccine

This table includes data for primary series and catch-up immunizations in previously unvaccinated children.

Age at First Dose	Primary Series	Booster Dose*
2-6 mos	3 doses, 6-8 wks apart	1 dose at 12-15 mos of age
7-11 mos	2 doses, 6-8 wks apart	1 dose at 12-15 mos of age
12-23 mos	2 doses, 6-8 wks apart	
≥24 mos	1 dose	

*The booster dose should be given at least 6 to 8 weeks after the final dose of the primary series.

Table E-2	Pneumococcal Conjugate Vaccine (PCV7) or 23-Valent Pneumococcal Polysaccharide (23PS) Vaccine for Children at High Risk of Pneumococcal Disease (Children with Sickle-Cell Disease, Asplenia, or HIV Infection)

Age	Previous Doses	Recommendations
≤23 mos	None	PCV7 as in Table E-1
24-59 mos	4 doses of PCV 7	1 dose of 23PS vaccine at 24 mo, at least 6-8 wks after the last dose of PCV7
		1 dose of 23PS vaccine, 3-5 yrs after the first dose of 23PS vaccine
24-59 mos	1-3 doses of PCV 7	1 dose of PCV7
		1 dose of 23PS vaccine, 6-8 wks after the last dose of PCV 7
		1 dose of 23PS vaccine, 3-5 yrs after the first dose of 23PS vaccine
24-59 mos	1 dose of 23PS	2 doses of PCV7, 6-8 wks apart beginning at least 6-8 wks after last dose of 23PS vaccine
		1 dose of 23PS vaccine, 3-5 yrs after the first dose of 23PS vaccine
24-59 mos	None	2 doses of PCV7 6-8 wks apart
		1 dose of 23PS vaccine, 6-8 wks after the last dose of PCV7
		1 dose of 23PS vaccine, 3-5 yrs after the first dose of 23PS

Adapted from Committee on Infectious Diseases, American Academy of Pediatrics: Policy statement: recommendations for the prevention of pneumococcal infections, including the use of pneumococcal conjugate vaccine (Prevnar), pneumococcal vaccine, and antibiotic prophylaxis, *Pediatrics* 106:362, 2000.

Index

Page numbers in italics indicate boxes and
illustrations, page numbers followed by t
indicate tables.

519